Dr. C. M. Wormington

PRIMARY CARE OPTOMETRY

Second Edition

Theodore P. Grosvenor, O.D., Ph.D.

PROFESSIONAL PRESS BOOKS
FAIRCHILD PUBLICATIONS
NEW YORK

Library of Congress Number 88-61666

ISBN 0-87873-084-2
Copyright © 1989 by Professional Press Books
Fairchild Publications Division of Capital Cities Media Inc.

Printed in the U.S.A.

Contents

Preface

Since the publication of the First Edition of *Primary Care Optometry* in 1982, our knowledge of vision and its disorders has continued to expand. As a result, the Second Edition of the text includes many major revisions and additions of new material.

Research in the development of refraction has occurred at a particularly rapid pace. In response to this, Chapter 2, "Epidemiology of Ametropia" is revised and updated, and a new chapter entitled "Myopia and Its Development" (Chapter 3) appears. Major areas addressed in new Chapter 3 include the prevalence of myopia as related to age, the classification of myopia, myopia progression, etiological factors, experimentally induced myopia, and attempts to control myopia.

With the ever-increasing role of diagnostic and therapeutic pharmacological agents in optometric practice, much of the material formerly included in Chapter 11 is now presented in expanded and updated Chapter 7, "The Ocular Health Examination." In new Chapter 7, the discussion of automated perimetry includes new instrumentation and techniques, such as indirect biomicroscopy with 60D and 90D lenses. As a result of the increasing emphasis on contrast sensitivity testing in recent years, this section is expanded and updated, with emphasis on clinical applications.

New Chapter 11, "Automatic Refraction and Biometry," includes information on the latest generation of objective and subjective auto-refractors and auto-keratometers, as well as a discussion of A-scan ultrasonic biometers (used for measuring axial distances within the eye). The major revision in Chapter 13, "Prescribing Ophthalmic Lenses," is an updated discussion of progressive addition lenses—a modality for the management of presbyopia that has been popular in Europe for some time but only recently has received large-scale acceptance in the United States.

Chapter 14, "Prescribing Contact Lenses," is revised to reflect this rapidly advancing area of optometric practice. Major additions appear in the discussions of hard gas-permeable, daily-wear lenses, toric contact lens fitting, monovision and bifocal fitting, management of keratoconus, and the fitting of extended-wear lenses—with emphasis on the use of high gas-permeability hard lenses for extended-wear fitting. The thoroughness of the information presented in Chapter 14 now rivals that of the author's

Contact Lens Theory and Practice (now out of print). In fact, Chapter 14 can serve as a "mini-textbook" in this important area of optometric practice.

The material on examining and prescribing for low-vision patients, formerly contained in two chapters, is combined here in Chapter 15, "Prescribing Optical Aids for Low Vision."

Primary Care Optometry is organized into three main sections. In Part One, Chapters 1–4, *basic science* material in the areas of optics, refraction, and binocular vision is presented. In Part Two, Chapters 5–11, *clinical procedures* (i.e., procedures employed while the patient is in the examining room) are covered. Part Three, Chapters 12–16, examines the procedures involved in *diagnosis and treatment.*

I am grateful to Dr. James Walters, for allowing access to an unpublished manuscript on the evaluation of automated perimeters; to Dr. David Loshin, for assistance in the area of contrast sensitivity testing; to Dr. David Perrigin, for assistance in the areas of photodocumentation, auto-refraction, and auto-keratometry; and to Dr. Tyler Thompson, University of Houston alumnus practicing in Little Rock, Arkansas, for granting permission to use data published in *Tyler's Quarterly Soft Contact Lens Parameter Guide.* I am indebted to Dean William R. Baldwin and Associate Dean Jerald Strickland of the University of Houston for their continuing encouragement.

Theodore Grosvenor
Professor of Optometry
University of Houston
Houston, Texas

Preface to the First Edition

Emphasis has been placed in recent years on the optometrist's role as a *primary care practitioner* or as a point of entry into the health-care system. Having once entered the health-care system, the patient may be found to require the services of secondary or tertiary care practitioners. The general practitioner of ophthalmology is usually considered a *secondary care practitioner*, caring for patients referred by both optometrists and general medical practitioners. However, the general ophthalmologist also serves many patients on a primary care basis, just as the optometrist does. A good example of a *tertiary care practitioner* in the eye-care field is the retinal surgeon, who depends on referrals from ophthalmologists and optometrists, seeing few, if any, patients on a primary care basis.

Optometry also has secondary and tertiary care practitioners. These practitioners usually serve those patients whose vision problems have a low prevalence or who belong to age groups or population groups having problems of a unique nature. Areas of secondary care optometry include the care of patients who lack binocular vision because of problems such as strabismus and amblyopia, vision care for children having reading or learning problems, rehabilitative care for patients having low vision, and some of the more highly specialized areas of contact lens fitting, including the fitting of scleral lenses and cosmetic lenses. Tertiary care areas in optometry are mainly the "frontier" areas, including such procedures as electroretinography, electro-oculography, visual evoked response testing, and contrast sensitivity testing. For example, the electro-diagnostic clinic at the University of Houston College of Optometry receives referrals not only from optometrists but from ophthalmologists, neurologists, and other medical practitioners.

As the title indicates, this textbook is intended for the student of primary care optometry. An in-depth coverage of secondary and tertiary care areas of optometry is clearly beyond the scope of a single volume. Fortunately, textbooks are available in ever-increasing numbers on subjects such as therapy for binocular vision problems, pediatric optometry, low-vision care, and contact lens practice.

ACKNOWLEDGMENTS

It is a pleasure to acknowledge the encouragement and assistance of those individuals who have made this textbook possible: Martin Topaz, who published my two contact lens textbooks; Peter Topaz, who encouraged me to write the "Optometry Reconsidered" column in the *Optometric Weekly* and later in the *Optometric Monthly;* and William Topaz, who has worked with me closely in the planning and publication of the manuscript. Also of great assistance was Mary Peterson Berry, who capably edited the manuscript. I am indebted to many colleagues for reading portions of the manuscript and making valuable suggestions for its improvement, including Drs. William Baldwin, Darrell Carter, Troy Fannin, Charles Haine, Knox Laird, William Long, David Perrigin, Sam Quintero, Jacob Sivak, James Walters, and George Woo.

PART ONE

Anomalies of Refraction and Binocular Vision

The four chapters in Part One are intended to provide the student with the background information necessary for an understanding of the examination procedures described in Part Two. No attempt has been made to provide an in-depth coverage of the optical system of the eye or of the neurophysiological aspects of binocular vision, as this is done in courses taught by visual science departments.

In the traditional optometry curriculum, a visual science course on the optical system of the eye is taught during the first year of the professional program, and the preclinic sequence begins during the second year. Under this system the four chapters in Part One may serve to a great extent as a review of previously covered visual science material. However, in those curricula in which the preclinic sequence is given prior to or concurrent with the visual science sequence, the chapters in Part One serve to introduce the student to the material covered in greater depth in later courses.

CHAPTER 1

Anomalies of Refraction

To understand the anomalies of refraction of the eye, brief discussions of the *optical system of the eye* and of *visual acuity* are necessary.

THE OPTICAL SYSTEM OF THE EYE

Sign Convention and Terminology

The following sign convention will be used in this textbook:

1. Light will be considered as traveling from left to right.
2. All distances (object distances, image distances, focal lengths, and so on) are measured from the lens.
   a. If measured in the direction in which light is traveling (from left to right), distances are considered positive.
   b. If measured in the direction opposite to that in which light is traveling (from right to left), distances are considered negative.
3. Divergent rays of light are considered negative, whereas convergent rays of light are considered positive.
4. Distances measured above the optic axis are considered positive, whereas distances measured below the optic axis are considered negative.

Referring to Figure 1.1, light diverges from an object, 0, and is therefore negative. It strikes a positive (i.e., converging) lens and is rendered positive. After leaving the lens, it converges toward the image, 0'. The object distance is negative because it is measured from the lens and in the direction opposite to that in which light is traveling; the image distance is positive because it is measured from the lens and in the same direction as that in which the light is traveling. It should be understood that a positive lens is one that causes rays of light to converge, whereas a negative lens is one that causes rays of light to diverge.

The distance from the lens to the object is specified by the lowercase letter l, and the distance from the lens to the image is specified by l'. All distances (object distance, image distance, focal lengths, and so on) are expressed in meters. Vergence of light, specified in diopters (D), is determined by finding the reciprocal of the appropriate object or image distance, specified in meters. Thus, the vergence of light in object space is specified by L, where $L = 1/l$; the vergence of light in image space is specified by L', where $L' = 1/l'$.

It is convenient to specify reciprocals by the use of an arrow ($\longrightarrow$). For example, we may state the following: 20cm $\longrightarrow$ 5.00D. This is a useful method of changing from centimeters to diopters, or vice versa. To convert distances to dioptral quantities, all that is necessary is to take the distance in centimeters and divide it into 100. Hence 20cm $\longrightarrow$ 100/20 $\longrightarrow$ 5.00D.

Consider a converging lens with an object situated at a distance of 50cm to the left of the lens, as shown

Figure 1.1 Sign convention (Grosvenor, 1963).

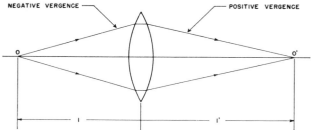

3

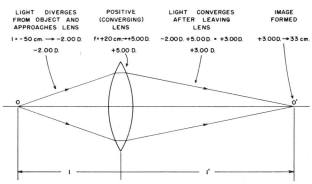

Figure 1.2   The step-along method (Grosvenor, 1963).

in Figure 1.2. Light from the object arrives at the surface of the lens with a divergence of 2.00D (100/50). Because it is divergent, the sign is negative and the vergence of the rays is therefore −2.00D. Assume that the converging lens has a secondary focal length (f′) of +20cm (i.e., F = 100/20 → 5.00D). Light leaving the lens, having arrived at the surface with −2.00D of vergence, is altered in its vergence by being converged 5.00D more than the original −2.00D of vergence; therefore, it now has (on leaving the lens) a vergence of +3.00D (as a result of adding −2.00 and +5.00D). The image is formed, therefore, at a distance of 33cm from the lens (+3.00D → 33cm). This is illustrated in Figure 1.2. It should be noted that no formula has been mentioned so far. The method by which the solution has been reached is known as the *step-along method*, which can be summarized by either of the following formulas:

$$F = L' - L \quad \text{or} \quad \frac{1}{f'} = \frac{1}{l'} - \frac{1}{l}$$

where F, L, and L′ are expressed in diopters, and f, *l*, and *l*′, are expressed in meters.

Using the first formula for this example, we have the following:

Given: L = −2.00D, F = +5.00D

To find: L′

L′ = F + L = +5.00D − 2.00D = +3.00D.

Using the second formula for the same example, we have:

Given: *l* − 0.50m, f′ = +0.20m.

To find: *l*′

$$\frac{1}{l'} = \frac{1}{f'} + \frac{1}{l} = \frac{1}{0.20} + \frac{1}{-0.50} = \frac{5 - 2}{1} = \frac{3}{1}$$

$$l' = +\frac{1}{3}\text{ m, or } +33\text{cm.}$$

The Schematic Eye

Given that the values of the corneal radii of curvature, the anterior chamber depth, the lens thickness and radii of curvature, and the axial length of the eye vary considerably from one eye to another, the optical system of the eye can best be described in terms of a "schematic eye," employing average values of these radii and distances.

Emsley (1953) describes an "exact" schematic eye designed by Gullstrand (see Figure 1.3). This schematic eye has the following values:

Indices of refraction: Cornea, 1.376; aqueous and vitreous, 1.336; lens cortex, 1.386; lens nucleus, 1.406.

Radii of curvature: Front and back surfaces of the cornea, 7.7mm and 6.8mm; front and back surfaces of the lens, 10.0mm and 6.0mm.

Focal lengths (measured from the corneal apex): Primary focal length, 15.70mm; secondary focal length, 24.38mm.

Axial distances: Corneal thickness, 0.5mm; distance from corneal apex to front lens surface, 3.6mm; distance from corneal apex to back lens surface, 7.2mm; distance from corneal apex to fovea (axial length of the eye), 24.0mm.

Principal planes and nodal points: Principal planes are located 1.35mm and 1.60mm from the corneal apex; nodal points are located 7.08 and 7.33mm from the corneal apex, and thus straddle the back surface of the lens. Definitions of *principal planes*, *nodal points*, and other terms can be found in the Glossary.

Refractive powers: Cornea, 43.05D; lens, 19.11D; complete eye, 58.64D. The refractive state of this schematic eye is 1.00D of hyperopia (note that the axial length of the eye is 0.38mm shorter than the secondary focal length). The values given here are for the unaccommodated

Figure 1.3   Gullstrand's "exact" schematic eye.

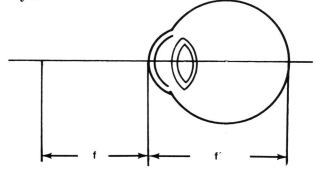

eye. During accommodation, changes occur in the position of the front surface of the lens, the radii of curvature of the lens, and in the lens power.

The Cornea and Tear Layer

More than two-thirds of the refraction of the eye is due to the cornea, the refracting power of which varies from as little as 36.00D to as much as 50.00D, although averaging approximately 43.00D (43.05D for the exact schematic eye). Although the index of refraction of the cornea is 1.3376, the keratometer (the instrument designed for measuring the refracting power of the cornea) is calibrated for an index of refraction of 1.3375 to take into consideration the refraction occurring at the back surface of the cornea. For a cornea having a radius of curvature of 7.7mm, the refracting power (using the index of refraction for which the keratometer is calibrated) is found to be

$$F = \frac{n-1}{r} = \frac{1.3375-1}{0.0077} = 43.83D.$$

The cornea owes its clear optical surface to the presence of the tear layer. The index of refraction of the tear layer is 1.336 (the same as that given by Gullstrand for the aqueous and vitreous), or very close to that of water. It is at the tear layer that light is first refracted, rather than at the cornea. The importance of the refraction taking place at the tear layer can be illustrated by calculating first the refraction taking place between air and the tear layer, and then the refraction taking place between the tear layer and the cornea. For a tear layer having a radius of curvature of 7.7mm, the refraction occurring at the air-to-tears interface is

$$F = \frac{1.336-1}{0.0077} = \frac{0.336}{0.0077} = 43.63D.$$

This equation shows that the tear layer accounts for almost all of the refraction ordinarily attributed to the cornea. Going one step further, if we assume the tear layer to be infinitely thin (with the result that the front surface of the cornea has the same radius of curvature as the front surface of the tear layer), the refraction taking place at the tears-to-cornea interface is

$$F = \frac{1.376-1.336}{0.0077} = \frac{0.040}{0.0077} = 5.19D,$$

which is only a small fraction of the refraction taking place between air and tears.

The refraction taking place between air and tears

is of little concern when the optometrist prescribes glasses, but when contact lenses are fitted, the contact lens often brings about a change in the tear layer curvature. When a hard contact lens is fitted, the lens tends to maintain its curvature while on the cornea; therefore, a contact lens having a steeper radius of curvature than that of the tear layer causes the tear layer radius to steepen, whereas a lens having a flatter radius of curvature than the tear layer causes the tear layer radius to flatten. However, when soft contact lenses are fitted, the lens usually conforms to the tear layer curvature.

The Crystalline Lens

The crystalline lens is located 3.6mm behind the cornea (in the schematic eye) and is immersed in the aqueous humor (in front) and the vitreous (behind). The index of refraction of the lens is considered to be 1.416, considerably greater than that of the cornea or of the aqueous and vitreous. The lens accounts for about one-third of the refraction of the eye; however, an important function is that of *accommodation*, or the ability to focus clearly for objects at different distances.

When the eye views a distant object, the lens is in a relaxed state and (if there is no refractive error or if corrective lenses are worn) a sharp image is formed on the retina. When the eye views a nearby object, the refracting power of the lens increases so that the image will again focus on the retina. Figure 1.4 shows that (*a*) for an object point located at

Figure 1.4 Accommodation for a near object: (*a*) Distant object with accommodation relaxed; (*b*) Near object with accommodation relaxed; (*c*) Near object with accommodation in play.

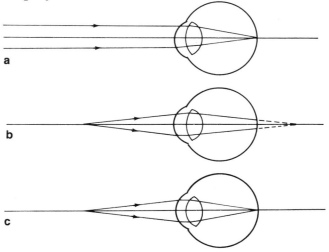

infinity, the optical system of the eye forms a point image on the retina; (*b*) for a point object located at some finite distance in front of the eye, the decreased vergence of the light within the eye causes the image of the object to be located behind the retina; and (*c*) with the correct amount of accommodation, the image of the object is again formed on the retina (in Figure 1.4c, the increased convexity of the lens denotes accommodation).

The Retinal Image

It is important to differentiate between the *optical image* and the *retinal image*. The optical image is the image formed by the optical system of the eye. It is always clearly focused, and it may or may not coincide with the retina. The retinal image, on the other hand, is the image formed on the retina, which may be either sharply focused or blurred. If the image formed by the eye's optical system is sharply focused on the retina, the optical image and the retinal image are one and the same. However, if the

optical image of a point object is not sharply focused on the retina, the retinal image will be a *blur circle*.

Blur circles

For a pupil of a given diameter, the size of the blur circle for a given object point varies with the distance of the optical image from the retina. As shown in Figure 1.5, the size of the blur circle increases with increasing distance of the optical image from the retina. On the other hand, if the pupil size is allowed to vary while the position of the optical image remains the same, the size of the blur circle increases or decreases as pupil size increases or decreases (see Figure 1.6).

It is important to understand that the concept of a blur circle applies only to *a point object*. For a line object, each point on the line is considered as forming a blur circle (unless the line is sharply focused on the retina), and for a two-dimensional object, each object point is again considered to form a blur circle. Blur circles formed by a line object and by a two-dimensional object are shown in Figures 1.7 and 1.8, respectively. It follows that for an out-of-focus eye, the clarity of an object (such as a letter on the visual acuity chart) depends on the size of the blur circle formed by each object point. This, in turn, depends on the distance of the optical image from the retina and on the size of the pupil.

Figure 1.5   Size of a retinal blur circle as related to the distance of the optical image from the retina.

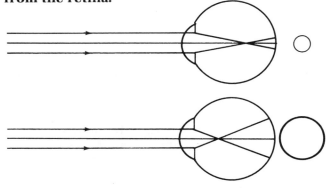

Figure 1.6   Size of a retinal blur circle as related to the pupil size.

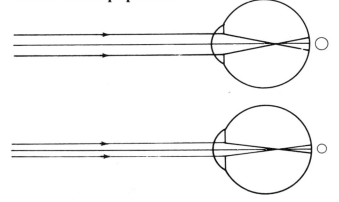

Figure 1.7   Blur circles formed by a line object.

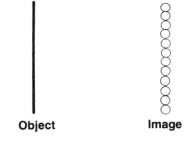

Figure 1.8   Blur circles formed by a two-dimensional object.

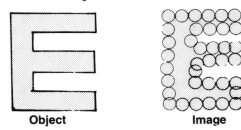

Accommodation

Accommodation is defined as the process by which the crystalline lens varies its focal length in response to changes in the vergence of incident light. Accommodation for a near object is illustrated in Figure 1.4.

Proof of the existence of accommodation

Prior to the 17th century, it was not known if it was necessary for the eye to change its focal power when viewing objects at varying distances. However, in 1619, Christopher Scheiner used a card containing two pinholes (now known as a *Scheiner disc*) to demonstrate the existence of accommodation (Moses, 1975). If the pinholes in such a card are separated by a distance less than the diameter of the subject's pupil (see Figure 1.9), an object that is not in focus on the retina will be seen *double* (in diplopia), whereas an object that is in focus on the retina will be seen *singly*.

While the subject looks at a distant object through the Scheiner disc, the distant object is seen as clear and single. However, if a small object such as a pin is interposed in the line of vision, close to the eye, the pin is seen as blurred and double (see Figure 1.10a). If the subject then concentrates on the pin, it is seen as clear and single but the distant object is blurred and double (Figure 1.10b). Scheiner's simple experiment demonstrates, therefore, that (1) distant and near objects cannot be simultaneously focused on the retina, and (2) a change in the dioptric power of the eye is therefore necessary to see clearly at various distances. However, Scheiner did not understand *how* the eye varied its dioptric power.

It remained for Thomas Young, in 1801, to demonstrate that the *lens* was responsible for accommodation. As described by Levene (1977), Young demonstrated that accommodation could not be caused by varying the refracting power of the cornea or by varying the axial length of the eye. He ruled out the cornea by immersing the eye in water, thus neutralizing the refraction of the cornea and demonstrating that accommodation could still take place. He then ruled out a change in the axial length of the eye by turning his eye inward toward the nose and placing a key behind the posterior pole of the eye (he could do this because his eyes were quite exophthalmic). The presence of the key behind the macular area caused him to see a *pressure phosphene*. He found that when he accommodated for a near object, the phosphene did not change in size, indicating that there was no change in the

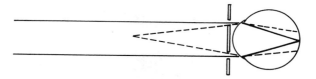

Figure 1.9   Sheiner's disc, or double-pupil. An object that is in focus is seen singly, while an object not in focus is seen in diplopia.

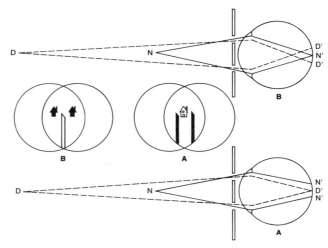

Figure 1.10   Demonstration of the existence of accommodation: (*a*) When focusing on a distant object through the Scheiner disc, a near object will be seen as blurred and double; (*b*) When focusing on a near object, the distant object will be seen as blurred and double (Moses, 1975).

length of the eye. Finally, Young demonstrated that the *lens* was responsible for accommodation by showing that an aphakic eye (one whose lens had been removed) was unable to focus on a near object.

The ciliary muscle

Young's experimentation was done prior to the time when the structure of the eye had been studied in detail by the use of the compound microscope, and as such he mistakenly concluded that the fibers of the lens were the muscle fibers responsible for accommodation. However, in 1847 Bowman and Bruke (each working independently) discovered the *ciliary muscle* and correctly identified it as being responsible for changing the power of the lens during accommodation. As shown in Figure 1.11, the ciliary muscle exerts its influence on the lens by

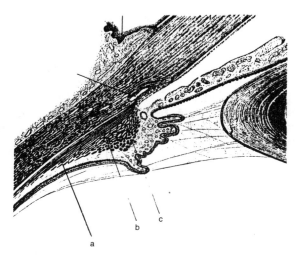

Figure 1.11   The ciliary muscle, showing (*a*) Longitudinal; (*b*) Radial; and (*c*) Circular fibers (Last, 1968).

means of the *zonular fibers* (also known as the suspensory ligament).

More recently, Fincham (1937) described the ciliary muscle as occupying most of the ciliary body and having the shape of a *prismatic ring*, with the base of the prism located anteriorly, close to the root of the iris. The ciliary muscle (Figure 1.11) is considered to have three types of fibers:

1. The *longitudinal* (meridional) fibers: long fibers having their origin at the scleral spur, just behind the corneoscleral junction, and inserting broadly into the elastic lamina in the equatorial portion of the suprachoroid.
2. The *radial* fibers: short fibers also apparently having their origin at the scleral spur, going backward (axially), and giving rise to circular fibers.

Figure 1.12   Fincham's reconstruction of the reticulated (radial) portion of the ciliary muscle (from E. F. Fincham, *The Mechanism of Accommodation*, London, Putman, 1937).

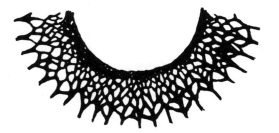

3. The innermost group of fibers, the *circular* fibers: having the action of a sphincter muscle.

Fincham preferred to call the radial portion of the muscle the *reticulated* portion, referring to it as an open network of muscle bundles interspersed with loose connective tissue. Fincham made a series of sections of the inner part of the ciliary muscle, and his diagrammatic reconstruction of the reticulum is shown in Figure 1.12.

The zonular fibers

The main group of zonular fibers inserts over a wide area into the lens capsule (thought to be a basement membrane secreted by the lens epithelium). These fibers are described by Moses (1975) as consisting of three bundles: (1) the *anterior* bundle, the strongest and thickest fibers, inserting into the anterior lens capsule and having the greatest effect for holding the lens in the unaccommodated (flattest) position; (2) the *equatorial* fibers, which are relatively small in number; and (3) the *posterior* fibers, which are large in number but relatively thin. Moses (1975) also describes a second group of zonular fibers made up of two subgroups: (1) fibers that form a dense meshwork on the inner surface of the ciliary body; and (2) fibers extending from the pars plana of the ciliary body into the vitreous, forming the *vitreous base*.

Changes taking place during accommodation

In 1855, Herman von Helmholtz used the Purkinje images (the "catoptric," or reflected images, formed by the cornea and lens) to determine the changes taking place during accommodation (1924, p. 454). He found that the third Purkinje image—formed by the front surface of the lens—became markedly smaller and moved forward during accommodation; whereas the fourth Purkinje image—formed by the back surface of the lens—became slightly smaller. He described the changes taking place in accommodation as follows:

1. The pupil constricts.
2. The pupillary margin of the iris and the anterior surface of the lens move forward.
3. The anterior surface of the lens becomes more convex.
4. The posterior surface of the lens becomes slightly more convex.

Two additional changes that take place, not described by Helmholtz, are:

5. Due to gravity, the lens sinks downward during accommodation (described by Hess, as cited in Moses, 1975).

6. The choroid moves forward. This can be demonstrated by placing a pin in the eye of an animal, just behind the ciliary body: the head of the pin will move backward during accommodation.

The mechanism of accommodation

On the basis of these changes, Helmholtz hypothesized that the natural shape of the lens is the relatively spherical *accommodated* form. When the lens is in the unaccommodated form the zonular fibers are taut (i.e., "on the stretch"), and therefore, hold the lens in its flattest (and thinnest) form. However, when the ciliary muscle contracts, acting as a sphincter muscle, it releases the tension on the zonular fibers, allowing the elastic lens capsule to increase its curvature and the lens to become thicker and more nearly spherical. Helmholtz considered the lens substance to be soft and easily molded by the elastic capsule, and so he proposed that presbyopia occurs due to a hardening of the lens substance with the result that it fails to respond to a relaxation of the zonular tension.

Fincham (1937) studied the lens capsule and demonstrated that its thickness is greater anteriorly than posteriorly, and that it is thicker at the equator (near the zonular attachments) than near the poles (see Figure 1.13). These variations in the capsular thickness cause the anterior surface of the lens to become *very highly curved* during accommodation—much more so than would be possible if the lens capsule had the same thickness throughout. This is an important contribution to the Helmholtz theory, as otherwise there would be no completely satisfactory explanation for the large increase in refracting power of the lens that occurs when the tension on the zonular fibers is released.

Figure 1.13 Fincham's representation of the lens capsule (E. F. Fincham, *The Mechanism of Accommodation*, London, Putman, 1937).

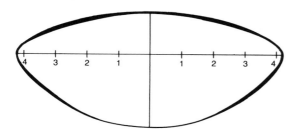

Range and amplitude of accommodation

Accommodation may be specified either in terms of *range of accommodation* or *amplitude of accommodation*. Both range and amplitude are based on the positions of the *far point* (the farthest point for which the eye can form a sharp image on the retina) and the *near point* (the nearest point for which a sharp image can be formed on the retina) of accommodation. Consider a young person with no refractive error (or whose refractive error is corrected by lenses) who has clear vision for an object at any point from infinity to a distance of only 10cm from the nose: the range of accommodation for this individual is infinity minus 10cm, which is still infinity; but the amplitude of accommodation, which is equal to the dioptric value of the near point of accommodation minus the dioptric value of the far point of accommodation, is 10.00D − 0, or 10.00D. Amplitude of accommodation, therefore, is a much more useful concept than range of accommodation.

Depth of Focus and Depth of Field

In a given situation, the retinal image of a fixated object may be acceptably sharp and clear even if the image is not sharply focused on the retina. For example, in testing visual acuity at 40cm, a small row of letters may appear to the patient to be in focus even though the optical image may be located at some distance in front of or behind the retina. The extent to which the image may be located in front of or behind the retina and still appear to be clear is referred to as the *depth of focus* of the eye; the extent to which the visual acuity chart may be moved toward or away from the patient (beginning with the position where the optical image is sharply focused on the retina) is referred to as the *depth of field* of the eye. These two concepts are illustrated in Figure 1.14.

Due to the extreme flexibility of accommodation exhibited by prepresbyopic patients, attempts to measure depth of focus or depth of field are seldom

Figure 1.14 The depth of focus and depth of field of the eye.

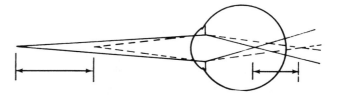

made in routine optometric practice. However, for a patient beyond the age of 55 or 60 years who is no longer able to accommodate, depth of field can be measured easily. If such individuals wear bifocals or reading glasses intended for a distance of 40cm, they may be able to maintain acceptably clear vision for distances ranging from 25 to 50 or 60cm. Because the depth of field increases with decreasing blur circle size, some older patients find that in sufficiently bright light (bringing about constriction of the pupil and a decrease in blur circle size), they may be able to read moderate-sized print without the aid of bifocals or reading glasses.

Aberrations of the Eye

Any optical system is subject to a number of aberrations. These include chromatic aberration and the monochromatic aberrations of spherical aberration, coma, oblique astigmatism, curvature of image, and distortion. *Chromatic aberration* occurs because ambient illumination is made up of radiation of many wavelengths, and depends on the material or materials of which the optical system is made. The presence of the monochromatic aberrations can be demonstrated only when chromatic aberration has been eliminated by the use of monochromatic light.

The aberrations of greatest concern for the human eye are chromatic aberration and spherical aberration. Coma, oblique astigmatism, curvature of image, and distortion are referred to as *oblique aberrations* because they are present only for light rays of oblique incidence. These oblique rays are imaged mainly on the peripheral retina, contributing relatively little to foveal vision, and therefore they are not discussed here.

Chromatic abberation

Chromatic aberration is present for an aperture of any size and can be considered either as axial chromatic aberration or as transverse chromatic aberration. *Axial chromatic aberration* refers to the fact that light of different wavelengths is focused at different points along the optic axis, and it can be demonstrated by refracting the eye, using light of various wavelengths (see Figure 1.15). Using this procedure, the Fraunhofer F (blue) line is refracted about 0.85D more than the Fraunhofer C (red) line (Emsley, 1953). *Transverse chromatic aberration* refers to the lateral spread, or dispersion, of images of different colors in the image plane. It is of little consequence in the eye, as the off-axial rays are received by off-foveal receptors.

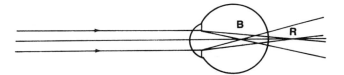

Figure 1.15 Axial chromatic aberration of the eye. Blue rays (B) have a shorter focal length than red rays (R).

The axial chromatic aberration of the eye can be easily demonstrated by the use of the bichrome test, described in Chapter 9. This test makes use of a chart having a red background on one side and a green background on the other. If a patient's myopia is undercorrected (or hyperopia overcorrected), letters on the red side of the chart appear more distinct than letters on the green side. As minus power is increased (or plus power decreased), a point will be reached at which letters on the red and green sides are equally distinct. Following this, a point will be reached at which letters on the green side are more distinct than those on the red side. For most patients the total chromatic aberration interval (from red more distinct to green more distinct) is from 0.50 to 0.75D.

Spherical aberration

As described by Emsley (1963), if a pinhole in a small card is moved vertically in front of the eye (see Figure 1.16), a horizontal line appears to move in the direction of movement of the pinhole. As shown in the figure, as the pinhole is moved upward, the somewhat blurred image of the horizontal line is below the macula and, therefore, is seen as moving upward.

The spherical aberration of the eye may also be

Figure 1.16 Spherical aberration of the eye as determined by observing a horizontal line through a pinhole in a moving card (Emsley, 1953). **The blurred image (O) is projected through the nodal point of the eye (N), with the result that the object appears to be located at O′.**

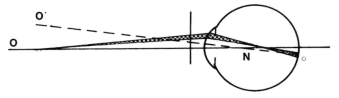

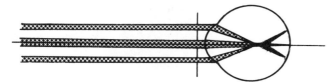

Figure 1.17   Spherical aberration of the eye as found by determining the refraction of the various zones of the eye's optical system.

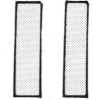 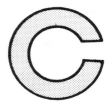

Figure 1.18   Konig bars and Landolt ring designed for measurement of visual acuity. For normal visual acuity, the width of a gap and of the bar or ring subtends an angle of 1 minute of arc.

demonstrated by refracting the eye, using a series of pinhole or doughnut-shaped apertures, each aperture confining incident light to a specific *zone* of the optical system. Using this procedure, rays of light from the more peripheral zones are refracted more than rays from the more central zones (see Figures 1.16 and 1.17), resulting in positive spherical aberration. As shown by Emsley (1963), for the Fraunhofer D (yellow) line, rays of light entering the pupil 2mm from the center are refracted approximately 1.00D more than those entering the axial portion of the pupil. Because the axial rays make a much greater contribution to the retinal image than the oblique rays (as shown by Stiles and Crawford, 1933), spherical aberration is of relatively little consequence. In the accommodated eye, negative spherical aberration occurs with the result that during partial accommodation spherical aberration is at a minimum.

VISUAL ACUITY

Visual acuity is defined as the *resolving power* of the eye, or the ability to see two separate objects as separate. It is often referred to as the *minimum separable* (as opposed to the minimum visible). It may be thought of as the ability to see a *gap*.

Early astronomers found that it was possible to resolve two stars as separate if the distance between the stars subtended an angle of at least 1 minute of arc. If the angular separation between the two stars was less than 1 minute of arc, most people would see them as one star rather than two. The "normal" resolving power of the eye was defined, therefore, as the ability to detect a gap with a width of 1 minute of arc.

In research, pairs of *Konig bars* are often used to determine visual acuity. As shown in Figure 1.18, these are pairs of black bars on a white background. For normal visual acuity, the width of each bar is 1 minute of arc, and the gap between them is also 1 minute of arc in width. The length of each bar is

usually five times the width, although the exact length is not critical. Imagine a chart with pairs of Konig bars of different sizes, the width of the gap always equal to the width of the bar. The smallest pair of Konig bars that can be resolved as two bars (rather than as one) gives a measure of the subject's visual acuity.

A *Landolt ring* (sometimes called a *Landolt C*), as shown in Figure 1.18, is a ring with a gap. For normal visual acuity, the width of the stroke and the width of the gap are each 1 minute of arc. With the Landolt ring, the subject is asked to tell in which part of the ring the gap is located—the upper, lower, left, right, upper left, and so on. The gap can be in any of eight positions so that if the subject is guessing there is only one chance in eight of a correct guess. A typical Landolt ring chart has several rows of rings, with gaps in different positions, starting with a large (6/60 or 20/200) ring and ending with a row of small (6/6 or 20/20) rings. Compared to the Landolt ring, the Konig bars have the obvious disadvantage that the gap can be oriented only in two directions (up and down or across), so the subject has a 50 percent chance of guessing correctly.

The universal method of measuring visual acuity involves the use of the Snellen acuity chart, as shown in Figure 1.19. A Snellen letter is a letter constructed so that the width of a stroke equals the width of a

Figure 1.19   The Snellen chart. Letter sizes are 6/60 (20/200), 6/30 (20/100), 6/24 (20/80), 6/18 (20/60), 6/12 (20/40), 6/9 (20/30), and 6/6 (20/20).

E
C B
D L F
P T E O
F Z B D E
O F L C T B
T F E O L F D E

gap. In most Snellen charts, letters are 5 units high and 4 units wide, although a few such charts use letters 5 units high and 5 units wide. The "best" Snellen letter is the letter E, in that it possesses three strokes and two gaps. Other letters such as L or T do not have a gap and, therefore, do not strictly meet the criterion for measuring visual acuity—the ability to see a gap. Even though these letters fail to meet this criterion, they are useful for measuring visual acuity. One advantage of the use of letters as compared to Landolt rings is that there are 26 letters to choose from, greatly reducing the possibility of the patient's guessing correctly. Another important advantage is that letters are familiar, and people have come to expect to read letters during a vision examination.

A *tumbling E chart* is often used for preschool children and illiterate patients. The letter E can be placed in any of four positions, and the child is asked to report which way the "legs" of the E point. Often the child is given a plastic or wooden letter E and is asked to hold the E in the same position as the one on the chart.

Specification of Visual Acuity

Visual acuity is specified in terms of the angular size of the gap for the smallest-sized letter the patient can identify. As already indicated, "normal" visual acuity (for an individual not requiring corrective lenses or with lenses, if required) is specified as the ability to detect a gap subtending 1 minute of arc. Refer to Figure 1.20; for any target distance, the linear width of the gap, x, for any given angular subtense, may be determined as follows:

$$\tan \Theta = \frac{x}{\text{distance}}.$$

For a target at 20 ft, or 6 m,

$$\tan \Theta = \frac{x}{20 \text{ feet}} \quad \text{or} \quad \frac{x}{6\text{m}},$$

and for a gap subtending 1 minute of arc,

$$x = 6(\tan \Theta)$$
$$= 6(0.000291)$$
$$= 0.001746\text{m}$$
$$= 1.746\text{mm}.$$

For a letter 5 units high, the letter height would be $5(1.746) = 8.73$mm.

Visual Acuity Notation

To measure visual acuity, one eye is occluded and the patient is asked to start at the top of the chart and read as many lines of letters as possible. The smallest line of letters read is then recorded. There are several methods of recording visual acuity.

Decimal acuity

Using the decimal system, "normal" visual acuity—the ability to detect a gap subtending 1 minute of arc—is given a value of 1.0. Decimal acuity decreases with increasing gap (or letter) size. For acuity to be one-half as good as 1.0, the letter would have to be twice as large. For visual acuity of 0.5, the letter size (for the smallest readable letter) would be 2(8.726), or 17.45mm; for visual acuity of 2.0, the letter size would be 8.726/2 = 4.363mm.

To construct a decimal acuity chart, the height of a letter for any given decimal acuity value can be determined by a simple relationship: height of letter = 8.726mm/decimal acuity. For a letter of a given height, decimal acuity = 8.726mm/height of letter. These relationships are used to derive the values shown in Table 1.1.

Although decimal acuity notation is seldom used clinically, it is a useful concept when acuity is plotted

Figure 1.20   Specification of visual acuity in terms of the tangent of the angle subtended by a gap in the letter E.

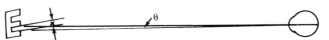

Table 1.1   Relationship between letter height, decimal acuity, and Snellen acuity.

Letter Height at 6m	Decimal acuity	Snellen acuity	
		Metric	English
4.4 mm	2.0	6/3	20/10
6.5 mm	1.33	6/4.5	20/15
8.7 mm	1.0	6/6	20/20
13.1 mm	0.67	6/7.5	20/30
17.5 mm	0.5	6/12	20/40
21.8 mm	0.4	6/15	20/50
43.5 mm	0.2	6/30	20/100
83.7 mm	0.1	6/60	20/200
174.5 mm	0.05	6/120	20/400

on a chart or on a graph designed to compare visual acuity to other variables.

Percentage acuity

If decimal acuity is multiplied by 100, the result is percentage acuity. Thus, a decimal acuity of 1.0 becomes 100 percent, a decimal acuity of 0.1 becomes 10 percent, and so on. Percentage acuity is not a useful concept and, in fact, can badly mislead patients. Some practitioners use percentage acuity when telling their patients how well (or how badly) they see. Consider a patient who, because of myopia, can only read the big *E* at the top of the chart. If the patient is told that he or she has only "5 percent vision," he will very likely think he is going blind. This procedure is not recommended.

Snellen acuity

The Snellen system of designating visual acuity was devised by Snellen in 1862, on the basis of the *Snellen fraction*, which is defined as follows:

$$\text{Snellen fraction} = \frac{\text{Testing distance}}{\text{Designation of smallest line read}}.$$

Perhaps a more scientific description of the Snellen fraction is the following:

$$\text{Snellen fraction} = \frac{\text{Testing distance}}{\text{Distance at which the smallest letter read subtends an angle of } 5' \text{ of arc}}.$$

The Snellen fraction may be stated in either *metric* or *English* units. Because visual acuity testing is almost always done at a distance of 6m (20 ft), the numerator of the Snellen fraction is almost always 6 (or 20) depending on whether the metric or English system is used. To convert decimal acuity into the Snellen fraction, it is necessary only to multiply the numerator of the Snellen fraction (6 or 20) by the reciprocal of the decimal acuity. Thus, for a decimal acuity value of 0.5, the denominator of the Snellen fraction would be

$$2(6) = 12 \quad \text{or} \quad 2(20) = 40;$$

and the Snellen acuity would be

$$6/12 \quad \text{or} \quad 20/40.$$

If the Snellen acuity is known, the corresponding decimal acuity may be determined by dividing the numerator of the Snellen fraction by its denominator. For example,

$$6/6 \text{ (or } 20/20) = 1;$$
$$6/30 \text{ (or } 20/100) = 0.2; \text{ and}$$
$$6/3 \text{ (or } 20/10) = 2.0.$$

The simplest way to convert English acuity to metric acuity is to convert the English Snellen fraction to decimal acuity and then convert decimal acuity to metric acuity. For example,

$$20/20 = 1.0 = 6/6;$$
$$20/200 = 0.1 = 6/60; \text{ and}$$
$$20/10 = 2 = 6/3.$$

The relationship between decimal acuity and Snellen acuity is illustrated in Table 1.1.

In communicating with patients, the Snellen fraction can be thought of as follows:

$$\text{Snellen fraction} = \frac{\text{Testing distance}}{\text{Distance at which a normal eye can see the smallest letter read}}.$$

Thus, if a patient asks a practitioner what is meant by saying that his or her visual acuity is 6/60 (or 20/200), one possible answer would be "The smallest letter that you can see at 6 meters (or 20 feet) can be seen by a normal eye at 60 meters (or 200 feet)."

Anatomical and Optical Bases for Visual Acuity

When we talk about visual acuity, we almost always mean foveal visual acuity; that is, acuity taken when the subject foveally fixates the letters on the chart. The central part of the fovea (the *fovea centralis*) is free of rods, having cones only, and is variously called the *rod-free area*, the *cone-pure area*, or the *central bouquet of cones*. In this area, each cone is thought to have its own "private line" (i.e., its own nerve fiber) to the visual cortex.

The angular size of the rod-free area is 54 minutes of arc (almost 1 degree) in diameter, subtended at the nodal point of the eye. The sun and moon each subtend an angle of about 30 minutes of arc; therefore, when you look at the moon (please do not look at the sun!), almost two moons would fit, side by side, in the rod-free area. We can also think of the rod-free area in terms of the size of the 6/60 (20/200) *E* on the Snellen chart. The 6/60 (20/200) *E* subtends an angle of 50 minutes of arc, so (as shown in Figure 1.21) it fits well into the rod-free area.

It is interesting to consider the resolving power

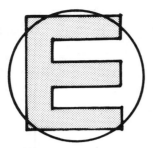

Figure 1.21   Retinal image of the 6/60 (20/200) _E_ as related to the rod-free area of the retina.

of the eye in relation to the dimensions of the _retinal mosaic_. Cohen (1975) gives the diameter of a foveal cone as 1.5μ. This corresponds to a visual angle, subtended at the nodal point of the eye, of 18 seconds of arc. Recall that the width of each stroke or gap of a 6/6 (20/20) _E_ is 1 minute of arc; we find that somewhat more than three rows of foveal cones fit into either a stroke or a gap of the retinal image of the 6/6 (20/20) _E_.

The resolving power of the eye can also be considered in relation to the _diffraction pattern_ formed on the retina. As astronomer Sir George Airy found in 1834, a point source of light is imaged by any optical system having a circular aperture as a _disk_ surrounded by a series of diffraction rings. For the optical system to resolve the images of two point sources (such as two stars), the minimum separation of the diffraction patterns formed by the two sources

Figure 1.22   Diffraction pattern formed on the retina by two point objects separated by an angular distance of 1 minute of arc.

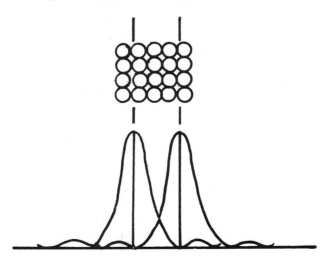

must be such that the center of one diffraction pattern falls on the first dark ring of the other. As given by Emsley (1963), for a circular pupil of radius _y_ and for light of wavelength (λ) in air, the radius of the first dark ring subtends at the nodal point an angle Θ, given by the expression,

$$\Theta = \frac{0.61\lambda}{y}.$$

For light having a wavelength of 555nm and for a 3mm pupil, the radius, Θ, of the first dark ring is 47 seconds, or slightly less than 1 minute of arc. This agrees with the observation that two stars can be seen as separate stars (or the two limbs of a letter _E_ can be seen as separate) if they are separated by an angular distance of 1 minute of arc (see Figure 1.22).

Intersubject Variation in Visual Acuity

It is found clinically that some people are capable of considerably better visual acuity than are others. In the absence of any refractive error (or with the patient wearing lenses to correct a refractive error) and in the absence of any eye disease, many people may be barely able to read the 6/6 (20/20) line, whereas others can easily read the 6/4.5 (20/15) or even the 6/3 (20/10) line. Many factors can contribute to this difference, including the following: (1) size of the retinal mosaic, (2) optical aberrations of the eye, (3) pupil size, (4) clarity of the optical media, (5) magnification of the retinal image, and (6) ability to interpret a blurred image.

These and other factors that may affect acuity tend to be distributed in the population (although not necessarily "normally" distributed), so the fact that everyone does not have the same "corrected" acuity should be no surprise. Other conditions that may be responsible for slightly lowered visual acuity are subclinical cases of amblyopia (defined as lowered visual acuity without obvious cause) and ocular diseases or degenerative conditions.

Variation with Retinal Location

Recall that in routine acuity testing, the patient fixates the letters on the chart using foveal vision. For retinal locations other than the fovea, what can we expect in the way of visual acuity? Some insight into this question may be obtained by considering the distribution of rods and cones in the retina, as shown in Figure 1.23. The broken line shows that there are about 150,000 cones per square millimeter at the center of the fovea, dropping down rapidly to

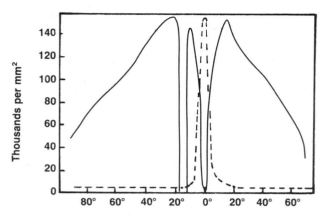

Figure 1.23 Osterberg's distribution of retinal rods and cones (from Pirenne, *Vision and the Eye*, London, Chapman and Hall, Ltd., 1967).

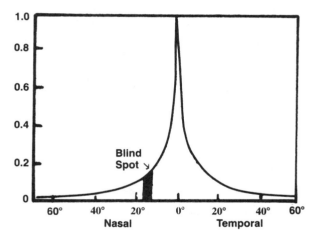

Figure 1.24 Visual acuity as a function of retinal location (F. H. Adler, *Physiology of the Eye*, 4th ed., St. Louis, Mosby, 1965).

only a few thousand per square millimeter at an angular distance of 10 degrees from the fovea. The rods, on the other hand, increase rapidly in concentration (beginning at the edge of the rod-free area), having their highest concentration about 20 degrees from the fovea and then gradually decreasing toward the periphery. On the basis of these distributions, one would expect a rapid lowering of visual acuity for nonfoveal retinal locations.

To determine a patient's visual acuity in a nonfoveal retinal location, it is necessary to provide a *fixation point* at some angular distance from the chart and to ask the subject to attempt to read the letters while looking at the fixation point. Most subjects find this to be a difficult task—trying to "see" something while looking somewhere else. Figure 1.24 shows that visual acuity indeed falls off quite rapidly

for nonfoveal locations, reaching 0.2 (6/30 or 20/100) at a point 10 degrees from the fovea and reaching 0.1 (6/60 or 20/200) at a point 20 degrees from the fovea.

Variation with Luminance and Contrast

"Standard" luminance for a visual acuity chart is considered to be a minimum of 10 foot-lamberts. If you are not accustomed to thinking in terms of foot-lamberts, the luminance of the page you are now reading is probably as high as 40 or 50 (or possibly even 100) foot-lamberts if you are in ordinary room lighting. As shown in Figure 1.25, increasing luminance to as high as 100 or even 1,000 foot-lamberts causes little increase in visual acuity, but reducing luminance to 1 foot-lambert or even 5 foot-lamberts causes a considerable visual acuity loss. Fortunately, levels of illumination ordinarily used in optometrists' examination rooms are high enough so that variation in luminance is not a factor of importance.

Contrast may be defined as the ratio of the difference between the maximum and minimal luminance of a test stimulus divided by the sum of the maximum and minimal luminance, or

$$\frac{L_{max} - L_{min}}{L_{max} + L_{min}}$$

In order to express contrast as a percentage, the ratio is multiplied by 100%. If we think of contrast as involving black letters on a white background, contrast can be reduced by having gray letters on a white background, black letters on a gray background, dark gray letters on a light gray background, and so forth. We can quantify contrast

Figure 1.25 Visual acuity as a function of illumination.

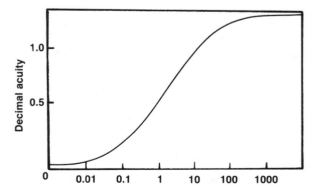

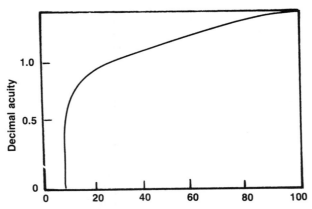

Figure 1.26 Visual acuity as a function of contrast.

by assigning a value of 100 percent when we have dark black letters on a pure white background, reducing contrast to 0 percent for gray letters on an equally gray background (in which case the letters would be invisible). As shown in Figure 1.26, visual acuity suffers with any decrease in contrast below approximately 90 percent. Methods of measuring *contrast* sensitivity are discussed in Chapter 7.

Variation with Pupil Size

The effect of pupil size on visual acuity depends on whether the eye's refractive error is corrected with lenses. As shown earlier, for an eye out of focus (i.e., the optical image does not coincide with the retina), the size of a blur circle on the retina for an object point increases with the distance of the optical image from the retina and with the size of the pupil. Therefore, decreasing pupil size for an out-of-focus eye (e.g., by increasing room illumination) tends to result in spuriously high visual acuity findings.

For an eye that has no refractive error or where the refractive error is corrected with lenses, visual acuity has been found to be best if pupil size is between about 2–5mm. If the pupil is much smaller than 2mm, diffraction effects tend to reduce visual acuity; whereas if the pupil is much larger than 5mm, spherical aberration may reduce acuity. Fortunately, at the illumination levels ordinarily used in visual acuity testing, most patients' pupils are within the 2–5mm range.

ANOMALIES OF REFRACTION

Emmetropia and Ametropia

Emmetropia is the "normal" refractive condition of the eye. In an emmetropic eye with accommodation

relaxed, parallel rays of light converge to a sharp focus on the retina (see Figure 1.27). An individual who is emmetropic would be expected to have good visual acuity (6/6 or better) at the 6m testing distance and, if accommodative amplitude is adequate, equally good visual acuity at the near testing distance of 40cm.

Ametropia is the general term for any refractive condition other than emmetropia, or a condition in which there is a refractive error or refractive anomaly. In an ametropic eye with accommodation relaxed, parallel rays of light fail to converge to a sharp focus on the retina. Categories of ametropia are myopia, hyperopia, and astigmatism.

Myopia

Myopia is the condition in which, with accommodation relaxed, parallel rays of light converge to a focus in front of the retina. If we assume that there is a "normal" axial length of the eye and a "normal" focal length for the eye's optical system, then myopia can occur in two extreme forms. As shown in Figure 1.28a, the axial length of the eye can be normal and

Figure 1.27 An emmetropic eye.

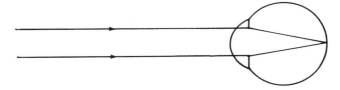

Figure 1.28 Myopic eyes: (*a*) Shorter than normal focal length of the eye's optical system; (*b*) Longer than normal axial length.

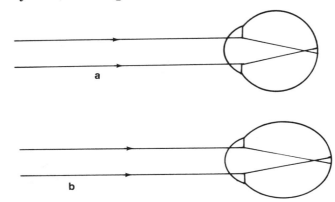

the focal length of the optical system shorter than normal; or the axial length of the eye can be longer than normal and the focal length of the eye's optical system normal (Figure 1.28b).

As shown by Sorsby, Benjamin, Davey, Sheridan, and Tanner (1957), small amounts of myopia are due to a combination of axial lengths and focal lengths within the ranges that are normal for the emmetropic eye. However, moderate and large amounts of myopia (about 4.00D or more) are due to the axial length being outside the normal limits.

Visual acuity in myopia

If we neglect the aberrations of the eye, an *emmetropic* eye can be considered as forming a

Figure 1.29 Relationship between uncorrected myopia and visual acuity. The dashed lines indicate 95 percent confidence limits. (Replotted from M. J. Hirsch, *Archives of Ophthalmology*, Vol. 34, p. 418, copyright 1948, American Medical Association).

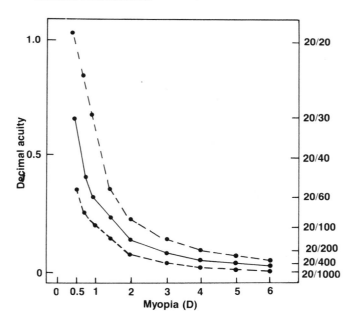

point image on the retina for each object point. However, if the eye is ametropic, the image formed for each object point will be a blur circle. As shown in Figures 1.5 and 1.6, the size of the blur circle formed by a myopic eye, for a distant object, depends on (1) the amount of myopia (the distance from the optical image to the retina) and (2) the size of the pupil. If we assume the pupil size to be constant, then the size of the blur circle formed by a myopic eye for a distant object and with accommodation relaxed depends solely on the amount of myopia. This means, of course, that uncorrected visual acuity is mainly a function of the amount of myopia.

However, in the clinical situation it is found that for a certain amount of myopia uncorrected visual acuity may vary widely from one individual to another. Factors responsible for these differences are: differences in pupil size from one patient to another; differences in illumination (which may be responsible for differences in pupil size); the tendency of some patients to squint, thus converting the pupil into a slit and possibly changing the curvature of the cornea; differences in the aberrations of the eye and the retinal gradient from one eye to another; and even the possibility that some patients make an effort to accommodate, thus blurring the vision more than would be the case otherwise. The relationship between uncorrected visual acuity and the amount of myopia, based on data published by Hirsch (1945), is shown in Figure 1.29. As the diagram shows, uncorrected acuity of a 1.00D myope can vary from approximately 20/30 to worse than 20/100, a difference of six lines of letters on the typical visual acuity chart.

How about the uncorrected myope's near visual acuity? As shown in Figure 1.30, if a 2.00D myope views an object at a distance of 50cm with accommodation relaxed, the object is in perfect focus (each object point forms a point image on the retina).

Figure 1.30   2.00D myope viewing an object at a distance of 50cm with accommodation relaxed.

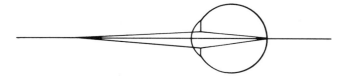

Far point and near point of accommodation

The *far point* of accommodation for a myopic eye, defined as the farthest object point for which an image point is focused on the retina, is always located at a finite distance in front of the eye. The *near point* of accommodation is the nearest object point for which an image point is focused on the retina, and is also always located in front of the eye. Therefore, a myopic eye has good visual acuity for objects located at the far point of the eye, at the near point of the eye, or at any point between the two.

Correction of myopia with lenses

Myopia may be "corrected" by means of a negative, or diverging, lens. The word *corrected* appears in quotation marks because the lens does not actually correct anything. All it does is enable the lens wearer to have clear vision while wearing the lens; once the lens is removed, the wearer's vision is back where it started. The same is true of lenses that "correct" hyperopia and astigmatism. Although *correct* is a poor term, it has been established in the literature and is used here.

The minus lens that corrects the myopic eye must be of such a power that the *secondary focal point* of the lens coincides with the far point of the eye. Figure 1.31 shows a myopic eye corrected with a spectacle lens and a contact lens. Note that the secondary focal length of the lens (f') is longer for the contact lens than for the spectacle lens. With a longer focal length, the refracting power of the contact lens is obviously less than that of the spectacle lens for the same eye.

Figure 1.31   A myopic eye: (*a*) Uncorrected; (*b*) Corrected with a spectacle lens; (*c*) Corrected with a contact lens (M_r = punctum remotum; A = spectacle plane; C = corneal plane; P = principal plane; d = distance between the spectacle lens and the cornea) (Grosvenor, 1963).

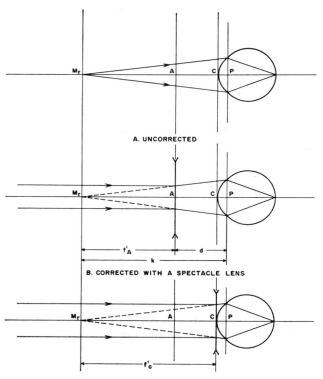

A. UNCORRECTED

B. CORRECTED WITH A SPECTACLE LENS

When a myopic eye is examined, the optometrist ordinarily does not attempt to determine the position of the far point of the eye. Instead, the power of the weakest minus lens that provides sharp distance visual acuity is determined. Assume that, for the patient considered in Figure 1.31, the refractive findings show that a −4.00D lens is required to obtain sharp visual acuity at distance. This means that the far point of the eye is located 0.25m, or 25cm, from the plane of the correcting lens (the trial lens or the lens used in the refractor).

What would be the power of a contact lens to correct the same eye? If we assume that the plane of the corneal apex is located 12mm to the right of the spectacle plane (and that the back surface of the contact lens is coincident with the corneal apex), then the focal length of the required contact lens is 25cm + 1.2cm = 26.2cm, and the power of the lens (expressing the focal length in meters) is

$$-\frac{1}{0.262} = -3.82D.$$

Therefore, to determine the power of the contact lens we: (1) find the focal length of the spectacle lens by taking the reciprocal of the power of the lens; (2) add to the focal length the distance from the spectacle lens (trial lens or refractor lens) to the cornea; and (3) find the power of the contact lens by taking the reciprocal of the distance found in step 2. The same result can be obtained by the use of the following formula:

$$F_{cl} = \frac{F_s}{1 - dF_s},$$

where F_{cl} = contact lens power, F_s = spectacle lens power, and d = the distance between the spectacle lens and the cornea. We can test this formula by substituting the values used in our example:

$$F_{cl} = \frac{-4.00}{1 - 0.012(-4.00)} = \frac{-4.00}{1.048} = -3.82D.$$

Axial myopia, ciliary spasm, and pseudomyopia

Once an individual begins to become myopic (which typically occurs during childhood), the amount of myopia tends to increase gradually with time, leveling off in the late teen years or the early twenties—thus, the term *progressive myopia*. When myopia "progresses," the progression is usually considered to be from an increase in the axial length of the eye. A theory developed by Young (1977) on the basis of research with monkeys but yet to be proved with humans, is that prolonged accommodation brings about a pressure increase in the vitreous chamber, which, in turn brings about an increase in the axial length of the eye.

Sato (1957) and other researchers have contended, however, that myopia occurs as a result of "ciliary spasm." As a result of prolonged accommodation, the ciliary muscle is thought to increase in tonicity to the point where it fails to fully relax when distance vision is attempted. In the beginning stages of myopia, the individual may complain that distance vision blurs following prolonged near work but that it clears up after a few minutes. This has given rise to the term *pseudomyopia*, which may be defined as a reversible form of myopia due to spasm of the ciliary muscle. The amount of myopia that is reversible (the pseudomyopia) is probably no more than 0.50 to 1.00D.

Those practitioners who have been successful in reducing or eliminating their patients' myopia by visual training have likely been working with pseudomyopes. There is evidence that, although myopia may begin in some individuals as pseudomyopia, after the elapse of some period of time the condition ceases to be reversible and eventually involves an increase in the axial length of the eye.

Night myopia

Many people are more myopic or less hyperopic in low illumination than in ordinary daytime illumination levels. This is because in low illumination there is insufficient stimulus to activate the eye's accommodative mechanism: for accommodation to relax completely when a person views a distant object, the object must have enough detail to form a sharp image on the retina. In low illumination sharp detail is lacking, with the result that accommodation tends to be "suspended" at an intermediate distance. An additional factor responsible for night myopia is the increased spherical aberration of the eye that occurs due to the increased pupil size in low illumination.

The presence of night myopia has important practical consequences for the optometrist. For example, one of the first symptoms of myopia in a young adult may be difficulty seeing for night driving. On the other hand, a hyperope who has just been given a correction for a small amount of hyperopia may find that although there are no problems with daytime vision, vision is blurred at night while wearing the correction. The amount of night myopia is usually no more than about 0.50D.

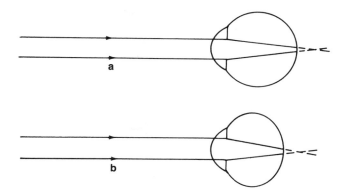

Figure 1.32 Hyperopic eyes: (*a*) Longer than normal focal length of the eye's optical system; (*b*) Shorter than normal axial length.

Hyperopia

Hyperopia (or hypermetropia) is the condition in which, with accommodation relaxed, parallel rays of light converge to a focus behind the retina. If we assume that there is a "normal" axial length and a "normal" focal length for the optical system, hyperopia can occur in two extreme forms. As shown in Figure 1.32, the axial length of the eye can be normal and the focal length of the optical system longer than normal, or the axial length can be shorter than normal and the focal length of the optical system normal.

As with myopia, it has been shown by Sorsby et al. (1957) that small amounts of hyperopia are due to a combination of axial lengths and focal lengths within the ranges that are normal for the emmetropic eye. However, moderate and large amounts of hyperopia (about 4.00D or more) are usually due to the axial length being shorter than that found in the emmetropic eye.

Visual acuity in hyperopia

Consider what happens when the hyperopic eye accommodates, as shown in Figure 1.33. In Figure 1.33a, the eye is viewing a distant object with accommodation fully relaxed, whereas in Figure 1.33b, the eye views the same object with accommodation in play. With the correct amount of accommodation, the image formed by the optical system of the eye coincides with the retina, and normal (6/6 or better) visual acuity is obtained. As compared to the uncorrected myope, whose distance visual acuity cannot be improved by accommodation, distance visual acuity of the uncorrected hyperope can be improved greatly by accommodation.

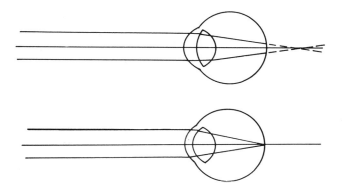

Figure 1.33 Hyperopic eye: (*a*) Viewing a distant object with accommodation relaxed; (*b*) Viewing distant object with accommodation in play.

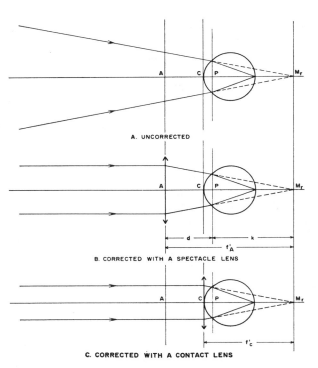

A. UNCORRECTED

B. CORRECTED WITH A SPECTACLE LENS

C. CORRECTED WITH A CONTACT LENS

Figure 1.34 A hyperopic eye: (*a*) Uncorrected; (*b*) Corrected with a spectacle lens; (*c*) Corrected with a contact lens (M_r = punctum remotum; A = spectacle plane; C = corneal plane; P = principal plane; d = distance between the spectacle lens and the cornea) (Grosvenor, 1963.)

The extent to which a hyperope's distance visual acuity can be improved by accommodation is limited only by the amplitude of accommodation. A young person having 3.00D of hyperopia and 10.00D of accommodation will have no difficulty accommodating enough to compensate for the hyperopia and achieve clear vision. However, an older person with the same amount of hyperopia and only 2.00D of accommodation would not be able to compensate fully for the hyperopia and would, therefore, not have clear distance vision.

Near visual acuity in hyperopia depends on the amount of hyperopia, the amplitude of accommodation, and the distance at which reading is attempted. Suppose an uncorrected 2.00D hyperope with 3.00D of accommodation attempts to read at a distance of 40cm. Because 2.00D of accommodation is needed to see clearly at infinity, only 1.00D is available to focus at a distance of 40cm. However, 2.50D of accommodation is necessary to focus at 40cm, so the patient lacks 1.50D of accommodation to accomplish the task, and near vision will be blurred.

Far point and near point of accommodation

The far point of accommodation for an uncorrected hyperopic eye (the farthest object point for which an image point is focused on the retina) is an *imaginary* point located behind the eye. As shown in Figure 1.34a, rays of light converging toward the far point are refracted in such a way that they are focused on the retina. However, such rays *do not exist*; this is consistent with the fact already

discussed—an uncorrected hyperope can have clear vision only by accommodating. The near point of accommodation for a hyperopic eye may be either a real object point located in front of the eye or an imaginary point located behind the eye.

Using the uncorrected 3.00D hyperope with 10.00D of accommodation as an example, the far point of this eye is located ⅓ meter, or 33cm, behind the spectacle plane; the near point is located 1/(10 − 3), or about 14cm, in front of the spectacle plane. For the 2.00D hyperope with only 3.00D of accommodation, the far point will be located ½ meter, or 50cm, behind the spectacle plane; and the near point will be located 1/(3 − 2), or 1m, in front of the spectacle plane. It is obvious that if the amplitude of accommodation is less than the amount of hyperopia, the near point of accommodation (as well as the far point) will be behind the eye, with the result that clear vision cannot be obtained even with maximum accommodation.

Correction of hyperopia with lenses

Hyperopia is "corrected" by means of a positive, or converging, lens. The correcting lens must be of such a power that the secondary focal point of the lens coincides with the far point of the eye. For a converging lens, the secondary focal point is located behind the lens. Figure 1.34 shows a hyperopic eye corrected by a spectacle lens and by a contact lens.

Note in Figure 1.34 that the secondary focal length of the correcting lens is shorter for the contact lens than for the spectacle lens, indicating that the power of the contact lens is greater than the power of the spectacle lens for the same eye.

An optometrist examines a hyperopic eye to determine the power of the strongest convex lens that will provide the patient with the best visual acuity. Let us assume that, for a given hyperopic eye examined with trial lenses or refractor lenses at a vertex distance of 12mm from the eye, the correction is found to be +5.00D. What correction would be required for a contact lens?

Referring to Figure 1.34, the secondary focal length, f', of the +5.00D correcting lens would be 20cm. But the secondary focal length of a contact lens for the same eye would be 12mm shorter, or 18.8cm. The power of the contact lens, therefore, would be the reciprocal of 18.8cm (stated in meters), or +5.32D.

Alternately, we can use the following formula:

$$F_{cl} = \frac{F_s}{1 - dF_s} = \frac{+5.00}{1 - 0.012(+5.00)} = +5.32D.$$

Latent versus manifest hyperopia

Many young hyperopes do such a good job of compensating for their hyperopia by accommodating that accommodation cannot be readily relaxed in a routine refractive examination. This condition, in which all or part of a patient's hyperopia is compensated for by the tonicity of the ciliary muscle, is known as *latent hyperopia.*

In a typical case, the optometrist may find that a young patient has 3.00D of hyperopia by retinoscopy (an objective test for determining the refractive error) but only 2.00D when subjective refraction is done. The 2.00D of hyperopia found in the subjective refraction represent the patient's *manifest hyperopia,* and the 1.00D that was compensated for by accommodation represents the latent hyperopia.

An individual with latent hyperopia may suffer severe asthenopia (eyestrain) until the hyperopia is found and corrected with appropriate lenses. As people age and their amplitude of accommodation decreases, latent hyperopia tends to become manifest. For this reason, some low hyperopes not requiring glasses (and not having enough latent hyperopia to cause symptons of asthenopia) find that, as the amplitude of accommodation gradually decreases with age, glasses are eventually required for clear and comfortable vision. The hyperopia was there all the time but became manifest only when the amplitude of accommodation decreased significantly.

Absolute versus facultative hyperopia

Absolute hyperopia is that hyperopia that cannot be compensated for by accommodation. For example, if a person has 3.00D of hyperopia and 1.00D of accommodation, the 2.00D of hyperopia that cannot be overcome by accommodation represent absolute hyperopia. The additional diopter of hyperopia that can be overcome by accommodation is *facultative hyperopia.* We therefore define facultative hyperopia as that hyperopia that can be overcome or compensated for by accommodation.

Facultative hyperopia and latent hyperopia should not be confused. Both apply to a relatively young individual with a reasonable amount of accommodation, but whereas facultative hyperopia can (at will) be compensated for by accommodation, latent hyperopia is hyperopia that the patient cannot help but compensate for by accommodation as a result of increased tonicity of the ciliary muscle.

Astigmatism

Astigmatism is a refractive condition in which the eye's optical system is incapable of forming a point image for a point object. This is because the refracting power of the optical system varies from one meridian to another. In *regular astigmatism* (which includes the great majority of cases), the meridian of greatest refraction and the meridian of least refraction are 90 degrees apart. The amount of astigmatism is equal to the difference in refracting power of the two principal meridians; in any other meridian, the amount of astigmatism is a function of the square of the sine of the angle between the meridian of least refraction and the meridian in question. (The meridians of greatest and least refraction are defined as the *principal meridians.*)

The cornea is usually the cause of clinically significant amounts of astigmatism, although the crystalline lens tends to cause astigmatism of small amounts. Most corneas are more steeply curved in the vertical meridian than in the horizontal meridian,

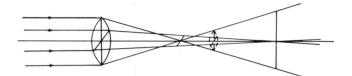

Figure 1.35 Refraction taking place at a toric surface: the conoid of Sturm.

causing the vergence of light to be greater in the vertical than the horizontal meridian. This condition is called *direct* or *with-the-rule astigmatism*. When the vergence of light is greater in the horizontal meridian than in the vertical meridian, the condition is called *indirect* or *against-the-rule astigmatism*. By convention, if the two principal meridians are more than 30 degrees away from 90 or 180 degrees, *oblique astigmatism* exists. Whereas a refracting surface having the same radius of curvature in all meridians is called a spherical surface, a refracting surface having differing radii of curvature in different meridians is called a *toric* surface.

Figure 1.35 shows how refraction takes place at a toric surface. Instead of a single point image being formed for each object point, the image consists of two *focal lines*, one parallel to each of the principal meridians; between the two focal lines the *circle of least confusion* is located. At any plane other than that containing one of the focal lines or the circle of least confusion, the image takes the form of a blur ellipse rather than a blur circle.

Clinical types of astigmatism

Astigmatism is classified in terms of the relationships of the two focal lines to the retina (with accommodation relaxed) as simple myopic astigmatism, simple hyperopic astigmatism, compound myopic astigmatism, compound hyperopic astigmatism, and mixed astigmatism. These are illustrated in Figure 1.36.

Figure 1.36 Clinical types of astigmatism: (*a*) Simple myopic, (*b*) Simple hyperopic, (*c*) Compound myopic, (*d*) Compound hyperopic, and (*e*) Mixed. Note that all diagrams indicate the presence of with-the-rule astigmatism.

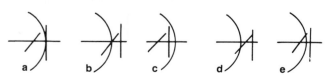

Simple astigmatism. With accommodation relaxed, if one focal line is located on the retina and the other is either in front of or behind the retina, the individual has simple astigmatism. If one focal line is on the retina and the other in front of the retina, the individual has *simple myopic astigmatism*, whereas if one focal line is located on the retina and the other is behind the retina, the condition is *simple hyperopic astigmatism*.

Compound astigmatism. With accommodation relaxed, if both focal lines are in front of the retina, the condition is called *compound myopic astigmatism*. If both focal lines are located behind the retina, the condition is called *compound hyperopic astigmatism*.

Mixed astigmatism. This occurs when, with accommodation relaxed, one focal line is located in front of the retina and the other behind the retina. The circle of least confusion, therefore, will be located close to the retina, giving the uncorrected eye reasonably good visual acuity (depending on the amount of astigmatism and the pupil size) without the necessity for accommodation.

Corneal, internal, and refractive astigmatism

As noted, the cornea is usually the source of clinically significant amounts of astigmatism. The amount of *corneal astigmatism*, along with the location of the meridians of least and greatest refraction, can be easily determined with a keratometer. The vast majority of corneas have with-the-rule astigmatism, the refracting power being greater in the vertical meridian than the horizontal; a small minority of corneas have against-the-rule or oblique astigmatism; and a small minority have no astigmatism.

As compared to corneal astigmatism, *internal astigmatism* is relatively small in amount, tends to vary little from one person to another, and is almost always against-the-rule (greatest refraction being in the horizontal meridian). The main causes of internal astigmatism are the toricity of the back surface of the cornea and the tilting of the crystalline lens. For a large population, the amount of internal astigmatism has been found to average 0.50D against the rule, varying from about zero to 1.50D against the rule. With-the-rule internal astigmatism is extremely rare. There is no clinical method of measuring internal astigmatism.

Refractive astigmatism (also called *total astigmatism*) is the astigmatism of the eye as determined by objective refraction (retinoscopy) or by subjective refraction. It includes both corneal and internal astigmatism. Thus, if both corneal and refractive astigmatism are known for a given eye, the internal astigmatism can be determined by means of the following simple formula: internal astigmatism = refractive astigmatism − corneal astigmatism.

In 1890, Javal proposed his now-famous rule for predicting the subjective astigmatism on the basis of the corneal astigmatism as determined by kera-tometry:

$$A_t = p(A_c) + k,$$

where

A_t = the total (refractive) astigmatism of the eye

A_c = the corneal astigmatism

p = approximately 1.25

k = approximately 0.50D against the rule.

As pointed out by Bannon and Walsh (1945), Javal made it clear that the rule was strictly empirical and that the constants p and k were only approximations.

Visual acuity in astigmatism

An uncorrected myope has poor visual acuity at distance but good visual acuity at near. An uncorrected hyperope can have good visual acuity at any distance if the amplitude of accommodation is sufficient. Although small amounts of astigmatism (0.50D or less) interfere little, if any, with visual acuity, there is no distance at which an uncorrected astigmat has a sharp retinal image.

If one or both of the focal lines are behind the retina (simple or compound hyperopic astigmatism), visual acuity can be improved to some extent by accommodating so that the circle of least confusion coincides with the retina. In mixed astigmatism visual acuity is relatively good, as discussed earlier, because the circle of least confusion is close to (and may even coincide with) the retina. However, if one or both of the focal lines are located in front of the retina (simple or compound myopic astigmatism), any attempts at accommodation will move the circle of least confusion even farther from the retina and thus make the retinal image even more blurred.

Correction of astigmatism with lenses

Simple astigmatism, in which the refraction in one principal meridian of the eye is myopic or hyperopic and the other is emmetropic, may be corrected by a cylindrical lens. This is a lens having no refracting power in one of the two principal meridians (the axis

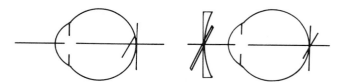

Figure 1.37 Correction of an eye having 1.00D of with-the-rule astigmatism (simple myopic astigmatism) with a spectacle lens.

meridian) and its maximum refracting power in the opposite meridian (the power meridian). For example, if a given eye has 1.00D of with-the-rule astigmatism (here we are talking about refractive, or total, astigmatism), it is evident that the refraction is 1.00D greater in the vertical meridian of the eye than in the horizontal meridian. This is shown in Figure 1.37. What is needed for this eye is a lens that decreases the vergence of light in the vertical meridian but has no effect in the horizontal meridian. The required lens has 1.00D of minus power (−1.00D) in the vertical meridian but no power in the horizontal meridian. The vertical meridian of the correcting lens is the power meridian, and the horizontal meridian is the axis meridian. If we think only of the vertical meridian, the situation shown in Figure 1.37 is exactly what would take place in the myopic eye.

Compound astigmatism, in which the refraction in both major meridians of the eye is either myopic or hyperopic, requires a toric lens for its correction. This is a lens having refracting power in both principal meridians, but more power in one principal meridian than in the other. For example, if a given eye is found to have 2.00D of myopia and, in addition, 1.00D of with-the-rule astigmatism, the refraction in the vertical meridian is not only 1.00D more than that in the horizontal meridian, but the vergence of light in the horizontal meridian is 2.00D greater than necessary for the formation of a sharp image of a distant object on the retina. This is shown in Figure 1.38. What is needed for this eye is a lens

Figure 1.38 Correction of an eye having 2.00D of myopia and 1.00D of myopic astigmatism (compound myopic astigmatism) with a spectacle lens.

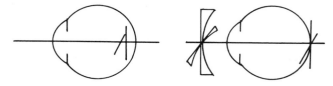

that decreases the vergence of light in the eye by 3.00D in the vertical meridian and 2.00D in the horizontal meridian. The cylindrical power of the lens is the same as for the preceding example (1.00D), and the axis and the power meridians are the horizontal and vertical meridians, as in the preceding example. In addition, however, the lens contains a spherical component (with 2.00D of minus power) to correct the eye's myopia.

It is obvious that we must have some method of notation—some method of specifying the powers of the spherical and cylindrical powers, together with the cylinder axes. This brings us to the topic of prescription writing.

Prescription Writing

If a patient has a spherical refractive error (myopia or hyperopia) only, the form in which the lens prescription is written is simple. For example, a two-diopter myope requires a minus-two-diopter sphere, so the prescription is written −2.00DS; a four-diopter hyperope requires a plus-four-diopter sphere, so the prescription is written +4.00DS.

If the patient has astigmatism only, the prescription must include both the cylinder power and the cylinder axis. In the example discussed above and illustrated in Figure 1.37, the lens prescription would be plano −1.00DC axis 180. If the patient has compound myopic astigmatism (i.e., both myopia and astigmatism), the lens prescription will include a spherical power, a cylinder power, and a cylinder axis. For the example illustrated in Figure 1.38, the lens prescription would be −2.00DS −1.00DC axis 180.

An example of a correction for simple hyperopic astigmatism would be +1.00DS −1.00DC axis 180. An example of a correction for compound hyperopic astigmatism would be +2.00DS −1.00DC axis 180. An example of a correction for mixed astigmatism would be +1.00DS −3.00DC axis 180.

Ordinarily the DS and the DC are omitted, and the letter x is substituted for the word axis, with the result that the above prescription would be written in the form +1.00 −3.00 x 180.

Transposition

When a cylindrical component is to be incorporated into a spectacle lens, it can be ground into either the front or back surface of the lens. Traditionally, front-surface cylinders have been used in single vision lenses and in Ultex-style one-piece bifocal lenses (which have the bifocal addition on the

back surface of the lens); and back-surface cylinders have been used on fused bifocals and on Executive-style one-piece bifocals (both of which have the bifocal additions on the front surface of the lens). However, back-surface cylinders have gradually become the "standard" for single-vision lenses because of the decreased amount of meridianal aniseikonia (difference in retinal image shape for the two eyes) that occurs when back-surface cylinders are used.

When a cylinder is to be ground on the front surface of a lens, the lens formula is written in the plus cylinder form; and the prescription for a back-surface cylinder is written in the minus cylinder form. To transpose the lens formula from one form to the other, a simple three-step rule is used:

1. Determine the new spherical power by algebraically adding the old spherical and cylindrical powers.
2. Change the sign of the cylinder.
3. Change the cylinder axis 90 degrees.

The following examples illustrate this rule. The minus cylinder formula +2.00 −1.00 x 180 converts to +1.00 +1.00 x 90, and the plus cylinder formula plano +1.00 x 60 converts to +1.00 −1.00 x 150.

To check the accuracy of transposition, power diagrams (also called optical crosses), as shown in Figures 1.39 and 1.40, may be drawn. In Figure 1.39, the first two crosses show the spherical and cylindrical components in minus cylinder form, the third cross shows the combined spherical and cylindrical powers, and in the final two crosses the spherical and cylindrical components are shown in the plus cylinder form. When working with power diagrams it is necessary to remember that the cylindrical component has its power in the meridian 90 degrees from the axis meridian.

Cylindrical lenses used in refracting (whether loose trial lenses or lenses mounted in a refractor) are available in either plus cylinder or minus cylinder forms. Although ophthalmologists usually use plus cylinders for refracting, optometrists usually use minus cylinders because they lend themselves more readily to the fogging method of refraction used by optometrists. Thus, ophthalmologists routinely write spectacle lens prescriptions in the plus cylinder form and optometrists routinely write them in the minus cylinder form.

When single-vision lenses were routinely supplied in the plus cylinder form, opticians "laying out" the lenses had to transpose optometrists' prescriptions for single-vision lenses, but not ophthalmologists'

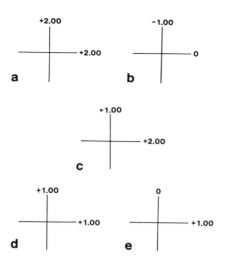

Figure 1.39 Power diagrams (optical crosses) showing the transposition of the formula +2.00DS −1.00DC *x* 180 to the plus cylinder form. Crosses (*a*) and (*b*) show the spherical and cylindrical components in the minus cylinder form; cross (*c*) shows the combined spherical and cylindrical powers; crosses (*d*) and (*e*) show the spherical and cylindrical components in the plus cylinder form.

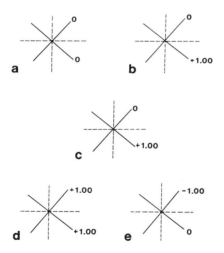

Figure 1.40 Power diagrams showing transposition of the formula +1.00DC *x* 50 to the minus cylinder form. Crosses (*a*) and (*b*) show the spherical and cylindrical components in the plus cylinder form; cross (*c*) shows the combined spherical and cylindrical components; crosses (*d*) and (*e*) show the spherical and cylindrical components in the plus cylinder form.

prescriptions. Because back-surface cylinders are now in general use, opticians have to transpose ophthalmologists' but not optometrists' single-vision prescriptions.

Anisometropia

For most people the spherical refractive error (the amount of myopia or hyperopia) is about the same for both eyes. However, if there is a significant difference in the spherical refractive errors for the two eyes, the individual is said to have *anisometropia*. As a general rule, anisometropia is considered to exist if the refraction differs by 1.00D or more for the two eyes. *Isometropia* is a seldom-used term indicating that the refractive error is the same for the two eyes. The term *antimetropia* indicates that a person is myopic in one eye and hyperopic in the other.

In separate studies involving school children, Blum et al. (1959) and Hirsch (1967) found the prevalance of anisometropia of 1.00D or more to vary from 2–6 percent, being lowest at age 5 and increasing during the school years. In Hirsch's (1967) study, some of the children had equal refractions in both eyes (isometropia) on entering school but developed anisometropia during the school years, whereas others had anisometropia when entering school but eventually became isometropic, and still others were found to be anisometropic on entering school and remained anisometropic.

Visual acuity in anisometropia

If an individual has *myopic* anisometropia, one expects the distance visual acuity in each eye to be lower than normal, the more myopic eye having the poorer visual acuity. If the amount of myopia in the less myopic eye is only 0.25 or 0.50D (a common occurrence) the visual acuity in that eye will be sufficiently good so that the patient may not be aware of a problem, even if the visual acuity in the more myopic eye is quite poor. On the other hand, in the case of *hyperopic* anisometropia, the visual acuity of both eyes will be relatively good as long as the patient has sufficient accommodation to focus on the letters on the acuity chart. In myopic and hyperopic anisometropia (or, for that matter, antimetropia) the individual may have no complaint of asthenopia (eyestrain) and the anisometropia may be discovered only during a routine vision examination. However, in some cases of hyperopic anisometropia, eyestrain may occur due to the fact that it is impossible for both eyes to focus simultaneously.

Because both eyes accommodate equally, an uncorrected anisometrope has the problem of never having sharply focused images on both retinas at the same time. For example, a person having 0.25D of myopia in one eye and 3.00D of myopia in the other will have a sharp retinal image for one eye for objects at a distance of 4m and a sharp retinal image for the other eye for objects at a distance of 33cm. When this occurs, the person gets into the habit of using the less myopic eye for distance vision and the more myopic eye for near vision. Although stereopsis (binocular perception of depth) is poor, such an individual has an advantage because in later years, bifocal lenses or reading glasses may not be necessary.

However, a person having 0.25D of hyperopia in one eye and 3.00D in the other eye has a more severe problem. The less hyperopic eye is used for distance vision, requiring only 0.25D of accommodation to achieve a clear retinal image; however, to use the more hyperopic eye for distance vision would require 3.00D of accommodation, and to use it for a reading distance of 40cm would require 5.50D of accommodation. The less hyperopic eye, therefore, never has a sharply focused image, so in early life a developmental anomaly known as *amblyopia* may occur.

Amblyopia

Amblyopia is a condition in which lowered visual acuity exists—even with the best corrective lenses—without an obvious cause. Although amblyopia can occur as a result of a wide variety of conditions, including various forms of toxicity and extreme malnutrition, when optometrists speak of amblyopia they usually mean *functional amblyopia*.

Functional amblyopia can occur as a result of uncorrected anisometropia or uncorrected astigmatism, in which case it is known as *refractive amblyopia*; or it can be a result of strabismus, in which case it is called, not surprisingly, *strabismic amblyopia*.

Presbyopia

As the crystalline lens grows, new fibers are constantly added in the outer part, or *cortex*, of the lens, while the older fibers are trapped in the inner *nucleus*. With the passage of time, the fibers in the nucleus become increasingly compressed and hardened by the constant addition of cortical fibers, resulting in a gradual decrease in the accommoda-

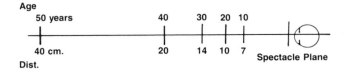

Figure 1.41   Increase in the near point of accommodation with age.

tive response to the contraction of the ciliary muscle. This decrease in accommodative ability is illustrated in Figure 1.41. As shown in this diagram, the near point of accommodation gradually recedes from about 7cm (2.75 inches) at age 10 to 20cm (8 inches) at age 40 and 40cm (16 inches) at age 50.

Presbyopia ("old-age sight") occurs when the near point of accommodation has receded to the point that it is difficult or impossible to accommodate sufficiently for reading or other close work. For most people, close work becomes difficult when the amplitude of accommodation is less than 5.00D (corresponding to a near point of accommodation—while wearing lenses to correct any distance refractive error—of 20cm). Presbyopia is relieved by convex lenses for near work, either in the form of reading glasses or bifocal lenses.

There is an old rule of thumb that a person will find close work to be comfortable if no more than one-half of the amplitude of accommodation must be used. If it is assumed that close work is done at a distance of 40cm, requiring 2.50D of accommodation, this rule of thumb tells us that a person having 5.00D of accommodation would require no reading glasses or bifocals; however, a person having 3.00D of accommodation should only have to routinely use 1.50D of accommodation and, therefore, should have a 1.00D addition in the form of a reading lens or bifocal.

Once presbyopia occurs, it gradually increases over a period of 10–12 years and then stabilizes. A presbyope typically requires a 1.00D reading addition in the early 40s, leveling off at about a 2.25 or 2.50D addition by about the age of 55. However, once presbyopia is evident, many emmetropes or low hyperopes undergo an increase in hyperopia after reading glasses have been worn for several months. For example, a 43-year-old emmetrope requiring +1.00D reading lenses may find that by the age of 45 the +1.00D lenses are no longer sufficient for close work but are just right for distance vision. This is sometimes referred to as the "hyperopia of presbyopia."

Study Questions

1. Define the following terms: (a) emmetropia; (b) myopia; (c) hyperopia; (d) astigmatism; (e) anisometropia; (f) presbyopia.

2. How do you differentiate between the optical image of the eye and the retinal image?

3. Give the "English" equivalent of each of the following metric visual acuities: (a) 6/30; (b) 6/120; (c) 6/12; (d) 6/60; (e) 6/45.

4. What is the amplitude of accommodation when (a) the far point of the eye is located 100cm in front of the spectacle plane and the near point is located 10cm in front of the spectacle plane? (b) the far point is located 200cm behind the spectacle plane and the near point is located at infinity?

5. Transpose each of the following spectacle prescriptions: (a) plano −1.00 x 180; (b) +1.50 −2.50 x 170; (c) +2.50 +1.00 x 75; (d) plano +1.00 x 10.

6. What effect does the shape of the lens capsule, as described by Fincham, have on the form of the lens during accommodation?

7. Give the following values for Gullstrand's "exact" schematic eye: (a) corneal radii; (b) thickness of the lens; (c) axial length; (d) indices of refraction of the aqueous, lens, and vitreous.

8. What would be the required power of a correcting lens if the far point of an uncorrected eye were located (a) 50cm in front of the spectacle plane? (b) 10cm in front of the spectacle plane? (c) 20cm behind the spectacle plane? (d) 400cm behind the spectacle plane?

9. If a patient has to walk toward the chart until he or she is 4 feet from it to see the 20/400 E, what is the patient's visual acuity (a) in the decimal system? (b) in the metric system? (c) in the English system?

10. If a patient's retinoscope finding (in which it is assumed that accommodation is completely relaxed) is +4.00DS and the subjective refraction is +2.50DS, what is the patient's (a) manifest hyperopia? (b) latent hyperopia?

11. A given patient has 5mm pupils in a dimly illuminated examination room but has 2mm pupils in a brightly illuminated examination room. How would the patient's acuity compare in bright as opposed to dim illumination if (a) the patient were a 5.00D uncorrected myope; (b) the patient were a 5.00D myope wearing an adequate spectacle correction?

12. If a patient is a 2.00D hyperope and has 3.00D of accommodation, (a) how much facultative hyperopia does the patient have? (b) how much absolute hyperopia does the patient have?

13. What correcting lens is required (a) if the far point for rays of light in the horizontal meridian is infinity and for rays in the vertical meridian is 200cm in front of the spectacle plane? (b) if the far point for rays in the horizontal meridian is located at 400cm in front of the spectacle plane and for rays in the vertical meridian is located 400cm behind the spectacle plane?

14. Using Javal's rule, what would be the expected refractive astigmatism for each of the following amounts of corneal astigmatism? (a) zero; (b) −1.00 x 180; (c) −1.00 x 90; (d) −2.00 x 180; (e) −2.00 x 90.

15. If a patient requires a −6.00D spectacle lens when refracted at a vertex distance of 12mm, what would be the required power of a contact lens for the same patient?

16. Using the rule of thumb concerning the prescribing of bifocal additions in presbyopia, what would be the required bifocal addition for a patient who, while wearing a +1.00DS correction for distance vision, was found to have a near point of accommodation of 33cm (a) for a 40cm reading distance? (b) for a 33cm reading distance?

17. For a patient who has a pupil 5mm or more in diameter, are the rays of light entering the peripheral portion of the pupil refracted more or less than the axial rays (a) in the unaccommodated eye? (b) in the maximally accommodated eye?

18. On the basis of the Purkinje images reflected from the front and back surfaces of the lens, what lens changes are known to occur during accommodation? On the basis of this and other

information, what *mechanism* did Helmholtz propose to account for accommodation?

19. Briefly describe the effects on visual acuity of (a) retinal location; (b) luminance; (c) contrast.

20. What effect does each of the following kinds of uncorrected astigmatism have on visual acuity? (a) simple myopic astigmatism; (b) simple hyperopic astigmatism; (c) mixed astigmatism.

CHAPTER 2

Epidemiology of Ametropia

HISTORICAL BACKGROUND

Although myopia and presbyopia were known to exist in ancient times, hyperopia was not generally recognized as a condition separate from presbyopia until late in the 19th century. The early history of the detection and measurement of refractive error has been reviewed by Levene (1977), whose quotation from Aristotle's *Problematica* illustrates the fact that Aristotle (384–321 B.C.) correctly differentiated between myopia and presbyopia:

> Why is it, that though both a short-sighted and an old man are affected by weakness of the eyes, the former places an object if he wishes to see it, near the eye, while the latter holds it at a distance? Is it because they are afflicted with different forms of weakness? For the old man cannot see the object; he therefore removes the object at which he is looking to the point at which the vision of the two eyes meet.... The short-sighted man, on the other hand, can see the object but cannot proceed to distinguish which parts of the thing at which he is looking are concave and which are convex ... but near at hand the incidence of light can be more easily perceived. (pp. 35–36)

There is no indication, however, that Aristotle understood the nature of ocular refraction and its anomalies.

Further understanding of the nature of myopia and presbyopia was not evident until almost 20 centuries later. As discussed by Levene (1977) and Hofstetter (1948), Francesco Maurolyco (1495–1575) theorized that errors of refraction were brought about by the crystalline lens. Johannes Kepler (1571–1630) described the optical system of the eye and the action of both concave and convex lenses. Father Christopher Scheiner (1575–1650) described the optics of the eye in more detail, discussing his measurements of the index of refraction of the ocular media and of the curvature of the cornea.

The first indication of an awareness of hyperopia was an account by William Wells (1757–1817) describing the use of convex lenses to correct his own hyperopia. This was followed by a description of hyperopia by James Ware (1756–1815), who, as quoted by Levene, referred to the work of Wells and then went on to say the following:

> There are also instances of young persons, who have so disproportionate a convexity of the cornea, crystalline, or both, to the distance of these parts from the retina, that a glass of considerable convexity is required to enable them to see distinctly not only near objects, but also those that are at a distance, and it is remarkable that the same glass will enable many such persons to see both near and distant objects. (p. 39)

When Donders wrote *On the Anomalies of Accommodation and Refraction of the Eye* (1864, reprinted 1972), he was distressed that many oculists of the period were still not aware of the existence of hyperopia and thought that presbyopia—rather than hyperopia—was the "opposite" of myopia.

An understanding of astigmatism came equally late in the course of events. Even though spectacles for the correction of presbyopia were in use as early as 1285, astigmatism had not yet been recognized as a clinical entity when, in 1764, Benjamin Franklin invented the bifocal lens. As described by Bannon and Walsh (1945), astigmatism was first mentioned in 1727 by Sir Isaac Newton, but it was Thomas Young who published, in 1800, the first description of astigmatism, which he found to be present in his own eye. The first lens to be ground for the correction of astigmatism was designed some 25 years later by the British astronomer Sir George Airy for correction of astigmatism in his own left eye. Donders described clinical procedures for the measurement of hyperopia, presbyopia, myopia, heterophoria, and strabismus, but he viewed astigmatism as a relatively rare abnormality, 1.00D or more occurring in only 1 out of 40 or 50 patients. Another half century passed before keratometry, retinoscopy, and subjective procedures for the measurement of astigmatism were developed to the point where they could be incorporated into the refractionist's examination routine.

PREVALENCE AND DISTRIBUTION

The prevalence and distribution of ametropia vary greatly with age. Refraction has been found to be normally distributed at birth, but early in infancy the majority of children are found to be somewhat hyperopic. During the school years children begin to become myopic in increasing numbers, with the result that the proportion of myopes in the population of 20-year-olds has reached 20 percent or greater. Relatively little change in refraction occurs in the early adult years, but by the age of 45 presbyopia has occurred, and for many people latent hyperopia begins to become manifest. Beyond the age of 55 or 60 there is a widening of the refractive error distribution curve, some people becoming increasingly hyperopic, some staying about the same, and others becoming myopic as a result of nuclear lens changes.

Astigmatism has been found to change relatively little with age. The majority of children and young adults have a small amount of with-the-rule astigmatism, but during the later adult years there is a tendency for with-the-rule astigmatism to decrease in amount and for against-the-rule astigmatism to increase.

Prevalence of Corrective Lens Wear

Readily comparable data indicating the prevalence of myopia, hyperopia, and astigmatism for unselected populations on the basis of age are difficult to obtain. Of the reports available in the literature, many involve clinical rather than unselected populations, and the criteria for myopia, hyperopia, and astigmatism vary from one report to another. However, the U.S. Department of Health, Education and Welfare has published data indicating the prevalence of corrective lens wear.

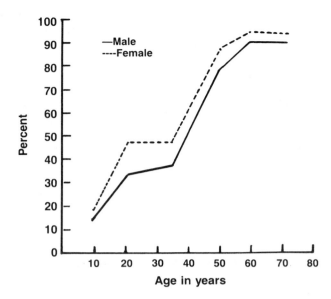

Figure 2.1   Percentage of U.S. population wearing corrective lenses, 1971–1972 (from *Characteristics of Persons with Corrective Lenses*, U.S. Department of Health, Education and Welfare, 1974).

Figure 2.1 shows the percentage of the U.S. population in various age groups wearing spectacles or contact lenses, based on a "national probability sample" population of 10,126 people examined during 1971–1972 as part of the Health and Nutrition Examination Survey conducted by the U.S. Department of Health, Education and Welfare (1974). The rapid increase in the percentage of people wearing corrective lenses between the ages of 10 and 20 undoubtedly is due mainly to the increasing number of children becoming myopic during their teenage years. On the other hand, there is evidence for the relative stability of refraction during the early adult years in the flattening of the curve between the ages of 20 and 40, and the steep rise in the curve between the ages of 40 and 50 years represents the universal onset of presbyopia during this period of life.

Figure 2.2 is taken from data presented in another publication of the U.S. Department of Health, Education and Welfare (1978). The figure indicates the proportions of individuals wearing minus as opposed to plus (spherical equivalent) spectacle or contact lenses. The graph is based on the neutralization of lenses brought to the examination center and reported to be worn for distance vision, so it apparently does not include subjects who wore lenses for presbyopia only. It is of interest that approximately equal numbers of people were found to wear plus

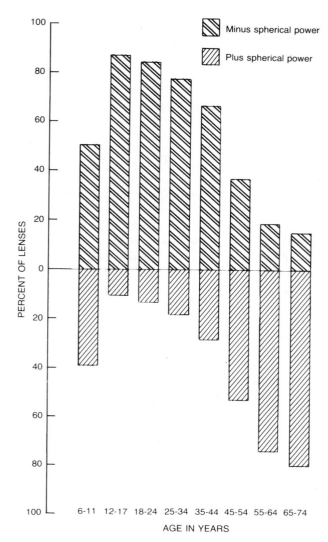

Figure 2.2 Percentages of individuals wearing minus as opposed to plus lenses (from *Refractive Status and Motility Defects of Persons 4–74 Years*, U.S. Department of Health, Education and Welfare, 1978).

and minus lenses at ages 6–11 and again at ages 45–54; and that while about 90 percent of 12–17-year-old lens wearers wore minus lenses, almost 90 percent of 65–74-year-old lens wearers wore plus lenses.

Distribution of Ametropia

The study of refractive error distribution most often quoted is that of Scheerer and Betsch, published in 1928 and 1929. According to Stenstrom (1948), their data included more than 12,000 clinical patients over

the age of 25 years for whom refraction was determined without a cycloplegic. The refractive error distribution curve for these patients, as compared with the theoretically determined binomial distribution curve, was published by Duke-Elder (1949) and is shown here in Figure 2.3. It is obvious that Scheerer and Betsch's distribution is much more "peaked," or *leptokurtic*, than the normal distribution curve, indicating that there are many more individuals with low refractive errors than would be the case for a normal distribution. The peak of the curve is at +0.25D, with almost 60 percent of the subjects falling between +0.75 and −0.25D.

Stenstrom (1948) analyzed the refractive error distribution data of Scheerer, Betsch, and other authors and concluded that the distribution of refractive errors in an adult population is not only leptokurtic but also skewed toward myopia. This

Figure 2.3 Refractive error distribution curve or Scheerer and Betsch (from S. Duke-Elder, *Textbook of Ophthalmology*, Vol. 4, St. Louis, Mosby, 1949, after Franchetti, in *Kurzes Hb d Oph*).

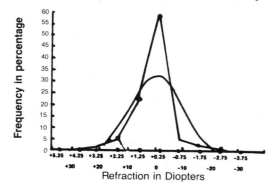

Figure 2.4 Magnified lower portion of Scheerer and Betsch refractive error distribution curve (from S. Duke-Elder, *Textbook of Ophthalmology*, Vol. 4, St. Louis, Mosby, 1949).

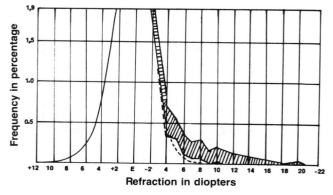

skew is not particularly apparent in Figure 2.3 but can be seen easily in Figure 2.4, which shows the lower part of the distribution curve more highly magnified. Duke-Elder (1949) pointed out that if the cases of myopia with degenerated fundi (the shaded area in Figure 2.4) are eliminated, the curve much more nearly approaches a normal distribution curve.

Distribution of Astigmatism

Few distribution curves for astigmatism have been published in optometric or ophthalmologic literature. Lyle (1971) published a distribution curve for corneal astigmatism for 1,208 eyes of patients of various ages seen in his optometric practice. This distribution curve is shown in Figure 2.5. Its general form is remarkably similar to the distribution curve for spherical ametropia, having its peak at 0.75D of with-the-rule astigmatism. Although Lyle did not plot the frequency of corneas having no astigmatism, Table 2 of Lyle's paper indicates that 36 eyes had spherical corneas. If a point representing these corneas had been plotted on the curve, it would have fitted nicely into the space between the two dashed lines.

Figure 2.5   Distribution of corneal astigmatism (from W. M. Lyle, "Changes in Corneal Astigmatism with Age," *American Journal of Optometry*, Vol. 48, pp. 467–478, 1971).

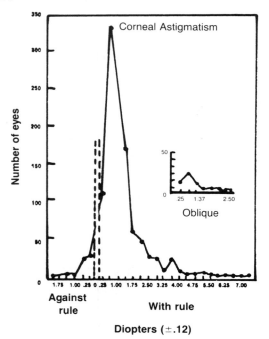

VARIABILITY OF THE EYE'S REFRACTIVE COMPONENTS

In attempting to understand the variability of the eye's refractive components, researchers have been limited by the technology available for the measurement of these components. An understanding of the variability in the refracting power of the cornea had to await Helmholtz's invention of the *keratometer*. Further, the invention of the *ophthalmophakometer* by Tscherning made it possible to determine the variability of the refracting power of the crystalline lens; and Rushton's development of the *X-ray method* for determining the *axial length* of the eye made it possible to determine the role of this important ocular component in the variation of ocular refraction. With the development of *ultrasound technology*, it is now possible to accurately measure all of the refractive components.

These technological advances and the subsequent growth in our knowledge of ocular refraction have been well documented by Duke-Elder (1949) and other authors. Arlt, in 1856, drew attention to the fact that highly myopic eyes were long and pear-shaped, showing thinning of the posterior portion of the sclera. Steiger, in 1913, used the Javal-Shiotz keratometer to measure the corneal refracting power of the eyes of 5,000 children and found that it varied from 39.00–47.00D. Steiger concluded that corneal refraction and axial length were independent and freely associated, and that chance combinations of corneal curvatures and axial lengths could bring about ametropia.

Tron used the ophthalmophakometer in 1934–1935 to establish that not only the corneal refracting power and axial length, but all of the components of refraction varied considerably from one eye to another. He plotted distribution curves for corneal radius, anterior chamber depth, lens thickness and radii, refractive indices, and axial length, and found that all components were normally distributed with the exception of axial length, which was found to be leptokurtic.

Stenstrom (1948) used Rushton's X-ray technique to study the refractive components of 1,000 selected subjects between the ages of 20 and 35. Other data collected by Stenstrom included static refraction at 10m, measurement of corneal radius with the Haag-Streit keratometer, measurement of the anterior chamber depth, and ophthalmoscopy to determine the presence of posterior conus (stretching and thinning of the sclera). He calculated correlation coefficients between refractive error and each of the components of refraction and found the following coefficients: depth of the anterior chamber, -0.34; axial length, -0.76; corneal radius, $+0.18$; and lens refracting power -0.00.

The minus sign in front of the correlation between refraction and axial length indicates that the greater the axial length, the greater the myopia. On the basis of these correlation coefficients, Stenstrom concluded that axial length is the most important factor in the determination of refraction and that most myopia is axial in nature.

Sorsby, Benjamin, Davey, Sheridan, and Tanner (1957) reported on an investigation of the emmetropic eye, determining the axial length by calculation based on other component data. They found that the emmetropic eye shows a wide range of axial lengths, corneal powers, and lens powers, the respective ranges being from 21–26mm, 38.00–48.00D, and 17.00–26.00D. For ametropia of less than $\pm4.00D$, Sorsby et al. observed that values for axial length, corneal power, and lens power were within the ranges found for the emmetropic eye and concluded that the ametropia was due to faulty correlation of individual components. However, for ametropia of more than $\pm4.00D$, axial length was almost always beyond the ranges found in emmetropia.

As a result of these findings, Sorsby et al. took issue with Steiger's assumption that there is free association between the components of refraction. They proposed a correlating mechanism that would account for a higher proportion of emmetropes in the general population than would be expected on the basis of free association. They argued that the emmetropic eye is not a haphazard combination of components but a well-coordinated organ.

Emmetropization

For a trait to be normally distributed, a large number of *independent variables* must be involved. For example, *height* is normally distributed, whereas *weight* (which depends mainly on height) is not normally distributed. The fact that *refractive error* is not normally distributed—there being more emmetropic eyes than would be found for a normal distribution—can be accounted for in that the variables making up the refractive state of the eye (corneal refracting power, anterior chamber depth, lens refracting power, and axial length) are *interdependent* rather than dependent variables.

Many researchers studying the components of refraction of the eye conclude that there is a process operating to produce a greater frequency of emmetropia than would be expected on the basis of chance. This process, known as *emmetropization*, is usually thought to involve one or more emmetropizing mechanisms. Such mechanisms have been proposed by Hirsch and Weymouth (1947), Sorsby et al. (1957), and others.

Hirsch and Weymouth (1947) reanalyzed Stenstrom's data, calculating partial correlation coefficients between the refractive components and the refractive state. Holding corneal radius and anterior chamber depth constant, they found that the correlation between axial length and refractive state was -0.87 rather than -0.76, as found by Stenstrom. They concluded that there can be no question that axial length is the most important variable and that the variation in the state of refraction is attributable to this element more than any other.

Holding axial length and anterior chamber depth constant, Hirsch and Weymouth (1947) found that the correlation between corneal radius and refractive state was $+0.70$, as compared to the correlation of $+0.18$ found by Stenstrom. Holding all other variables constant, they found the correlation between anterior chamber depth and refractive state to be $+0.25$ rather than Stenstrom's -0.34. As a result of their analysis, Hirsch and Weymouth proposed two mechanisms to account for the process of emmetropization. One mechanism involves the axial length and the anterior chamber depth, and the other involves axial length and corneal curvature. More recently, a mechanism involving axial length and the refracting power of the lens has been suggested.

They proposed that as the eye increases in axial length, tending to bring about myopia, the depth of the anterior chamber increases, tending to bring about a decrease in myopia. As for the cornea, as the axial length increases, the cornea tends to flatten, and corneal flattening likewise tends to bring about a decrease in myopia. Hirsch and Weymouth concluded that about $\frac{1}{2}$ of the variance in refractive error is due to axial length, $\frac{1}{4}$ is due to corneal curvature, $\frac{1}{20}$ to the depth of the anterior chamber, and the remaining $\frac{1}{5}$ is divided between measurement errors and variations in crystalline lens and refractive indices.

In their study of the emmetropic eye, Sorsby et al. (1957) pointed out that from birth to adult life the eye grows about 8mm in axial length (from an average of about 16–24mm), which involves a reduction in refracting power of 20.00 to 30.00D. They proposed that changes in corneal curvature and crystalline lens power can act as correlating mechanisms to maintain the eye at or near emmetropia.

Sorsby et al. (1957) suggested that the mechanism involving corneal curvature is simply a mechanical one, involving the tendency for the cornea to flatten as the eye grows. However, for the mechanism involving the crystalline lens, they proposed the existence of a biological mechanism in which the optic vesicle acts as the "organizer" of the overlying ectoderm. That is, it first causes it to form a lens, and then a continuation of the same "organizing" process by the retina (derived from the optic vesicle) may determine the shape and curvature of the lens after birth.

A more detailed emmetropizing mechanism has been offered by Van Alphen (1961). He submitted Stenstrom's data to factor analysis and concluded that three factors existed: the first factor involved corneal curvature and axial length and was labeled the *size factor*; the second involved axial length, anterior chamber depth, and lens power and was called the *stretch factor*; and the third factor, the *derailment factor*, involved all variables and was explained by too little, just enough, or too much stretch. Van Alphen suggested that the stretch factor and not the size factor ultimately determines the refraction (this is equivalent to saying the size, in itself, is unimportant, in that both a mouse and an elephant can be emmetropic).

Van Alphen (1961) proposed that the ciliary body and the choroid form an elastic envelope that limits the stretch of the sclera by counteracting part of the intraocular pressure, and that the macula supplies information regarding focus to the brain, which in turn feeds back information concerning the necessary degree of stretch. Van Alphen summed up his theory by saying that the eye is essentially self-focusing, that emmetropia is produced by subcortical control of the tonus of the ciliary muscle, and ametropia is caused by factors that interfere with the mechanism.

Hofstetter (1969) suggested that emmetropization may not be a biological process at all, but can be accounted for entirely on the basis of mathematics. He called attention to the fact that *radial dimensions* are used both for the dioptric and the structural appraisal of the eye, and argued that by using a "universal" schematic eye (Figure 2.6) it would be possible to construct an assortment of emmetropic eyes. A frequency distribution of all such eyes would produce an infinitesimally slender vertical line, the absolute limit of leptokurtosis. However, small varia-

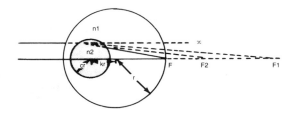

Figure 2.6   Hofstetter's universal schematic eye (from H. W. Hofstetter, "Emmetropization: Biological Process or Mathematical Artifact?" *American Journal of Optometry*, Vol. 46, pp. 447–450, 1969).

tions in the values of the refractive components would be expected to cause the slight dispersion of refractive errors away from perfect leptokurtosis.

What can we conclude about emmetropization?

Whatever mechanism or mechanisms (if any) account for emmetropization, the process seems to work reasonably well in view of the findings of Sorsby et al. (1957). They found that refractive errors up to ±4.00D, in which the values for axial length, corneal power, and lens power were all within the ranges found for the emmetropic eye, accounted for 98 percent of all refractions. Only for the 2 percent having ametropia of more than ±4.00D has the process completely failed, these eyes having axial lengths beyond the range found in emmetropia or low ametropia.

CHANGES IN REFRACTION WITH AGE

Refraction in Premature Infants

The presence of high myopia in premature infants was first identified as associated with *retrolental fibroplasia*, a condition occurring in premature infants due to the administration of oxygen. However, Fletcher and Brandon (1955), in a study of 462 premature infants, found that myopia is found in all premature infants, whether or not they are afflicted with retrolental fibroplasia. They found that for premature infants weighing more than 1,700g (3.74 lbs) at birth, fundi were mature and the amount of myopia varied from 0–6.00D, fluctuating little and becoming stationary by the end of 4–10 weeks. For the premature infants weighing less than 1,250g (2.75 lbs) at birth, the fundi were immature and the eyes exhibited from 10.00–20.00D of myopia, which fluctuated as much as 20.00D during the ensuing weeks and became stabilized near zero at the end of approximately one year.

Fledelius (1981) reports changes in refraction and eye size for 137 eighteen-year-old Danes, approximately half of whom had a low birth weight (below 2,000g) and half who were full-term controls. For emmetropes and myopes it was found that the eyes of low birth weight subjects had more steeply curved corneas and shorter axial lengths than those of full-term subjects. A number of reports concerning low birth weight children have been reviewed by Goss (1985), who concludes that, because such eyes have more steeply curved corneas and shorter lengths than those of full-term children, the myopic eye of a premature infant is an *underdeveloped* eye. Further, Goss notes that such cases suggest myopia may be caused by a *clouding of the media*, a consequence of retinopathy of prematurity.

Refraction of the Newborn

For the first half of the 20th century it was believed that all babies were born with several diopters of hyperopia, which they "outgrew" by the age of 5 or 6 years. As discussed by Hirsch (1963b), this belief was the result of a study published in 1892 by Herrnheiser, who used an ophthalmoscope to measure the refractive state of 1,930 infants and found that all but two had from 1.0–6.00D of hyperopia. Herrnheiser's results were later reported by Steiger (1913) together with some of his own results, and they were reported again by Wibaut (1926) with the result that they were often incorrectly attributed to Wibaut. As Hirsch pointed out, no other investigator has found a distribution like Herrnheiser's.

One of the first large-scale studies of refraction in newborn infants since Herrnheiser's time was reported by Cook and Glasscock (1951). They used retinoscopy with atropine cycloplegia to determine the refraction of 1,000 eyes of newborn infants. Their refractive error distribution varied greatly from that of Herrnheiser, extending from 11.00 to 12.00D of myopia to 11.00 to 12.00D of hyperopia. Their data for 370 eyes of white infants have been plotted by Hirsch (1963b) and are reproduced in Figure 2.7 (solid line). In this distribution the modal group, which includes 20 percent of the subjects, is in the +1.00 to +2.00D interval.

More recently, Goldschmidt (1968) reported that he used atropine cycloplegia to refract 356 Danish infants (having a birth weight in excess of 2,500g) from 2–10 days old, and found a normal distribution

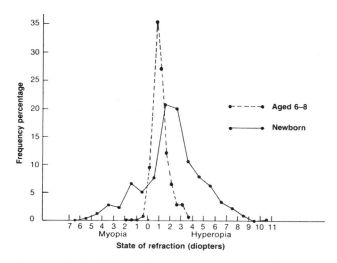

Figure 2.7   Refractive error distribution for newborn infants (Cook and Glasscock, 1951) **and for children aged 6–8** (Kemph, Collins, and Jarman, 1928) (calculated and redrawn by M. J. Hirsch, *Vision of Children*, Chilton, 1963).

of refraction ranging from approximately 8D of hyperopia to 7D of myopia. Goldschmidt notes that considerable development of the eyes occurs during the last few months of pregnancy and the first few months of life, with the result that the developmental "age" of an infant may have an effect on the refraction at birth. He refers to a report of Gleiss and Pau (1952), who followed the refraction of premature babies and concluded that, during the last few months of pregnancy, the degree of hyperopia increases and the degree of myopia decreases (assuming that the conditions of growth were the same whether the babies were born or were still *in utero*). Goldschmidt (1968) considers the question of whether it is possible to predict the adult refractive state on the basis of refraction at birth. He suggests that, in the majority of cases the amount of congenital myopia decreases and may even disappear altogether. This finding is consistent with that of Fletcher and Brandon (1955); that is, in some cases the myopia of prematurity stabilizes near zero by the end of the first year of life.

Changes During Preschool Years

Sorsby, Benjamin, and Sheridan (1961) concluded that the growth of the eye during infancy is extremely rapid, its adult size being reached by the age of 3 years. They point out that the length of the globe increases an average of 5mm between birth and the age of 3 years, whereas between the ages of 3 and 13 years the increase in axial length averages only a total of about 1mm, or an average of 0.1 mm per year.

Unfortunately, little data are available for children between the first few months of life (when they can be examined in well-baby clinics) and the age of 5 or 6 (when they can be examined in kindergartens or schools). Kemph, Collins, and Jarman (cited in Hirsch, 1963b) obtained refractive data on a group of 333 children from 6–8 years old. Their data are shown in Figure 2.7 (dashed line). The refractive error distribution indicates that by the ages of 6–8 emmetropization has taken place, the great majority of the children being in the emmetropic group, having its peak at 1.00D of hyperopia.

More recently, Mohindra and Held (1981) refracted 400 full-term infants between birth and age 5 using "near retinoscopy" (a procedure in which noncycloplegic retinoscopy is done at a distance of 50cm in a dark room with the child watching the retinoscope light, with −1.25D added to the spherical component at neutrality). For children aged 0–4 weeks they found a bell-shaped distribution of refraction, ranging from −14D to +12D, gradually

narrowing to a range of −3D to +4D at age 129–256 weeks (see Figure 2.8). These results demonstrate that the process of emmetropization is evident during the first year of life.

Changes During School Years

The belief that all children are hyperopic was reinforced by a study published by Slataper (1950), based on data on several thousand clinical patients. Using spherical equivalent refraction, Slataper found that the average refraction was +2.32D at birth, increasing to +3.93D at age 7, and then decreasing at the rate of about 0.25D per year. Slataper was apparently unaware that a clinical population varies greatly from an unselected population, in that most infants and young children who visit an ophthalmologist's office are brought there because of strabismus that is often accompanied by high hyperopia.

In a study of 1,432 unselected children, Sorsby, Benjamin, and Sheridan (1961) found that the mean ocular refraction, under cycloplegia, decreased from +2.33D at age 3 to +0.93D at age 14 for boys, and from +2.96D at age 3 to +0.64D at age 15 for girls.

Figure 2.8   Narrowing of the distribution of refraction during the first 5 years of life, demonstrating that the process of emmetropization is evident very early in life. In group 0–4 weeks the data of Cook and Glasscock (1961) is included (broken line and circles); adult data are from Sorsby et al. (1960) (diagram from Mohindra and Held, 1981).

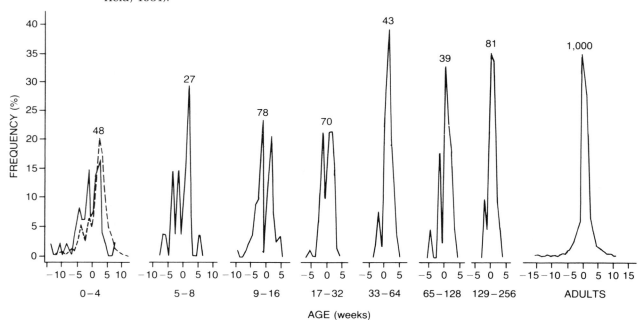

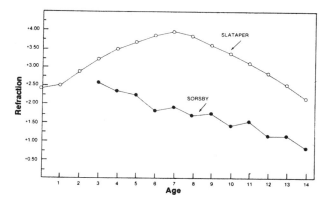

Figure 2.9 Refractive error data for children: Slataper's (1950) data compared with data of Sorsby et al. (1961) (redrawn from F. J. Slataper, *Archives of Ophthalmology*, Vol. 43, pp. 466–481, copyright 1950, "Age Norms in Refraction and Vision," American Medical Association; and A. Sorsby et al., *Refraction and Growth of the Eye from the Age of 3*, 1961, with permission of the Controller of Her Majesty's Stationery Office, London).

Figure 2.9, showing Slataper's data compared to the average of Sorsby's data for boys and girls, clearly indicates the excessive amount of hyperopia found in Slataper's clinical population. It should be noted that Sorby's data for 6-to-8-year-old children show a mean refraction of about +2.00D as compared to less than +1.00D for the Kemph, Collins, and Jarman data shown in Figure 2.7. Factors that may partially account for this difference are differences in the depth of cycloplegia used in the two studies and the difference in the subject populations (English children versus American children).

The studies of Slataper and of Sorsby et al. have the disadvantage of not furnishing information about individual children: they are *cross-sectional studies*, involving one set of findings on each of a large number of subjects. As opposed to this type of study, a *longitudinal study* is one in which each subject is examined repeatedly over a period of years, making it possible to determine the changes taking place in an individual's refractive state with the passage of time.

Hirsh (1961) used retinoscopy to refract a group of children in Ojai, California, twice each year throughout the first eight grades of school. Although 1,200 children were included in the study when it began, complete data were available on only about 500 children by the time they had reached the eighth grade.

In one of his earlier reports on the study, Hirsch

(1961) concluded that during the first six years of school, 84–90 percent of the children showed a refractive change in a linear fashion; for the remaining 10–16 percent, refraction changed in a curvilinear manner. Most of those varying in a linear fashion changed in the direction of becoming more myopic or less hyperopic as they grew older (the direction shown in both Slataper's and Sorsby's studies). Only a small minority changed in the direction of more hyperopia or failed to change at all.

Figure 2.10 shows two typical curves. The upper curve is that of a child who decreased at the rate of about 0.06D of hyperopia per year, from 1.00D of hyperopia at age 6 to 0.50D at age 12. The lower curve shows the change in refraction for a child who was emmetropic at age 7 but increased in myopia at the rate of about 0.50D per year for the following 5 years.

In a later report, Hirsch (1964) analyzed the changes in refraction separately for children who were myopic, emmetropic, and hyperopic when entering school. He arrived at the following results: (1) of four children who were myopic at ages 5–6,

Figure 2.10 Curves showing change in refraction with age for individual children (redrawn from M. J. Hirsch, "A Longitudinal Study of Refractive State of Children During the First Six Years of School," *American Journal of Optometry*, Vol. 38, pp. 564–571, 1961).

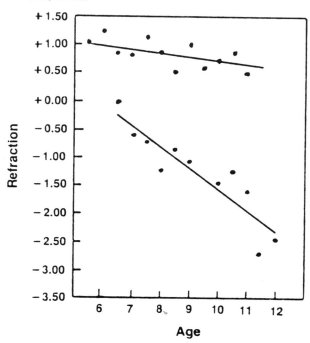

all were still myopic at ages 13–14; (2) of 185 children who were emmetropic at ages 5–6, 86 had become myopic, 84 were still emmetropic, and 15 were hyperopic at ages 13–14; and (3) of 72 children who were hyperopic at ages 5–6, only two became myopic by ages 13–14, whereas 16 became emmetropic and 54 were still hyperopic.

On the basis of these data, Hirsh (1964) concluded the following:

1. If a child has any myopia at all at ages 5–6, the myopia will remain and will probably increase.
2. If a child has hyperopia in excess of +1.50D at ages 5–6, it is likely the child will remain hyperopic, or nearly so, by ages 13–14.
3. If a child has a spherical refraction between +0.50 and +1.25D at ages 5–6, the child has the greatest chance of being emmetropic at ages 13–14.
4. A child having a spherical refraction between zero and +0.50D at ages 5–6 has a high probability of becoming myopic by the age of 13–14; the probability is even greater if against-the-rule astigmatism is present. (These conclusions are summarized in Table 2.1.)

Sorsby and Leary (1970) reported on a longitudinal study of refraction and its components in which 129 children were examined on two or more occasions between the ages of 3 and 21 years. Their data for 25 myopic children are of particular interest. Figure 2.11, based on their Tables 12 and 13, shows a high correlation between rates of change of axial length and of refraction, each increase in axial length of 0.10mm being accompanied by an

increase in myopia of about 0.17D per year. For example, a child whose axial length increases 0.10mm per year has an increase in myopia of 0.17D per year, whereas a child whose axial length increases 0.40Dmm per year has an increase in myopia of about 0.70D per year. Figure 2.12, based on the same tables, shows no systematic relationship between yearly rate of change of lens power and rate of change of refraction. On the basis of these two diagrams we may conclude that, for these 25 myopes, the increase in myopia is primarily due to the increase in axial length.

Figure 2.11   Relationship between rates of change of axial length and refraction (plotted from data of A. Sorsby and G. Leary, *A Longitudinal Study of Refraction and its Components During Growth*, Her Majesty's Stationery Office, London, 1970).

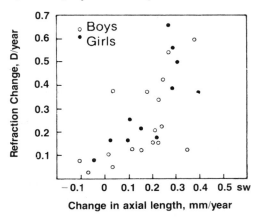

Figure 2.12   Relationship between rates of change of lens power and refraction (plotted from data of A. Sorsby and G. Leary, *A Longitudinal Study of Refraction and its Components During Growth*, Her Majesty's Stationery Office, London, 1970).

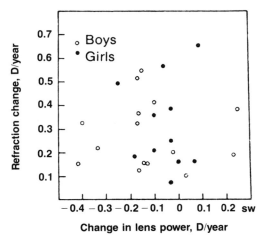

Table 2.1   Conclusions on the basis of the Ojai study (Hirsch, 1964).

Refraction at ages 5–6	Prediction for ages 13–14
Myopia	Myopia will remain and will probably increase
Hyperopia in excess of +1.50D	Child will likely remain hyperopic
Between +0.50 and +1.25D	High probability of being emmetropic at ages 13–14
Between 0.00 and +0.50D	High probability of being myopic at ages 13–14
Between 0.00 and +0.50D and against-the-rule astigmatism	An even higher probability of becoming myopic by ages 13–14

There appear to be few, if any, studies of refraction occurring during the late teenage years. However, there is good reason to believe that the trends apparent during childhood continue into the late teen years and level off by the age of 20 or 21. Most hyperopes change little during this period; increasingly fewer emmetropes become myopic, and those who are already myopic tend to level off in the amount of myopia. Changes in astigmatism during this period are relatively small.

Changes in the Young Adult

The literature on refraction contains few studies of refractive change during the 20s and 30s. One study involving this age group was reported by Morgan (1958). A nonvisually selected group of subjects was examined at age 13 and again at age 33. Morgan's subjects included 51 women and 44 men, and data were reported separately for the two groups. Mean data for keratometric astigmatism, refractive astigmatism, and equivalent sphere refraction are shown in Table 2.2.

Inspection of Table 2.2 indicates that changes in mean refraction during the 20-year period were very small. Equivalent sphere refraction for females changed 0.22D in the direction of less hyperopia or more myopia during this period, as compared to a change of only 0.04D, in the same direction for males. Changes in mean astigmatism were similarly small.

In an effort to obtain a more complete picture of changes in refraction during the adult years, a questionnaire was published in the *Optometric*

Table 2.2   Mean refraction at ages 13 and 33 (Morgan, 1958).

	Age 13	Age 33
Females		
Keratometric astigmatism	0.69 WR[a]	0.91 WR
Refractive astigmatism	0.14 WR	0.26 WR
Equivalent sphere	+0.09D	−0.13D
Males		
Keratometric astigmatism	0.41 WR	0.58 WR
Refractive astigmatism	0.08 WR	0.03 WR
Equivalent sphere	+0.39D	+0.35D

[a]WR = with-the-rule.

Weekly (Grosvenor, 1977a), requesting readers to indicate their own refractive corrections at 5-year intervals between the ages of 15 and 45. By the time the data were analyzed, 191 questionnaires had been returned, 111 of which contained complete data for ages 20 through 40. Of these 111 subjects, 109 were males, one was female, and one failed to specify sex.

Refraction for the most plus meridian of the right eye was tabulated for each of the 111 subjects at ages 20, 25, 30, 35, and 40 (Grosvenor, 1977b). Mean refraction and standard deviation at each age level are shown in Figure 2.13. During the 20-year period, mean refraction decreased from −0.08 to −0.18D, and the standard deviation increased from 1.47D at age 20 to 1.92D at age 40.

Refractive error distribution curves for ages 20 and 40 are shown in Figure 2.14. Comparison of these two distribution curves indicates that, although a certain amount of "deemmetropization" took place

Figure 2.13   Mean refraction and standard deviation, ages 20–40 (T. Grosvenor, "A Longitudinal Study," Part 1, *Optometric Weekly*, Vol. 68, 1977b).

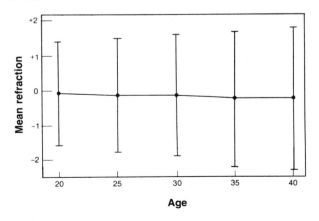

Figure 2.14   Refractive error distribution curves, ages 20 and 40 (T. Grosvenor, "A Longitudinal Study," Part 1, *Optometric Weekly*, Vol. 68, 1977b).

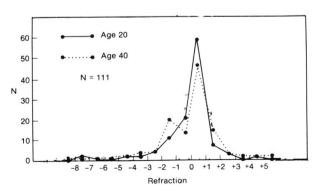

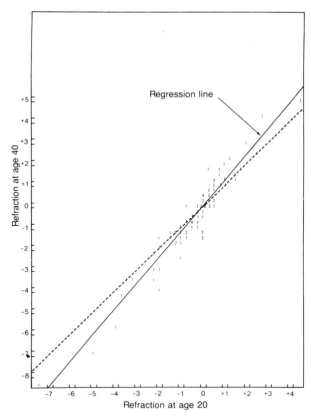

Figure 2.15 Scatterplot of refractive data, ages 20–40 (T. Grosvenor, "A Longitudinal Study," Part 4, *Optometric Weekly*, Vol. 68, 1977b).

1. In the emmetropic region of the graph, the small amount of scatter, together with the fact that the origin of the regression line is at −0.03, indicates that a subject who was emmetropic at age 20 could be expected to be emmetropic or near-emmetropic at age 40.

2. In the myopic region of the graph, the fact that the regression line moves away from the broken line toward increasing myopia indicates that the more myopic a subject was at age 20, the greater increase in myopia might occur by age 40.

3. In the hyperopic region of the graph, the fact that the regression line moves away from the broken line in the direction of increasing hyperopia indicates that the more hyperopic a subject was at age 20, the greater increase in hyperopia was likely to occur by age 40.

How can we explain the observations that myopes tend to become more myopic and hyperopes tend to become more hyperopic? Possible explanations are that the increase in myopia is due to continued stretching of the posterior segment of the already stretched myopic eye, and that the increase in hyperopia possibly is due to the further relaxing of accommodation in an already hyperopic eye, allowing latent hyperopia to become manifest. It is also possible that, because the subjects included in the study are not representative of the population as a whole, trends shown in the data are not necessarily typical of those found in an unselected population or even of those found in a typical clinical population.

Refractive Changes in the Older Adult

Presbyopia

The onset of presbyopia is ordinarily considered to occur when the amplitude of accommodation has

during the 20-year period, the percentage of subjects in the emmetropic group (plano to +0.87D) decreased only from 53 percent at age 20 to 40 percent at age 40.

To analyze the data in terms of the changes for individual subjects, the data were plotted in the form of a scatterplot, as shown in Figure 2.15. Each subject's refraction at age 20 was plotted along the x-axis and refraction at age 40 plotted along the y-axis (Grosvenor, 1977c). If all subjects' refractive states had remained the same during the 20-year period, all data points in Figure 2.15 would have fallen on the broken line, which represents a perfect correlation between refraction at ages 20 and 40. The correlation coefficient for the subjects' data was found to be 0.955, and the regression line (the solid line) was found to have a slope of 1.22 and a y-intercept of −0.03. The relationship between the regression line necessary for a perfect correlation (the broken line) and the actual regression line (the solid line) can be described as follows:

Table 2.3 Donders's table showing amplitude of accommodation as related to age (Borish, 1970).

Age (in years)	Amplitude	Age (in years)	Amplitude
10	14.00D	45	3.50D
15	12.00	50	2.50
20	10.00	55	1.75
25	8.50	60	1.00
30	7.00	65	0.50
35	5.50	70	0.25
40	4.50	75	0.00

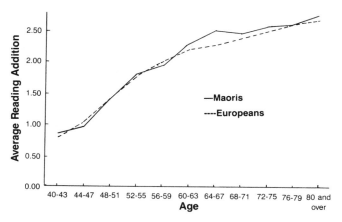

Figure 2.16 Average reading addition as related to age (from T. Grosvenor, "Refractive Error Distribution in New Zealand's Polynesian and European Children," *American Journal of Optometry*, Vol. 47, pp. 355–361, 1970a).

decreased to 5.00D or less. According to Donders's table of accommodative amplitude as related to age, shown in Table 2.3, this level has been reached by the age of 40, and the amplitude continues to decrease until the age of 75, when it reaches zero. However, it has been shown by Ong, Hamaski, and Marg (1956) that amplitude of accommodation reaches zero as early as age 54, and what appears to be accommodation after this age is due to the eye's depth of focus. Data comparing reading additions for Maoris and Europeans in New Zealand (Grosvenor, 1965) show that the average addition is +0.75D at ages 40–43, increasing to +2.00D at ages 56–69, and to +2.50D at ages 68–71 (Figure 2.16).

Spherical ametropia

Refractive data for 820 patients over the age of 45 were reported by Hirsch (1958). Although these patients were examined in a private optometric practice and cannot be considered unselected

subjects, Hirsch pointed out that they are fairly representative of the general population, since by the age of 45 most people find it necessary to have some help with either distance or near vision. Of the 820 subjects, 460 were women and 360 were men.

Hirsch found that the median refractive state increased from +0.18D at ages 45–49 to +1.02D over the age of 75; the dispersion in refractive state increased markedly with age. As shown in Table 2.4, hyperopia of +1.13D or more increased from 16 percent at ages 45–49 to 48 percent at ages 70–74; myopia of −1.13D or more was relatively constant at about 7 percent from ages 45–64 but increased to 15 percent over the age of 75. The increase in the prevalence of myopia in the older subjects was due to the presence of nuclear lens changes affecting approximately 10 percent of this group. Hirsch warned that, in view of the increased prevalence of both hyperopia and myopia beyond the age when +2.00 or +2.25D addition is required, practitioners should not tell such patients that "this is the last lens change we shall have to make."

Are there mechanisms for emmetropization in the adult eye?

Although a number of emmetropizing mechanisms have been described for the developing eye, little attention has been given to the possibility that emmetropizing mechanisms may be present in the adult eye. If we neglect those eyes that develop myopia (either during childhood or during the later years of life), we may conclude that a large proportion of eyes change relatively little in spherical refraction throughout adult life. As already noted, Hirsch (1958) found that after age 55 most eyes tend to remain the same or to change in the direction of increasing hyperopia. Therefore, it is reasonable to propose the existence of one or more emmetropizing mechanisms in the adult eye.

Table 2.4 Spherical ametropia as a function of age (Hirsch, 1958).

Age (in years)	Incidence of ametropia		
	Hypermetropia	Emmetropia	Myopia
45–49	16.3%	77.2%	6.7%
50–54	23.5	70.4	6.2
55–59	35.4	59.3	5.0
60–64	40.1	52.3	7.4
65–69	43.9	43.9	12.3
70–74	47.7	43.8	8.8
75 and over	47.9	36.9	15.3

It has been known since the time of Donders (1864) that the lens becomes thicker with increasing age due to the constant addition of new lens fibers, resulting in a gradual reduction in the depth of the anterior chamber. This, in the absence of other changes, has the effect of moving two converging lenses closer to one another and, therefore, tends to change the refraction of the eye in the direction of *myopia*. Donders incorrectly assumed that the lens gradually becomes flatter with age. If this were true, the flattening of the lens would change the refraction of the eye in the direction of hyperopia, thus compensating for the decrease in anterior chamber depth. However, it has been reported by Brown (1974) that the lens actually steepens in the process of becoming thicker with age. Because the shallowing of the anterior chamber and the steepening of the lens would both drive the eye in the direction of myopia, we must look elsewhere for a compensatory mechanism that tends to stabilize the refraction of the eye with increasing age. An obvious candidate for this mechanism is a shortening of the eye.

Grosvenor (1985; 1987b) analyzed the cross-

Table 2.5   Mean values of ocular refraction and refractive components of subjects having ocular refraction between 0.00 and +2.00 D. (Data from Sorsby, Benjamin, Davey, Sheridan and Tanner, 1957 and Sorsby, Sheridan and Leary, 1962).

Age group	Mean age	Subjects M	Subjects F	Ocular refract (D)	Corneal power (D)	Ant Ch depth (mm)	Lens power (D)	Power of eye (D)	Axial length (mm)
0–9	7	24	25	+1.1	43.3	3.4	21.4	60.7	23.4
10–19	13	24	24	+0.6	42.8	3.6	19.8	58.8	24.1
20–29	23	27	19	+0.6	42.8	3.5	19.9	58.9	24.1
30–39	36	15	20	+0.7	43.6	3.2	20.2	59.8	23.8
40–49	44	32	33	+0.9	43.4	3.3	21.0	59.9	23.6
50 & older	55	13	15	+0.9	43.3	3.2	20.9	60.8	23.5

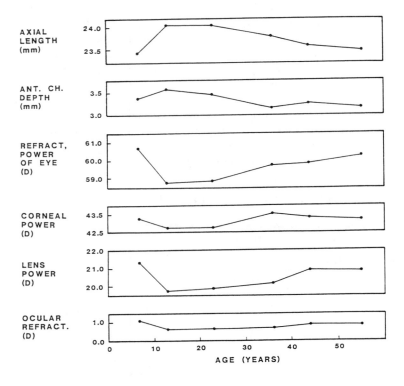

Figure 2.17   Mean values of ocular refraction and refractive components, by 10-year age groups, for subjects whose spherical equivalent refraction was between plano and +2.00D (data from Sorsby, Sheridan, Davey, Benjamin, and Tanner, 1957; and Sorsby, Sheridian, and Leary, 1962).

sectional refractive component data published in two separate monographs by Sorsby et al. (1957; 1962) using only those subjects whose spherical refraction was between plano and +2.00D. He found that the axial length of the eye appears to decrease with increasing age. As shown in Table 2.5 and Figure 2.17, mean axial length for the Sorsby et al. subjects increases from 23.4mm at ages 4–9 years to 24.1mm at ages 20–29 years, then gradually decreases to 23.5mm at age 50 and older. In addition, the mean refracting power of the eye decreases from 60.7D at ages 4–9 years to 58.9D at ages 20–29 years, then increases to 60.8D by age 50 and over. These data suggest the presence of an emmetropizing mechanism in the adult eye—the axial length decreases to compensate for the increase in the refractive power of the eye (the latter being due to an increase in the refracting power of the cornea and the lens).

Because Sorsby et al. (1957; 1962) *calculated* axial length on the basis of equations that assume unchanging indices of refraction for the ocular media, it is possible that the apparent decrease in axial length could have been due to changes in indices of refraction of the media with age. However, cross-sectional population studies making use of *ultrasound* measurements (Francois and Goes, 1971; Leighton and Tomlinson, 1972) have also shown an apparent decrease in the axial length of the eye with age. As for possible index changes, Leighton and Tomlinson noted that, although ultrasound measurements are based on assumed indices of refraction, the method has the advantage that errors due to possible index changes tend to cancel each other out. That is, an increase in the density of the lens increases ultrasound speed and underestimates the lens thickness and axial length; a decrease in the index of the vitreous due to liquefaction decreases the ultrasound speed and overestimates the vitreous depth and axial length of the eye.

CHANGES IN ASTIGMATISM WITH AGE

Eye practitioners have long known that astigmatism changes relatively little during much of the life span, tending to change toward the against-the-rule direction in the later years. Until recently only rather sketchy information was available concerning changes in astigmatism during the early years of life. As a result of a number of studies published during the past decade, however, a clearer picture is now emerging.

Astigmatism at Birth

It is unfortunate that many of the studies of refraction at birth and in early infancy have not reported information concerning astigmatism. However, information now available concerning astigmatism during the first year of life indicates that both the prevalence and the amount of astigmatism are relatively high at birth, decreasing significantly during the preschool years. This is not unexpected in view of the fact that spherical ametropia has a wide distribution at birth, which narrows considerably during the first few years of life as the process of emmetropization becomes established.

The Preschool Years

One of the first studies of the prevalence of astigmatism in preschool children to be published in recent years is Woodruff's (1971). He reported that for 631 children between the ages of 1 and 6 years the prevalence of astigmatism (0.75D or more) was only 3 percent at age 2 increasing to 10 percent at age 6. Most of this was with-the-rule astigmatism. Curiously, no subsequent study has shown trends similar to those reported by Woodruff. Mohindra and Held (1981), in the study noted earlier in which near retinoscopy was used to refract 400 full-term infants and children between birth and age 5, found the prevalence of astigmatism (1.00D or more) to be 30 percent for children 0–4 weeks of age, peaking at about 60 percent at 17–32 weeks, and reducing to about 40 percent at 129–256 weeks (2.5–5 years). Mean cylinder power was found to decrease from about 2.25D at age 0–4 weeks to about 1D at 129–256 weeks.

Studies by Gwiazda et al. (1984), Dobson et al. (1984), and Howland and Sayles (1984)—all published in the same issue of *Investigative Ophthalmology and Visual Science*—showed trends similar to those of Mohindra and Held (1981). Gwiazda et al. (1984) used the near retinoscopy procedure to refract 1,000 children from early infancy to 6 years of age, and found the prevalence of astigmatism (1.00D or more) to be about 50 percent during the first year of life and decreasing to about 20 percent at age 5. Before age 4.5 years most of the astigmatism was in the against-the-rule direction, but beyond that age most was with-the-rule. Dobson et al. (1984) reported on cycloplegic retinoscopy data for 281 children from birth to age 9.5 years, all of whom had 1.00D or more of astigmatism. They found that the great majority of subjects refracted during the first year of life had against-the-rule astigmatism, whereas the majority of 6–9-year-olds had with-the-rule astigmatism. Dobson et al. concluded that against-the-rule astigmatism predominates before age 3.5, whereas with-the-rule astigmatism predominates after age 3.5. Howland and Sayles (1984) refracted 312 infants and preschool children using a method called *photorefraction*, in which a fiber-optic light source forms an image on the subject's retina, which is photographed. Measurements were subsequently taken from the photograph to determine the refraction of the eye. They found a prevalence of astigmatism (1D or more) during the first year of life of approximately 60 percent, reducing to almost zero by ages 5–6 years.

The changes in astigmatism during the preschool years can be summarized by quoting a statement made by Howland and Sayles, which compares their results to those of the Gwiazda et al. (1984) and Dobson et al. (1984) studies:

> The major similarities of the 3 studies are: (1) all studies report a preponderence of against-the-rule astigmatism over with-the-rule astigmatism in the first 4.5 years of life, and (2) the three studies . . . all show a uniform decrease with increasing age during the first 3–5 years of life. (1984, p. 98)

Finally, the findings of the three studies are in agreement with the concluding statement of Gwiazda et al.:

> If a child does not have astigmatism in infancy, he or she is unlikely to acquire it at a later age, at least up to 4–6 years of age. (1984, p. 91)

The School Years

Most of the data on astigmatism during the school years shows a low prevalence of clinically significant astigmatism during this period, with relatively little change in either prevalence or amount. In a visual screening program in elementary schools conducted in Orinda, California, in which refraction was done by retinoscopy, Blum et al. (1959) found that the prevalence of astigmatism of 1D or more increased gradually from about 2 percent at age 6 to 3 percent at age 14.

In a longitudinal study of refraction, Hirsch (1963a) also found little change in astigmatism during the school years. Using a criterion of 0.75D or more, he found the prevalence of astigmatism to increase from 4.2 percent at age 6.5 to 6 percent at age 12.5. Almost all of the astigmatism found by Hirsch was with-the-rule: the prevalence of against-the-rule

astigmatism was 0 percent at age 6.5 and only 0.3 percent at age 12.5. Hirsch concluded that large changes of astigmatism do not occur during the school years, and that "if a child is going to have marked astigmatism it will be present when he enters school."

The Early Adult Years

Astigmatism, as well as spherical ametropia, tend to change little during the early adult years. In Morgan's (1958) longitudinal study of refraction at ages 13 and 33, he found that both mean corneal astigmatism and mean refractive astigmatism changed little during this period. For males, mean refractive astigmatism increased from 0.15D–0.26D with-the-rule during the 20-year period; whereas for females, mean refractive astigmatism decreased from 0.08D–0.03D with-the-rule. In a retrospective longitudinal study of the refraction of 111 optometrists, Grosvenor (1977d) also found relatively little change in astigmatism. A total of 61 subjects (55 percent of the sample) had no change in astigmatism between the ages of 20 and 40 years, whereas the prevalence of with-the-rule astigmatism increased 14 percent and that of against-the-rule astigmatism increased 14 percent during the same period. It was concluded that changes in astigmatism between ages 20 and 40, for this subject population, did not occur in any regular predictable manner.

The Later Adult Years

A number of studies confirm the observation that against-the-rule astigmatism increases in older patients while with-the-rule astigmatism decreases. Lyle (1971) has reported on changes in keratometric astigmatism for 1,208 eyes of patients seen in his optometric practice in Winnipeg, Manitoba, over a 28-year period. Lyle found that the prevalence of against-the-rule astigmatism (of 0.12D or more) increases from 6 percent at ages 41–50 to 27 percent at age 61 and over. His data indicate that the amount of astigmatism gradually decreases for eyes having with-the-rule astigmatism and gradually increases for eyes having against-the-rule astigmatism. Further, Lyle found no evidence that indicates the axis rotated from a horizontal to a vertical position. Hirsch (1959b) reported on subjective astigmatism data for 1,606 eyes of patients over the age of 40 seen in his practice in Ojai, California. Hirsch found that during the 40-year span between the ages of 40 and 80, the average change in astigmatism was 1.00D in the against-the-rule direction, or an average of 0.25D every 10 years.

The changes in astigmatism with age could result from changes in corneal astigmatism, internal (i.e., nonkeratometric) astigmatism, or both. Although Lyle's (1971) data concerns changes in corneal astigmatism and Hirsch's (1959b) data concerns changes in refractive astigmatism, a study involving both corneal and refractive astigmatism (allowing for the calculation of internal astigmatism) remained to be done. Such a study was done by Anstice (1971), who reported on corneal, refractive, and internal astigmatism findings for the right eye of each of 621 patients, whose ages ranged from 5 to over 75 years, and who were examined in a New Zealand optometric practice. Anstice's data indicate that beyond the age of 35, both corneal and refractive astigmatism change in the against-the-rule direction at the rate of approximately 0.20D every 10 years. Anstice points out that the practical value of this finding is the following: if the practitioner has difficulty obtaining accurate retinoscopic or subjective cylindrical data on an older patient, Javal's rule can be used to arrive at a tentative cylindrical correction, since it is the corneal rather than the internal astigmatism that changes with age.

Baldwin and Mills (1981) reported on a retrospective longitudinal study of patients between 30 and 70 years of age who were examined in the optometric practice of Ryer and Hotaling in New York. They selected records of patients who were examined over a 40-year span and who were between the ages of 30 and 70 years, having eyes whose principal meridians were within 10 degrees of vertical and horizontal. For the 34 eyes meeting their criteria, Baldwin and Mills tabulated data for the first examination beyond the age of 40 (at an average age of 51.2 years) and the last examination (at an average age of 65.3 years). Both mean corneal astigmatism and mean refractive astigmatism changed in the against-the-rule direction during the 15-year period: mean corneal astigmatism was 0.38D with-the-rule at the first examination and 0.07D with-the-rule at the last examination; mean refractive astigmatism was 0.24D against-the-rule at the first examination and 0.76D against-the-rule at the second examination. These results differ from those of Anstice in that the change in corneal astigmatism did not entirely account for the change in refractive astigmatism. Baldwin and Mills note that, because there was a change of 0.52D in refractive astigma-

tism but only 0.31D in corneal astigmatism, there must have been a change in mean noncorneal astigmatism of 0.21D. However, they conclude that

> This study supports the hypothesis that steepening of the horizontal meridian of the cornea, beginning in the middle life and continuing throughout the remainder of life, accounts for most, if not all, changes in refractive astigmatism typical of this age period. (Baldwin and Mills, 1981, p. 210)

What Causes Age Changes in Astigmatism?

On the basis of data concerning astigmatism at various stages of life, it may be concluded that a typical child is born with against-the-rule astigmatism that decreases markedly during the preschool years and results in a small amount of with-the-rule astigmatism during the school years. This astigmatism changes little during the early adult years, begins to decrease gradually during the 30s, reduces to zero, and eventually becomes against-the-rule astigmatism.

Age changes in astigmatism are consistent with the following hypothesis:

1. Against-the-rule astigmatism that tends to occur at birth may be due to a "sagging" of the cornea of the still-developing globe.
2. The small amount of with-the-rule astigmatism that develops during the preschool years occurs as a result of the rather stiff upper tarsal plate constantly exerting pressure on the horizontal meridian of the cornea, particularly in the case of an eye that has low ocular rigidity. With the passage of time, this results in with-the-rule corneal astigmatism.
3. As the upper tarsal plate begins to lose its rigidity in middle life and beyond, the horizontal meridian is allowed to steepen so that the cornea again assumes an approximately spherical shape (as shown in the Baldwin and Mills [1981] data), resulting in a small amount of against-the-rule refractive astigmatism.

HEREDITARY AND ENVIRONMENTAL FACTORS

If a child is going to have clinically significant hyperopia or astigmatism, it is present at birth or at a very early age. It is normally assumed, therefore, that these refractive conditions are hereditary in nature. On the other hand, because myopia is seldom present at birth but in most cases apparent only after several years of schooling, many researchers conclude that it occurs as a result of environmental rather than hereditary influences. However, those who believe that myopia occurs as a result of hereditary factors point out that a trait does not have to be present at birth to be inherited. Thus, ocular refraction has not escaped the "nature versus nurture" controversy.

The Role of Heredity

The assessment of the role of heredity in the determination of the refractive state of the eye is complicated, because the refractive state is the result of a number of interrelated refractive components. The inheritance of refractive components is discussed by Francois (1961), who points out that it is likely that several genetic factors contribute to the refraction of the eye—each of the components probably being inherited independently of the others and possibly transmitted according to different patterns of heredity.

The inheritance of refractive anomalies is discussed at some length in two major textbooks, *Ophthalmic Genetics* (Sorsby, 1970) and *Heredity in Ophthalmology* (Francois, 1961). Sorsby concludes that all refractive states including myopia are genetically determined and that myopia and hyperopia can occur in dominant and recessive forms. Francois cites the work of Steiger as indicating that low myopia and low hyperopia can be considered as variations within the normal limits of the binomial distribution, and refers to additional studies indicating that these conditions are inherited as dominant characteristics, whereas myopia and hyperopia of 6.00D and over are inherited either as dominant or as recessive characteristics.

Wixson (1958) compared refractive findings for 10 pairs of identical twins, 6 pairs of fraternal twins, and 10 pairs of same-sex siblings. He found that correlation coefficients for spherical equivalent refraction were +0.99 for the identical twins, +0.67 for the fraternal twins, and +0.54 for the siblings. He concludes that the closer the genetic ties between individuals, the greater the similarity between both the type and range of refractive error. Sorsby, Sheridan, and Leary (1962) also studied refraction in twins, using as subjects 78 pairs of identical twins, 40 pairs of same-sex fraternal twins, and a control group of 48 unrelated same-sex pairs. They found

that, for ocular refraction in the vertical meridian, 70.5 percent of the identical twins had close agreement in refraction (no differences exceeding 0.50D), while 30 percent of the fraternal twins and 29 percent of the control group pairs had similarly close agreement.

Hirsch and Ditmars (1969) analyzed data concerning the refractive states of both parents of each of 258 myopic children. They found that the higher the myopia possessed by the children, the greater the percentage of parents who were also myopic; they reported a rank-order coefficient of correlation for degree of myopia and percentage of myopic parents to be +0.89 ($p = 0.01$).

Astigmatism

Wixson (1958), Francois (1961), and others provide evidence that astigmatism is genetically determined. In the twin study noted earlier, Wixson found the correlation coefficients for refractive astigmatism to be +0.93 for identical twins, +0.07 for fraternal twins, and +0.47 for the control group of same-sex siblings. Francois states that "the only certain data about the inheritance of refraction concerns corneal refraction and astigmatism" (1961, p. 191). He quotes several studies and concludes that astigmatism is generally transmitted as an autosomal dominant and is known to be transmitted through several generations. He reports that concordant hyperopic astigmatism in identical twins has been found by many authors, but that discordance has been found to be the rule in fraternal twins.

Environmental Factors

Although the role of environmental factors in myopia has been a lively topic of discussion for many years, few if any authors have suggested that environmental factors are of importance in hyperopia. The great majority of children are hyperopic when entering school and few progress significantly in hyperopia during the school years.

For astigmatism, the pronounced changes in corneal toricity that can occur as a result of contact lens wearing have stimulated an interest in the role of environmental factors in this refractive anomaly.

One of the first proponents of the theory that myopia can be caused by excessive use of the eyes for near work was Ware (cited in Young, 1977). Ware observed in 1813 that there was a considerable amount of myopia among the officers of the Queen's Guard in England, most of whom were literate, but little myopia among the enlisted men, most of whom were illiterate. Donders (1864, reprinted 1972) proposed that myopia occurs as a result of prolonged tension on the eyes during close work and is due to an elongation of the visual axes.

Young and his co-workers have reported on a number of investigations designed to demonstrate the relationship between near work and myopia. In one study, Young, Beattie, Newby, and Swindal (1954) found a much higher prevalence of myopia among residents of Pullman, Washington, where a large proportion of residents were engaged in academic and clerical pursuits, than among residents of the surrounding area, most of whom were engaged in agriculture.

The roles of heredity and environment in the refraction of 41 Eskimo family units in Point Barrow, Alaska, were investigated by Young, Leary, Baldwin, West, Box, Harris, and Johnson (1969). They found the average refraction to be +1.69D for the 82 parents and +0.33D for the 115 children. They also found that correlations between parents and children were not significantly different from zero, but that correlations between siblings were high and significant. They interpreted the results as indicating that there is no major hereditary component involved in the development of myopic refractions among the offspring, while there is a strong environmental component operating to create sibling correlations. The proposed environmental component was compulsory schooling leading to a considerable amount of reading among the children.

Studies of the development of myopia in monkeys reported by Young (1967a) indicate that the development of myopia is related to the conditions under which the monkeys are reared. Young found that laboratory monkeys were considerably more myopic than wild monkeys, and monkeys kept indoors in cages developed more myopia than monkeys kept outside in pens. (The development of myopia in terms of hereditary and environmental factors is discussed more fully in Chapter 3.)

Environmental Factors in Astigmatism

There is no doubt that the files in many optometrists' offices contain information that, if tabulated and analyzed, would demonstrate the hereditary nature of astigmatism. The reports of Wixson (1958) and Francois (1961) noted earlier provide convincing evidence of the role of heredity in astigmatism. However, evidence is gradually accumulating regarding environmental influences on astigmatism. The fact that astigmatism changes in a predictable

manner with age, that both hard and soft contact lenses can bring about changes in astigmatism, and that variations in astigmatism exist among racial groups must be considered to fully understand the etiology of astigmatism.

The tendency of both hard and soft contact lenses to cause changes in corneal astigmatism is well documented. A typical case in which astigmatism is caused by the wearing of hard contact lenses is reported by Janoff (1976), who found that during a 12-year period of contact lens wear a patient's corneal astigmatism increased in the with-the-rule direction 2.50D in one eye and 3.25D in the other. Numerous verbal reports by contact lens practitioners indicate that 2.00D or more of with-the-rule astigmatism can be caused by hard lenses in just a few years, and that this astigmatism is usually not reversible.

Hartstein and Becker (1970) reported not only on the development of with-the-rule astigmatism but also on the development of keratoconus while wearing contact lenses. These investigations determined ocular rigidity by comparing Shiötz tonometer readings with 5.5 and 10g weights for a group of hard contact lens wearers. They found that patients who developed with-the-rule corneal astigmatism had lower ocular rigidity than those who did not develop astigmatism; those patients who developed keratoconus while wearing contact lenses had still lower ocular rigidity findings. Changes in astigmatism with soft contact lenses were reported in a study (Grosvenor, 1975a) in which 24 patients were fitted with lathe-cut soft contact lenses; two of the patients were found to have an increase in corneal astigmatism on the order of 0.75D in the with-the-rule direction. In both cases the patients were subsequently fitted with more loosely fitting lenses and the astigmatism eventually returned to normal.

Many studies show that the prevalence of corneal astigmatism varies considerably both between and within racial groups. One such study is that of Lyle, Grosvenor, and Dean (1972), who studied the prevalence of corneal astigmatism in unselected groups of Indian children in northern Saskatchewan and in Brantford, Ontario, and in an unselected group of Caucasian children in Kitchener, Ontario. They found that the mean corneal astigmatism in the northern Saskatchewan Indian children was significantly higher than that of the Caucasian children and considerably higher than that of the Brantford Indian children. They pointed out that the two Indian groups differed in that the Brantford Indians had lived an urbanized life for several generations, whereas the Saskatchewan Indians still carried on a rural, "Indian-like" way of life. They proposed that the increased astigmatism in the Saskatchewan Indians may be accounted for on the basis of inadequate nutrition: the present generation of these Indians is greatly influenced by the white man's diet, and it is believed that their nutrition has suffered greatly from a diet low in protein and high in carbohydrates, including refined sugar.

The key to these variations of astigmatism—changes with age, changes with contact lens wearing, and variation within racial groups—may be *ocular rigidity*. It has been suggested (Grosvenor, 1976g) that whether or not a given cornea has astigmatism may be a function of the relationship between corneal rigidity and the pressure exerted by the tarsal plate in the upper lid. The cornea is a portion of an inflated sphere, the inflation being a result of the intraocular pressure. If no outside pressures were acting on the cornea, one would expect it to be spherical, having the same radius of curvature in all meridians. One possibility is presented by the contraction of the extraocular muscles, in that the four rectus muscles have their insertions within 5–10mm of the corneoscleral junction. However, Fairmaid (1959) found that convergence of the eyes resulted in only a clinically insignificant increase in the radius of curvature in the horizontal meridian of the cornea and a corresponding decrease in the radius of curvature in the vertical meridian.

The suggestion that eyelid pressure can cause astigmatism is not a recent one, having been made in the 19th century by Snellen and Birch-Hirschfield, as reported by Gullstrand (1924) and by Duke-Elder (1970). The effect of retracting the eyelids on corneal astigmatism was investigated by Wilson, Bell, and Chotai (1982), who performed keratometry on 18 subjects while the lids were held apart by the use of a speculum. They found that for corneas having more than 1.00D of with-the-rule astigmatism, retraction of the lids had the effect of reducing the amount of astigmatism. They note that their results are comparable to those of Masci (1965), who also found a reduction in the toricity of with-the-rule corneas when the lids were retracted. Wilson et al. conclude that the pressure exerted on the eyeball by the eyelids is a major factor influencing astigmatism.

Contact lens practitioners classify their patients as having "tight" or "loose" eyelids, and find that eyelids inevitably "loosen" as part of the aging process. Many patients in the presbyopic age group have great difficulty learning to remove hard lenses, because their eyelids are so loose and flabby. Young people, on the other hand, tend to have "tighter" eyelids and therefore have little trouble in flipping off their hard lenses.

The relationship between ocular rigidity and lid pressure can be considered to operate in the following manner. A child born with no corneal astigmatism or with against-the-rule corneal astigmatism would be expected to develop a small amount of with-the-rule astigmatism during childhood, due to the bandlike pressure of the upper tarsal plate that is exerted across the horizontal meridian of the cornea during blinking. Later in life, as the rigidity of the upper tarsal plate gradually decreases, the amount of with-the-rule corneal astigmatism would be expected to decrease, with the result that against-the-rule internal astigmatism becomes manifest.

If eyelid pressure can cause astigmatism, why doesn't *every* child develop corneal astigmatism? The great majority of children *do* develop with-the-rule corneal astigmatism, but in most cases the amount is so small that all or most of it is negated by internal astigmatism. However, those few children having a combination of low ocular rigidity and normal or high eyelid pressure would develop large amounts of with-the-rule astigmatism, which would be expected to be reduced considerably in later years, when the lids exert less pressure on the cornea.

The effect of a hard contact lens would be to magnify the pressure exerted by the upper tarsal plate, thus greatly increasing the flattening of the horizontal meridian of the cornea. Soft contact lenses, particularly the large, thick, lathe-cut lenses that are no longer in general use, could also be expected to magnify the pressure of the upper tarsal plate on the cornea.

As for the high degrees of corneal astigmatism found in the Saskatchewan Indians, it is possible that a link between poor nutrition and low corneal rigidity may eventually be found. Obviously, much additional information is needed to confirm the proposition that with-the-rule astigmatism occurs as a result of the pressure of the upper tarsal plate on the horizontal meridian of the cornea.

Etiology of Presbyopia

The following changes are known to take place in the crystalline lens during accommodation: the anterior pole of the lens moves forward and the anterior surface becomes markedly more convex; the posterior pole remains fixed in position but the posterior surface becomes slightly more convex; and the lens tends to sink downward due to gravity.

Although early investigators had difficulty determining whether the ciliary muscle acted as a dilator muscle or a sphincter muscle, Helmholtz (1924) correctly concluded that it acts as a sphincter muscle and that in the unaccommodated state the zonular fibers are kept "on the stretch," holding the lens in its flattest form, whereas in the accommodated state the contraction of the ciliary muscle releases the tension of the zonular fibers and allows the lens to assume a more nearly spherical shape.

As described earlier, Fincham (1937) concluded that the lens capsule is relatively thin at the anterior and posterior poles and at the equator, but somewhat thicker in the peripheral zones of the anterior and posterior surfaces (see Figure 1.13). He proposed that when the ciliary muscle contracts, "the zonule gives up some of its stretch and the elastic capsule, under the freedom now given it, presses upon the soft lens substance and moulds it into the accommodated form by compressing it at the equator and in those regions where the capsule is thickest, allowing it to bulge in the thinner parts" (p. 70).

Lens fibers continue to be formed throughout life, and as they are formed (just underneath the lens capsule), the older fibers are compressed into what becomes the nucleus of the lens. The nucleus thus becomes increasingly less elastic with age, with the result that the response of the lens to the released tension of the zonule, in attempted accommodation, is gradually diminished. Therefore, it is possible that the decrease in accommodation occurring with age is entirely due to the decrease in the elasticity (i.e., sclerosis) of the lens.

It has been proposed, however, that presbyopia may be due to a loss of power of the ciliary muscle. Finchan (1937) entertained this possibility but rejected it on the basis that it seems unlikely that the ciliary muscle should have begun to lose power at the relatively early age at which the near point of accommodation begins to recede. In addition, he referred to a 40-year-old subject whose lens substance had been absorbed, leaving an empty lens capsule. When the subject attempted to accommodate, Finchan observed a great change in the form of the lens capsule, which convinced him that the ciliary muscle was quite active in the absence of lens substance to offer resistance to it.

Many investigators, particularly Van Hoven (1959) and Morgan (1954), have presented arguments for and against the proposition that presbyopia may be due, at least in part, to a loss of ciliary muscle power. However, there can be little doubt that the major cause of presbyopia is the gradual loss in elasticity of the crystalline lens—loss of ciliary muscle power, if it occurs at all, most likely occurs as a result of the increased hardening of the lens.

ADDITIONAL EPIDEMIOLOGICAL CONSIDERATIONS

The refractive state of the eye has been found to vary with such epidemiological considerations as race, reading ability, intelligence test scores, academic achievement, and personality traits.

Racial Variations

Many investigators have reported findings that appear to show racial variations in refraction. Many of these reports have been reviewed by Post (1962) and Baldwin (1964). On the basis of his review of numerous studies concerning refraction of people of various races, Post proposed that these differences are not racial differences but rather are due to the relaxation of natural selection in more advanced societies. Racial and ethnic groups whose refraction has been investigated include blacks, Orientals, East Indians, Melanesians, Polynesians, Jews, and American Indians.

Blacks

In a report based on vision screenings conducted by University of Houston optometry students, Reber (1964) reported that the prevalence of myopia for 2,578 American children screened (both Caucasian and black) was 13 percent, but for the 213 black children included in the study, the prevalence of myopia was only 8 percent. Post (1962) compared refractive error distributions for Gabon blacks and three groups of Caucasians (British, German, and Swedish), and found that the Caucasians had an obvious excess of both myopia and hyperopia as compared to the Gabon blacks. He pointed out that the blacks (as well as Eskimos, also included in the same study) engaged primarily in hunting and food gathering and not in agriculture or animal husbandry.

Orientals

Numerous studies indicate a high prevalence of myopia in Japanese, Chinese, and other Oriental children. Post (1962) reported that twice as many Japanese as American children aged 6–11 years

Table 2.6 Prevalence of myopia for children of various races in Hawaii (Data of Crawford and Hamman, reported by Baldwin, 1964).

Racial group	Number studied	Percent of myopes
Chinese	5,621	17%
Korean	490	13
Japanese	41,684	12
Caucasian	5,353	12
Spanish	193	9
Portuguese	6,562	7
Filipino	9,732	7
Puerto Rican	1,764	4
Part Hawaiian	20,375	4
Hawaiian	2,758	3

failed a visual acuity test. The criterion for failure was 20/70 or worse. Baldwin (1964) reported on a study by Crawford and Hamman, who investigated the refraction of a large, nonselected sample of school children in Hawaii. Their findings, shown in Table 2.6, show the highest prevalences of myopia for Chinese, Korean, Japanese, and Caucasian children. In another study reported by Baldwin (1964), Dzen tabulated the refraction of 576 consecutive Chinese and 574 consecutive Caucasian patients examined in the Peking University Medical College. He found a prevalence of myopia of 52 percent for Chinese and 20 percent for Caucasians. The disagreement found from one study to another is due, at least in part, to differing criteria for the presence of myopia and to differing age distributions.

East Indians

Post (1962) summarized the data from a number of studies of refractive error of East Indians and found that among Brahmans (Indians of the highest caste), the rates of myopia were very close to those of Caucasians, but among non-Brahmans the rates were considerably lower.

Melanesians

Rose (1964), a New Zealand optometrist, examined some 2,000 Fijian army recruits while stationed in Suva during World War II and found no myopia at all. He reported that these recruits were pure Melanesian and had undergone little admixture with Caucasians and almost none with Indians.

Garner et al. (1985; 1986) performed noncyclo-plegic retinoscopy on Melanesian children in the Vanuatu islands (formerly the New Hebrides), and found little myopia. In the 1985 study, 977 school children between the ages of 6 and 17 years were examined, and the prevalence of myopia greater than 0.25D was found to be only 1.3 percent. In the 1986 study, in which 788 school children were examined, the spherical equivalent refraction (right eye), for 763 (96.8 percent) of the children was found to be between +1.00D and −0.25D, with 23 (2.9 percent) having myopia greater than 0.25D, 2 (0.3 percent) having hyperopia greater than 1.00D, and 2 (0.3 percent) having refractive astigmatism greater than 1.00D. The prevalence of myopia was found to increase with age, being 0.8 percent for primary school pupils and 6.5 percent for secondary school pupils.

Polynesians

The refractive error distributions of Polynesian and Caucasian children were compared (Grosvenor, 1970b) using the modified clinical screening technique for children in two New Zealand high schools. Of a total of 973 children, 683 were Caucasian and 290 were Polynesian. The refractive error distributions (see Figure 2.18) indicate that the Polynesian children had a greater frequency of emmetropia (from −0.25D to +0.50D) and lower frequencies of both myopia and hyperopia than the Caucasian children.

Figure 2.18 Refractive error distributions of 683 Caucasian and 290 Polynesian children in New Zealand (Grosvenor, 1970b).

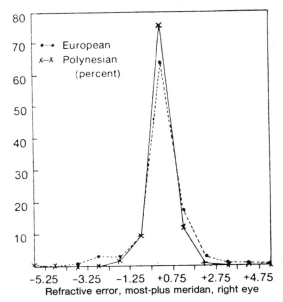

Refractive error, most-plus meridan, right eye

Jews

In a study cited by Post (1962), "defective vision" was compared for Jewish and non-Jewish boys. It was found that defective vision (20/40 or worse) was present for 40 percent of the Jewish boys of all ages, whereas the failure rate for non-Jewish boys increased from 14 percent at ages 8–9 to 28 percent at ages 13–14. In a study by Sorsby (cited by Baldwin, 1964), 33 percent of Jewish children aged 10–14 were found to be myopic, as compared to 25 percent for non-Jewish children in the same age range and in the same community.

American Indians

Studies of refraction comparing American Indians with Caucasians show that some groups of Indian children have a much greater prevalence of with-the-rule astigmatism than Caucasian children. The study of Lyle, Grosvenor, and Dean (1972) is described earlier. Additional studies involving American Indians are discussed in a paper by Grosvenor (1976g).

The Role of Natural Selection

As mentioned earlier, Post (1962) proposed that the higher prevalence of visual defects in more developed societies is not due to racial factors but to a relaxation of the pressure of natural selection. He points out that primitive people must traverse unmarked wildlands in the never-ending quest for food, and that the penalty for any members of the tribe who do not see the enemy before the enemy sees them may be sudden death, while there is a relaxation of selection pressure in the more developed societies that are not primarily engaged in hunting and food gathering. If it is assumed that mating in a primitive society occurs as soon as puberty permits, it is clear that many cases of myopia would not become manifest until after the tribesmen had already reproduced their kind. In such cases, selection pressure would be nonexistent. However, it is a well-known fact that in today's society, children who are going to become *high* myopes begin to show signs of myopia as early as age 5 or 6, and by puberty they may have uncorrected visual acuity of 20/200 or 20/400. Thus, it seems reasonable that in a primitive society the elimination of potentially high myopes would have the effect of removing the gene pool for all myopia.

Refractive State and Reading Ability

Many studies have been conducted to determine what relationship, if any, exists between refractive state and reading ability. Many of the studies have been poorly designed, poorly controlled, and have failed to specify criteria for myopia, hyperopia, and astigmatism. The interpretation of the results of these studies is complicated by the fact that reading ability is known to depend on numerous factors. Poor reading ability has been traced to such factors as poor intelligence, poor health, neurological problems, mixed dominance or mixed laterality, developmental anomalies, intellectual deprivation, poor teaching, emotional and psychological disorders, perceptual-motor anomalies, and hyperactivity—in addition to refractive and binocular vision anomalies (Carter, 1970).

One of the most widely quoted studies relating refractive anomalies to reading ability was published by Eames (1948), who compared refractive and binocular vision anomalies for 1,000 reading failures and 150 unselected children. He reported that the prevalence of myopia was the same (4 percent) for both the reading failures and the unselected children, but that the prevalence of hyperopia of 1.00D or more was 43 percent for the reading failure group but only 13 percent for the unselected group. In a study involving 336 children examined over a 4-year period, Kelly (1957) found that 43 subjects having a moderate or high "myopic tendency" during the 4-year period had above-average scores on reading speed, comprehension, and reading proficiency, all significant at the 0.05 confidence level. He also reported that the 46 students with the best reading averages for the 4-year period had a high "myopic tendency," significant at the 0.0005 confidence level.

In a review of 18 studies concerning the relationship between myopia and reading ability, Francis (1973) reported that myopia was found to be associated with reading success in 14 of the studies, whereas no significant relationship was found in the other four studies. After reviewing 24 studies relating hyperopia to reading ability, Francis reported that 18 of the studies found that hyperopes tended to have difficulty in reading, while 6 found no significant relationship. It is of interest that in none of the studies reviewed by Francis was it found that hyperopes were more successful readers than myopes.

In the study reported by Kelly (1957), lateral phoria findings were measured at distance and at near using the Keystone Telebinocular. Students who were exophoric at distance or at near had reading scores falling within the normal range, but students who were esophoric at distance or near were significantly low in both intelligence test scores and in reading scores. Kelly's most interesting data concerns the combined effects of refractive state and lateral phoria findings on reading scores. Children having a "myopic tendency," whether exophoric or esophoric, tended to have above-average reading scores. As for children having a "hyperopic tendency," those having esophoria at near had mean reading scores that were significantly low in vocabulary, comprehension, and proficiency, whereas those who were exophoric at near were "almost as good as the myopes" in their reading scores.

Uncorrected ametropia

In comprehensive vision screening programs, often most of the children found to have hyperopia are "newly discovered" hyperopes and thus are not wearing corrective lenses. Even those children whose hyperopia may have been previously diagnosed may not have glasses, or if they have them they may not wear them because a schoolteacher or nurse has told them that they "don't see any better with the glasses than without them." Experience in conducting vision screening programs also indicates that a large proportion of children with myopia are also in the "newly discovered" category.

The fact that a large proportion of hyperopic children do not wear corrective lenses is of particular importance. Not only do these children have to accommodate sufficiently to compensate for the distance at which the reading material is held, but they also have to accommodate an additional amount to overcome the hyperopia. For a normal accommodative convergence/accommodation (AC/A) relationship (discussed in Chapter 4), the use of this additional accommodation makes the child esophoric at near, requiring the use of *negative fusional vergence* to keep from seeing double. For example, a child having 2.00D of uncorrected hyperopia has to accommodate 2.50D for a 40cm reading distance plus 2.00D to overcome the hyperopia. For a "normal" 6/1 AC/A ratio, and if the child is orthophoric at distance, this additional 2.00D of accommodation brings into play 12 prism diopters (Δ) of accommodative convergence, requiring the use of 12Δ of negative fusional vergence to maintain single binocular vision.

The 2.00D myope, on the other hand, has to accommodate only 0.50D (assuming the child is uncorrected) for a 40cm reading distance. Although the amount of accommodative convergence associated with 0.50D of accommodation is insufficient to maintain single binocular vision, the uncorrected myope has no difficulty learning to make use of

proximal convergence to maintain single binocular vision. In summary, uncorrected hyperopia is a decided *detriment* to maintaining clear, single binocular vision at the reading distance, whereas uncorrected myopia is a decided *asset*.

Refractive State and Intelligence Test Scores

The relationship between refractive state and intelligence test scores has been studied by a number of investigators. Without exception, the findings indicate a tendency for myopes to achieve higher scores on these tests than hyperopes. The findings should come as no surprise if it is understood that many intelligence tests are, to a great extent, tests of reading ability.

Hirsch (1959a) reported on a study in which the refraction of 554 schoolchildren between the ages of 6 and 14 was determined by retinoscopy, and refractive errors were compared to intelligence test scores. Correlation coefficients between refractive state and intelligence test scores were found to be -0.04 for 6-to-9-year-old children, -0.21 for 10-to-13-year-old children, and -0.24 for 14-to-17-year-olds. The minus sign in the correlation coefficient indicates that higher intelligence test scores tend to be associated with myopia. The coefficients for the older two groups were significant (at the 0.01 and 0.001 levels, respectively), whereas the coefficient for the younger children was not significant. The younger children were given the Stanford-Binet test, which is administered to the children individually, whereas the older children were given the California Test of Mental Maturity, a group test that involves the visual perception of fine detail. Hirsch proposed that the significant correlations found with the older children could be due to the fact that the California test, requiring fast and accurate visual perception, gave the myope an advantage and put the hyperope at a disadvantage. Hirsch emphasized the fact that the relationship between refractive state and intelligence test scores was not a strong one and had little predictive value: the highest correlation obtained (-0.24), when squared, is about 0.06, indicating that about 6 percent of the variability in intelligence test scores is associated with variation in refraction.

Young (1963) reported on a group of 251 children who were tested on both the Stanford-Binet test and the California Test of Mental Maturity. He agreed with Hirsch that there was a higher correlation between refractive error and paper-and-pencil tests of intelligence than between refractive error and a test that requires a minimum of reading. Young rejected the idea that there is a relationship between refractive state and intelligence, but he favored the idea of a relationship between refractive state and reading ability.

A study involving 707 intermediate school-children in New Zealand (Grosvenor 1970a) compared refractive data to results obtained on the Otis Self-Administered Test, a "verbal" test that had been administered by a school official. Myopes (−1.00D and more) were found to have significantly higher Otis scores than hyperopes (+1.00D and more). The Raven Matrix test, a nonverbal test of intelligence, was subsequently administered to 290 of the same children, and the relationship between this test and refractive error was found not to be significant. Because the Raven Matrix test requires the perception of fine detail but does not require reading, it was concluded that the trend for myopes to score higher than hyperopes on the Otis test was not the result of superior vision for fine detail but of superior reading ability.

Therefore, it appears that a myopic child has two advantages over a hyperopic child in taking a self-administered intelligence test that requires reading. The child has (1) an advantage in taking the test itself, in that reading is likely easier than for the hyperope, as well as (2) the advantage of having previously acquired more information, through reading, than the hyperope. It should be emphasized, as Hirsch notes, that this relationship is not a strong one and cannot be used to predict intelligence test scores on the basis of refractive error.

Refractive State vs. Perceptual Skills and Learning Difficulties

The relationship between refractive state and perceptual skills has been investigated by Rosner and Gruber (1985) by comparing results of perceptual skills screening tests to refractive error. As noted by these authors, screening tests for visual and auditory perceptual skills are routinely administered to patients between the ages of 5 and 12 years examined at the University of Houston Optometry Clinic. Any one of three visual perceptual skills tests may be used—the Developmental Test of Motor Integration (VMI), the Rutgers Drawing Test, or the Test of Visual Analysis Skills (TVAS)—each of which assesses the child's ability to copy a geometric design, to identify its separate parts, and to map the relations among those parts. The Test of Auditory Analysis Skills (TAAS), which provides an index of the child's

analytical aptitudes with respect to identifying the phonemic features of spoken words, was administered to all of the children.

Comparing refractive status to the results obtained on visual and auditory perceptual skills tests for 710 children examined during a 7-month period, Rosner and Gruber (1985) found a significant relationship between refraction and visual perceptual skills test results. The tests were passed by 95 percent of myopic children (more than −0.50D) but only by 18 percent of hyperopic children (more than +1.25D), with the results for the emmetropic children falling somewhere between. However, the auditory perceptual skills test was passed by the majority of children, regardless of refractive status. Rosner and Gruber conclude that the findings support the hypothesis that hyperopes are much more likely to lag in the development of visual perceptual skills than are emmetropes or myopes, and that this is probably an outcome of the hyperopia. As for the evidence that myopes' visual perceptual skills appear to be better than those of the other two groups, they suggest that myopes may signal their condition even before it manifests by displaying better than age-appropriate visual perceptual skills.

In a subsequent study, Rosner and Rosner (1987) compared visual characteristics of children with and without learning difficulties. Data were tabulated from the case records of 757 children (aged 6–12) examined during a 14-week period, 261 of whom were diagnosed as having learning difficulties. The prevalence of myopia (−0.50D or more) was found to be 19 percent for the learning difficulty (LD) children as compared to 54 percent for the children having no learning difficulties (NLD). Further, the prevalence of hyperopia (+1.00D or more) was 54 percent for the LD children as compared to 16 percent for the NLD children, and the prevalence of astigmatism was about the same for both groups. There was no apparent relationship between learning difficulties and vergence/accommodation infacility, strabismus, or amblyopia. Rosner and Rosner conclude that the data strongly support the proposition that hyperopia appears to be associated with learning difficulties, and corroborates earlier reports of a close relationship between visual perceptual skills and elementary school achievement.

Refractive State and Personality

Perhaps the earliest observation that personality characteristics of myopes differ from those of emmetropes and hyperopes was that made by Thorington who, as reported by Baldwin (1964), remarked in 1900 that myopes were introverted and shy, had few friends, and preferred indoor activities. A more recent observation was that of Gesell, Ilg, and Bullis (1949), who reported that "the pronounced myope . . . gathers all experience unto himself and is in consequence better oriented within himself, but not so facilely oriented to his physical or social milieu" (p. 286).

The first investigation designed for the purpose of relating refractive error to specific personality traits was that of Schapero and Hirsch (1952), who administered the Guilford-Martin Temperament Test to 119 optometry students and compared the results to spherical equivalent refractive error. These researchers concluded that myopes tended to have inhibited dispositions and overcontrol of emotions, tended to be inert and disinclined to motor activity, but scored high in social leadership. Hyperopes tended to have happy-go-lucky, carefree dispositions, tended to engage in vigorous activity, but scored high in social passiveness. Schapero and Hirsch warned that the degree of association was so slight as to be of no predictive value. Additional studies showing relationships between myopia and personality traits have been reported by Van Alphen (1961); Young, Singer, and Foster (1975); and Shultz (1960).

In a study reported by Grosvenor (1980a), the Minnesota Multiphasic Personality Inventory (MMPI) was administered to 70 third-year optometry students. Of the 64 students for whom complete data were available, 46 (or 72 percent) were myopes, and only 3 subjects (5 percent) had 1.00D or more of hyperopia. Of the 10 MMPI scales, significant correlations were found for female subjects on only 2 of the scales, and no significant correlations were found for male subjects. In a study reported earlier by Shultz (1960) using the MMPI, a significant relationship was found on only 1 of the 10 scales.

In discussing his results, Grosvenor (1980a) suggests that perhaps the "conventional wisdom" that myopes are shy and introverted should be called into question. Observations that myopes are shy and introverted may well apply less to "corrected" myopes than to uncorrected myopes: inability to succeed at baseball and other games or the inability to recognize one's classmates on the playground may well be causes of shy and introverted behavior.

For the first few children who appear in the classroom wearing glasses (these are the children who will become the highest myopes), the correction of myopia with glasses is sure to be greeted by shouts of "four eyes," further reinforcing previously acquired introvertive patterns. In contrast, children who will become myopic later in their school years or even in college (the moderate and low myopes) are spared this embarrassment, for glasses are commonplace in the upper grades of school and college.

Even the higher myopes, once they have survived the ravages of elementary school, have reason to face the world more confidently than their myopic parents did. Whereas previous generations of myopic high school and college students were forced to wear "ugly" glasses or to view the world dimly— a choice preferred by some myopes—the present-day availability of fashion frames and contact lenses may well remove the major cause of shyness and introversion.

The preceding discussion is consistent with the contention that myopia is the cause rather than the result of personality traits. To the extent that personality traits may cause myopia or to the extent that myopia and personality traits may spring from a common underlying factor, the conventional wisdom of myopia may retain a degree of validity.

Study Questions

1. According to an HEW study, at what age group (a) do approximately 90 percent of corrective lens wearers wear plus lenses? (b) do approximately 90 percent of corrective lens wearers wear minus lenses?

2. Why did Sorsby disagree with Steiger's theory that the components of ocular refraction are freely associated?

3. How did the refractive error distribution for newborn babies reported by Cook and Glasscock differ from that reported by Herrnheiser?

4. On the basis of data reported by Hirsch and others, how does the refractive error distribution change beyond the age of 45 (a) for spherical refraction? (b) for astigmatism?

5. Describe the refractive error distribution curve found by Scheerer and Betsch for 12,000 patients over the age of 25. How can this curve be made to look more nearly like a normal distribution curve?

6. According to Hirsch, children having a refractive error in what range at ages 5–6 would be most likely at ages 13–14 years to be (a) hyperopic? (b) emmetropic? (c) myopic?

7. According to Van Alphen's theory of emmetropization, how is the amount of stretch of the eye controlled?

8. At what period of life (a) does relatively little change in refractive error occur over a period of about 20 years? (b) does refractive error distribution first appear to be markedly leptokurtic? (c) do a high percentage of people become myopic?

9. According to Sorsby and his co-workers, how many millimeters does the eye grow in axial length (a) from birth to age 3 years? (b) from 3 years to 13 years?

10. How can you account for the following findings by Hirsch and Weymouth, reanalyzing Stenstrom's refractive data by using partial correlations: (a) the correlation between corneal radius and refractive state was found to be +0.70 as compared with the +0.18 found by Stenstrom; (b) the correlation between anterior chamber depth and refractive state was found to be +0.25 rather than Stenstrom's −0.34.

11. Discuss why uncorrected hyperopia tends to make reading difficult for a child, whereas uncorrected myopia tends to make reading easy.

12. On the basis of what evidence did Fincham conclude that presbyopia is caused by a loss in elasticity of the crystalline lens rather than by loss of power of the ciliary muscle?

13. What evidence indicates the possibility of environmental influences in astigmatism?

14. In view of the fact that myopes tend to score higher on intelligence tests than emmetropes or hyperopes, what evidence is there that this tendency for higher scores does not indicate that myopes are more intelligent than hyperopes or emmetropes?

15. Which of the refractive components of the eye (including corneal radius, anterior chamber depth, lens radii of curvature and thickness, refractive indices, and axial length) did Tron find not to be normally distributed?

16. Summarize the changes in refraction that would typically occur—for an individual who does not become myopic during the school years—during the following periods of life: (a) from birth to age 6; (b) from ages 6–20; (c) from ages 20–45; (d) beyond age 45.

17. Summarize the changes in refraction that would typically occur—for an individual who becomes myopic during the school years—during the following periods of life: (a) from birth to age 6; (b) from age 6–20; (c) from age 20–45; (d) beyond age 45.

18. What condition is necessary for a trait to be normally distributed? Does this condition apply to refractive error?

19. Discuss the concept of "developmental age" at birth in terms of the development of refractive state.

20. Discuss the possible emmetropizing mechanisms that may be present in the adult eye.

CHAPTER 3

Myopia and Its Development

It is appropriate to ask the question, "Why should we be concerned about the development of myopia but not about the development of hyperopia or astigmatism?" There are several reasons for this apparent inconsistency:

1. Although clinically significant hyperopia and astigmatism are each present in 2–4 percent of children when entering school, neither of these refractive anomalies increases in prevalence during the school years and neither has a tendency to progress with the passage of time.
2. The fact that hyperopia and astigmatism fail to increase in prevalence during the school years tends to point to hereditary factors, minimizing the probability that environmental influences are involved.
3. Although myopia is present in only about 2 percent of children when entering school, its prevalence increases markedly during the school years. Further, once a child becomes myopic, the condition tends to progress rapidly for a period of several years.
4. The fact that myopia usually develops only after several years of schooling suggests the possibility of environmental influences.
5. Myopia has been shown to be associated with significant ocular and visual morbidity, including retinal detachment, glaucoma, and choroidal and retinal degeneration.

PREVALENCE OF MYOPIA AS RELATED TO AGE

During the past several years an increasing amount of data has become available concerning the prevalence of myopia at various stages of life, particularly during the early years.

Myopia at Birth and in Early Childhood

The available information concerning the prevalence of myopia at birth and in early childhood is discussed in Chapter 2 and summarized in Table 3.1. Recall that, although the older studies (published during the latter part of the 19th century) found that

Table 3.1   Prevalence of myopia for children from birth to ages 6–8.

Age (years)	Source	Subject	Criterion	Prevalence (percent)
Birth	Cook & Glasscock (1951)	Caucasian	Any myopia	24%
Birth	Goldschmidt (1969)	Danish	Any myopia	25
Birth	Mohindra & Held (1981)	Boston area	Any myopia	50
5–6	Hirsch (1952)	Los Angeles	−1.00D or more	1
6	Blum et al. (1959)	Orinda, CA	−0.50D or more	2
6	Hirsch (1964)	Ojai, CA	−0.50D or more	2
6–8	Kemph et al. (1928)	Caucasian	Any myopia	2
7–8	Laatikainen & Erkkila (1980)	Finnish	−0.50D or more	2
7	Mantajarvi (1983)	Finnish	−0.25D or more	1

all children were born with hyperopia, more recent studies show a wide range of refraction at birth (Cook and Glasscock, 1951; Goldschmidt, 1969) which is thought to be due to the fact that there is a wide range in the maturity of the development of the eye; eyes not completely developed at birth tend to be myopic, whereas more completely developed eyes tend to be emmetropic or hyperopic. It is now understood that the myopia found in premature (low birth weight) infants is due not to axial elongation but to an underdevelopment of the eye, the eye having a steep cornea and an underdeveloped, relatively spherical lens (Fledelius, 1981; Goss, 1985).

It appears that during the first few months of life the process of emmetropization occurs rapidly (Mohindra and Held, 1981), with the result that by the end of the first year few children are found to be myopic. Many studies show that by the age of 5 or 6 years, only about 2 percent of children have myopia of 0.50D or more (Kemp et al., 1928; Blum et al., 1959; Hirsch, 1964; Laatikainen and Erkkila, 1980; Mantajarvi, 1983).

The School Years

It is known that many children who are emmetropic when entering school become myopic during the school years. This is shown by the data summarized in Table 3.2. Much of this data is based on an extensive report published by the U.S. Department of Health, Education and Welfare (1978) concerning the refractive status and motility defects of more than 20,000 people between the ages of 4 and 74 years,

who constituted a "national probability sample" of the United States population. Although the prevalence of myopia is not given as such in the report, it can be estimated by cross-reference to two of the report's tables. On the basis of the information summarized in Table 3.2, a conservative estimate would be that the prevalence of myopia of 0.50D or more increases in a relatively linear manner from about 2 percent at age 6 to about 20 percent at age 20.

The Early Adult Years

Data concerning the prevalence of refractive errors for adults are not easily found because people in this age group are not readily available for visual screening tests. However, data from a number of sources are summarized in Table 3.3. Attention should be called to the high prevalences of myopia reported by Fledelius (1983), who investigated refractive data for 1,306 adult Danes referred to a hospital eye clinic from other hospital departments for ophthalmic evaluation of general disease (but not eye disease). Although patients diagnosed as diabetic were not included in the study, it is possible that the unusually high prevalence of myopia may reflect an unrecognized form of selection.

On the basis of the information summarized in Table 3.3, it may be conservatively estimated that the prevalence of myopia (of 0.50D or more) reaches a peak of about 30 percent between the ages of 20 and 40 years, after which it begins to decrease

Table 3.2 Prevalence of myopia during the school years.

Age (years)	Source	Subject	Criterion	Prevalence (percent)
6–11	U.S. Dept. of Health, Education and Welfare (1978)	NPS[a]	Wearing a correction[b]	6%
13–14	Hirsch (1952)	Los Angeles	−1.00D or more	5
13–14	Hirsch (1952)	Los Angeles	−0.25D or more	23
14	Blum et al. (1959)	Orinda, CA	−0.50D or more	15
14	Hirsch (1964)	Ojai, CA	−0.50D or more	12
14–15	Laatikainen & Erkkila (1980)	Finnish	−0.50D or more	22
15	Mantajarvi (1983)	Finnish	−0.25D or more	23
12–17	U.S. Dept. of Health, Education and Welfare	NPS[a]	Wearing a correction[b]	26

[a]National probability sample of United States population aged 4–74 years.
[b]Currently wearing a correction (glasses or contact lenses) for myopia.

Table 3.3   Prevalence of myopia during the early adult years.

Age (years)	Source	Subject	Criterion	Prevalence (percent)
18–24	U.S. Dept. of Health, Education and Welfare (1978)	NPS[a]	Wearing a correction[b]	33%
20–30	Borish (1970)	Jackson (1932) Tassman (1932) data	> −0.50D	22
25–34	U.S. Dept. of Health, Education and Welfare (1978)	NPS[a]	Wearing a correction[b]	34
26–35	Fledelius (1983)	Hospital patients	−0.25D or more	41
30–40	Borish (1970)	Jackson (1932) and Tassman (1932) data	> −0.50D	16
35–44	U.S. Dept. of Health, Education and Welfare (1978)	NPS[a]	Wearing a correction[b]	31
36–45	Fledelius (1983)	Hospital patients	−0.25D or more	33

[a]National probability sample of United States population aged 4–74 years.
[b]Currently wearing a correction (glasses or contact lenses) for myopia.

Table 3.4   Prevalence of myopia during the later adult years.

Age (years)	Source	Subject	Criterion	Prevalence (percent)
45–49	Hirsch (1958)	Optometric patients	−1.13D or more	7%
40–50	Borish (1970)	Jackson (1932) and Tassman (1932) data	> −0.50D	14
45–54	U.S. Dept. of Health, Education and Welfare (1978)	NPS[a]	Wearing a correction[b]	32
46–55	Fledelius (1983)	Hospital patients	−0.25D or more	26
55–64	U.S. Dept. of Health, Education and Welfare (1978)	NPS[a]	Wearing a correction[b]	18
56–65	Fledelius (1983)	Hospital patients	−0.25D or more	26
65–74	U.S. Dept. of Health, Education and Welfare (1978)	NPS[a]	Wearing a correction[b]	16
> 66	Fledelius (1983)	Hospital patients	−0.25D or more	14
> 70	Borish (1970)	Jackson (1932) and Tassman (1932) data	> −0.50D	21
> 75	Hirsch (1958)	Optometric patients	−1.13D or more	15

[a]National probability sample of United States population aged 4–74 years.
[b]Currently wearing a correction (glasses or contact lenses) for myopia.

because of the tendency for some of the low myopes to lose their myopia, rejoining the emmetropic group.

The Later Adult Years

Data concerning the prevalence of myopia in the later adult years are summarized in Table 3.4. Hirsch (1958), using a criterion of −1.13D or more for myopia, found that the percentage of myopic patients increased from 6.7 percent at ages 45–49 to 15.3 percent beyond age 75. Hirsch attributed this increase to the presence of nuclear lens changes, affecting about 10 percent of the older subjects. It is of interest that the prevalence of myopia reported by Hirsch for ages 45–49 is only about one-fourth of that reported by the U.S. Department of Health, Education and Welfare (HEW) for subjects of the same age, whereas the prevalence reported by Borish (1970) was only about one-half that reported by HEW. However, different criteria were used. Because more than half of all myopes have less than 1.13D of myopia, Hirsch would have found a much higher prevalence of myopia had he used −0.25D or −0.50D as a criterion.

On the basis of the information shown in Table 3.4, it is likely that beyond the age of 45 years the prevalence of myopia of 0.50D or more continues to decline due to some of the low myopes joining the emmetropic or hyperopic ranks, but increases somewhat in the later years of life due to the presence of nuclear lens changes, as suggested by Hirsch (1958).

Population Differences in the Prevalence of Myopia

In any discussion of the prevalence of myopia we must consider that the prevalence of refractive anomalies varies widely from one geographical, racial, or occupational group to another. Baldwin (1967) has reviewed much of the literature concerning the prevalence of myopia in various racial and occupational groups. One of the most interesting studies cited by Baldwin was that of Crawford and Hammar (1949), who screened 50,000 schoolchildren of various racial groups living in Hawaii. They found that the percentage of children having myopia ranged from about 3 percent for Hawaiian (Polynesian) children to 12 percent for Caucasian children and 17 percent for Chinese children.

Recent studies have reported vastly differing prevalences of myopia for various population groups. Garner et al. examined 977 Melanesian schoolchildren (1985) between the ages of 6 and 17 in the Pacific Island nation of Vanuatu, followed by the examination of an additional 788 children (1986). They found only 1.3 percent (1985) and 2.9 percent (1986) to have myopia greater than 0.25D. At the other extreme, alarmingly high prevalences of myopia have been reported in the Republic of China (Taiwan). Ko (1984) reported prevalences of myopia in the cities of Taipei and Koahshiung of 28 percent in primary school students, 67–71 percent in junior high school students, and 81–89 percent in senior high school students. In addition, he reported the prevalence of myopia in medical school students at National Taiwan University to be 91.5 percent, with the peak of the refractive error distribution curve being between 4.00 and 4.99D, and with 95 percent having an axial length greater than 24mm. In another report, Lin et al. (1987) stated that 75 percent of Taiwanese people have myopia, and half of them

have myopia of more than 3D. Lin credited the high prevalence of myopia to school examinations in Taiwan, which are highly competitive and require students to study 9–10 hours per day.

Post (1962) has suggested that what appear to be racial variations in the prevalence of refractive error are not racial variations at all but are due to the relaxation of natural selection. Assembling the data from a large number of studies, Post found that the prevalence of refractive error was the lowest in groups engaged primarily in hunting and food gathering, higher in groups engaged primarily in agriculture, and still higher in industrialized groups.

Even within a single racial or ethnic group, the prevalence of myopia has been found to vary greatly with occupation. Baldwin (1967) reviewed the results of 6 studies in which the prevalence of myopia was compared for near workers and those not engaged in near work. Inspection of Baldwin's bar graphs indicates that the mean prevalence of myopia for near workers was approximately 33 percent as compared to 15 percent for non-near workers. In a recent study of a group of United States Air Force Academy cadets, O'Neal and Connon (1986) reported a prevalence of myopia of 44.2 percent on entrance into the program, increasing to 53.7 percent during the third year.

CLASSIFICATION OF MYOPIA

Since the time of Donders, many systems for the classification of myopia have been proposed, many of which have been based on observed or assumed etiological factors. Donders (1864), who believed that myopia occurred as a result of prolonged use of the eyes for close work, classified myopia into three categories on the basis or rate of progression:

1. Stationary myopia, usually of low degree, not progressing throughout the life span.
2. Temporarily progressive myopia, progressing only during the early years of life.
3. Permanently progressive myopia, of high degree by the age of 15 years and continuing to progress throughout life. In discussing the latter form of myopia, Donders commented that "it is rare at 60 years of age to find a tolerably useful eye" (p. 349).

Steiger, writing in 1913, was the first researcher to propose that errors of refraction are based on biological variability. Using the Javal-Shiotz keratometer to measure the corneal refraction of 5,000 children, Steiger found that corneal power varies widely from one child to another, and concluded that the refraction of the eye depends on a "free association" between corneal refracting power and axial length. As Goldschmidt (1968) has noted, Steiger believed that the entire range of myopia should be considered as an etiological entity, determined genetically, and that classification into subcategories is unnecessary.

Duke-Elder (1949) has classified myopia into just two categories:

1. Simple myopia, occurring as a result of normal biological variability, making its appearance between age 5 and puberty, with its progression tending to stabilize after adolescence.
2. Degenerative myopia—the degenerative changes occurring particularly in the posterior segment of the globe—is relatively rare, but frequently leads to visual disability and not infrequently to blindness.

Emphasizing the inhomogeneity of myopia, Hirsch (1950) used the methodology of inferential statistics to analyze refractive data from the eyes of 562 adults having myopia of 1.00D or more. His analysis, done separately for each sex, resulted in three distribution curves that he termed the *alpha, beta,* and *gamma* groups:

1. The distribution for the alpha group followed a normal distribution curve, including emmetropes and hyperopes as well as myopes, having a theoretically derived peak at +0.50D and a tail in the myopic region extending to about −5.00D, and was considered by Hirsch to represent normal biological variability.
2. The beta group is represented by a second normal distribution curve, the myopia probably being hereditary.
3. The gamma group is a small group, extending from about −9.00D to −15.00D, which Hirsch described as including those cases formerly considered as malignant, pathological, degenerative, or congenital.

In their classical investigation of the emmetropic eye, Sorsby et al. (1957) described both myopia and hyperopia in two broad categories, based on the relationships between the components of refraction:

1. Refractions between plano and ±4.00D, accounting for about 98 percent of all refractions in their sample, in which the components of refraction are found to be within the same ranges as those of the emmetropic eye but less highly coordinated than in the emmetropic eye.
2. Refractions greater than ±4.00D, in which the

axial length is almost always beyond the range found in the emmetropic eye.

As a result of an epidemiological study of myopia in Denmark, Goldschmidt (1968) proposed the existence of three types of myopia, classified on the basis of both the degree of myopia and the age of onset:

1. Low myopia, the most frequent type of myopia, principally genetically determined, developing during the first 20 years of life, progressing steadily and rarely exceeding 6–9D.
2. Late myopia, developing after the cessation of bodily growth, seldom reaching higher degrees, and seemingly related to excessive close work.
3. High myopia, either genetically or environmentally determined, frequently having an early onset and capable of reaching excessive degrees, causing severely reduced vision and degenerative changes in the eye over a period of years.

Defining myopia as "expansion glaucoma," brought about by an increase in intraocular pressure, Kelly (1981) described three types of myopia, classified on the basis of etiology:

1. Self-inflicted vitreous glaucoma (simple myopia) due to blockage at the zonular level, accounting for 90 percent of myopia, occurring because the ciliary body, during accommodation, pulls forward on the thick anterior vitreous, concentrating the zonule and closing the zonular gap.
2. Active anterior chamber glaucoma (malignant myopia) due to the presence of a retinoschisis-like membrane blocking the trabecular area, accounting for 5 percent of myopia.
3. Inactive glaucoma (congenital myopia) due to an intraocular pressure rise *in utero.*

In *The Myopias, Basic Sciences and Clinical Management,* Curtin (1985) introduced a system of classification based on etiology, degree of myopia, and time of onset:

1. Physiologic myopia (low or simple myopia), developing postnatally because of a correlation failure between the total refracting power of the eye and a normal axial length.
2. Intermediate myopia (medium or moderate myopia), due to an expansion of the posterior segment of the globe in excess of normal ocular growth, subdivided into congenital, childhood, and late myopia.
3. Pathologic myopia, defined as the ocular disease in which a number of serious complications are associated with elongation of the eye.

Classification on the Basis of Age-Related Prevalence and Age of Onset

Many of the classification systems just described combine degree of myopia with the assumed etiological factors and with age of onset. A system of classification of myopia has recently been proposed by Grosvenor (1987a). Based on readily available and easily verifiable information, including age-related prevalence and age of onset, it makes no assumptions concerning the etiology of the various categories of myopia. The proposed system is based on the available data concerning the prevalence of myopia during the preschool years (Table 3.1), the school years (Table 3.2), the early adult years (Table 3.3), and the later adult years (Table 3.4).

Grosvenor's (1987a) classification system, as illustrated in Figure 3.1, includes four categories: (1) congenital myopia (diagonal cross-hatching at the bottom of the graph); (2) youth-onset myopia (vertically cross-hatched portion of the graph); (3) early adult-onset myopia (horizontal cross-hatching); and (4) late adult-onset myopia (diagonal cross-hatching, upper right portion of the graph).

1. *Congenital myopia.* Although many children are born with myopia (particulary those with low birth weight), most of these children lose their myopia during the first year of life (Mohindra and Held, 1981). Therefore, this classification includes only children whose myopia persists throughout infancy and is present when entering school. The prevalence of this form of myopia, which is usually of sufficient amount to persist throughout life, is about 2 percent.

2. *Youth-onset myopia.* This form of myopia has its onset during the period from about the age of 6 through the teenage years. During this period, the prevalence of myopia (of 0.50D or more) increases from about 2 percent at age 6 to about 20 percent at age 20. A large percentage of youth-onset myopes have a relatively small amount of myopia (particularly those who became myopic after the age of 12), many of whom will become emmetropic or even hyperopic in later years, with the result that the prevalence of this form of myopia would be expected to decrease during the adult years.

3. *Early adult-onset myopia.* This form of myopia has its onset during the period from age 20 to about age 40 and brings the prevalence of myopia (of 0.50D or more) to about 30 percent during this period of life. Many of those will have only a small amount of myopia and will become emmetropic or even hyperopic in their later years.

4. *Late adult-onset myopia.* This form of myopia has its onset beyond the age of 40, with the prevalence gradually increasing in the later years of life.

Figure 3.1 Proposed classification system for myopia, based on age-related prevalence and age of onset: categories are congenital myopia; youth-onset myopia; early adult-onset myopia; late adult-onset myopia (Grosvenor, 1987).

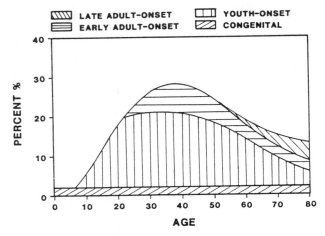

MYOPIA PROGRESSION

Unlike hyperopia or astigmatism, once myopia is found to exist, it tends to progress. For example, data from Hirsch's (1963) longitudinal study of refraction between the ages of 5–6 and 13–14 years indicated that hyperopia tends to decrease by a small fraction of a diopter per year during this period, whereas myopia tends to increase on the order of 0.50D per year. Myopia occurring during the adult years, on the other hand, tends to progress at a slower rate.

Progression of Myopia in Children

The progression of juvenile myopia has been studied by Goss and Winkler (1983), who used as subjects 299 patients selected from three optometric practices. All of the subjects had at least 0.50D of myopia and had been refracted on at least four occasions between the ages of 6 and 24 years. Graphs were plotted, showing the amount of myopia versus

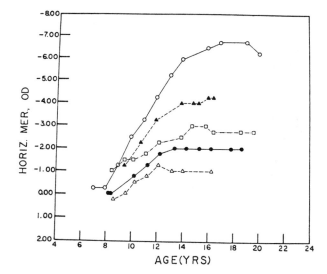

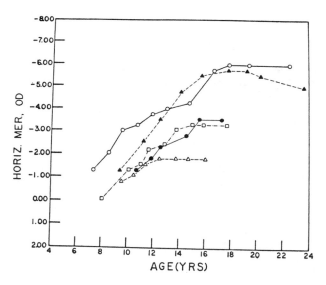

Figure 3.2   Progression of myopia with age, showing that progression tends to level off in the middle or late teen years. Upper graph, data for 5 girls; lower graph, data for 5 boys (Goss and Winkler, 1983).

age (see Figure 3.2), and it was found that in most cases the myopia tended to increase in a linear manner into the middle or late teen years, then leveling off.

Goss and Winkler (1983) used two methods to determine the mean change in refraction during the period of progression: averaging the results for the two methods, mean progression rates were 0.42D per year for males and 0.48D per year for females.

Four methods were used to determine the "age of cessation"; that is, the age at which the myopia ceased to progress. Averaging the results obtained by two of these methods, the mean age of cessation was approximately 16 years for males and 15 years for females. There was a considerable amount of variation in the cessation age, the standard deviation being about 2 years for both males and females.

In a report on a 3-year study of the use of bifocal lenses for the control of myopia conducted at the University of Houston, Grosvenor, Perrigin, Perrigin, and Maslovitz (1987) found mean rates of progression of 0.30D per year for wearers of single-vision lenses, 0.34D per year for wearers of +1.00D add bifocal lenses, and 0.32D per year for wearers of +2.00D add bifocal lenses. Graphs for each of the 124 subjects show the progression on the basis of semiannual refractions (spherical equivalent refraction, right eye) for the 3-year period (see Figures 3.3 through 3.8). Inspection of these graphs indicates that for both sexes and all three treatment methods, (1) subjects who entered the study prior to age 12 with 2D of myopia or more tended to progress at a rapid rate—as high as 1.00D per year—whereas (2) subjects who entered the study beyond the age of 12 with no more than 1D of myopia tended to progress slowly or not at all. There were, of course, exceptions to this general rule.

Both the Goss and Winkler (1983) data and the Grosvenor et al. (1987) data tend to confirm the observation that the earlier a child becomes myopic, the more rapidly the condition tends to progress. Consequently, a child who becomes myopic at an early age (by age 6 or 7), is in "double jeopardy," in that he or she will not only have more years in which to progress prior to cessation (at age 15 or 16 ± 2 years) but will be likely to progress at a significantly faster rate than if the myopia had presented itself at a later age.

As noted in Chapter 2, the data of the longitudinal study of refraction and its components by Sorsby and Leary (1970) indicated a strong relationship between the progression of myopia and increase in axial length, but a weaker relationship between the progression of myopia and change in crystalline lens power. In a second report on the Houston study of bifocal lenses for the control of myopia (referred to above), Young and Leary (1987) reported that for those children whose myopia remained constant during the 3-year study, the values for the components of refraction remained constant; but when myopia progressed, it was accompanied by an increase in both axial length and vitreous depth.

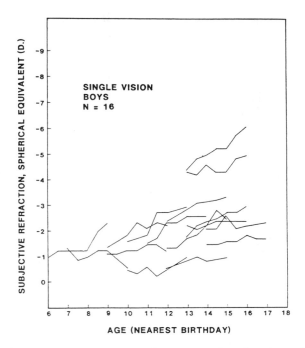

Figure 3.3 Progression on the basis of semiannual refractions for a 3-year period, for boys wearing single-vision lenses (Grosvenor, Perrigin, Perrigin, and Maslovitz, 1987).

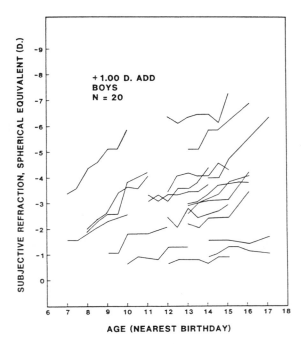

Figure 3.5 Progression on the basis of semiannual refractions for a 3-year period, for boys wearing +1.00D add bifocals (Grosvenor, Perrigin, Perrigin, and Maslovitz, 1987).

Figure 3.4 Progression on the basis of semiannual refractions for a 3-year period, for girls wearing single-vision lenses (Grosvenor, Perrigin, Perrigin, and Maslovitz, 1987).

Figure 3.6 Progression on the basis of semiannual refractions for a 3-year period, for girls wearing +1.00D add bifocals (Grosvenor, Perrigin, Perrigin, and Maslovitz, 1987).

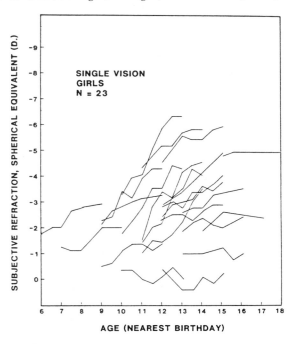

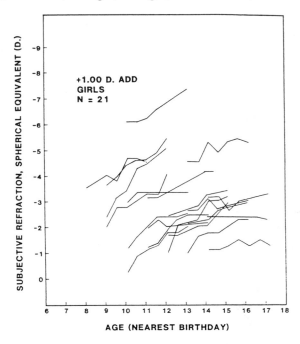

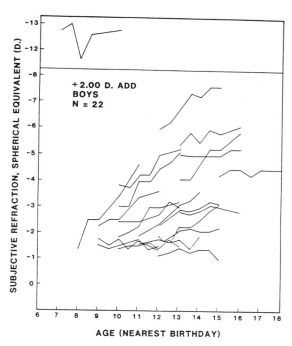

Figure 3.7 Progression on the basis of semiannual refractions for a 3-year period, for boys wearing +2.00D add bifocals (Grosvenor, Perrigin, Perrigin, and Maslovitz, 1987).

Figure 3.8 Progression on the basis of semiannual refractions for a 3-year period, for girls wearing +2.00D add bifocals (Grosvenor, Perrigin, Perrigin, and Maslovitz, 1987).

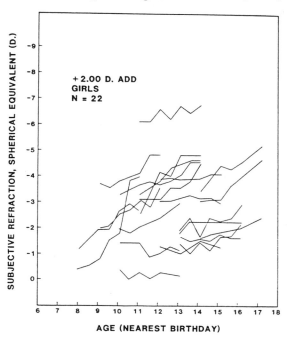

Progression of Myopia in Young Adults

It is the experience of most practitioners that myopia tends to progress slowly in the adult years. In the longitudinal study of refraction between the ages of 20 and 40 years described in the previous chapter (Grosvenor, 1977c), mean progression for subjects who were myopic at age 20 was about 1D during the 20-year period, or 0.05D per year.

The records of 108 adult myopes, gathered from five optometric practices, were studied by Goss, Erickson, and Cox (1985). The criteria for inclusion in the study included three or more examinations beyond 18 years of age. In analyzing the progression of myopia for these patients, Goss et al. placed each patient in one of three categories: (1) adult stabilization (68 percent of males and 89 percent of females), in which there was a rapid increase in myopia during early adolescence followed by stabilization in adulthood; (2) adult continuation (a less prevalent form), again involving a rapid increase in myopia during the adolescent years but with a slower rate of progression during the adult years; and (3) adult acceleration (the least prevalent form), in which the rate of progression accelerates after adolescence (which also includes adult-onset myopia).

Goss et al. (1985) reported that for 32 of the subjects on whom three or more refractions and keratometer measurements were recorded beyond 18 years of age, the rate of change in myopia (D/year) and in corneal radius (mm/year) were determined. It was found that for 20 such subjects in the first group (adult stabilization), the corneal radius increased (flattened) for 11 subjects, decreased (steepened) for 11 subjects, and did not change at all for one subject. However, for the second and third groups (adult continuation and adult acceleration), the corneal radius decreased (steepened) for all subjects: for these two groups the mean increase in myopia was 0.12D per year, whereas the mean decrease in corneal radius was 0.012mm per year. According to the authors' calculations, a decrease in corneal radius of 0.012mm should account for an increase in myopia of approximately 0.06D, indicating that the corneal steepening could have accounted for approximately half of the myopia progression for these subjects.

As a result of further analysis of their data, Goss and Erickson (1987) reported the following relationships between refractive change and corneal change: (1) for 100 patients between the ages of 6 and 15 years, there was no significant relationship between progression of myopia and change in corneal radius; and (2) for 37 patients beyond the age of 18 years, there was a positive relationship between progression of myopia and corneal steepening, accompanied by a tendency for astigmatism to increase in the with-the-rule direction. The authors concluded that the ocular component mechanism responsible for young adulthood myopia progression in many patients is an increase in power (steepening) of the anterior surface of the cornea.

ETIOLOGICAL FACTORS IN MYOPIA

Myopia is one of the many conditions—along with hypertension, diabetes, strabismus, and others—that cannot be traced to a single-gene mode of inheritance or to a strictly environmental cause, and therefore may be considered to be of *polygenic*, or *multifactorial*, origin. Although studies (discussed in the previous chapter) have shown that identical twins have similar refractive errors and that myopia tends to "run in families," these studies seldom rule out the possibility that environmental factors are involved. Studies that appear to show that myopia occurs as a result of prolonged reading, on the other hand, seldom rule out the possibility that genetic factors are involved.

Congenital versus Acquired Myopia

All reported studies of *congenital* myopia—myopia present at birth or at a very early age and persisting throughout life—have found it to be present in no more than 1 or 2 percent of the population. Even though it is congenital, this form of myopia is not necessarily hereditary. For example, myopia occurring in premature (low birth weight) infants as a result of underdevelopment of the eye, would not normally be considered as hereditary.

Acquired myopia, on the other hand, is a much greater problem because almost one-third of the population in an industrialized society (and as many as two-thirds in some population groups) will become myopic after several years of schooling or during the adult years. It is understandable, then, that a large amount of attention has been given to discovering the cause of acquired myopia.

What Causes Acquired Myopia?

In *On the Anomalies of Accommodation and Refraction of the Eye* (1864), Donders proposed that myopia occurs as a result of prolonged tension on the eyes during close work and elongation of the visual axes:

> How then is this prolongation explained? Three factors may here come under observation: 1. Pressure of the muscles on the eyeball in strong convergence of the visual axes; 2. Increased pressure of the fluids, resulting from accumulation of blood in the eyes in the stooping position; 3. Congestive processes in the fundus oculi, which, leading to softening, even in the normal, but still more under the increased pressure of the fluids of the eye, give rise to extension of the membranes. That in increased pressure the extension occurs principally at the posterior pole, is explained by the want of support from the muscles of the eye at that part. (p. 343)

Ciliary spasm and the lens

In spite of Donders's succinctly stated hypothesis, many vision practitioners—prior to the availability of clinically useful methods for measuring the length of the eye—believed that *spasm of the ciliary muscle* was the cause of acquired myopia. This belief was due, at least in part, to the fact that a common presenting symptom by individuals who become myopic as young adults (for example, college students) is that their distance vision blurs after prolonged close work but clears up after a few minutes. This condition was considered to be *pseudomyopia*, due to ciliary spasm; and if the condition progressed to a clinical (constant) myopia, it was thought that the ciliary spasm had become a permanent condition. Although not often stated as such, the hypothesis of many clinicians was that congenital myopia was due to elongation of the eye, but acquired myopia was due to ciliary spasm, occurring as a result of prolonged accommodation.

Sato (1957), one of the most ardent proponents of the idea that myopia was due to ciliary spasm, studied the development of myopia in Japanese schoolchildren. He concluded that myopia was acquired as a result of accommodative spasm followed by hypertrophy of the ciliary muscle, with no concurrent change in axial length. If A-scan ultrasonography had been available to Sato, he would surely have found that the development of myopia was accompanied by an increase in the axial length of the eye.

Accommodation and axial elongation

As a result of Stenstrom's (1948) study, making use of the X-ray method of measuring axial length, together with Sorsby's (1957) study in which axial length was calculated, and later studies making use of A-scan ultrasonography, researchers interested in acquired myopia began to look for mechanisms to account for an increase in axial length of the developing eye. Although accommodation was still considered by many to be the "culprit," attention was turned toward determining how accommodation could bring about an increase in the length of the eye.

The possible role of accommodation in causing myopia has been emphasized by Kelly et al. (1975), who refer to myopia as "juvenile expansile glaucoma," a self-inflicted condition brought about by excessive near work that results in an increase in intraocular pressure followed by an expansion of the vitreous chamber of the eye. Kelly (1981) described myopia as occurring due to a blockage of the flow of aqueous within the eye, estimating that 90 percent of myopia is due to a blockage of aqueous flow in the zonular area, due to the sphincter muscle pulling forward on the thick anterior vitreous during accommodation, blocking the zonule, and closing the zonular gap. Kelly found the intraocular pressure of myopic subjects, when measured by applanation tonometry, to be significantly elevated when measured in the morning.

Other researchers, however, have implicated elevated *vitreous* chamber pressure (rather than anterior chamber pressure, as measured by clinical tonometry) as being the cause of myopia. Using cats as subjects, Coleman and Young (1972) simultaneously measured anterior chamber and vitreous chamber pressure during accommodation. They used manometry in each chamber and found a pressure gradient consisting of a decrease in anterior chamber pressure accompanied by an increase in vitreous chamber pressure. Young (1975) made use of a surgically implanted radiosonde transducer to measure changes in the vitreous chamber pressure of the pigtail monkey during accommodation. On the basis of ambient pressure, the transducer (a small drum, about the size of an aspirin tablet) amplifies or depresses the signal from a radio frequency source outside the eye. The pigtail monkey has a strong eye-contact response and will look at the eye of a human as long as the human looks at the monkey. Using the experimenter's eyes as a stimulus for accommodation for the monkey (seated in a restraining chair), it was found that the vitreous chamber pressure increased in a linear fashion as the experimenter moved from a distance of 6m to within 30cm of the monkey's face.

To account for these results, Young (1981) hypothesized that the anterior hyaloid membrane, which separates the vitreous chamber from the posterior chamber, can act as a differentially permeable membrane, having the potential of blocking the normal movement of fluid from the vitreous chamber to the posterior (aqueous) chamber during strong accommodation. In more recent experimentation with the radiosonde transducer, Young and Leary (1987) reported that the monkey's vitreous pressure was found to be 12mm Hg for a fixation distance of 6m, and 24mm for a fixation distance of 20cm, but remained constant if the fixation distance was not changed.

Increased pressure within the eye and the application of heat were shown to be responsible for the development of myopia by Maurice and Mushin (1966), who placed rabbits in a heated box while bringing about an increase in intraocular pressure. The heated box caused the animals' body temperature to increase to 41–43 C°, and the intraocular pressure was raised to 100mm Hg by passing air into the anterior chamber. From 0.75 to 1.50D of myopia developed by the twelfth day, and the authors assumed that the cause of the myopia was a stretching of the sclera. Citing the Maurice and Mushin report, Hirsch (1972) noted that coughing increases the intraocular pressure, and suggested that any disease that involves both coughing and an increase in body temperature may supply the mechanism for myopia. Such diseases could be measles, scarlet fever, and whooping cough.

The role of the ciliary body and choroid

The emmetropization mechanism proposed by Van Alphen (1961) (see Chapter 2) has interesting implications for the production of myopia. Van Alphen suggested that the ciliary body and the choroid form an elastic envelope that limits the stretch of the sclera by counteracting a part of the intraocular pressure, and that the macula supplies information regarding focus to the brain, which in turn feeds information back to the Edinger-Westphal nucleus concerning the degree of stretch necessary to maintain emmetropia (i.e., to keep the retinal image in focus). If for any reason the mechanism fails, inadequate tonus of the choroid-ciliary body envelope would allow the eye to stretch excessively, resulting in myopia. Van Alphen summed up his theory (1967) by saying that the eye is essentially self-focusing, emmetropia being produced by subcortical control of the tonus of the ciliary muscle; and that ametropia is caused by factors that interfere with or "derail" the mechanism.

In a later article, Van Alphen (1986) reported on

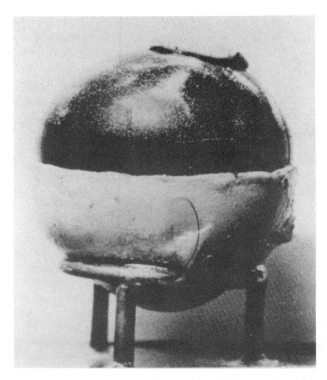

Figure 3.9 Van Alphen found that during inflation, the choroid expanded in the anterioposterior direction (as shown by the absence of the yellow PbO) indicating that the ciliary body rather than the choroid was stretching (Van Alphen, 1986).

experiments that reinforced the importance of ciliary muscle tone in maintaining emmetropia. Human eyes were enucleated within 24 hours after death, the posterior sclera (behind the equator) was removed, and the eye was mounted in a ring and inflated with saline via a 19-gauge needle. The eyes were mounted with the cornea facing downward, and yellow PbO powder was dusted on the exposed choroid and used as a marker to analyze the choroidal expansion that occurred when the eye was inflated. During inflation, the choroid expanded in an antero-posterior direction, assuming an ellipsoidal shape; as the choroid expanded, the brown surface of the choroid and the yellow PbO zone (Figure 3.9) clearly delineated the area of the choroid that was progressively emerging from the anterior sclera, with increasing inflation pressure. Before breaking, the PbO-free zone measured between 2.9 and 4.1mm, with a mean of 3.4mm. These results—similar for 32 eyes ranging in age from 1 day to 68 years—indicated that the greatest deformation of the

posterior segment resulted from changes in front of the equator, in the area occupied by the ciliary body. Other experiments, in which other portions of the sclera were removed, confirmed the fact that the stretching that occurred when the eye was inflated was due to a stretching of the *ciliary body* rather than the choroid. Van Alphen concluded that this experimentation demonstrated that the tonus of the ciliary muscle determines the tension in the choroid, which ultimately determines the axial length of the eye.

The concept of "emmetropization at near"

An interesting application of this theory (not suggested by Van Alphen) is based on the concept of the macular feedback mechanism maintaining a state of emmetropia *relative to the fixation distance.* During the evolution of the species, the mechanism must have functioned to maintain emmetropia for remote and intermediate fixation distances— distances that were of importance in terms of survival.

However, in modern society, with the increased use of much closer fixation distances, it might be supposed that the mechanism would function in such a manner as to maintain emmetropia for these closer distances. This concept would mean that the emmetropizing mechanism, rather than being "derailed" when myopia occurs, would simply be performing as it was designed to perform, adapting to the closer fixation distances. A possible consequence of this "emmetropization at near" hypothesis is that when minus lenses are worn, causing the image of a remote object to be focused on the retina, if the individual does a large amount of close work the emmetropizing mechanism must begin all over again, adapting to the close fixation distance. This concept has been expressed by Kelly (1983), who refers to minus lenses as "dangerous distance glasses," believing that once they are prescribed, additional myopia is bound to result.

The role of the extraocular muscles

In a theoretical analysis based on engineering principals, Greene (1980, 1981) evaluated the stresses experienced by the posterior sclera by accommodation, convergence, vitreous pressure, and the extraocular muscles. He argued that the vitreous pressure increases caused by accommodation are small in magnitude, and because they are created by a shell (the choroid) that resides inside the sclera, the stress increase is not transmitted to the sclera; whereas the vitreous pressure increases caused by convergence can be quite large in magnitude and are transmitted directly to the sclera. Greene concluded that the mechanical effects of convergence completely dominate those created by accommodation, even though both occur simultaneously when the eyes focus on a very close target. His calculations showed that the total stress experienced by the posterior sclera is the sum of the stresses induced by intra-ocular pressure and by the oblique muscles. This led Greene to conclude that the posterior pole of the sclera (the region between the two oblique muscle attachments) is subject to tensile stresses higher than those at any other locale on the globe. This theory, therefore, could account for the posterior staphyloma that occurs in high myopia.

The role of the cornea

Although refractive component studies have demonstrated the dominant role of axial length in determining the refractive state of the eye, the role played by the cornea has been less obvious. Stenstrom (1948) found a correlation between refractive error and axial length of −0.76, and a correlation between refractive error and corneal radius of only +0.18. However, when Hirsch and Weymouth (1947) reanalyzed Stenstrom's data by holding axial length and anterior chamber depth constant, they found the correlation between refractive error and corneal radius to be +0.70. Sorsby et al. (1957) found that emmetropic eyes tended to have a favorable relationship between axial length and corneal power (a relatively long eye would have a relatively flat cornea). When ametropia occurred, there was almost always an unharmonious relationship (a relatively long eye with the cornea too steep to maintain emmetropia). Interestingly, the Sorsby et al. data showed that the lens almost always supplied the correct power to maintain relative emmetropia. If significant ametropia was present in an eye with an axial length outside the normal range, the cornea was usually "at fault"—not flattening sufficiently to maintain emmetropia.

The work of Goss and his co-workers demonstrated that the cornea cannot be overlooked as a possible cause of myopia. As noted earlier, Goss and Erickson (1987) found that there was no significant relationship between progression of myopia and change in corneal radius for myopes between the ages of 6 and 15 years, but for myopes beyond the age of 18, progression of myopia tended to be accompanied by corneal steepening.

What does it all mean?

How can we attempt to rationalize all of these sometimes conflicting causative factors for acquired myopia? They may be summarized—and rationalized—as follows:

1. Ciliary spasm. Although ciliary spasm is often present in the early stages of myopia, there is solid evidence that youth-onset myopia virtually always involves an eye whose axial length is too long for the corneal power. Only limited longitudinal data have been published, however, on the role of the lens in adult-onset myopia.

2. Anterior chamber pressure versus vitreous chamber pressure. The fact that anterior chamber pressure is found to be significantly elevated in young myopes when measured in the morning (Kelly, 1981), is not necessarily in conflict with the fact that vitreous chamber pressure is found to increase during accommodation (Coleman and Young, 1972; Young, 1975, 1981, 1987). The obvious approach to this dilemma is to measure, in the same myopic subject or group of subjects, the vitreous chamber and anterior chamber pressure during accommodation, as well as the anterior chamber pressure at various times of day, with accommodation at rest. Although it is desirable to use humans rather than monkeys for the vitreous chamber pressure measurements, this is not possible because the radiosonde transducer must be surgically implanted in the vitreous.

3. Application of heat and intraocular pressure increase. Although this experiment, performed on rabbits (Maurice and Mushin, 1966) would not be appropriate for human subjects, there's no reason to believe that the results would be different for humans. Hirsch's (1972) suggestion—that diseases involving coughing in the presence of a fever may supply the mechanism for myopia—appears to be reasonable.

4. Inadequate tonus of the choroid-ciliary body envelope. Backed up by strong evidence, Van Alphen's hypothesis (1961, 1986), unlike other theories and hypotheses, offers a well-defined mechanism that not only accounts for the normal growth of the emmetropic eye but also explains the occurrence of myopia when the emmetropizing mechanism fails. Van Alphen's more recent experimentation (1986), showing that the ciliary body stretches as much as 3–4mm when vitreous chamber pressure is increased, is particularly convincing. An intriguing application of Van Alphen's hypothesis is that eyes having poorly developed macular areas, as in ocular or oculo-cutaneous albinism, tend to develop high refractive errors.

5. *High tensile stresses at the posterior pole.* Greene's (1980, 1981) conclusion that the sclera at the posterior pole is subject to higher tensile stresses than any other locale of the globe, predicts the occurrence of posterior scleral thinning and ectasia found in high myopia. The various types of posterior staphyloma described by Curtin (1981) occur in just the area outlined by Greene—that area between the insertions of the superior oblique and inferior oblique muscles. Further, there is no conflict between Greene's conclusion and Van Alphen's finding—that the ciliary body stretches in an anterio-posterior direction when the intraocular pressure is increased—if one considers the development of myopia as a continuum in which an early, beginning stage and a late, end-stage can be identified:

a. In the beginning stage of myopia (or even before clinical myopia is present) the ciliary body begins to lose its tone, allowing the globe to begin to elongate axially.

b. As the globe continues to elongate and the tensile stresses applied to the posterior sclera gradually increase (as witnessed by the presence of crescent formation followed by chorioretinal atrophy and other changes), the posterior sclera continues to weaken in response to these stresses with the result that, in cases of extreme axial lengthening, a posterior staphyloma (the end stage) may develop.

Curtin and Karlin (1972) have tabulated the percentages of eyes having various posterior fundus changes on the basis of axial lengths. Their graphs show, for example, that for eyes having axial lengths of 27mm, crescent formation is found in 95 percent of eyes, chorio-retinal atrophy is found in 40 percent of eyes (age 40 or older), and posterior staphyloma is found in about 4.8 percent of eyes. The prevalence of posterior staphyloma reaches about 70 percent for eyes having axial lengths of 33mm.

6. *Steepening of the cornea.* Although adult myopia (especially adult-onset myopia) has been considered by many to have a different etiological basis than youth-onset myopia, the finding by Goss, Erickson, and Cox (1985)—that progression of adult myopia is sometimes associated with corneal steepening—comes as somewhat of a surprise. For example, Adams (1987), using himself as a subject, argues that adult-onset myopia is due to an increase in axial length rather than to corneal steepening. However, more data are needed to fully understand the basis of adult myopia. A 3-year longitudinal study of changes in refraction and the refractive components of young adults is currently underway at the University of Houston.

How Does Congenital Myopia Differ from Acquired Myopia?

Relatively little has been written about congenital myopia—myopia that is present at birth and persists throughout life. This is undoubtedly due, in part, to the prevalence of this form of myopia being no more than about 2 percent. However, it is also due to the fact that this form of myopia, often being high in amount, tends to be associated in later life with degenerative changes and therefore is more likely to be categorized as *degenerative* myopia.

Duke-Elder (1949) included *congenital axial myopia* as one of three categories of degenerative myopia, the other two categories being developmental degenerative myopia and myopia acquired with disease. He described this form of myopia as not usually coming under observation until the second or third year of life, commenting that "In a number of these cases the myopia remains stationary, but in others it progresses and may result at an early stage in a double detachment of the retina. In some cases the vision is good; in others it is subnormal" (pp. 4314–16). It should be understood that, in Duke-Elder's time, the condition now known as retinopathy of prematurity (due to the use of oxygen for premature babies) with its attendant myopia, was unknown. As noted earlier in the chapter, this form of myopia is due not to axial elongation of the eye but to the eye having a steep cornea and a small, underdeveloped and relatively spherical lens (Fledelius, 1981; Goss, 1985). Although few statistics are available, it is likely that congenital myopia (except for those relatively milder premature cases, which revert to emmetropia in the early months of life) is usually relatively high in amount.

The relation between myopia and astigmatism in congenital and early-onset myopia was investigated by Fulton, Hansen, and Petersen (1982). From the records of 5,032 hospital patients, they selected the records of 298 patients whose ages ranged from birth to 10 years, having 0.25D of myopia or more in one or both eyes. Fulton et al. reported that the mean spherical equivalent refraction of their subjects for 2-year intervals beginning at birth (0–1, 2–3, 4–5, 6–7, 8–10 years, respectively) was approximately −4D, −8D, −7.5D, −10D, and −6D. Although the authors stated that "there was no age-related increase in the degree of myopia for the group as a whole" (p. 299), the apparent lack of progression could result partially from (1) the fact that the data are cross-sectional, rather than longitudinal, and (2) the possibility that the data represented a large amount of "self-selection," since the parents of a pre-school infant or child would not be likely to suspect that anything is wrong unless the child's vision loss was relatively extreme.

Fulton et al. (1982) plotted separate distributions of myopia for (1) subjects having less than 1D of astigmatism and (2) subjects having astigmatism of 1D or more. They found that the mean amount of myopia ranged from 0.50–3.00D or greater (depending on age) for those having astigmatism of 1D or more. In addition, they plotted separate distributions of myopia for (1) subjects having oblique astigmatism and (2) subjects having with- or against-the-rule astigmatism. They found that the mean amount of myopia was greater, at every age, for the subjects having oblique astigmatism. The authors postulated that the presence of astigmatism, by degrading pattern vision, may influence the course of the development of myopia. Commenting that the mechanisms by which these astigmatic errors could encourage the development of myopia are not apparent, the authors noted that astigmatic errors do blur pattern vision, and they speculated that obliquely oriented cylindrical axes may especially blur the nearly symmetrical human face "that is so important in a young child's visual world."

It should be understood that the cause-and-effect relationship proposed by Fulton et al. (1982) required the tacit assumption that the astigmatism was present *before* the myopia developed: Unfortunately there appeared to be no evidence, for their subjects, supporting this assumption. An alternative hypothesis is that their subjects' myopia and astigmatism developed concurrently and prior to birth (because the authors labeled myopia present prior to age 6 as "congenital") when no visual stimulation was present.

It is of interest, however, that Hirsch (1964), in his discussion of myopia that develops during the school years, found that against-the-rule astigmatism was often present prior to the appearance of the myopia.

EXPERIMENTALLY INDUCED MYOPIA

Two experimental approaches have been taken in inducing myopia in monkeys and other animals:

1. The visual environment is manipulated, either by placing the animal in a particular posture or position or by restricting the distance at which objects may be viewed.
2. The eye itself is manipulated to alter the visual stimulus as, for example, by suturing the eyelids of one or both eyes.

Manipulation of the Visual Environment

Much of the early work in this area has been reviewed by Young (1967) and Criswell and Goss (1983). As noted by Young, animal experimentation on myopia began when Levinsohn presented a paper to the Medical Society of Berlin in 1912. Levinsohn believed that myopia results from the pull of the eye on the optic nerve when the eye is held in a downward position, so that the anterio-posterior axis of the globe is oriented vertically. To test this theory, Levinsohn placed young dogs, cats, and rabbits in boxes, and oriented the boxes in such a way that at least one eye would be positioned with the anterio-posterior axis vertical. The animals were kept in this position for 6 hours per day for 5–6 months. Some change toward myopia was found to occur, but Levinsohn turned to the use of monkeys as experimental subjects. The monkey was placed in a box that was oriented on a table so that the face plane was parallel to the floor, with the result that after a few months, myopia was found to occur and to increase as long as the experiments were carried on. As noted by Criswell and Goss (1983), three monkeys were kept in this position: one of them developed 14–15D of myopia after 9 months, the second developed 7–9D of myopia after 1 year, and the third developed 1–2D of myopia after 4 weeks. Intraocular pressure did not increase during the experiment, and Levinsohn concluded that the myopia was axial in nature because ophthalmoscopic examination revealed the presence of conus at the optic disc.

More recently, Young (1961) reported on experiments with monkeys in which the visual environment was carefully controlled. He immobilized six pigtail monkeys for a period of one year in an upright restraining chair by means of a plywood collar, with the visual environment limited to a distance of 38cm (15 in.) by a plywood hood, painted white. The open top of the hood was illuminated by diffuse fluorescent light, passing through a translucent cloth. Five additional monkeys, serving as a control group, were placed in restraining chairs but hoods were not placed over their heads. During the experiment, retinoscopy was performed biweekly for both the experimental and the control animals. The refraction of the experimental animals increased from an average of −0.29D at the beginning of the experiment to an average of −1.12D at the end of one year. For the control animals, the refraction increased only from an initial average of −0.54D to a final average of −0.58D. The increase in myopia in the experimental animals persisted for 18 months following the removal of the hoods.

In a later report (1967), Young's results indicated that the development of myopia is related to the conditions under which the monkeys are reared. Laboratory monkeys were found to be considerably more myopic than wild monkeys, and monkeys kept indoors in cages developed more myopia than animals kept outside in pens.

Manipulation of the Eye to Alter the Visual Stimulus

Lid-suture myopia in monkeys

In the first reported experiment in which unilateral lid-suturing resulted in the development of myopia, the occurrence of the myopia was an unexpected event. During an investigation of monocular visual deprivation in monkeys, Hubel et al. (1975) found that the eye in which the lids had been closed by lid-suturing since birth developed a high degree of myopia.

This experiment was followed by a study by Wiesel and Raviola (1977) in which unilateral and bilateral lid fusion was performed on ten macaque monkeys (*M mulatta* or rhesus, and *M arctoides* or stump-tail) at various times after birth. Under general anesthesia, the margins of both the upper and lower lids were excised lateral to the lacrimal papilla, and the cut surfaces of the lids were brought together by silk sutures from the lateral canthus to the lacrimal papilla. The sutures were removed 1–2 weeks after surgery, at which time the lids had fused and appeared as a thin, translucent diaphragm that attenuated light by about 0.5 log unit. After variable periods of time (from 19 days to 26 months) the lids were surgically opened, two drops of one-percent homatropine were instilled, and the refraction of both eyes was determined by retinoscopy. In

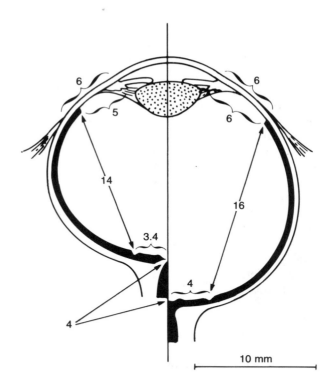

Figure 3.10 Posterior segment of the lid-sutured eye compared to that of the normal eye (Wiesel and Raviola, 1977).

addition, the corneal refraction was measured by keratometry and the fundus was examined. After completion of the experimentation, the animals were perfused with 10 percent formalin, the eyes were enucleated, and the axial length was measured.

Of the eight animals submitted to unilateral lid-suturing, the difference in refraction of the sutured eye and the normal eye ranged from 0D for a mature rhesus monkey to −13.5D for a 2-week-old rhesus monkey. For the animal sutured at 2 weeks, corneal diameters and the distance from the rectus muscle insertions to the limbus were the same for both eyes. However, (1) the axial length of the sutured eye was 21 percent longer than that of the normal eye, (2) the distance from the fovea to the optic disc was 18 percent greater for the sutured eye than for the normal eye (see Figure 3.10), and (3) the posterior sclera was thinner for the sutured eye than for the normal eye. To establish whether the induced myopia was due to the fact that only one eye was sutured, an additional animal was sutured bilaterally at the age of 5 weeks, with the result that 11D of myopia was found to be present in both eyes. Wiesel and Raviola (1977) suggested that, because the refractive error is larger when lid fusion is performed early in life, this type of myopia represents a derangement of the development of the eye.

Von Norden and Crawford (1978) sutured the lids of macaque monkeys, but the sutured eyes of their animals failed to consistently develop myopia. Of the 13 animals unilaterally or bilaterally sutured, only 4 eyes were found to have as much as 7.50 to 13.75D of myopia after varying periods of lid closure, and the others were found to have only low myopia or even hyperopia. Von Norden and Crawford reported that they had used a different lid-suturing technique than that used by Wiesel and Raviola, which may have accounted for the difference in results.

Reviewing their work over a period of several years, Raviola and Wiesel (1985) have described the following experiments:

1. To investigate the possibility that *mechanical or thermal factors* resulting from lid fusion may be responsible for the development of myopia, two rhesus monkeys with lid fusion were reared in the dark (Raviola and Wiesel, 1978). At the end of the period of deprivation, the sutured and normal eyes had identical refraction (+2D) and identical axial length. When a monkey raised in the dark for 10 months was kept for an additional 9 months in a lighted environment, the sutured eye increased in length and developed 3D of myopia whereas the open eye remained 2D hyperopic. Mechanical or thermal factors were not sufficient to induce excessive eye growth, the crucial determinant being *abnormal visual input*.

2. Abnormal visual input was provided by an alternate procedure, the cornea of one eye of each of two neonatal monkeys being rendered opaque by injecting a suspension of fine polystyrene beads into the corneal stroma (Wiesel and Raviola, 1979). After one year, the eyes with the opaque corneas were 1.0–1.22mm longer than the open eyes, corresponding to a difference in refraction of −4 to −5D. This result, together with the fact that there was no lengthening of the eye when the lids were sutured and the animal was reared in the dark, enable the conclusion that the *nervous system* is involved in experimentally induced myopia.

3. It can be argued that if *accommodation* is responsible for lid-fusion myopia, the daily use of atropine should prevent myopia from occurring. The lids of one eye of each of four neonatal stump-tail monkeys were sutured, leaving a small opening for the daily instillation of 1 percent atropine sulfate ointment for a period of up to one year, with the result that the atropine prevented the sutured eyes from increasing in length. However, when the same procedure was used for three rhesus monkeys, the atropine failed to prevent the sutured eyes from lengthening. Raviola and Wiesel (1985) suggested two possibilities for this: (a) atropine may not be effective in the rhesus monkey, or (b) there may be one neural mechanism operating to induce myopia in the stump-tail monkey and a second neural mechanism operating in the rhesus monkey.

4. Using a second method to study the role of accommodation, the ciliary ganglion was removed from the orbit of one rhesus monkey, interrupting the parasympathetic innervation to the ciliary muscle. After one year of lid fusion the closed eye was 10D more myopic than the open eye and the vitreous depth was 2mm greater. Raviola and Wiesel (1985) concluded that this finding confirms the results of the atropine administration, ruling out accommodation as a factor in lid-suture myopia in the rhesus monkey, and supports the idea that two separate mechanisms may be present: (a) in the stump-tail monkey the lengthening of the eye may be a neural event initiated by *accommodation*, whereas (b) in the rhesus monkey, the lengthening of the eye may also be a neural event, initiated not by accommodation but by the *retina* itself.

5. The role of the *sympathetic nervous system* in the development of lid suture myopia was investigated by unilateral removal of the superior cervical ganglion and bilateral lid suturing, whereas the role of the *sensory nerve supply* was investigated by unilateral section of the trigeminal nerve and unilateral lid-suturing. For both procedures—in both the rhesus and the stump-tail monkeys—the surgical procedures failed to prevent the lengthening of the sutured eye. Raviola and Wiesel (1985) concluded that neither the sympathetic nor the sensory nerve supply to the globe is involved in the development of lid-suture myopia.

6. An additional possibility is that the distortion of visual input may act *locally* on the eye, disturbing normal eye growth. When both optic nerves of a stump-tail monkey were sectioned at the optic chiasm and the lids of one eye were sutured, no elongation of the eye resulted. However, when this procedure was used with three rhesus monkeys, the sutured eye lengthened 1.6–2.6mm, and 4 to 9D of myopia was induced. Raviola and Wiesel (1985) concluded that this finding suggests the existence of a local mechanism (due to the retina) contributing to the development of lid-suture myopia in the rhesus monkey but not in the stump-tail monkey.

As a result of these experiments, Raviola (1987) has suggested a hypothesis having a moleculer basis: (1) the retina is designed to operate on the basis of *contrast*, and (2) when contrast is destroyed, there must be some mechanism that responds to the lack of contrast, perhaps a change in the release of a neurotransmitter-modulator (e.g., one of the *polypeptides*). The result would be a much higher concentration of the polypeptides in the retina (amacrine cells) in the sutured eye than in the open eye. According to Raviola, the first task is to *find the molecule* and the second is to *find how the molecule works*.

Optically induced anisometropia in kittens

To study the effect of form deprivation on refractive error while avoiding the effects of light deprivation or potential mechanical and thermal effects, Smith, Maguire, and Watson (1980) reared kittens fitted with anisometropia-inducing goggles. Nine kittens were reared in the dark for 28 days after eye-opening. On the 29th day the kittens received 2–3 hours of visual experience each day while wearing lightweight plastic goggles. Each of eight kittens wore a plano lens on the left eye and a strong minus lens (from −10 to −16D), inducing a large amount of anisometropia, on the right eye; a control kitten wore plano lenses on both eyes. At 12 weeks of age, the refractive state was measured using a Bausch & Lomb Ophthalmetron and the axial length was measured using A-scan ultrasonography.

The mean refraction of the normal eyes (wearing plano lenses) was found to be +1.06D, whereas the mean refraction of the deprived eyes was −1.12D. For five of the eight deprived kittens, the axial length differed for the two eyes, the deprived eye being longer than the normal eye. For the control kitten, as well as for two light-reared controls, refraction and axial length were similar for the two eyes. Smith et al. (1980) noted that the refractive error changes were similar to those found in form-deprived animals, which had undergone either lid fusion or corneal opacification, and because mechanical or thermal changes were ruled out, the key factor in the development of the myopia appeared to be the blurred retinal image. Because form deprivation led to myopia in the absence of light deprivation, the authors proposed that the area centralis, which is highly susceptible to a defocused image, is somehow involved in the process of emmetropization.

Using hard gas-permeable contact lenses rather than goggles, anisometropia was induced in nine kittens by Nathan, Crewther, Crewther, and Kiely (1984). The right eye of each kitten was fitted with either a plano lens or no lens at all, and the left eye was fitted with one of the following contact lenses: +6D (three kittens), −3D (one kitten), −6D (one kitten), −8D (one kitten), −11D (two kittens) and −16D (one kitten). The lenses were fitted at 3 weeks of age after experiencing a normal visual environment, and were worn for a period of 8 hours each day after which the kitten was placed in a dark room for the remainder of the 24-hour day. During the period of lens wear (which varied from 1–18 months), the following measurements were regularly made: (1) the axial distances within the eye were measured by means of A-scan ultrasonography, and (2) refraction was measured by either retinoscopy or the use of an ophthalmoscope (the ophthalmoscope was used because the anesthetic used prior to refraction—intramuscular ketamine chloride and xylazine—caused corneal drying that made retinoscopy difficult).

The results of the Nathan et al. (1984) study failed to indicate a consistent pattern of differences in axial length and refractive error between the two eyes. In most cases, the differences in axial length between the normal and deprived eyes were no more than 0.02–0.04mm (no greater than the accuracy that may be expected with this procedure). Further, differences in refraction between the two eyes were no more than 0.25D (an implied accuracy that is surprising, in that direct ophthalmoscopes normally are fitted with lenses no weaker than 1D). The one kitten fitted with a −16D contact lens on the left eye wore the lens for 4 months, after which the refraction of both that eye and the normal right eye was −0.50D. The authors concluded that kittens are not useful laboratory animals for studying the induction of myopia by retinal image degradation.

The differences between the results of the Smith et al. (1980) study and the Nathan et al. (1984) study are striking. At the end of the period of lens wear, in the Smith et al. study, the eye wearing minus powered lens was an average of 2D more myopic and 0.8mm longer than the fellow eye. In the Nathan et al. study, the eye wearing the powered lens (either plus or minus) had, in almost all cases, exactly the same refraction (to the nearest 0.25D) and the same axial length (within the 0.02–0.04mm accuracy expected for this measurement). The differences in experimental design, which may account for these differences, include the following:

1. An important difference is the fact that in the Smith et al. study the kittens were reared in darkness for a period 28 days following eye-opening, prior to the visual experience with goggles; while in the Nathan et al. study the kittens were reared in a normal visual environment for the first 3 weeks of life, prior to the fitting of the contact lenses. From the time of eye-opening until the contact lenses were fitted, a significant amount of development must have taken place in the kittens' cortical and subcortical visual pathways. This development would be more difficult to reverse than if the kittens had been kept in the dark prior to the fitting of the lenses, delaying (or inhibiting) normal neural development.

2. The fact that one of the kittens in the Nathan et al. study was observed on two occasions to have 5D of myopia while wearing a *plano* contact lens, indicating that the lens had been fitted too steeply, introduces the possibility of another major difference in the design of the two studies. Whereas the kittens in the Smith et al. study wore the same pair of goggles (with the same minus-powered lens) for the duration of the study, Nathan et al. reported that over the period of ocular growth, several lens sizes (back surface radius of curvature 5.8–7.3mm) were required. With each change in lens curvature, the power of the lens-eye system would change abruptly, and would then change gradually (in the opposite direction) with the growth of the eye, until the next lens was fitted, with the result that the eye would have experienced a variety of lens powers during the experimental period.

3. An additional difference is that in the Smith et al. study the kittens were given 2–3 hours of visual experience each day for a period of 8 weeks, whereas in the Nathan et al. study the kittens were given 8 hours of visual experience each day for periods varying from approximately 1 month to 18 months. Perhaps the number of hours of visual experience each day is not as important as the fact that the visual input was degraded (by the goggle lens or contact lens) during all visual experience. As for the additional months of visual experience in the Nathan et al. study, it is possible that much of this occurred at a time well beyond the critical period for vision development.

Deprivation in chicks

Like many other birds, chickens have two foveas (see Figure 3.11), one located in the upper retina for "frontal" vision tasks such as pecking at grain or other food, and the other located in the nasal retina

for vision in the lateral field. In a series of experiments with chicks, Wallman et al. (1978, 1981) found that if newly hatched chicks are fitted with transparent plastic occluders that restrict their field of view to the frontal field, as much as 20 to 40D of myopia can be produced in only a few weeks. The induced myopia was associated with both an axial length increase and corneal flattening, and it was thought that a part of the myopia may have occurred due to lenticular changes.

Wallman et al. (1981) suggested that the rapid development of myopia with brief periods of frontal vision may have been related to the fact that chicks appear to use their frontal field for very close (2–5cm) visual inspection that precedes pecks, and that the deprivation of the lateral visual fields usually employed in distance vision may encourage more close vision. To evaluate the possibility that accommodation played a role in producing the frontal field myopia, Wallman et al. sectioned the ciliary nerve of one eye just behind the ciliary ganglion and did a "sham" operation on the fellow eye, in which the ciliary nerve remained intact. For 24 chicks, the mean refraction of the nerve-cut eyes was −4D compared to a mean refraction of −22D for the fellow eyes. The authors noted that the susceptible period for refractive changes resulting from their experimental manipulations coincided with the

Figure 3.11 Chicks have two foveas, one located in the upper retina for frontal vision such as pecking, and another located in the nasal retina for the lateral field (Hodos and Kuenzel, 1984).

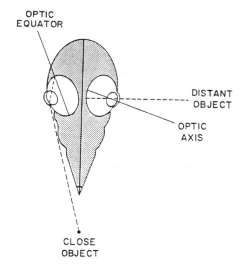

period during which the eye grows in such a way as to bring about emmetropization. They proposed that the mechanism for this growth toward emmetropia is probably the same as that responsible for frontal vision myopia, and that the mechanism uses accommodation or accommodative demand as an error signal to regulate the harmonious growth of the globe.

Changes in the shape of the chick eye due to the use of goggles have been reported by Hodos and Kuenzel (1984), who fitted one eye of 2-day-old chicks with either of two kinds of goggles—hemispherical plastic goggles (designed to degrade both the frontal and lateral fields) and crescentic goggles (designed to degrade the frontal field only). Both groups of chicks were exposed to 14 hours of light and 10 hours of darkness for 12–25 days, after which the chicks were killed, the eyes were removed, fixed and photographed, and the photographs were measured in the equatorial and axial directions. The eyes that had worn the hemispherical goggles were found to be longer in both the equatorial and the axial directions (by an average of 1.09mm and 0.33mm, respectively), whereas those that had worn the crescentic goggles were found to be longer only in the equatorial direction (by an average of 0.49mm).

Because the crescentic goggles (which degraded frontal vision only) resulted in a significant increase only in the equatorial diameter of the eye, Hodos and Kuenzel (1984) suggested that the results reported by Wallman et al. (1978, 1981) were due *not* to the fact that the chicks were permitted frontal vision but to the fact that *their lateral vision was obscured*. That is, the lack of normal neural input from the lateral visual field (see Figure 3.12) may have been responsible for the lengthening of the eye in the direction of the optic axis, which corresponds to the visual axis for the lateral field. Hodos and Kuenzel proposed that the existence of "equatorial myopia"

in the absence of axial myopia suggests that birds may have a mechanism for selective accommodation in the frontal and lateral fields.

In a more recent paper, Wallman et al. (1987) reported on experiments designed to test the suggestion of Hodos and Kuenzel that different regions of the eye could become myopic independently. Newly hatched chicks were raised with white plastic occluders placed over the eyes, designed to (1) totally deprive the animal of form vision, (2) deprive only the nasal retina, or (3) deprive only the temporal retina (see Figure 3.13). The occluders were removed at 2 weeks and at 6 weeks of age, and refraction was done by means of a Hartinger Refractometer, under

Figure 3.13 The direction of the lengthening of the vitreous chamber corresponded to the visually deprived area of the retina. Averages traced from photographs; in each drawing, the dotted line is the deprived eye and the solid line is the control eye for the same animal (Wallman et al., 1987).

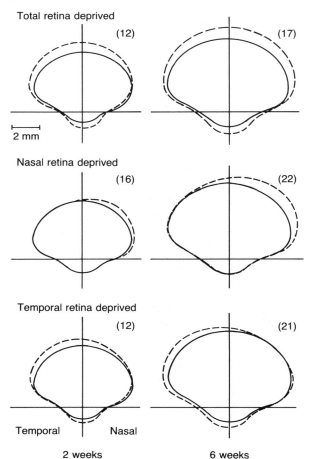

Figure 3.12 White plastic occluders were designed *(a)* to totally deprive the eye of form vision; *(b)* to deprive only the nasal retina; *(c)* to deprive only the temporal retina (Wallman et al., 1987).

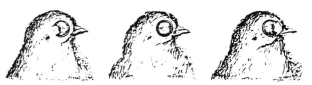

cycloplegia. Local differences in refraction were evaluated by taking measurements along three different lines of sight: along the optic axis, 30 degrees nasal to the optic axis, and 30 degrees temporal to the optic axis. In all cases the retinal area that was found to be significantly myopic was the area that had been visually deprived. In eyes in which the nasal retina was visually deprived, only the nasal retina became severely myopic; in eyes in which the temporal retina was visually deprived, only the temporal retina became severely myopic; and eyes with total form deprivation became myopic in all three retinal regions.

To determine the nature of the vitreous chamber elongation of the deprived eyes, Wallman et al. (1987) enucleated and photographed the postmortem eyes. As shown in Figure 3.13, it was found that the direction of the lengthening of the vitreous chamber corresponded to the visually deprived area of the retina—nasal-retina deprived eyes lengthened nasally, temporal-retina deprived eyes lengthened temporally, and totally deprived eyes lengthened symmetrically. The authors noted that these results imply that regions of the retina can control the growth of the subjacent sclera. Further, they concluded that local myopia occurs because of a lack of sufficient local retinal activity.

The results of their experimental work led Wallman et al. (1987) to suggest that vitreous chamber elongation and myopia may occur in humans as a result of prolonged reading because of the following "peculiarities of the printed page":

1. Printed text material contains mainly small features (i.e., high spatial frequencies), whereas most scenes in everyday life are made up of features varying widely in size (containing a broad range of spatial frequencies). Nonfoveal neurons, having large receptive fields, cannot resolve individual letters, so they respond to the average luminance level, as if the letters were not there. Only at the fovea will the responses change greatly as the eyes are moved across the page.
2. The range of luminances present on the printed page is much smaller than that experienced in typical outdoor scenes, resulting in a lower level of neural activity.
3. Reading material is achromatic whereas most real life scenes contain a variety of colors. The most numerous retinal ganglion cells show a transient response to achromatic stimuli but a slowly decaying response to colored stimuli, so the cell's response would be expected to fade very rapidly after each eye movement.

Wallman et al. concluded that, although local ocular factors are sufficient to produce local growth and myopia, it is possible that other factors including accommodation may also be important both in emmetropization and in the etiology of myopia.

In another experiment, the level of retinal activity of a group of chicks wearing translucent occluders was artificially increased by supplementing the room illumination with a 10 cycle-per-second stroboscopic light (Wallman and Gottlieb, 1987). Eyes reared with stroboscopic illumination showed 2D of myopia in the deprived regions, compared to 13D of myopia for eyes wearing translucent occluders but reared without stroboscopic illumination. This result reinforces the hypothesis that decreased retinal activity leads to vitreous chamber lengthening and myopia.

Clinical Implications of Experimental Myopia Research

What implications do the results of this experimentally induced myopia research have for the clinician? How can these research results assist the clinician in the management of myopic patients? Although employing widely differing methods to produce their results, the experiments that have been successful in producing axial elongation and myopia have the following factors in common:

1. Before the experiments began, the animals were allowed to have little or no visual experience in a normal, illuminated environment.
2. The experiments were conducted during the critical period for the development of refraction—the period in which the process of emmetropization becomes established—for the species in question. For humans this process is evident during the first few months of life and is well established by the end of the first year (Mohindra and Held, 1981), whereas for chicks the variability in refraction declines sharply near hatching and then much more slowly for a period of 8 weeks (Wallman et al., 1981).
3. The experimental procedure involved degrading the visual stimulus for one or both eyes by greatly reducing or eliminating visual form (i.e., contrast) but without materially reducing illumination.

If we accept Van Alphen's hypothesis (1961, 1986)—that the refractive state of the eye is regulated by a self-focusing mechanism, the macula providing information concerning focus to the brain, and this information being fed back by parasympathetic fibers to the choroid-ciliary body envelope that regulates the stretch of the eye—and if we also accept the premise that the macula has something to send to the brain only if there is *contrast* in the visual stimulus, then the results of the experiments can be accounted for on the basis that the eye was deprived of form vision at a crucial time for the development of refraction.

Levinsohn, who induced myopia by placing animals in boxes so that their eyes were directed toward the floor, apparently supplied no information concerning the visual stimulus provided by the floor. However, if the floor contained little or nothing by way of contrast, his results could have been due entirely to visual form deprivation. The fact that the visual axes were directed downward may have been completely irrelevant. Young's monkeys (1961) were provided with a visual stimulus consisting of a white plywood hood at a distance of 38cm. The fact that the monkeys became myopic must, therefore, have been due to form deprivation. Although one might suggest that the monkeys became myopic because they "accommodated" for the 38cm distance, the stimulus had most of the characteristics of a *ganzfield*, which, under normal circumstances, allows accommodation to assume its resting state.

The only unexpected finding in the Raviola and Wiesel (1985) experiments was that lid-suture myopia in the rhesus monkey appears to be solely due to the retina, without involving accommodation. However, recall that Van Alphen (1986) found, when an eye was inflated to increase intraocular pressure with the posterior sclera removed, that the eye elongated due to a *lack of tonus* in the ciliary muscle. Is it possible, therefore, that myopia develops not because of something that the ciliary muscle does but because of something that it does not do? Lack of ciliary tonus would explain the fact that the rhesus monkey develops lid-suture myopia in spite of the instillation of atropine, in spite of the sectioning of the parasympathetic supply to the eye, and in spite of the sectioning of the optic nerve.

The Smith et al. (1980) study demonstrated that optical blur, like blurring due to lid fusion, could cause axial elongation and myopia. Further, because mechanical and thermal factors were ruled out, Smith et al. pointed to the involvement of the area centralis in the process of emmetropization. The fact that Nathan et al. (1984) failed to produce axial elongation on a consistent basis, using contact lenses to provide optical blur, may be due to the kittens being allowed to experience a normal visual environment until 3 weeks of age or to the contact lenses not producing a sufficient amount of optical blur.

The studies involving chicks reported by Wallman et al. (1981, 1987) and by Hodos and Kuenzel (1984) have resulted in an entirely new theory concerning the cause of myopia in humans. Although Wallman et al. (1978, 1981) originally thought that restricting newly hatched chicks to their frontal visual fields produced myopia by encouraging close-up vision, Hodos and Kuenzel (1984), because of their own findings, speculated that myopia occurred in the Wallman study because the lateral vision had been restricted. Subsequently, Wallman et al. (1987) found that, when only a part of the retina was deprived, the lengthening of the eye corresponded to the portion that had been deprived. They suggested that the myopia occurred because of strictly *local factors*, not necessarily involving the accommodative system.

Is reading a form of visual deprivation?

The suggestion by Wallman et al. (1987), that human myopia occurring as a result of prolonged reading may be due to *an absence of neural activity*, adds an entirely new concept to the development of myopia. Because printed material fails to stimulate retinal photoreceptors other than those in the macular area, these authors suggest that reading is a form of visual deprivation. Their hypothesis is based on the observations that printed text material (1) involves only high spatial frequencies, (2) provides a restricted range of luminances, and (3) is achromatic, causing rapidly fading transient responses rather than the more slowly decaying sustained responses.

Finally, the finding that local retinal factors appear to cause myopia in chicks tends to reinforce the finding of Raviola and Wiesel (1985) that, for the rhesus monkey, myopia appears to result from retinal factors rather than from accommodation. Thinking again in terms of the Van Alphen (1986) theory—concerning the retina in the afferent portion of the feedback loop and the ciliary body in the efferent portion—is it possible that the experimentally induced myopia in the rhesus monkey and the kitten occurs because of interference with the retinal portion of the loop, whereas that in the pig-tail monkey and the chick occurs because of interference with the ciliary portion of the loop?

The possibility that reduced retinal activity may cause myopia presents vision practitioners with a new challenge—that of providing therapeutic measures that increase the level of retinal activity in myopic (or not-yet-myopic) children—or even that of modifying the printed page to increase its potential for retinal activity. In any event, there is ample evidence that accommodation plays a role in the development of myopia. Hence, it is reasonable to believe that patient management procedures that reduce the necessity for accommodation should prove to be effective in the control of myopia. Such procedures are discussed in the following section.

ATTEMPTS TO CONTROL MYOPIA

Since early in the present century, attempts have been made by many vision practitioners (both optometrists and ophthalmologists) to control or arrest the progression of myopia. Most of the procedures advocated for myopia control have been based on the supposition that *accommodation* is what causes myopia to progress, and that if the necessity for accommodating can be reduced or eliminated, the progression of myopia will slow down or stop. Procedures that have been advocated for the control of myopia have included undercorrection, visual training, the use of bifocals, the use of atropine or other cycloplegic drugs, the use of contact lenses, and various surgical procedures.

Any procedure for the control of juvenile myopia should be evaluated in view of the fact that the progression of myopia tends to level off during the teenage years, no matter what form of treatment is applied. As noted earlier, Goss and Winkler (1983) reported that myopia ceased to progress at a mean age of approximately 15 years for females and 16 years for males. They also reported a large amount of variability in the age of cessation. The standard deviation for the cessation age was 2 years, but some myopes ceased to progress as early as age 11 or 12, with others continuing to progress until age 20 or beyond.

Undercorrection

During the past half century, many practitioners have recommended *undercorrection* as a method of controlling the progression of myopia. The recommended amount of undercorrection has usually been in the neighborhood of 0.50–0.75D. To my knowledge, no controlled studies making use of undercorrection have been reported. Goss (1984) reported on

a study involving *overcorrection* of myopia. The results of the study were negative.

The Bates Method of Eye Exercises

When examining 1,500 schoolchildren in 1903 in Grand Forks, North Dakota, Bates (1920), an ophthalmologist, found that some of the children failed the Snellen visual acuity test on the first trial but passed it on the second or third trial. One of the teachers was so impressed with the improvement in acuity on repeated testing that she asked Bates to allow her to place a Snellen chart permanently in her classroom. The children were instructed to read, at least once every day, the smallest row of letters they could see from their seats, covering each eye in turn with the palm of the hand in such a way as to avoid pressure on the eyeball. The Snellen chart was subsequently used in all of the public schools in Grand Forks for a period of 8 years, and Bates (1920) reported that during this period myopia was reduced from 6 percent to 1 percent. Unfortunately, Bates gave no details of the amount of myopia possessed by the children or the "before" or "after" acuities. In addition to Snellen chart reading, Bates recommended practice in central fixation, "palming" (covering the eyes with one's hands and attempting to "see black"), and sun gazing as methods of improving vision not only for myopes but for everyone. Peppard, Corbett, and the author Aldous Huxley not only popularized Bates's procedures but enlarged on them (Grosvenor, 1980b). Not surprisingly, there has never been any scientific evidence that these procedures are of any help in controlling myopia.

Optometric Visual Training

During World War II, many optometrists were consulted by myopic men who requested visual training in order to be accepted by (or to remain in) one of the armed services. Optometrists who tried to help these patients, therefore, were not simply attempting to control the progression of myopia but to reduce it in amount or to eliminate it altogether. Although the stated goal for such training programs was the reduction of myopia, the success or failure of such a program was usually determined by whether or not there was an improvement in *visual acuity*. When improvement in visual acuity is the only criterion used, one may conclude that the patient has simply learned to interpret a blurred image. An additional interpretation, not often recognized by optometrists who engaged in this kind of training, was that the patient memorized the letters on the Snellen chart. The typical program involved both training and testing sessions, and in most cases the same Snellen chart was used for all testing sessions.

In 1944, a study known as the Baltimore Myopia Control Project was conducted. The Curtis Publishing Company financed the project and recruited the 111 subjects. The training procedures were conducted by optometrists and technicians under the sponsorship of the American Optometric Association, and the results were evaluated by staff ophthalmologists of the Wilmer Institute at Johns Hopkins Hospital. Subjects for the study were unselected, having refractive errors from −0.50 to −9.00D and ranging in age from 9–32 years. Although none of the many reports indicated the nature of the training procedures, the average number of training sessions was reported to be 25, over a 13-week period.

The official ophthalmological report concerning the study was written by Woods (1945), and the official optometric report was written by Ewalt (1946). Although neither of these reports provided data on the reduction in the measured amount of myopia as a result of the visual training, Ewalt published visual acuity graphs that indicated (on visual inspection) an average improvement in visual acuity of about two lines of letters. Carl Shepard (1946), a well-known optometric educator of the period, summarized the Woods and Ewalt reports and concluded that "as a demonstration of control of myopia, in the face of data reported by the Wilmer Institute, but not by the AOA bureau, it must be admitted to be a complete failure. It has shown that optometry cannot control myopia" (p. 135).

Biofeedback Training

In recent years a number of authors have reported on the use of various *biofeedback* training procedures for the control of myopia. Such procedures commonly involve a method of relaxing (and measuring) accommodation, and make use of an auditory signal to indicate to the subject that accommodation is changing in the correct (or incorrect) direction. With some exceptions, those who advocate this form of training present their results in terms of improvement in *visual acuity* rather than in terms of reduction of myopia. No large-scale, controlled studies of biofeedback training have been reported.

Trachtman (1978) published a report of the results of biofeedback training on a 30-year-old myope, involving seven sessions that totaled 34 minutes. Feedback was in the form of a tone whose frequency increased as the subject's accommodation (myopia) decreased. Trachtman reported a reduction in myopia of 1.05D in the Badal optometer system, while clinical findings indicated a reduction in myopia of approximately 1D (from a spherical equivalent refraction, right eye, of −1.00D before training to 0.00D after training) with an improvement in unaided acuity from 20/50−2 to 20/30−2. The author gave no indication of the permanence of the training effects.

In a study involving 17 subjects between the ages of 20 and 46 years, Balliet, Clay, and Blood (1982) used an automated optometer system for biofeedback training, with buzzers indicating the "correct" and "incorrect" responses. The mean improvement in visual acuity, after 38 training sessions, was 3.4 lines (from 20/213 to 20/44). No data concerning reduction in myopia were reported. Rosen, Schiffman, and Myers (1984) reported on one of the few studies in which the subjects were refracted before and after the training procedures. The 29 subjects, aged 19–47 years, were divided into three groups: 10 subjects received behavioral training plus feedback, 10 subjects received behavioral training only, and 9 subjects received no training. The training consisted of viewing Landolt rings at gradually increasing distances; the feedback was in the form of verbal reinforcement. The authors published graphs of their results, which indicated (1) a mean improvement in visual acuity for the experimental subjects from about 20/300 to 20/150, and (2) a mean *increase* in myopia of about 0.2D for the experimental subjects who received feedback, as compared to a slight decrease in myopia for the other two groups of subjects.

Trachtman's (1978) biofeedback instrumentation was employed by Berman (1985), who used as subjects 16 myopic patients between the ages of 9 and 37 years. Visual acuity was measured, binocularly, using American Optical and Bausch and Lomb acuity charts, both at the beginning and at the end of each training session. Seven training sessions were given, each session consisting of 10 minutes of training, 10 minutes of rest, and a further 10 minutes of training. Mean improvement in visual acuity for the 16 subjects was from 20/90 to 20/35. There was no indication of the permanence of the visual acuity improvements. Data concerning change in refractive error were not given.

In another study using Trachtman's (1978) instrumentation, Gallaway, Pearl, Winkelstein, and Scheiman (1987) administered biofeedback training to 12 myopic subjects between the ages of 23 and 42 years, nine of whom completed the training sessions. Although there were no changes in refractive error, some of the subjects showed an improvement in visual acuity. Because the training procedure required repeated visual acuity measurements, Gallaway et al. suggested that the improvement in visual acuity may have been due to a learning effect in the measurement of visual acuity rather than to the biofeedback training. They concluded that additional research was needed to determine the usefulness of biofeedback training of accommodation as a means of visual acuity enhancement and myopia reduction.

The Use of Bifocals

The belief that myopia is brought about by prolonged accommodation has caused some practitioners and researchers to suggest that bifocals may slow down its progression by reducing the accommodative demand. Although the optometric literature contains numerous reports of the use of bifocal lenses for the control of myopia, reports of controlled studies making use of bifocals are few. Five large-scale studies have been reported in recent years. The authors of two of these studies found that bifocals had no effect on the progression of their subjects' myopia, whereas the authors of two studies found that bifocals *were* effective in controlling myopia, and the author of one study found that bifocals were effective in controlling the myopia of subjects having certain near-point findings.

Mandell (1959) reported on rates of progression of myopia for 59 myopes fitted with bifocals and 116 myopes fitted with single-vision lenses. He concluded that bifocals failed to eliminate or reduce the progression of myopia beyond what might be expected to occur on a chance basis. However, the average age of Mandell's subjects when entering the study was 17.1 years for the single-vision group and 14.3 years for the bifocal group, with many of the single-vision lens wearers being over the age of 20 when entering the study. Because it is well known that myopes over the age of 17 (and certainly those over the age of 20) will progress very slowly no matter what is done, Mandell's conclusion that bifocals had no effect on the progression of myopia should be interpreted with extreme caution. Unless single-vision and bifocal groups are matched on the

basis of age, sex, and amount of myopia when entering the study, the results of this (or any other) study cannot be considered as conclusive.

Roberts and Banford (1967) reported on a study involving 85 myopes wearing bifocals and 396 single-vision lens wearers seen in their optometric practice during a 14-year period. During this period, the bifocal wearers progressed an average of 0.314D per year, whereas the single-vision lens wearers progressed an average of 0.407D per year. Even though the authors found this difference to be statistically significant, it was so small (0.093D per year) that if the same rate of change took place for a 5-year period of bifocal wearing, at the end of this period the child would be, on the average, only about 0.50D less myopic than if bifocals had not been worn.

Oakley and Young (1975) reported on a study involving 544 children between the ages of 6 and 15. Bifocal lenses were prescribed with a 0.50D undercorrection at distance and with a +1.50 or +2.00D addition with the segment line splitting the patient's pupil. Annual rates of myopia progression were found to average 0.50D for single-vision wearers and 0.04D for bifocal wearers. The authors attributed the success of their study to the very high bifocal position; however, because all refractions were performed by the same refractionist, they noted the possibility of a bias in favor of the bifocal wearers. In this study the bifocal and single-vision groups were matched on the basis of beginning refractive error, age, and sex.

The records of three optometric practices in the central United States were analyzed in a retrospective study reported by Goss (1986). Included in the analysis were the records of 112 myopes aged 6–15 years, 60 of whom were fitted with bifocals and 52 with single-vision lenses. The mean rates of myopia progression were 0.37D per year for the bifocal wearers and 0.44D per year for the single-vision lens wearers. The difference was not statistically significant. However, the differences in progression rates were found to be statistically significant for two groups of subjects: (1) those with near-point esophoria (mean progression of 0.34D per year for bifocals and 0.54D per year for single vision), and (2) those with near-point cross cylinder nets of +0.50D or more (mean progression of 0.25D per year for bifocals and 0.48D per year for single vision). Goss made the point that if bifocals are prescribed for young myopes with the idea of providing comfortable vision for those who are esophoric or have high cross cylinder nets at near-point, there may be the added advantage of a decrease in progression.

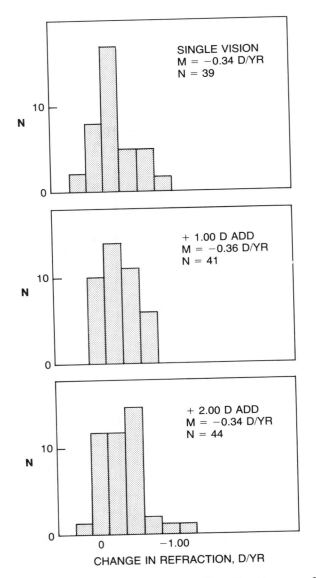

Figure 3.14 Frequency distributions of mean changes in spherical equivalent refraction, right eye, for subjects wearing single vision lenses, +1.00D add bifocals and +2.00D add bifocals for a period of 3 years (Grosvenor, Perrigin, Perrigin, and Maslovitz, 1987).

In a 3-year randomized clinical trial recently completed at the University of Houston, each of 212 myopic children between the ages of 6 and 15 years was fitted with single vision-lenses, +1.00D add bifocals, or +2.00D add bifocals (Young, et al., 1985; Grosvenor, et al., 1985). Subjects were placed in one of the three treatment groups on the basis of a table of random numbers, and were matched on the basis of sex, initial age, and initial amount of myopia. Two

teams of researchers conducted the study: (1) an evaluation team whose members were responsible for the evaluation of each subject prior to inclusion in the study and at the end of each year, and (2) a patient care team whose members were responsible for the fitting of the single-vision or bifocal lenses and for all follow-up care. Executive bifocals were used, in polycarbonate plastic, and were fitted so that the dividing line was 2mm below the center of the pupil. The criterion for the subjective end-point, for both single-vision and bifocal wearers, was "maximum plus or minimum minus power for best visual acuity."

In the report by the patient care team, Grosvenor, Perrigin, Perrigin, and Maslovitz (1987) stated that for the 124 subjects who remained in the study for the entire 3-year period, mean rates of myopia progression were 0.34D per year for single-vision lens wearers, 0.36D per year for +1.00D add bifocal wearers, and 0.34D per year for +2.00D add bifocal wearers. The small differences in mean rates of progression (0.02 per year) were found not to be statistically significant. To determine if the near-point phoria had any effect on the tendency of bifocals to control the progression of myopia, mean progression of myopia was tabulated for the three treatment groups on the basis of whether the subject was esophoric, orthophoric, or exophoric at the near-point. Mean rates of progression for esophoric subjects were found to differ little for subjects wearing single-vision lenses, +1.00D add bifocals, or +2.00D add bifocals, being 0.33, 0.37 and 0.30D per year, respectively. These results, therefore, fail to confirm the finding of Goss (1986), that bifocals tend to have a favorable effect in reducing the rate of myopia progression for patients who are esophoric at the near-point.

Grosvenor et al. (1987) proposed that lack of a significant effect of the bifocals on the progression of myopia may have been due to the fact that once the eye has begun to elongate, the scleral tissue is stretched and thinned to the extent that it loses much of its resiliency and will continue to elongate, even in the presence of normal intraocular pressure. If this is the case, bifocals would be expected to have a significant effect on the progression of myopia only if they were worn before the eye began to elongate. This would mean that bifocals would have to be worn before the onset of myopia.

Because it was shown by Hirsch (1964) that children at the greatest risk for the development of myopia are those who have no more than 0.50D of hyperopia at the age of 5 or 6 years, particularly if they also have against-the-rule astigmatism, children

83

Table 3.5 Comparison of results of bifocal studies (from Grosvenor, Perrigin, Perrigin, and Maslovitz, 1987).

Study	Age	Treatment	Mean Change
Mandell (1959)	Mean 17.1	Single vision	(see below)[a]
	Mean 14.3	Bifocals	(see below)[a]
Roberts & Banford (1967)	<17	Single vision	−0.41D/year
	<17	Bifocals	−0.36D/year
Oakley & Young (1975) (Native Americans)	6–21	Single vision	−0.37D/year
	6–21	Bifocals	−0.11D/year
Oakley & Young (1975) (Caucasians)	6–21	Single vision	−0.52D/year
	6–21	Bifocals	−0.02D/year
Goss (1986)	6–15	Single vision	−0.44D/year
	6–15	Bifocals	−0.37D/year
Grosvenor et al. (1987)	6–15	Single vision	−0.34D/year
	6–15	+1.00D add	−0.36D/year
	6–15	+2.00D add	−0.34D/year

[a]Mean changes in refraction were not reported, but it was concluded that bifocals did not eliminate or reduce the progression of myopia.

who fit this description could be fitted with bifocals (with plano uppers) or with reading glasses and followed during their elementary school years. A problem with this approach, however, is convincing parents (as well as children) of the necessity of wearing glasses even though no refractive error or visual problem exists.

The results of all of the studies discussed here are summarized and compared in Table 3.5. The data presented in the right-hand column of the table (entitled "Mean Change") show that only the Oakley and Young (1975) study resulted in what might be considered to be a clinically significant difference (i.e., 0.25D per year or more) between rates of progression with bifocals and single-vision lenses.

The Use of Atropine

Because myopia is considered by some practitioners to occur as a result of accommodation, a number of cycloplegic agents, including atropine, scopolamine, and tropicamide, have been used in attempts to control myopia. However, the use of a cycloplegic agent in a large-scale study presents a number of problems. There must be some provision for subjects to see for reading and other close work. This can be accomplished by providing subjects with bifocal lenses or, for relatively low myopes, by having them remove their glasses while reading. A second problem is that of retaining subjects in the study. Daily instillation of the drug is a nuisance, and the lack of accommodation is an inconvenience even if bifocals are worn. The constant mydriasis causes sensitivity to sunlight, and some subjects develop allergic reactions (such as allergic dermatitis) and other side effects.

In a study reported at the 1964 International Myopia Congress and described by Young (1965), Bedrossian compared 24 myopic children with a control group of 20 myopic children of the same age and with myopia progressing at the same rate. Each member of the experimental group was given one drop of atropine every day, in one eye only, for a period of a year, after which atropine was instilled in the other eye (only) for an additional year. Bedrossian found that the myopia stabilized in the atropinized eye during the year in which the atropine was used, whereas the nonatropinized eye continued to progress at about the same rate as before. He concluded that over the 2-year period, each eye progressed about half as much as it would have progressed without the use of atropine. In a second study reported by Young (1965), Gastin used scopolamine on 106 myopic children (apparently with no control group) for more than a year. Bifocals were prescribed to permit reading and other close work. Gastin reported that all the children's myopia progressed before the study began, but progression ceased with the scopolamine treatment.

Other studies involving the use of cycloplegics have been reported by Gimbel (1973) and Abraham (1966). Gimbel used atropine in a controlled study lasting 3 years. Although few subjects finished the study, he reported that the yearly average progression was 0.41D for the control group but that there was no progression at all for the atropinized group.

Abraham (1966) reported on a study in which 1 percent tropicamide was instilled daily, at bedtime, in the eyes of 68 myopes from 7 to 18 years of age, with 82 myopic children serving as a control group. During an observation period averaging 18 months, the mean changes in refraction for the treated subjects were −0.44D for both males and females; while for control subjects the mean changes were −0.92D for males and −0.77D for females.

Brodstein et al. (1984) reported on a study in which both bifocals and atropine were used in an effort to control the progression of myopia. The experimental group consisted of 435 subjects, each of whom wore +2.25D add bifocals and was given one drop of 1 percent atropine every morning in each eye; while the control group consisted of 146 subjects wearing single-vision lenses. The age range of the subjects was not reported, although one of the tables indicates that some of the subjects were "under 8" and others were "over 16" years of age. All refractions were done under cycloplegia. The mean period of follow-up for the experimental subjects was 33 months while under treatment and 22 months post-treatment, whereas the mean period of follow-up for control subjects was 79 months. Results for the 253 subjects who completed the study were reported in terms of change in myopia in diopters per month, on the basis of age of onset of myopia and age during the study. Combining the data for all age groups, mean annual rates of progression were found to be:

Experimental group, during treatment:	0.16D per year
Experimental group, post-treatment:	0.30D per year
Control group:	0.25D per year.

Brodstein et al. acknowledged the potential for error occasioned by the fact that follow-up refractions were done under a weak cycloplegic (Mydriacyl) for the control group but under a strong cycloplegic (atropine) for the experimental group.

Studies Using Timolol

Another approach to the control of myopia progression involves the use of timolol mileate, a beta-blocker used for the management of glaucoma. This drug has the advantage of reducing intraocular pressure without causing miosis, and does not require as frequent instillation as pilocarpine or other pressure-reducing drugs. A pilot study was reported by Goldschmidt, Jensen, Marushak, and Ostergaard (1985), in which ten children (7–12 years of age) with severe progressive myopia were treated for 12 months with timolol maleate 0.25 percent eyedrops twice daily. For those children whose intraocular pressure reduced during the treatment period, the rate of myopia progression was found to reduce also. No serious side-effects were observed.

In a subsequent study, the daily instillation of timolol maleate was used in a clinical trial involving 51 experimental subjects and 51 controls (Jensen, 1987). One of the criteria for inclusion in the study was myopia of 1.25D or more. At the end of 2 years there was a mean decrease in intraocular pressure of 2–3mm Hg for the experimental group but there was no difference in the rate of myopia progression for the two groups.

Contact Lenses

Whether contact lenses are effective in the control of myopia has been a matter of controversy ever since Morrison (1956) reported that he had fitted a large number of young myopes with contact lenses who after a period of more than 2 years showed no progression. Morrison's patients ranged from 7–19 years of age and were fitted with polymethyl methacrylate (PMMA) lenses from 1.62–2.50D, flatter than the flattest corneal meridian. Morrison suggested that the lack of progression could have been due to a flattening effect on the cornea, an interference or effect on metabolism of the cornea, or other factors.

As noted earlier, any procedure for the control of juvenile myopia should be evaluated in view of the fact that the progression of myopia tends to level off during the teenage years no matter what is done, as documented by Goss and Winkler (1983) who found a mean cessation age of 15 years for females and 16 years for males. In addition, any suggestion that *contact lenses* can control the progression of myopia must be considered in the light of (1) the tendency of practitioners to *overcorrect* a myopic contact lens wearer, and (2) a number of well-documented, *time-dependent* changes in corneal curvature and refraction of wearers of PMMA contact lenses.

In response to the reports of Morrison and other practitioners, Bailey (1958) called attention to the following factors, all of which tend to result in an overcorrection of a myopic contact lens wearer:

1. Flattening of the cornea (which can occur even when the alignment method of fitting is used).
2. A possible reduction in anterior chamber depth due to corneal flattening, with a consequent decrease in the axial length of the eye.
3. Overcorrection of the myopia due to the presence of photophobia during the initial and subsequent refractions while wearing the lenses.
4. Settling of the lens on the cornea, reducing the tear layer thickness.
5. Effective power error, due to failure to take effective power difference into consideration when ordering the contact lenses.
6. Ophthalmometer "error," caused by using an ophthalmometer (keratometer) to verify the finished lenses.
7. The practitioner's tendency to overlook an overcorrection of myopia in follow-up examinations.

Bailey (1958) made the point that these factors could, in combination, be responsible for an overcorrection of as much as 1.50D. He also noted that a typical myope levels off at about 3.00D of myopia, and that if contact lenses are first fitted when a power of −1.50D is required, an overcorrection of 1.50D will assure that the power of the lenses will not have to be increased until the myopia has reached −3.00D.

The time-dependent changes in corneal curvature and refraction due to PMMA contact lens wear have been studied by Rengstorff (1967, 1969a, 1969b, 1971). They include a diurnal variation in corneal curvature and refraction, changes in corneal curvature and refraction with long-term wear, and changes in corneal curvature and refraction on discontinuation of contact lens wear. These changes, described in some detail in Chapter 14, can have the following effects:

1. Because the cornea tends to steepen during lens wear and flatten after lens removal, refractive findings taken immediately after lens removal tend to show more myopia than those taken in the morning, prior to lens wear.
2. Because the cornea tends to gradually flatten with long-term lens wear, refractive findings taken after a year or more of lens wear tend to show less myopia than those taken prior to lens wear.
3. Because the cornea flattens considerably in the first few days after discontinuation of lens wear (reversing to about the prefitting curvature after several weeks of nonwear), refractive findings

taken during this period show less myopia than those taken immediately after lens removal.

The literature concerning the use of contact lenses for myopia control is confined almost entirely to PMMA lenses. However, although there is reason to believe that gas-permeable hard lenses may be effective in the control of myopia, there has been no evidence that soft (hydrogel) lenses are effective in myopia control. Whereas myopia control may be considered in terms of arresting or retarding the rate of progression of juvenile myopia, as described in Morrison's (1956) report, it may also be considered in terms of procedures designed to reduce the amount of existing myopia, known as *orthokeratology*.

Controlling the progression of juvenile myopia

Soon after Morrison's (1956) early report, a number of practitioners reported that they, too, had found that contact lenses arrested the progression of myopia. Most of these reports were concerned with only a small number of patients and were written at a time when contact lenses were relatively large, thick, and fitted flatter than the corneal apex. One of the first studies conducted since the development of smaller, thinner lenses was the prospective study of Baldwin et al. (1969). These investigators reported refractive data on 65 myopes between the ages of 7 and 13 years, 42 of whom were fitted with contact lenses and 23 fitted with glasses. During a period of approximately one year, mean progression was found to be 0.49D for the contact lens wearers as compared to 0.38D for the spectacle wearers. However, at the beginning of the study the contact lens wearers had a higher mean amount of myopia than the spectacle wearers, so one would expect them to progress at a faster rate. Further, axial length measurements showed that axial length changes were associated with age, not with contact lens wear.

In another prospective study, Kelly et al. (1975) fitted 57 subjects with Ruben offset lenses with an "apex-clear tear-pool" who wore their lenses for a period of 4 years. They reported that myopia was arrested for 22 (38 percent) of the subjects. The ages of the subjects were not given.

Of all of the studies reported in the literature, the most definitive was carried out by Stone and her colleagues (1973, 1976). The study made use of a control group and an effort was made to match subjects in the experimental and control groups in regard to the initial amount of myopia. The age range of the subjects was chosen to embrace the period of life when myopia is most likely to progress. The study was of sufficiently long duration and the time of testing was specified in relation to the time of lens removal. As stated in Stone's first report (1973), the experimental group was made up of 84 contact lens wearers (53 males and 32 females) and the control group was made up of 40 spectacle wearers (18 males and 22 females). Members of the experimental group were fitted with lenses having a diameter of 9.2mm or smaller and an optic zone of 7.0mm or smaller, fitted "just steeper than the flattest keratometer reading."

Upon completion of the 5-year study, Stone (1976) reported keratometric and refractive data taken immediately after lens removal. The mean increase in myopia for the contact lens wearers was 0.50D (averaging the horizontal and vertical findings) for the 5-year period, or 0.10D per year, whereas the mean increase in myopia for the spectacle wearers was 1.75D, or 0.35D per year. Corneal changes were much less than the changes in refraction—mean corneal refracting power decreasing about 0.50D for contact lens wearers and 0.12D for spectacle wearers during the 5-year period.

In discussing the results, Stone (1976) made the point that not all of the difference in progression of myopia for the two groups of subjects could be accounted for by *corneal flattening* (i.e., the difference in mean corneal flattening for the two groups was less than 0.50D, whereas the difference in mean increase in myopia was 1.65D per year). Further, Stone concluded that, because the effects of contact lenses on the progression of myopia cannot be due entirely to corneal flattening, it is possible that contact lenses may cause an effect on the *axial elongation* of the eye. Unfortunately, axial length was not measured.

With the completion of Stone's (1976) study, the following questions remained unanswered:

1. How *permanent* is the stabilization of myopia due to the wearing of contact lenses?
2. Do contact lenses have an effect in slowing down the axial *elongation* of the eye?
3. Are *gas-permeable* contact lenses effective in stabilizing the progression of myopia?

A study making use of silicone-acrylate, gas-permeable hard contact lenses is in progress at the University of Houston (Perrigin, Quintero, Perrigin, and Grosvenor, 1987). One hundred myopes between the ages of 10 and 13 years were fitted with Paraperm "O$_2$ Plus" silicone-acrylate lenses, fitted by the alignment ("on K") method, to be worn for a period of 3 years. Subjects for the recently completed bifocal study will serve as a control group. Two teams of researchers are conducting the study—an evaluation team and a patient care team. The evaluation team refracts each candidate for the study and measures the axial length of the eye, using ultrasound, prior to enrollment in the study and at yearly intervals for the duration of the study. The patient care team supervises the fitting and follow-up care. At the time of this writing, 58 subjects have completed one year in the study. Mean changes in refraction, corneal refracting power, and axial length for these subjects were as follows:

Refraction:	0.06D more myopia
Corneal power:	0.20D decrease (flatter)
Axial length:	0.06mm longer

The mean increase in myopia was just half that of the control subjects, matched for age and amount of myopia (0.40D per year). There was a large amount of variability among subjects: change in refraction ranged from 0.75D less myopia to 1.75D more myopia; change in corneal power ranged from 0.75D decrease to 0.25D increase; and change in axial length varied from 0.5mm shorter to 1.2mm longer. These preliminary results indicate that silicon acrylate, gas-permeable contact lenses tend to flatten the wearer's corneas, as PMMA lenses do, thus apparently reducing the rate of progression of myopia.

Orthokeratology

The usual procedure in orthokeratology is to fit succeedingly flatter PMMA lenses, with an attempt to bring about a reduction in myopia through a flattening of the cornea. Once the practitioner believes a maximum of flattening has taken place, the patient's wearing time is reduced, with the intention that the reduction in myopia will persist with the reduced wearing schedule (i.e., the wearing of "retainer" lenses). Even though the aim of orthokeratology is that of reducing the amount of myopia, the practitioner usually evaluates the success of the procedure in terms of improvement in unaided *visual acuity*. Although there is a large body of literature on the subject, most of it consists of reports by practitioners who tend to be biased toward orthokeratology (or to their own particular variation of orthokeratology).

Two large-scale, controlled clinical trials of orthokeratology have been reported. Kerns (1976,

1977, 1978) reported on a study in which he took an objective position, not advocating the use of ortho-keratology but investigating it in a scientific but clinically oriented basis. Using as subjects conventional contact lens wearers (26 eyes) and experimental (orthokeratology) wearers (36 eyes) who were fitted with larger, thicker, and flatter lenses to "initiate" orthokeratology changes. After a period of some-what more than a year, mean changes for the experimental group were:

Refraction in horizontal meridian: 1.06D less myopia (SD ±0.98D).

Refraction in vertical meridian: 0.68D less myopia (SD ±0.90D).

Refractive astigmatism (w-rule): 0.42D increase (SD ±0.74D).

The mean changes were such as to bring about a reduction in myopia but with induced with-the-rule astigmatism. Kerns pointed out that the standard deviations were so high that it would not be possible to predict that changes comparable to the mean changes would occur with any given patient. Even the patient typified by the mean values would have, at the end of the study, approximately 1.00D less spherical error but 0.50D more astigmatism than before the study began. Kerns reported that the limiting factor in inducing corneal flattening is the "sphericalization" of the cornea, which occurs when the corneal apex becomes sufficiently flat so that it has the same radius of curvature as the periphery. No data were given concerning the permanence of the orthokeratology changes.

In another large-scale clinical trial, Polse et al. (1983) fitted 80 subjects (40 experimental and 40 control) with contact lenses and followed them for 18 months. Experimental (orthokeratology) subjects were fitted with larger and thicker lenses, and fitted flatter than control subjects. This was a randomized clinical trial in which even the subjects did not know which group they were in. "Mock" lens changes were made for the members of the control group and real changes were made for members of the orthokera-tology group. Myopia reduced an average of 1.00D for the experimental subjects as compared to 0.50D for the control subjects. Polse et al. did not find the with-the-rule astigmatism reported by Kerns, and commented that this was because they monitored lens fit and made sure the lenses were well centered on the wearers' corneas (instead of "riding high"). They found that the reduction in myopia was not permanent, requiring the use of retainer lenses to perpetuate the effect. Also, vision was variable from day to day. There were no clinically significant adverse effects, but the orthokeratology patients required more visits due to complications than the control subjects.

What can we conclude about orthokeratology? For a low myope, orthokeratology may bring about sufficient reduction in myopia so that contact lenses do not have to be worn on a regular basis. However, contact lenses usually have to be worn on a part-time basis, as *retainers*, to maintain the reduction in myopia and improvement in visual acuity.

Surgical Procedures

A surgical procedure known as *radial keratotomy* has received a large amount of media attention. The National Eye Advisory Council has expressed grave concern regarding this procedure, which is being adopted on a large scale in this country even though reports concerning the procedure have not provided an adequate basis on which to assure the public of its safety and efficacy (*AOA News*, July 1, 1980). Radial keratotomy is only one of a series of surgical procedures that are advocated for the control of myopia. Other procedures include scleral resection, scleral reinforcement, crystalline lens removal, and refractive keratoplasty.

Scleral resection, as reported by Borley and Tanner (1964), was described by Muller in 1903. It involves the excision of a band of sclera for the purpose of shortening a highly myopic eye. Although originally intended for eyes having detached retinas, it has occasionally been used in cases of high myopia where no detachment exists.

Scleral reinforcement is an operation in which fascia or donor sclera is grafted onto the back of the eyeball to reinforce the sclera at the posterior pole. The graft may be in the form of either a vertically oriented strip about 7mm wide or a cruciate graft placed beneath the inferior and superior oblique muscles and beneath all tendons so to fit the sclera as snugly as possible. This procedure also has seen only occasional use.

Crystalline lens removal has been reported in the literature, from time to time, as a "cure" for high myopia. A major problem with this procedure is that myopic eyes have an increased risk of retinal detach-ment and other complications after lens removal.

Refractive keratoplasty, a technique developed by Barraquer (1964), involves removing a slice of the patient's cornea. This slice is then frozen and placed on a lathe (while frozen). It is cut to the required shape to correct the patient's refractive error and then sutured back onto the patient's cornea. This technique is not widely used.

Radial keratotomy was first described by Sato, Akiyama, and Shibata (1953). They made use of partial thickness, radially oriented incisions in the anterior and posterior surfaces of the cornea, each incision extending from the corneoscleral junction to the pupillary zone, allowing for a 6mm clear central zone. The subsequent scars had the effect of flattening the apical portion of the cornea, thus reducing the patient's myopia. The reduction in myopia for 32 patients ranged from 1.50 to 7.00D, with the average being 3.00D. The authors reported that within 2 months after surgery, fine radial lines could be seen under strong focal illumination in a dark room, but they were unseen under ordinary light.

Fyodorov and Durnev (1979) reported the use of radial keratotomy on 60 eyes of 30 patients whose myopia ranged from −0.75 to −3.00D. These surgeons used 16 radial incisions on the anterior corneal surface only, approaching three-fourths of the thickness of the cornea. In all cases the central corneal curvature flattened from 5.00–6.00D within 3 or 4 days after the surgery, but then it began to steepen, stabilizing by the third postsurgical month. After stabilization, 29 eyes were found to be emmetropic, 21 were still myopic but of a lesser amount than before surgery, and 10 were hyperopic. The longest follow-up period reported by Fyodorov and Durnev was from 2–3 years for 13 of the original 30 subjects (although in an addendum to the article they reported having performed a total of 676 procedures). Because the surgical process purposely weakens the structure of the peripheral portion of the cornea, one may question whether the weakened cornea can be expected to maintain its integrity throughout the patient's lifetime. During the years following Fyodorov and Durnev's reintroduction of radial keratotomy, this procedure rapidly became a popular form of treatment for myopia even though a controlled clinical trial of the procedure had not yet been carried out.

Waring et al. (1985) reported on the first-year results of a 9-center clinical trial known as the Prospective Evaluation of Radial Keratotomy (PERK) study. The study was designed to investigate the safety, efficacy, predictability, and stability of a single, standardized surgical technique of radial keratotomy. The study involved 435 patients, ranging in age from 21–58 years (with a mean age of 35 years), having bilateral physiological myopia from −2.00D to −8.00D equivalent sphere, and refractive astigmatism of 1.50D or less. The surgical procedure involved the use of eight radial incisions and provided an optical zone of 4.0mm for eyes having from 2.00 to 3.12D of myopia, 3.5mm for eyes having from 3.25 to 4.37D of myopia, and 3.0mm for eyes having from 4.50 to 8.00D of myopia. Radial keratotomy was done on only one eye of each subject. At the end of one year after surgery, 34 percent of the subjects had a spherical equivalent refractive error between +0.50 and −0.50D, and 49 percent had uncorrected visual acuity of 20/20 or better.

Patients who have undergone radial keratotomy often complain of fluctuating vision, their uncorrected vision worsening during the course of the day. The diurnal variations in refraction, corneal curvature, and visual acuity of patients who took part in the PERK study were reported by Schanzlin et al. (1986). Only those PERK study patients who had complained about fluctuating vision were included in the study. Patients were examined 3 months after surgery and 1 year after surgery, first between 7 and 8 A.M. and again between 7 and 8 P.M. The mean diurnal changes 1 year after surgery were as follows: refraction, a mean increase of 0.42D of myopia; corneal refraction, a mean steepening of 0.42D; and uncorrected visual acuity, a mean loss of 5.3 letters, or about one line of letters. These diurnal changes varied little from the changes occurring 3 months after surgery. The authors speculated that, because the scars that heal the radial incisions do not reconnect the collagen stromal fibers from end to end, radial keratotomy may cause a permanent loss of the structural integrity of the cornea. To illustrate this point, they cited two cases in which the cornea ruptured through radial keratotomy incisions 1 year after successful surgery.

A number of cases of visual impairment following radial keratotomy were described by O'Day et al. (1986). Of a total of 13 patients with visual impairment seen in their consultative ophthalmological practice, seven patients experienced complications of surgery or drug treatment but not unique to radial keratotomy, whereas 11 experienced complications unique to radial keratotomy (four patients having complications in both categories). In the first category were two cases of optic atrophy due to trauma during retrobulbar injection, one retinal detachment, two cataracts, one endophthalmitis, and one corneal ulcer. In the second category there was a failure to reduce the myopia of four patients, a marked undercorrection of myopia for three patients, and an overcorrection (resulting in significant hyperopia) for five patients.

Study Questions

1. What evidence exists that suggests the myopia occurring in monkeys after lid-suturing is due to visual deprivation rather than to other factors?

2. Discuss the concept of "emmetropization at near."

3. What evidence exists that indicates myopia is (a) genetically determined? (b) environmentally determined?

4. What evidence exists that indicates acquired myopia is caused by (a) an increase in corneal refractive power, (b) an increase in lens refracting power, and (c) an increase in the axial length of the eye?

5. What is the approximate prevalence of myopia at each of the following ages in an industrialized society: (a) at birth; (b) at ages 5–6; (c) at ages 14–15; (d) at ages 20–30; (e) at ages 40–50; (f) beyond the age of 60.

6. Discuss the population differences that have been reported in the prevalence of myopia.

7. How rapidly would you expect a child's myopia to progress if it was first apparent at (a) age 7 and (b) age 12?

8. Discuss the possible etiological factors of myopia occurring in (a) newborn infants; (b) primary schoolchildren; (c) young adults; (d) older adults.

9. What evidence is there to support Van Alphen's hypothesis that during growth, the length of the eye is controlled by the stretch of the ciliary body and choroid acting as an elastic envelope, counteracting a part of the intraocular pressure, in response to macular feedback to cortical or subcortical centers?

10. As proposed by Greene, what is the role of the extraocular muscles in the development of myopia?

11. How does congenital myopia tend to differ, in cause as well as in severity, from acquired myopia?

12. Discuss the experiments in which myopia was induced in monkeys by having them hanging downward, looking at the floor, or seated in restraining chairs wearing hoods. What were the results of these experiments and what were the likely causes of the results?

13. What evidence is there that experimentally induced myopia (due to lid-suturing or other procedures) may have a different mechanism in the rhesus monkey as opposed to the stump-tail monkey?

14. What is the evidence for Wallman's theory that myopia may be due to a lack of retinal activity in (a) chicks and (b) humans?

15. Discuss and evaluate each of the following procedures used to control myopia: (a) Visual training (including biofeedback training); (b) bifocal lenses; (c) contact lenses used for the stabilization of juvenile myopia; (d) contact lenses used for the reduction of myopia; (e) atropine and other pharmacological agents; (f) surgical procedures.

CHAPTER 4

Anomalies of Binocular Vision

For efficient single binocular vision to occur, the retinal images for the two eyes must be in good focus and of similar size and shape. In addition, the eyes must be capable of aligning themselves in such a manner that the retinal images of a fixated object can easily be placed and maintained on the foveae of the two eyes. In the discussion of normal binocular vision that follows, the eyes are considered free of errors of refraction and binocular vision, and all sensory and motor pathways subserving vision are assumed intact.

SENSORY ASPECTS OF BINOCULAR VISION

Vision Direction and Corresponding Retinal Points

In *Researchers in Binocular Vision*, Ogle (1950) reviews the theory of corresponding retinal points developed by Muller, Lotze, Hering, Panum, and other 19th-century investigators. According to Lotze, each light-sensitive element in the retinal mosaic has a specific *local sign:* when a particular retinal element is stimulated, the individual experiences a specific subjective visual direction with respect to the directionalization of the fovea.

Hering (1879) spoke of the *principal visual direction* as the subjective direction associated with the fovea when a given object is fixated. A foveally fixated point is interpreted by the individual as being "straight ahead," and objects in the visual field are experienced as being located above, below, to one side, and so on, of the foveally fixated point. Each retinal element, therefore, has its own subjective visual direction, and the visual field for a steadily fixating eye may be considered a mosaic that corresponds point for point (although inverted and

reversed by the optical system of the eye) with the retinal mosaic.

The kind of subjective visual direction described here, in which the primary visual direction is associated with the fovea, is often referred to as *oculocentric* directionalization, or visual direction with respect to the *eye*. *Egocentric* directionalization, on the other hand, is visual direction with respect to the *head*. If fixation movements are made while the head remains motionless, oculocentric directionalization (for each fovea) does not change, but egocentric directionalization does change.

The Binocular Visual Field

When the eyes steadily fixate a point in the "straight ahead," or primary, visual direction, the visual fields for the two eyes overlap (as shown in Figure 4.1)

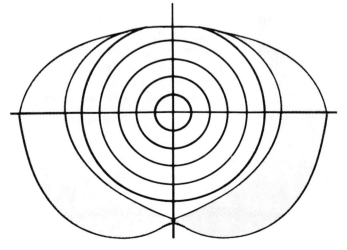

Figure 4.1 The binocular visual field. The shaded areas are the monocularly seen temporal crescents.

except for the temporal crescents (imaged on the nasal retinas). The binocular field of vision has a radius, extending from the fixation point, of approximately 60 degrees, or a diameter of approximately 120 degrees. For a given fixation point, each point within the binocular visual field is considered to be imaged on a point on each of the two retinas. These points (one on each retina), therefore, have the same visual direction and are known as *corresponding retinal points*. An additional attribute of a pair of corresponding retinal points is that they share the same "cortical image," giving rise to the phenomenon of *fusion*, or *unification*.

In summary, corresponding points may be defined as pairs of points, one in each retina, having the same visual direction and sending their nerve impulses to the same point in the visual cortex.

The Horopter

The concept of corresponding retinal points is illustrated in Figure 4.2. In this diagram the point F, the fixation point, is imaged on the two foveae, f and f'. Similarly, the peripheral point P is imaged on the peripheral retinal points p and p', and the point Q is imaged on the retinal points q and q'. For a given fixation point, all points in object space that form images on pairs of corresponding retinal points form an imaginary surface known as the *horopter*. In Figure 4.2, the curved line HH' is a trace, in the horizontal plane, of the horopter associated with the specific fixation point, F.

It should be understood that the horopter is an *imaginary* two-dimensional surface, centered on the fixation point, that moves with the eyes. In the majority of methods used to determine an observer's horopter, measurements have been made only in the horizontal plane. It has been shown by Ogle (1950) that if corresponding retinal points for the two eyes are symmetrically placed, the shape of the horopter is a circle (known as the Vieth-Muller circle), which passes through the fixation point and the centers of the entrance pupils of the two eyes (see Figure 4.3). However, when the horopter is determined experimentally, it is found to have a much flatter curvature than that of the Vieth-Muller circle. For short fixation distances, it is *concave* toward the observer; for longer distances, it is *convex* toward the observer; and for a distance of about 1m (the "abathic" distance), it is in the form of a flat plane. The fact that the experimentally determined horopter does not coincide with the Vieth-Muller circle has been interpreted to indicate that the

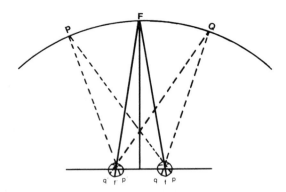

Figure 4.2 Corresponding retinal points and the horopter.

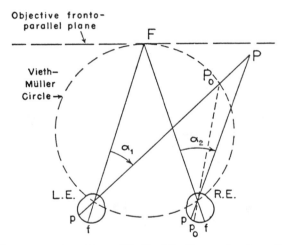

Figure 4.3 The Vieth–Muller circle: the theoretical shape of the horopter that would result if corresponding retinal points for the two eyes were symmetrically placed (Ogle, 1950, p. 16).

separation of corresponding retinal points is unequal on the nasal and temporal halves of the retina.

Ogle (1950) described a number of methods of experimentally determining the horopter. The method that is most commonly used and that provides the most consistent results, is that of determining the positions of points (in the horizontal meridian) that appear to lie in a frontoparallel plane located at the distance of the fixation point. This is known as the *apparent frontoparallel plane* method. The frontoparallel plane is considered a vertical plane, passing through the fixation point that is parallel to the vertical plane containing the line connecting the centers of the pupils of the two eyes (the base line). The apparatus used for determining the apparent frontoparallel plane horopter consists of a number of vertically oriented rods that can be

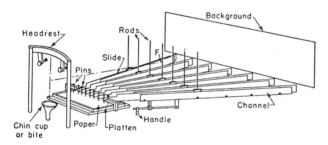

Figure 4.4 Ogle's apparatus for determining the apparent frontoparallel plane horopter (Ogle, 1950, p. 20).

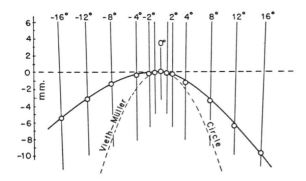

Figure 4.5 Horopter data for one observer. Vertical dimensions have been increased tenfold (Ogle, 1950, p. 25).

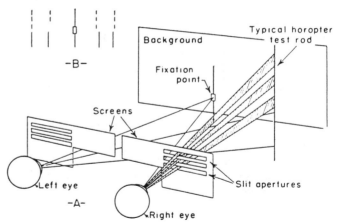

Figure 4.6 "Nonius" or vernier horopter apparatus, designed to determine the identical visual direction horopter (Ogle, 1950, p. 37).

forth, using the criterion that the upper and lower half of each rod are seen in identical directions. (For the interested reader, these and other methods are described in more detail in Chapters 3 and 4 of Ogle's [1950] text.)

Sensory Fusion

The term *sensory fusion* refers to the process by which the images formed on the retinas of the two eyes are combined into a single percept. *Unification* is often used as a synonym for sensory fusion. Ogle (1950) included anatomic, physiologic, and psychologic mechanisms as components of the fusional process without implication as to the nature of the phenomenon and spoke of "cortical images" (fiber synapses) in rather localized regions of the occipital cortex. There is disagreement over whether, once the nerve fibers from corresponding retinal points "meet" in the visual cortex, fusion of the two images takes place strictly on a physiological basis or whether a "psychic" response is involved.

Panum's Fusional Areas

In 1856, Panum demonstrated that within certain limits fusion was possible when the two retinal images of an object were not formed on corresponding retinal points. In the stereoscopic target shown in Figure 4.7, the two vertical lines presented to the left eye have a constant separation, whereas those presented to the right eye may be varied. Within limits, the subject sees only two vertical lines,

moved toward or away from the observer. As shown in Figure 4.4, the channels through which the rods move are oriented so that they all extend from the center of the interpupillary base line. Ogle has described two horopter apparatuses, each containing 13 rods, one for use at distances of 20, 40 and 75cm and another for use at a distance of 1m. The data for one of his observers are shown in Figure 4.5.

The method that is the most theoretically correct is that of determining the position of each of a number of points (in the horizontal meridian) so that the subjective visual directions of the images formed on the two retinas are identical—the *identical visual direction* method. The identical visual direction criterion is more difficult for an observer to apply than the apparent frontoparallel plane criterion. As shown in Figure 4.6, the upper nasal and lower temporal fields of view of each eye are occluded, and the upper temporal field for each eye is provided with horizontal apertures so that the upper part of each rod appears to consist of several short sections. With this apparatus, the subject makes a vernier or "nonius" alignment as each rod is moved back and

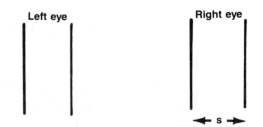

Figure 4.7 Stereoscopic target for measuring the horizontal extent of Panum's fusional areas. Eye for which separation is variable is indicated by s.

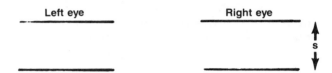

Figure 4.8 Stereoscopic target for measuring the vertical extent of Panum's fusional areas. Eye for which separation is variable is indicated by s.

but if the separation of the lines seen by the right eye is increased beyond a certain point, three lines are seen. This target can be used only to measure the horizontal extent of Panum's fusional areas: their vertical extent can be measured by means of the target shown in Figure 4.8.

Ogle (1950) reported that the horizontal dimension of Panum's fusional areas was somewhat greater than the vertical dimension. He found that the horizontal dimension varied with peripheral visual angle. Averaging his data for three subjects, the horizontal width of Panum's areas was approximately 8 minutes of arc for a visual angle of 1 degree, increasing to 12 minutes of arc for a visual angle of 4 degrees and to 25 minutes of arc for a visual angle of 12 degrees.

The existence of Panum's fusional areas means that corresponding retinal points are far from being points. Using Østerberg's figure of 147,300 foveal cones per square millimeter, an 8-minute-wide fusional area located 1 degree from the center of the fovea would encompass almost 300 cones; using a figure of about 140,000 rods per square millimeter at a distance of about 12 degrees from the center of the fovea (see Figure 1.23), a 25-minute-wide fusional area would include approximately 2,300 rods. In both cases the number of receptors would be increased by virtue of the eyes' micronystagmus movements, the fine, oscillating movements that the eyes make during fixation.

Physiological Diplopia

Because of Panum's fusional areas, the horopter is not a surface but a *solid*, as shown in Figure 4.9. Points located within the *region of single binocular vision* (indicated in the diagram) form images within Panum's areas for the two eyes and, therefore, are seen singly. However, if an object point is located in front of or behind the region of single binocular vision (while the subject fixates the point F), double vision occurs. This is known as *physiological diplopia*.

In everyday life we are aware of the presence of physiological diplopia only under the most extreme conditions. For example, if one fixates on the windshield wiper when riding in an automobile, an object seen on the road ahead—such as another car—may appear to be double, whereas fixating on a distant object may make the windshield wiper appear to be double.

Ogle (1950) made the point that there is a distance beyond which all fixated objects have their images falling entirely within Panum's fusional areas, with the result that no doubling of images occur. He calculated that for an interpupillary distance of 64mm, this distance is about 20m, or 60 feet.

Retinal Disparity and Stereopsis

When an object point fails to stimulate corresponding retinal points for the two eyes, it is said to stimulate disparate (noncorresponding) points. The resulting stimulus situation is known as *retinal disparity*. For large amounts of retinal disparity, diplopia results (the physiological diplopia described above). However, for small amounts of retinal disparity, the individual usually experiences a form

Figure 4.9 The horopter as a solid. Ordinates are magnified twofold (Ogle, 1950, p. 42).

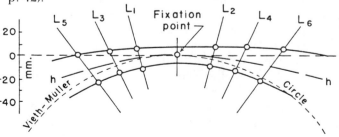

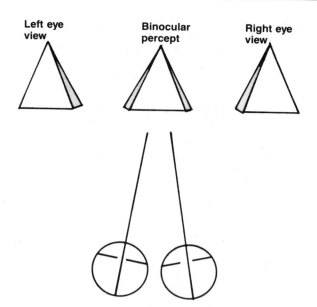

Figure 4.10 Stereoscopic perception of depth. The two eyes see the pyramid from slightly different angles, causing noncorresponding (disparate) retinal points to be stimulated, with the result that the pyramid appears to be solid.

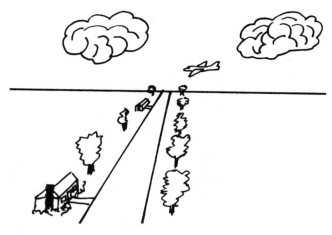

Figure 4.11 Monocular clues for the perception of distance.

of binocular vision in which points closer or farther away from the fixation point (in front of or behind the horopter solid) are perceived as being in three dimensions, or in depth. This is the well-known stereoscopic depth, or *stereopsis* ("solid vision").

Stereoscopic perception of depth exists because the two eyes are separated in space (see Figure 4.10). It varies with the interpupillary distance and can be enhanced by increasing the interpupillary distance artificially, as may be done with prism binoculars or with a stereoscopic range finder. Ogle (1950) has defined stereopsis as "a specific experiential response—a sensation—directly arising from physiologic stimuli in the same sense that the color red is an experience arising from the excitation of the retina by light of a particular wavelength" (p. 135). He further described stereoscopic vision as having a physiologic basis founded on the anatomic organization of the visual apparatus; he characterized stereopsis as being *innate*, whereas the monocular clues to the perception of depth are empirical clues that must be *learned*.

Accommodation and convergence

Although less powerful than stereopsis due to retinal disparity, *accommodation* and *convergence*

also serve as clues for the perception of depth or distance. Like stereopsis, accommodation and convergence are considered to be innately determined, requiring little or no learning.

Monocular clues for the perception of distance

The *monocular clues* for the perception of depth or distance are illustrated in Figure 4.11. They include *size* (a large object is interpreted as being closer than a small object), *overlay* (an object that blocks another object is interpreted as being the closer of the two), *geometrical perspective* (typified by a road or railroad tracks converging toward the horizon), *aerial perspective* (objects high above the horizon are interpreted as being closer than objects near the horizon), and *light and shadow*. The monocular clues require learning, and as such are sometimes referred to as *empirical clues*. They are also known as the "picture-painting" clues, because they are used by artists in conveying the illusion of distance.

MOTOR ASPECTS OF BINOCULAR VISION

Movements of the eyes can be described in terms of *conjugate* or *version movements*, in which both eyes move in the same direction (to the right, to the left, upward, or downward), or in terms of *disjunctive* or *vergence movements*, in which the eyes move toward one another (convergence) or away from one another (divergence).

Conjugate Movements

Except for vertical movements, conjugate movements involve the action of different muscles for the two eyes. For example, in a movement to the right (dextroversion), the muscles responsible are the right lateral rectus and the left medial rectus; a movement to the left (levoversion) requires the opposite combination. The muscles involved in making the movement are called *yoke muscles*, and their innervation has been described by Hering's law, which states that in all voluntary conjugate movements of the eyes, equal and simultaneous innervation flows from the oculogyric centers to the muscles concerned in establishing the direction of gaze. Conjugate movements may be either *saccadic* movements or *following* (pursuit) movements.

A *saccadic movement* is a fast, abrupt movement initiated by a sudden increase in innervation to the muscles concerned. This increase in innervation is followed by a steady firing of the agonist muscles and an accompanying reduction in firing of the antagonist muscles (Sherrington's law of reciprocal innervation). For a saccadic movement to the right, the antagonists are the left lateral rectus and the right medial rectus (see Figure 4.12).

According to Burde (1975), saccadic movements are thought to be mediated by the eyefields in the frontal lobe (area 8) and can occur with a speed as high as 400 degrees per second. Saccadic movements can occur (1) as voluntary refixation movements, (2) as involuntary or random movements, or in response to visual or auditory stimuli, (3) as the fast phase in nystagmus, (4) as the rapid eye movements occurring in sleep, (5) as microsaccades, and (6) in pursuit movements faster than 45 degrees per second.

A *following* (pursuit) *movement* is a slower conjugate movement made to keep the image of a moving object on or near the fovea or to keep the image of a stationary object on or near the fovea as the head moves. According to Burde (1975), following movements are mediated by the visual association area located in the parieto-occipital junction (area 19) and occur accurately only to velocities of 30 degrees per second. As already indicated, saccadic movements are used in following objects faster than 45 degrees per second.

Vergence Movements

Convergence is a much more highly developed function than divergence, its total amplitude being approximately ten times that of divergence. In converging toward the nose, as in the familiar "push-up" test for convergence, the eyes may converge as much as 60 degrees (100Δ); however, the total amount of divergence that can be stimulated by the use of base-in prisms is only about 6 degrees (10Δ).

Vergence movements are made in a rather constant and random basis during daily life (as conjugate movements are, also), as objects at different distances attract one's attention. Eye movements often contain both a conjugate and a vergence component, as in using asymmetric convergence when changing fixation from a distant object straight ahead to a near object located to one side. The stimuli for vergence movements include (1) changes in accommodation (*accommodative convergence*), (2) retinal disparity (*disparity convergence*, or *fusional convergence*), and (3) awareness of nearness of an object (*proximal convergence*).

Burde (1975) describes *convergence movements* as involving a gradual increase in the activity of the medial rectus muscles, reaching a maximum and gradually declining, with the lateral rectus muscles showing reciprocity throughout the movement (see Figure 4.13). He describes two types of electromyographic activity for *divergence:* the first type involves a saccadic burst of firing in both the lateral and medial rectus muscles followed by reciprocal excitation and inhibition of agonists and antagonists, respectively; the second involves an immediate

Figure 4.12 A conjugate movement to the right. Agonists (+) are the right lateral rectus and the left medial rectus muscles; antagonists (−) are the right medial rectus and the left lateral rectus muscles.

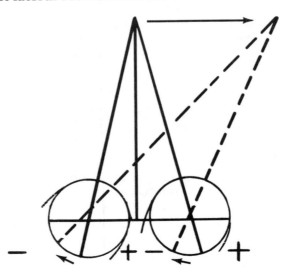

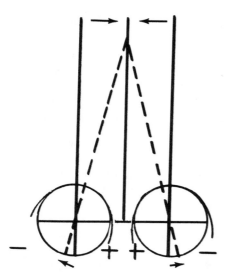

Figure 4.13 A convergence movement. Agonists (+) are the two medial rectus muscles; antagonists (−) are the two lateral rectus muscles.

saccadic burst of activity to the lateral rectus muscles with a concomitant inhibition of the medial rectus muscles and followed by irregular activity of both muscles.

Vergence movements occur with a velocity of approximately 20 degrees per second.

Motor Fusion

Sensory fusion has already been defined as the process by means of which the images formed on the retinas of the two eyes are combined into a single percept. The term *motor fusion*, on the other hand, refers to the vergence movements made by the eyes in response to retinal disparity and having the result of obtaining or maintaining images on corresponding retinal points so sensory fusion may take place.

Ogle (1950) described motor fusion in terms of what he called the *fusion compulsion:* if a prism, base-out, is suddenly placed in front of one eye while a distant object is fixated, two objects are seen momentarily, but (if not too far apart) they suddenly move toward one another and coalesce, as if attracted to one another by a magnetlike force. An observer would note that the eye made a sudden inward (vergence) movement. This movement, as described by Ogle, takes place for the purpose of preventing double vision.

ACCOMMODATION

Accommodation is the process by means of which the optical system of the eye varies its focal length in response to visual stimuli. This process is mediated by the ciliary muscle and involves an increase in the vergence of light brought about by the crystalline lens. (The mechanism of accommodation is described in Chapter 1.) Accommodation may be specified either in terms of the *accommodative stimulus* or the *accommodative response.* In clinical work we must deal with the stimulus to accommodation because we have no method of knowing, at any given moment, the accommodative response.

The Accommodative Stimulus

Accommodation may be stimulated in either of two ways: (1) by placing the test object at a distance closer than infinity (in practice, closer than 6m) or (2) by the use of minus lenses. Either of these procedures has the effect of increasing the vergence of the rays of light in the eye. Whichever method is used, the stimulus to accommodation (like the refractive state of the eye) is specified in terms of the *diopter.*

Assuming that a given eye has no refractive error or that the refractive error is compensated by lenses, an object located at an infinite distance would form a sharp image on the retina without the need for accommodation. However, if an object is placed at a distance of 40cm from the eye's spectacle plane (note that object distances, for specification of accommodation, are measured from the spectacle plane located 13mm in front of the corneal apex), rays of light from the object would diverge and, if no accommodation took place, would focus at an imaginary point behind the eye. However, with sufficient accommodation, the rays will focus on the retina. The amount of accommodation required is 1/0.40D, or 2.50D. Note again that the 2.50D is the stimulus to accommodation.

For the same eye, instead of moving the test object to a distance of 40cm from the spectacle plane, another way to stimulate 2.50D of accommodation would be to allow the test object to remain at infinity and to place a −2.50D lens in the spectacle plane of the eye. The stimulus to accommodation indicated in Figure 4.14 is the same: 2.50D. The two methods may be used in combination. For example, a test object may be placed at a distance of 1m, stimulating 1.00D of accommodation, and a −2.00D lens may be placed in front of the eye, stimulating an additional

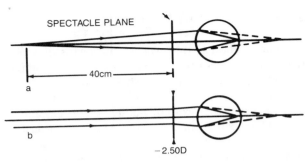

Figure 4.14   Stimulating accommodation by (a) placing the test object at a distance closer than 6m, or (b) placing the test object at 6m and placing a minus lens in front of the eye. In both cases, the vergence of the light rays between the spectacle plane and the eye is the same (dashed lines show the vergence of the light rays in the eye with accommodation relaxed; solid lines show the vergence with accommodation in play).

2.00D for a total of 3.00D stimulus to accommodation.

The Accommodative Response

The *haploscope*, an instrument used in research but not ordinarily used clinically, provides us with a method of measuring the accommodative response. With this instrument, a tiny point of light is used as a stimulus for one eye, and the 20/20 line of a Snellen acuity chart at a distance of 20 feet is used as a stimulus for the other eye. Using the "fogging method" (the equivalent of placing convex lenses in front of the eyes), the vergence of light on the retina is so great that artificial myopia is created, and the use of excessive accommodation will only blur the target further. As the amount of "fog" is gradually decreased, the point of light (which originally was a blurred blob) will gradually clear up and appear as a sharp point. At that moment, the operator can determine the amount of accommodation in play.

Lag of Accommodation

In a given clinical situation, for a stimulus to accommodation of 2.50D, the accommodative response may be only 1.50D. The difference (1.00D in this case) is known as the *lazy lag of accommodation*. Typically, people do not accommodate more than is necessary to form an acceptably distinct image on the retina.

The fact that a patient accommodates only 1.50D for a line of letters at a distance of 40cm means that he or she is accommodating for a point at a distance of 67cm rather than 40cm. The line of letters is acceptably distinct, even though accommodation is postured for a plane 27cm farther away than the card on which the letters are printed and it is 1.00D out of focus.

The lag of accommodation depends on the depth of focus of the eye (if we think of the retina) or on the depth of field (if we think of object space). (These concepts are described in Chapter 1 and demonstrated in Figure 1.14.) For a given eye, the depth of focus varies with pupil size and the size of the object of regard. The smaller the pupil, the greater the depth of focus; the larger the object for a given size of pupil, the greater the depth of focus. One way to minimize the effects of depth of focus is to avoid using illumination so high as to unduly constrict the patient's pupil (a 40-watt bulb at a distance of about 2 feet from the reading card is adequate). In addition, the letters should be as small as possible consistent with the patient's visual acuity, and the practitioner should admonish the patient to keep the letters in sharp focus.

It is possible, by means of *dynamic retinoscopy* (described in Chapter 8), to determine a patient's lag of accommodation. However, the lag of accommodation found in dynamic retinoscopy applies only to that particular testing situation. There is no clinical method for monitoring the lag of accommodation while performing tests of binocular visual function.

CONVERGENCE

Convergence of the eyes is measured in terms of the *prism diopter*. The prism diopter is a tangent measurement rather than an arc measurement (degrees and radians are arc measurements), 1Δ being equal to a tangent displacement of 1cm at a distance of 1m. Referring to the top portion of Figure 4.15, if a patient having an interpupillary distance of 6cm converges to the midline to fixate a point at a distance of 1m, each eye will turn inward 3Δ (displacement of 3cm at a distance of 1m) for a total of 6Δ of convergence for both eyes.

For distances other than 1m, the number of prism diopters of convergence is determined by multiplying the displacement by the reciprocal of the testing distance in meters. Thus, when the eyes converge to the midline at a distance of 50cm, and the interpupillary distance is 6cm, the convergence

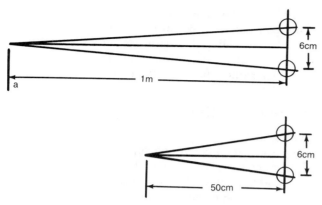

Figure 4.15 Patient having an interpupillary distance of 6cm converging to the midline (*above*) at a distance of 1m, and (*below*) at a distance of 50cm.

required for each eye is 3(2) = 6Δ or a total of 12Δ for both eyes (see the bottom portion of Figure 4.15). If, on the other hand, the eyes converge to the midline at a distance of 6m, for an interpupillary distance of 6cm each eye would converge 3(1/6) = 0.50Δ, or a total of 1Δ for both eyes.

Specification of Convergence

Convergence is specified in relation to the *center of rotation* of the eye rather than in relation to the spectacle plane. Although it has been shown that the center of rotation of the eye is not a single point and varies considerably from one eye to another, the center of rotation is usually considered to be located

Figure 4.16 Specification of stimulus to accommodation (2.50D) and stimulus to convergence (15Δ) for a 40cm distance, for a patient having an interpupillary distance of 64 mm.

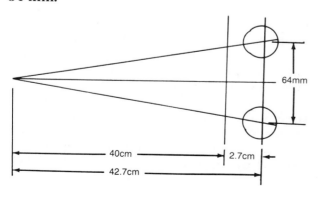

14mm behind the corneal apex, or 27mm behind the spectacle plane.

Clinical testing distances are specified in terms of distance from the *spectacle plane:* scales on "reading rods" attached to refractors are calibrated in terms of distance from the spectacle plane, so when a near-point card is placed at a 40cm distance, the stimulus to accommodation is 2.50D, but the stimulus to convergence must be determined on the basis of a distance of 40cm + 2.7cm (see Figure 4.16), or 42.7cm.

For the calculation of accommodation and convergence stimuli for a testing distance of 40cm, the patient's interpupillary distance is often assumed to be 64mm. When this is assumed, the required convergence (again referring to Figure 4.16) for each eye is equal to 3.2 (1/0.427) = 7.49Δ. Rounding to 7.5Δ, the convergence required for both eyes is 15Δ.

Fixation Disparity

Although an individual may have acceptably clear vision in spite of a lag of accommodation of 1.00D or more, the patient may underconverge or overconverge only a small amount without diplopia occurring. This underconvergence or overconvergence with respect to the plane of regard, called *fixation disparity*, is measured in minutes of arc and depends on the size of Panum's fusional areas. Ogle (1950) described fixation disparity as resulting in a slippage of the cortical images with respect to one another. He pointed out that the cortical images remain preceptually fused as long as this cortical disparity is less than the relevant dimension of Panum's fusional areas.

Carter (1957, 1980) described fixation disparity as a minute strabismus, existing in the presence of normal retinal correspondence and normal single binocular vision. As shown in Figure 4.17, fixation

Figure 4.17 Fixation disparity: (*a*) exo fixation disparity (underconvergence), and (*b*) eso fixation disparity (overconvergence).

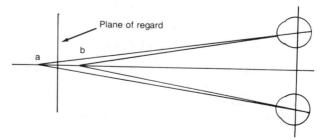

disparity in which the eyes underconverge in relation to the plane of regard is called *exo fixation disparity*, whereas fixation disparity in which the eyes overconverge is called *eso fixation disparity*.

CLASSIFICATION OF VERGENCE MOVEMENTS

In 1893, Maddox provided the first description and classification of vergence movements of the eyes. In discussing Maddox's concepts, Morgan (1980) commented that they were based on clinical experience rather than on controlled experimentation, and were influenced by the work of Donders, Hering, Prentice, and other researchers during that period. Maddox described four components of convergence: tonic convergence, reflex (or fusional) convergence, accommodative convergence, and voluntary convergence.

Tonic Convergence

Maddox stated that if all innervations to the ocular muscles were to cease, the anatomical position of rest of the eyes would be one of considerable divergence, and he described *tonic convergence* as being responsible for moving the eyes from the position of anatomical rest to a more convergent position. This latter position is described as the physiological position of rest, or the *phoria position*, and it is the position taken by the eyes when no stimuli to fusion are present. Morgan (1980) pointed out that Maddox identified two nonvisual causes of tonic convergence: the tonus exhibited by the ocular muscles and the persisting activity of converging information. Morgan described the "converging information as what we would now call the central control mechanism of convergence, having a tonic activity of its own and being affected by conditions such as sleep, drowsiness, alcohol, and anesthetic agents" (p. 538). Deficient tonic convergence would result in exophoria, whereas excessive tonic convergence would result in esophoria.

Fusional (Reflex) Convergence

Maddox described *fusional convergence*, or *reflex convergence*, as compensating for any excess or deficit in tonic convergence, identifying retinal disparity as its stimulus, and also indicating a constant utilization element or conditioned response from constant use. Because fusional "convergence" would have to be "divergent" for an individual with esophoria, Morgan (1980) prefers the term *fusional vergence* rather than fusional convergence.

Accommodative Convergence

Stating that distance vision required the use of only tonic and reflex convergence, Maddox described a form of convergence, *accommodative convergence*, as an additional kind of convergence used in near vision. As indicated by Morgan, accommodative convergence is a function not necessarily of the *amount* of accommodation but of the *effort* of accommodation: it is increased when accommodation is made more difficult by the use of atropine and decreased when accommodation is made easier by the use of eserine.

Voluntary Convergence

Maddox described *voluntary convergence* as convergence due to the knowledge that an object is nearby. This component of vergence is usually referred to as *proximal convergence* and has also been described as psychic convergence and as convergence due to the awareness of nearness.

CLINICAL MEASUREMENT OF THE FOUR CONVERGENCE COMPONENTS

Of the four components of convergence described by Maddox, fusional vergence and accommodative convergence most easily lend themselves to clinical measurement. Fusional vergence may be stimulated by the use of prisms, which induce retinal disparity by deviating the rays of light either temporalward (base-out) or nasalward (base-in). Accommodative convergence may be brought into play by stimulating accommodation, either by the use of a near-testing distance or by the use of minus lenses.

Tonic convergence cannot be measured directly but can only be inferred on the basis of the physiological position of rest, or phoria position, of the eyes during distance fixation. Proximal convergence also is incapable of direct measurement. Its existence can be inferred only indirectly on the basis of other findings. (Further discussion of the components of convergence can be found in Chapters 10 and 12.)

The AC/A Ratio

It has been shown by Fry (1937), Hofstetter (1945), and other investigators that each diopter of accommodation is accompanied by a specific amount of convergence. This convergence, brought into play with accommodation, is the accommodative convergence described in the previous section; the relationship between accommodative convergence and accommodation is known as the *AC/A ratio*.

If an individual is emmetropic or if any refractive error is compensated with lenses, the stimulus to accommodation for a distant object is zero. If, when a person fixates a distant object, the visual axes are parallel when all stimuli to fusion are eliminated (the condition of orthophoria), the stimulus to convergence is also zero. On the other hand, when an object at a distance of 40cm is fixated, the stimulus to accommodation for this individual will be 2.50D, and the stimulus to convergence, assuming an interpupillary distance of 64mm, will be 15Δ. The "normal" AC/A ratio, therefore, is equal to

$$\frac{\text{Accommodative convergence}}{\text{Accommodation}} = \frac{15}{2.5} = \frac{6}{1}.$$

Note that (for the individual who is emmetropic and orthophoric at distance) the AC/A ratio will have a "normal" value only if 2.50D of accommodation is accompanied by 15Δ of accommodative convergence. If 2.50D of accommodation is accompanied by only 10Δ of accommodative convergence,

$$\frac{\text{AC}}{\text{A}} = \frac{10}{2.5} = \frac{4}{1}$$

and if 2.5D of accommodation is accompanied by 20Δ of accommodative convergence,

$$\frac{\text{AC}}{\text{A}} = \frac{20}{2.5} = \frac{8}{1}.$$

Stimulus AC/A versus response AC/A

As already noted, in routine clinical work we have no way of knowing the patient's state of accommodation (i.e., the accommodative response). We have information concerning only the *stimulus* to accommodation as provided by the test object distance, the use of minus lenses, or both. The *stimulus AC/A ratio* (or *clinical AC/A ratio*), therefore, is defined as the ratio between accommodative convergence and the stimulus to accommodation. The *response AC/A ratio* can be determined only when it is possible to measure the accommodative response by means of a haploscope, and it is defined as the ratio between accommodative convergence and the accommodative response. (The AC/A ratio is discussed further in the following section on binocular vision anomalies.)

BINOCULAR VISION ANOMALIES

Binocular vision anomalies can be considered in terms of two broad categories: (1) anomalies in which binocular vision is maintained, but often at the cost of a considerable amount of stress; and (2) anomalies in which binocular vision is absent.

Anomalies of binocular vision in which fusion is maintained include heterophorias (usually simply called *phorias*), anomalies of fusional vergence, fixation disparity, and anomalies of accommodation. Many of these anomalies occur in association with a deficiency or an excess of accommodative convergence, and when this occurs an easily recognizable *binocular vision syndrome* may be present. When binocular vision is absent, the condition is known variously as strabismus, heterotropia, or squint. Strabismus may be accompanied by one or more of a variety of adaptive phenomena, including suppression, amblyopia, eccentric fixation, and anomalous retinal correspondence.

Heterophoria

In *Treatise on the Motor Apparatus of the Eyes*, George T. Stevens (1906) coined the word *heterophoria*, defining it as a "latent deviation of the eyes," in contrast to *heterotropia*, which is a manifest deviation of the eyes.

The phoria position

The *phoria position*, or the *physiological position of rest*, is the position that the visual axes take with respect to one another in the absence of all stimuli to fusion. For the majority of people, for distance fixation the visual axes are parallel or slightly divergent in the phoria position but, due to the presence of tonic convergence stimuli, they are less divergent than in the *anatomical position of rest*.

Unless an individual has strabismus, when a distant object is viewed the visual axes will be parallel, being "aimed" at the object of regard within the limits of fixation disparity (which, as we have seen, is limited to only a few minutes of arc.) This accurate aiming of the visual axes occurs as a result of information provided by retinal disparity. However, if retinal disparity information is temporarily removed—a process known as *dissociation* of the eyes—the eyes will assume the phoria position.

Dissociation

One of the simplest methods of dissociating the eyes is to place a cover, or occluder, in front of one eye. If this is done while a person is fixating a distant object, the covered eye will deviate outward (*exophoria*), inward (*esophoria*), upward or downward (*hyperphoria*), or will remain in its original position (*orthophoria*). If an observer looks behind the cover, no movement of the eye will be seen unless the phoria is about 3 or 4Δ or more (phoria measurements, like all measurements involving the vergence of the eyes, are made in terms of prism diopters). If the occluder is quickly removed, the eye will return to its original position. Again, an observer will be able to see the movement only if the movement is 3 or 4Δ or more.

The positions taken by the visual axes of the two eyes when one eye is occluded are shown in Figure 4.18a (for exophoria) and in Figure 4.18b (for esophoria).

The alternating cover test

Although it is possible to observe the covered eye to determine whether it turns outward or inward under cover, a much more effective method of determining the presence of a phoria is for the practitioner to repeatedly move the occluder from one eye to the other and to observe the eye that has just been uncovered. If the eye that has just been uncovered turns inward it must have been deviating outward when under cover, and therefore exophoria exists. Similarly, if the eye that has just been uncov-

ered turns outward it must have been deviating inward when under cover, and therefore esophoria exists.

Although the *alternating cover test* is described here as a test for the detection of a phoria, in reality an inward movement of the just-uncovered eye indicates the presence of either exophoria or exotropia, and an outward movement of the just-uncovered eye indicates the presence of either esophoria or esotropia. In clinical practice, the *unilateral cover test* (described in a later section on strabismus) is used to detect the presence of a tropia. (The clinical application of the alternating and unilateral cover tests is described in Chapter 6.)

Other methods of dissociating the eyes

Other methods of dissociating the eyes include the use of a vertical prism, a Maddox rod, and red and green filters.

Vertical prism. The use of a moderate amount of vertical prism, either base-up or base-down (see Figure 4.19), is a convenient method of dissociating the eyes. Once the eyes are dissociated, horizontal prisms can be used to measure the lateral phoria. Horizontal prism, either base-in or base-out, can also be used to dissociate the eyes. Once the eyes have been dissociated (usually with base-in prism), vertical prisms can be used to measure the vertical phoria. (Phoria measurement by means of prisms is described in Chapter 10.)

Maddox rod. A Maddox rod is a series of parallel glass or plastic rods that spread out the light from a small spot source into a streak perpendicular to the orientation of the Maddox rod. As shown in Figure 4.20, when a horizontally oriented Maddox rod is placed in front of one eye, the patient will see the spot source of light with the uncovered eye and a vertical streak with the eye that sees through the Maddox rod. Horizontal prism power may then be added in front of the uncovered eye until the spot and the vertical streak coincide. To measure a vertical phoria, the Maddox rod, oriented vertically, is placed in front of one eye, the patient sees a horizontal streak; vertical prism is then added in front of the other eye until the spot and the streak coincide. A problem with the use of a Maddox rod to measure lateral phorias is that the patient may localize the streak of light as if it were at a closer distance than the distance of the light source, with the result that Maddox rod phorias tend to be in error in the direction of increased esophoria.

Figure 4.18   Positions taken by the visual axes when one eye is occluded: (*a*) exophoria, (*b*) esophoria.

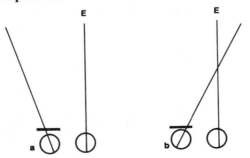

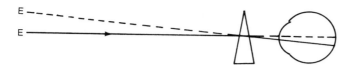

Figure 4.19 Dissociation of the eyes by means of a vertical prism. A base-down prism causes light rays to be deviated downward (toward the base), with the result that the test object is seen as being displaced upward (toward the apex).

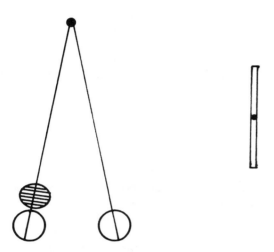

Figure 4.20 Dissociation of the eyes by the use of a Maddox rod. The patient fixates a spot of light, and the eye with the horizontally oriented Maddox rod sees the spot as a vertical streak. If there is no lateral phoria, the streak is seen to go "through" the spot.

Red and green filters. Sometimes called *anaglyphs*, red and green lenses are sometimes used in combination with red and green test objects. Normally the red lens is used in front of the right eye, and the stimuli are red and green flashlights of projectors. The right eye will see only the red spot of light and the left eye only the green spot. Anaglyphs are not often used for the measurement of phorias, but they are used mainly in the diagnosis of strabismus.

Crossed and uncrossed diplopia

When a patient has a lateral phoria, the diplopia experienced when the eyes are dissociated may be either a crossed diplopia or an uncrossed diplopia. An understanding of the concept of crossed versus uncrossed diplopia requires familiarity with the

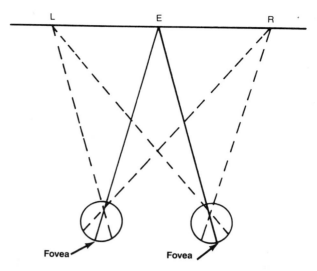

Figure 4.21 For the steadily fixating eye, objects seen in the left half of the visual field are imaged on the right half of each retina; objects seen in the right half of the visual field are imaged on the left half of each retina.

relationship between the retinal image and the visual field.

Figure 4.21 shows the two eyes steadily fixating the letter *E*, which is imaged on the foveas of the two eyes. The visual field in the plane of the lines of sight and the fixation point is represented by the line connecting the letters *L* and *R*. Due to the crossing of all light rays at the nodal point of each eye, the images of *L* for the two eyes are located in the right half of each retina, and the images of *R* are located in the left half of each retina. The retinal image, therefore, is just the reverse of the visual field: all objects seen to the right of the fixation point are imaged on the left half of the retina, and all objects seen to the left of the fixation point are imaged on the right half of the retina.

Crossed and uncrossed diplopia are illustrated in Figures 4.22 and 4.23. In both cases, a base-down dissociating prism has been placed in front of the right eye, and the patient has been instructed to fixate the lower letter *E*—the one seen by the left eye. For the exophoric patient shown in Figure 4.22, the letter *E* is imaged to the right of the fovea of the right eye and thus is seen as being in the left visual field (i.e., to the left of the *E* that is seen by the fixating eye), resulting in crossed diplopia.

For the esophoric patient shown in Figure 4.23, the letter *E* is imaged to the left of the fovea of the

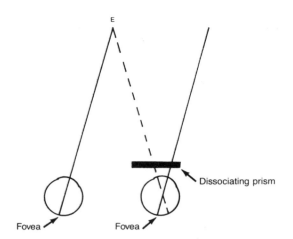

Figure 4.22   Crossed diplopia, in exophoria. The letter *E* is imaged on the right half of the right retina and is therefore seen as being in the left visual field.

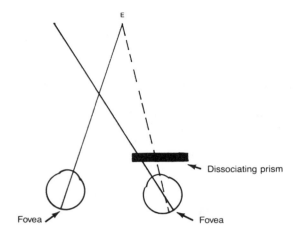

Figure 4.23   Uncrossed diplopia, in esophoria. The letter *E* is imaged on the left half of the right retina and is therefore seen as being in the right visual field.

right eye and, therefore, is seen as being in the right visual field (to the right of the *E* seen by the fixating eye), resulting in uncrossed diplopia.

Fusional Vergence Anomalies

Referring to Stevens' (1906) original definition, a phoria is a latent deviation of the eyes, whereas a tropia is a manifest deviation. What is it that prevents a latent deviation from becoming manifest? The answer is the ability to make fusional movements on the basis of disparity information. The importance of the ability to make fusional movements may be demonstrated by using as an example the development of functional (as opposed to paralytic) strabismus.

In children, an important risk factor in the development of functional strabismus is the presence of uncorrected hyperopia. For example, if a child has 4.00D of uncorrected hyperopia and has a normal, 6/1, AC/A ratio, the use of 4.00D of accommodation (to focus the eyes for distance vision) brings into play 6(4.00), or 24Δ of accommodative convergence, in that each diopter of accommodation brings into play 6Δ of accommodative convergence. Assuming that the visual axes would be parallel, for distance vision with accommodation completely relaxed, the expected distance phoria finding with accommodation in play would be 24Δ of esophoria. In the presence of 24Δ of esophoria, the eyes will remain straight only by the continuous use of 24Δ of negative fusional vergence.

Although the compulsion to fusion, as described by Ogle (1950), is very strong—recall that Ogle compared it to a magnetic force—a constant and continuous need for the use of 24Δ of negative fusional vergence may eventually result in the latent deviation becoming manifest. This example illustrates the statement made earlier: that the difference between a phoria and a tropia is fusional vergence.

Measurement of positive fusional vergence

Fusional vergence movements may be measured by the use of ophthalmic prisms. As already demonstrated (see Figure 4.19), a large amount of prism placed in front of one eye, while the eyes fixate a distant object, will bring about dissociation of the eyes. This occurs because the retinal disparity brought about by the prism is so great that it is impossible for the eyes to make a fusional movement. However, if a small amount of prism is placed in front of one eye, disparity will be sufficiently small that fusional movements will be possible.

In practice, a small amount of prism is placed in front of *each eye* as shown in Figures 4.24 and 4.25. As shown in Figure 4.24, when a small amount of base-out prism is placed in front of each eye while a distant object is fixated, the images on the two retinas will be displaced in a temporal direction. This temporalward displacement requires a convergence movement to keep the images on the foveae and thus maintain single binocular vision. If the amount of

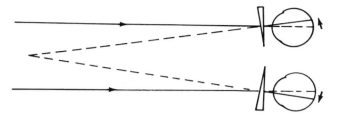

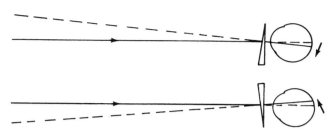

Figure 4.24 Positive fusional vergence movement brought about by a small amount of base-out prism.

Figure 4.25 Negative fusional vergence movement brought about by a small amount of base-in prism.

base-out prism before each eye is gradually increased, the amount of convergence in play will increase and will continue to do so until the disparity is so great that no additional disparity convergence is possible. When that point is reached, either of two things will occur: (1) all convergence effort will cease, and the eyes will diverge back to the phoria position with the consequent appearance of diplopia; or (2) additional convergence may be called into play by the use of accommodative convergence, with the result that, as additional base-out prism is added, single vision will be maintained but vision will be blurred because the accommodative mechanism has been thrown out of focus. The point will eventually be reached at which no additional accommodative convergence is available, so the eyes will diverge back to their phoria position and diplopia will occur.

The next step in the procedure, once a break has been reported, is to gradually reduce the amount of base-out prism before the two eyes until single vision is once again reported. This part of the procedure is called the *recovery finding.* The whole procedure is spoken of as the *base-out to blur, break, and recovery.* This test is done at both the 6m distance, as just described, and the standard 40cm near testing distance. The appropriate stimulus for the procedure is a vertical line of 20/20 letters (for both the 6m and 40cm distances). (More specific details on the performance of this test are given in Chapter 9.)

Measurement of negative fusional vergence

If a small amount of base-in prism is placed in front of each eye while a distant object is fixated, the images on the two retinas will be displaced in the nasal direction, as shown in Figure 4.25. This displacement requires a divergence movement to keep the images in the two foveae and maintain single binocular vision. If the amount of base-in

prism in front of each eye is gradually increased, the amount of divergence (negative fusional vergence) in play will increase until a further increase is impossible. When this point is reached, the eyes will converge back to their phoria position, and diplopia will occur.

Recall that in the base-out vergence test, fusional vergence could be supplemented by accommodative convergence, with the result that single vision could be maintained at the expense of clarity. However, in the base-in vergence test at distance, it is expected that accommodation is completely relaxed throughout the test (because any existing ametropia is corrected by appropriate lenses). Therefore, no accommodation can be relaxed, and no accommodative divergence can be employed. However, if a patient should report a blur during the base-in vergence test at distance, it would indicate that accommodation was not completely relaxed by the lenses being worn and the correction may require more plus lens power or less minus power.

Once the break is reported, the amount of base-in prism is gradually reduced until single vision is again reported. This sequence of tests is known as the *base-in to break and recovery.* The test is also done at the 40cm testing distance, but at this distance a blur is expected. At 40cm the stimulus to accommodation is 2.50D, so once the limit of negative fusional vergence has been reached, additional divergence is possible by relaxing accommodation and accommodative convergence. When a break occurs following a blur, it indicates the limit of relaxation of accommodation.

Measurement of vertical fusional vergences

Vertical fusional vergences (often incorrectly called vertical ductions) are measured by slowly increasing the amount of vertical prism in front of

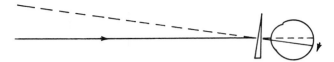

Figure 4.26 Vertical fusional vergence movement brought about by a small amount of vertical prism.

one eye until a break is reported. As shown in Figure 4.26, placing a small amount of base-down prism in front of one eye causes the eye to turn upward to maintain single binocular vision. Thus, base-down prism is used to measure *supravergence* for each eye, and base-up prism is used to measure *infravergence*. In measuring vertical vergences, no blur is expected, as vertical prism has no effect in stimulating accommodation; therefore, only the break and recovery are recorded.

Fusional vergence demand and reserve

For any given testing distance, fusional vergence may be considered in terms of either *demand* or *reserve*. The positive and negative fusional vergence tests discussed above, measured with base-out and base-in prisms, respectively, are tests of fusional vergence reserve. The demand on fusional vergence, on the other hand, is a function of the heterophoria. Exophoria requires the use of positive fusional vergence demand, whereas esophoria requires the use of negative fusional vergence.

For example, if a patient has 6Δ of exophoria at a given testing distance, single binocular vision is maintained only by the constant use of 6Δ of positive fusional vergence. The phoria, therefore, places a demand of 6Δ on positive fusional vergence. Similarly, a patient having 4Δ of esophoria at a given testing distance must make use of 4Δ of negative fusional vergence to maintain single binocular vision; the 4Δ is the demand on negative fusional vergence as a result of the esophoria.

In making a clinical diagnosis, fusional vergence reserve (the base-out or base-in vergence finding) must be evaluated in terms of the fusional vergence demand (due to the phoria)—the greater the fusional vergence demand, the greater must be the reserve. Sheard (1930, reprinted 1957) suggested that, for the patient to enjoy comfortable binocular vision, the fusional vergence reserve should be equal to twice the fusional vergence demand. (Sheard's criterion and other criteria used in prescribing for patients with binocular vision problems are discussed in Chapter 12.)

Fixation Disparity

Fixation disparity, as described earlier, is a small amount of convergence or divergence that may be present, relative to the plane of regard, when an object is fixated. As described by Ogle (1950), fixation disparity occurs because disparate images on the two retinas can be fused if the images fall within Panum's fusional areas, and can be considered as a slippage of the cortical images from the two retinas with respect to one another. Ogle stated that the angular value of fixation disparity is a measure of the degree to which the images have slipped—in the same sense that Panum's area pertains to a cortical area within which disparate images are fused.

Ogle measured fixation disparity by means of the test stimulus shown in Figure 4.27. All parts of the stimulus were viewed binocularly with the exception of the vernier target in the center. The letters surrounding the vernier target served as a *fusion lock* for the maintenance of single binocular vision. The vernier lines were polarized so the upper (fixed) line was seen only by one eye and the lower (movable) line seen only by the other eye. As the subject looked at the upper vernier line, the operator flashed on the lower vernier line for a fraction of a second, after which the subject reported whether the lower line was to the right or the left of the upper line. By this means, the movable line was adjusted until it appeared to be directly under the upper line. The angle of separation of the two vernier lines, when they appeared to the subject to be lined up, indicated the subject's fixation disparity.

Ogle (1950) also measured the heterophoria of

Figure 4.27   Ogle's apparatus for measuring fixation disparity at a distance of 30cm (K. N. Ogle, *Researches in Binocular Vision*, Saunders, 1950).

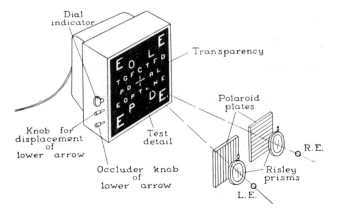

each subject and found that, for the majority, the fixation disparity and the phoria were in the same direction; that is, a subject having eso fixation disparity would be found to have esophoria, whereas a subject having exo fixation disparity would be found to have exophoria. Ogle described fixation disparity as a measure of the muscular imbalance between the two eyes while fusion is maintained (as compared to a phoria, which may be described as a measure of the muscular imbalance in the absence of fusion). Values of fixation disparity found by Ogle ranged from more than 15 minutes of eso disparity (for a highly esophoric subject) to about 20 minutes of exo disparity (for a highly exophoric subject), but in the great majority of cases there were no more than about 5 minutes of eso or exo disparity.

Variation of fixation disparity with forced vergence

Using the procedure just described, Ogle (1950) measured fixation disparity for a group of subjects at distances of 2.5m and 30cm under conditions of forced convergence and divergence. Prism power was presented in fixed amounts, alternating between base-in (to force divergence) and base-out (to force convergence); fixation disparity measurements were made for amounts of prism varying by 2Δ (base-in at distance) or 4Δ (base-out at distance, and base-in and base-out at near). A graph was plotted for each subject, showing how fixation disparity varied with vergence demand. In each graph, forced vergence was plotted along the x-axis (divergence plotted to the left and convergence to the right); fixation disparity was plotted along the y-axis, in minutes of arc (eso fixation disparity was plotted above the y-axis and exo fixation disparity below the x-axis).

Ogle found that the subjects fell into four distinct groups. Figure 4.28 shows an example of each. The majority of subjects had curves similar to that identified as Type I. For these subjects, fixation disparity varied in a constant manner throughout the middle portion of the curve, tending to level off with larger amounts of forced divergence or convergence. Ogle interpreted these curves as indicating that "for these subjects the cortical images from the two eyes increasingly slip and the fusion of these images becomes increasingly less exact as the prism power increases, until finally diplopia occurs (1950, p. 78).

For the second group of subjects (see the Type II curve in Figure 4.28), fixation disparity changed little over a wide range of prism power, then suddenly made a large change at one or both of the extremes (when a large amount of base-in or base-out prism

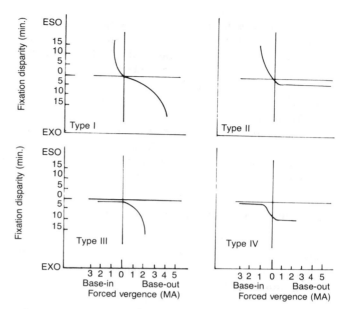

Figure 4.28   Examples of Ogle's four types of fixation disparity curves (redrawn from K. N. Ogle, *Researches in Binocular Vision*, Saunders, 1950).

was introduced). Type III curves, in many cases, were little different from Type II curves, but differed from them in that the data tended to approach a constant value more gradually. For subjects having Type IV curves, fixation disparity changed with forced vergence only within a narrow interval, and outside the interval leveled off at nearly constant values. These subjects were found, by other tests, to have poorly developed binocular coordination.

In discussing these curves, Sheedy (1980a) commented that the Type I curve is the most common type, occurring in about 60 percent of the population, and is usually associated with an asymptomatic patient. Types II, III, and IV occur in 25, 10, and 5 percent, respectively, of the population and are most often associated with a symptomatic patient.

Clinical application of fixation disparity testing

Fixation disparity testing was not applied clinically until more than a decade after Ogle's (1950) pioneering work, when Mallett (1964, 1966), Grolman (1966), and Borish (1978) introduced clinical fixation disparity tests. However, these tests were not designed to measure fixation disparity but to determine the amount of prism necessary to eliminate it. This procedure—the determination of the

base-in or base-out prism power necessary to eliminate fixation disparity—is the measurement of the
associated phoria. As compared to the ordinary
dissociated phoria, the associated phoria is a
measurement taken while both eyes are fixating and
while peripheral clues to fusion are present.

The first clinical instrument designed to measure
fixation disparity, called the *Disparometer,* has been
described by Sheedy and Saladin (1977) and by
Sheedy (1980a, 1980b). (The clinical use of fixation
disparity is discussed in Chapters 10 and 12.)

Anomalies of Accommodation

Anomalies of accommodation include *presbyopia,
spasm of accommodation, fatigue of accommodation, insufficiency of accommodation,* and *paralysis
of accommodation.*

Presbyopia

Although often discussed in conjunction with
errors of refraction, presbyopia is actually an
anomaly of accommodation brought about by
changes in the structure of the crystalline lens with
age. The occurrence of presbyopia is a universal
phenomenon, just as certain to occur as "death and
taxes."

As described in Chapter 2, the crystalline lens
continues to grow throughout life. As new fibers are
formed in the outer cortex of the lens, older fibers
are compressed into the inner nucleus. As a result,
the nucleus becomes increasingly less elastic with
age, and the lens substance gradually loses its ability
to change shape as the ciliary muscle contracts.
Moreover, it is possible that with increasing age the
ciliary muscle loses some of its power to contract.

As shown in Figure 4.29, based on Donders's
(1864) table, the amplitude of accommodation
decreases gradually from 14.00D at age 10 to about
4.50D at age 42 and to 0.00D at age 70. It is likely
that amplitude shown beyond the age of 55 is largely
the result of the depth of focus (depth of field) of the
eye. As a general rule, clear, comfortable vision for
sustained near work is possible as long as no more
than one-half of the amplitude of accommodation
must be used. Because the usual reading distance for
most adults is about 40cm, requiring 2.50D of
accommodation, presbyopia is said to be present
when the amplitude of accommodation has reached
5.00D or less.

The need for reading glasses or bifocal lenses
varies greatly from one person to another: factors
such as occupation, hobbies, and arm length are all

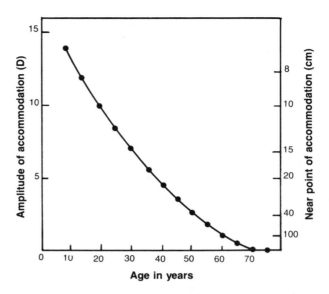

**Figure 4.29   Amplitude of accommodation
as related to age, based on Donders's (1864)
table.**

of importance. Most people begin to need some help
with their close work at some time between the ages
of 40 and 45 years. When presbyopia first becomes
manifest, the reading addition is usually about 1.00D
in power. During a period of about 10 years, the
addition must gradually be increased in power,
usually leveling off at a power of +2.25 to +2.50D.

Spasm of accommodation

Recall that a latent hyperope is an uncorrected
hyperope who compensates for the hyperopia by
accommodation; a pseudomyope is an emmetrope
who, due to overaccommodation, experiences
blurred distance vision. Each of these conditions
may, but does not necessarily, involve spasms of
accommodation.

Borish (1970) described latent hyperopia as either
tonic, involving a relatively fixed state of accommodation, or *clonic,* in which a temporary "cramping"
or spasm of the ciliary muscle occurs. The excessive
amount of accommodation required in uncorrected
hyperopia may often result in complaints of
eyestrain, or asthenopia. The treatment for latent
hyperopia is the prescription of convex lenses of
sufficient power to make the continual use of accommodation unnecessary.

The pseudomyope typically complains that
following a prolonged period of reading or other
near work, distance vision is blurred for a while but
gradually clears up. Often, convex lenses prescribed

for close work only will relax accommodation to the extent that distance vision will remain clear. However, if the myopia has become constant and apparently irreversible, concave lenses may be required for distance vision.

Fatigue of accommodation

An individual with a normal amplitude of accommodation may complain of eyestrain or fatigue accompanying close work. Upon examination, the practitioner may find the patient to have a lag of accommodation. This condition is often associated with a low AC/A ratio, so a large exophoria may be present at the 40cm testing distance. This condition has been referred to by Heath (1959) as *false convergence insufficiency*. A combination of accommodative facility training and convergence training is usually sufficient not only to relieve the patient's symptoms but, in many cases, to cause a decrease in the near exophoria finding.

Insufficiency of accommodation

Occasionally a patient will have a markedly lowered amplitude of accommodation for his or her age. The cause may be either physiological or pathological. In some cases the condition may be a matter of *fatigue*, as discussed above, and it may respond to accommodative facility training.

An *uncorrected myope* may have a lowered amplitude of accommodation: this is because little or no accommodation has been required for close work. Once the myopia has been corrected with appropriate lenses, the patient will then have to make use of the normal amount of accommodation for near work, and the amplitude of accommodation will quickly increase to within the normal range.

Paralysis of accommodation

Paralysis of accommodation is a relatively rare condition in which there is an inability to focus for near work and, in some cases, a dilated pupil. Duke-Elder (1947) has listed the following causes of paralysis of accommodation:

1. Congenital defects.
2. Paralysis by cycloplegic drugs.
3. Paralysis of infective origin.
4. Paralysis associated with degenerative conditions affecting the brain stem.
5. Paralysis occurring in metabolic toxemias.
6. Paralysis due to exogenous poisons.
7. Paralysis due to involvement of the third nerve trunk, anywhere in its course.
8. Paralysis due to diseases of the eye affecting the ciliary body, such as cyclitis and glaucoma.
9. Traumatic paralysis due to a concussion injury.
10. Hysterical paralysis.

Duke-Elder has noted that paralysis by *cycloplegic drugs* is the most common cause, occurring not only by accidental instillation of drugs into the conjunctival sac but also by contamination of the fingers by the drug or due to the effects of the drug taken internally.

Treatment of paralysis of accommodation is, of course, directed toward the cause. However, plus lenses will be needed for near work, just as for a presbyope, unless or until the condition is alleviated.

Anomalies of Accommodative Convergence

As discussed in a previous section, the "normal" AC/A ratio is said to be 6/1; that is, each diopter of stimulus to accommodation brings into play 6Δ of accommodative convergence. For an individual who is orthophoric at 6m and has an interpupillary distance of 64mm, the total amount of convergence required at a distance of 40cm from the spectacle plane is 15Δ, (remember that convergence findings are specified in regard to the *center of rotation* of the eye, which is located 27mm behind the spectacle plane). Thus, with a 6/1 AC/A ratio, the total convergence demand for the 40cm distance would be supplied by accommodative convergence:

$$\frac{AC}{A} = \frac{15}{2.5} = \frac{6}{1}.$$

This being the case, the individual would be orthophoric at 40cm (as well as at 6m), and no fusional vergence would be required to maintain single binocular vision at that distance.

Clinical experience has found that it is desirable to have an AC/A ratio somewhat lower than "normal." For example, a patient who is orthophoric at distance and has only 10Δ of accommodative convergence in play at 40cm will have the following AC/A ratio:

$$\frac{AC}{A} = \frac{10}{2.5} = \frac{4}{1}.$$

The fact that only 10Δ of accommodative convergence are available at 40cm means that, to make up the total of 15Δ of convergence, 5Δ of *positive fusional vergence* must be used.

The fact that 5Δ of positive fusional vergence

must be used at the 40cm distance means that the patient exhibits 5Δ of exophoria at that distance. As compared to *negative fusional vergence*, positive fusional vergence is a well-developed function, and most patients have little difficulty maintaining as much as 5Δ of positive fusional vergence for long periods.

Negative fusional vergence, however, is not a well-developed function, and its use, even in small amounts, may be a source of asthenopia. Negative fusional vergence will be required for a patient who has esophoria at 40cm; and esophoria at this distance is often accompanied by a high AC/A ratio (i.e., by excessive accommodative convergence). Consider a patient who is orthophoric at distance and has 20Δ (rather than the "required" 15Δ) of accommodative convergence at 40cm. The AC/A ratio would be

$$\frac{AC}{A} = \frac{20}{2.5} = \frac{8}{1}$$

and the patient would have 5Δ of esophoria (20Δ − 15Δ) at 40cm. This esophoria would require the use of 5Δ of negative fusional vergence at 40cm to avoid diplopia.

To summarize, it is desirable for a patient to have a small amount of exophoria at 40cm, so (assuming orthophoria at 6m) it is desirable for the AC/A ratio to be somewhat less than 6/1. As a matter of convenience we may consider the "normal" range for the AC/A ratio as being between 4/1 and 6/1, with AC/A ratios below 4/1 considered "low," and those above 6/1 considered "high."

If the AC/A ratio is abnormally low, the condition is known as *convergence insufficiency;* an abnormally high AC/A ratio is known as *convergence excess.* (Diagnosis and treatment of anomalies of accommodative convergence are discussed in Chapters 10 and 12.)

STRABISMUS

Recall that strabismus is a manifest deviation of the eyes (as compared to a phoria, which is a latent deviation). Strabismus may be manifest in just one eye as a *unilateral strabismus* or in either eye as an *alternating strabismus.* Unilateral strabismus is designated in terms of the deviating eye. If the right eye turns outward, the condition is *right exotropia;* if the left eye turns inward, it is *left esotropia;* and if the right eye turns upward, the condition is called *right hypertropia.*

Strabismus is classified in terms of constancy,

being a *constant strabismus* if it occurs at all times and *intermittent* if it occurs only part of the time. If it occurs at only one testing distance (at 6m but not at 40cm, or vice versa), it is called *periodic strabismus.*

Strabismus also may be classified in terms of *comitancy* and *etiology*. Strabismus is called *concomitant* if the angle of squint is the same in all directions of gaze, and is *incomitant* if the angle differs in different directions of gaze. As for etiology, strabismus may be either *functional* or *paralytic.* Functional strabismus is always concomitant and may be due to a preexisting condition (or combination of conditions), such as an uncorrected refractive error, an abnormally high or low AC/A ratio, or a deficiency in fusional vergence. Paralytic strabismus is typically incomitant, although long-standing cases tend to develop comitancy. *Congenital paralytic strabismus* is usually due to an ocular muscle anomaly, such as a long or short muscle or a misplaced muscle insertion or tendon. *Acquired paralytic strabismus* is more apt to be due to a lesion affecting one or more of the oculo-motor nerves or nuclei of origin.

Detection and Measurement of Strabismus

If a patient has a large angle of deviation (i.e., 20 degrees or more), the strabismus is so obvious that no special testing procedure is required for its detection. For smaller angles of deviation, specific procedures are necessary for the detection (and also measurement) of strabismus. Two of the most commonly used methods are the *unilateral cover test* and the *corneal reflex test.*

The unilateral cover test should not be confused with the already described alternating cover test used for the detection and measurement of a phoria. In the alternating cover test, the occluder is alternately placed in front of one eye and then in front of the other, the movement of the occluder being so fast that binocular vision is not allowed to take place. However, in the unilateral cover test (also called the *cover-uncover test*), one eye is covered for a second or so, after which both eyes are allowed to fixate the target before the fellow eye is covered. It should be understood that the alternating cover test does not distinguish between a phoria and a tropia. For example, a movement inward of the right eye, when the cover is moved from the right eye to the left eye, indicates the presence of either an exophoria or an exotropia. However, if any movement at all is noted in the unilateral cover test to be described, it indicates the presence of a tropia.

The Unilateral Cover Test

Consider a patient with a constant right exotropia: the right eye deviates outward at all times with respect to the left eye. If an occluder were placed in front of the deviating eye while a distant object was fixated, the fixing eye would undergo no movement. Likewise, if the occluder were removed from in front of the deviating eye, no movement of the fixing eye would occur. The fixing "good" eye fixated the target before, during, and after the occlusion of the deviating eye.

However, after both eyes have remained uncovered for a few seconds, if the occluder is now placed in front of the fixing eye while a distant object is fixated, the deviating eye will be seen to turn inward to take up fixation, and it will remain in this position as long as the "good" eye is occluded; it will return to its outward-deviating position only when the occluder is removed. Upon removal, the fixing eye will be seen to take up fixation, while the deviating eye turns outward.

Similarly, in right esotropia the left eye will make no movement whatsoever when the right eye is covered and then uncovered. When the left, fixing, eye is covered, however, the right eye will turn outward to take up fixation and will remain in that position as long as the "good" eye is covered, turning inward once again when the fixing eye is uncovered.

In summary, occluding the deviating eye has no effect on the position of the fixing eye, but occluding the fixing eye causes the deviating eye to take up fixation and then, when the occluder is removed, to return to its position of deviation. The positions of the two eyes in exotropia and esotropia are shown in Figures 4.30 and 4.31.

Both the alternating cover test and the unilateral cover test may be used not only to detect, but also to measure a phoria or a tropia. This is done with individual square prisms or a prism bar. These procedures will be discussed in Chapter 5.

The Corneal Reflex Test

The corneal reflex test provides a second method for the detection and measurement of strabismus. The examiner faces the patient at a distance of approximately 40cm, holding a penlight or other small, bright source of light. The patient is instructed to look at the light; the examiner, while viewing directly

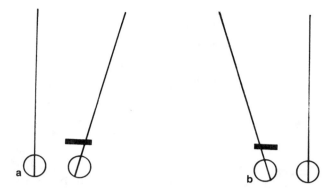

Figure 4.30 Right exotropia (*a*) with occluder placed in front of the deviating eye; (*b*) with occluder placed in front of the fixing eye. The "bad" eye fixates only when the "good" eye is occluded.

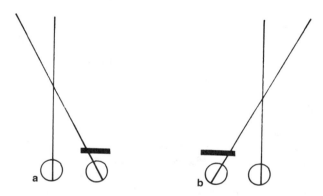

Figure 4.31 Right esotropia (*a*) with occluder placed in front of the deviating eye; (*b*) with occluder placed in front of the fixing eye. As with exotropia, the "bad" eye fixates only when the "good" eye is occluded.

over the light source, notes the positions of the reflections of the light source in the two eyes.

If no tropia exists, the corneal reflexes will be in the same positions for the two eyes. Ordinarily they will be positioned slightly nasal (about 0.5mm) to the center of the pupil. If exotropia exists, the corneal reflex will be displaced inward from the center of the pupil. If esotropia exists, the reflex will be displaced outward. The position of the corneal reflex of each eye is shown in Figure 4.32 for exotropia and esotropia.

Using the corneal reflex test, the examiner may either *estimate* (Hirschberg method) or *measure* (Krimsky method, using prisms) the angle of

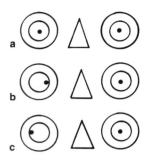

Figure 4.32   The corneal reflex test: (a) no strabismus (each reflex is approximately 0.5mm nasal to the center of the pupil); (b) right exotropia; (c) right esotropia.

strabismus. It should be understood, however, that measurements made with a light source as a fixation object may suffer from the fact that a light source is not an adequate stimulus to accommodation. Serious measurements of the angle of strabismus should be done with a small line of letters or (for infants and young children) with a picture involving fine detail as an accommodative stimulus.

Adaptations to Strabismus

A strabismic patient is beset by two concurrent problems: *diplopia* and *confusion.* As shown in the upper diagram in Figure 4.33 when the "good" eye foveally fixates an object (a house, in this case), the object is imaged on a nonfoveal area of the deviating eye, resulting in diplopia. At the same time, whatever

Figure 4.33   Diplopia and confusion in right esotropia: (a) the stimulus situation; (b) what the patient sees. The objects seen by the strabismic eye are shaded. Note that the house is imaged on the left side of the retina of the right eye, so it is seen to the right of the "real" house: this is uncrossed diplopia.

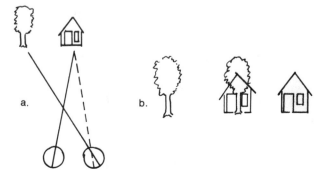

object happens to be on the foveal line of sight for the deviating eye (a tree, in this case) will appear to occupy the same position in space as the house, causing confusion. Assuming that the house and the tree are the only objects in the patient's visual field, the patient's percept is that shown in the right hand diagram of Figure 4.33. Two houses and two trees are seen, with the "middle" images of the house and the tree coinciding.

When strabismus is present at birth or develops early in life, the problems presented by diplopia and confusion are often solved by the development of one or more of a number of adaptive mechanisms. These adaptations include suppression, amblyopia, eccentric fixation, and anomalous retinal correspondence.

Suppression

Suppression is a phenomenon in which there is a cortical inhibition of the information arriving from specific regions of the retina of the deviating eye. The regions in which suppression areas develop are the macular area (thus avoiding confusion) and the peripheral area of the retina corresponding to the direction of fixation for the normal eye (thus avoiding diplopia). According to Parks (1979), macular and peripheral suppression differ in that macular suppression exists in both binocular and monocular vision, whereas peripheral suppression exists only in binocular vision.

One of the simplest methods of testing for suppression involves the use of the *Worth Dot test.* As shown in Figure 4.34, this test is comprised of four illuminated disks: two green, one red, and one white. The test may be presented at any distance, while the patient wears red/green glasses (the red lens is routinely worn on the right eye) in addition to his or her own spectacle correction, if any. The test is presented in a semidarkened room, and the patient is asked to report how many dots are seen. (This test should not be referred to in the patient's presence as the "4–Dot" test, as this gives the patient a strong clue as to how many dots should be seen!) Possible responses follow:

1. *Two dots*, both red, indicate suppression of the left eye.
2. *Three dots*, all green, indicate suppression of the right eye.
3. *Four dots*, two red and two green, indicate normal binocular vision (no suppression and no diplopia).
4. *Five dots*, two red and three green, indicate diplopia.

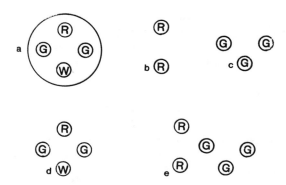

Figure 4.34 The Worth Dot test: (*a*) the stimulus; (*b*) two dots, indicating suppression of left eye; (*c*) three dots, indicating suppression of right eye; (*d*) four dots, normal; (*e*) five dots, indicating diplopia.

Parks (1979) pointed out that if a small area of foveal suppression exists (in what he calls the *monofixation syndrome*), the patient may report the presence of either two or three dots, indicating suppression, when the test is presented at a distance of 6m. However, if the patient is asked to walk slowly toward the test, a point will be reached at which four dots are seen. This is because the foveal scotoma encompasses the four-dot stimulus when presented at the 6m distance, but at some closer distance the angular separation of the dots is greater than the size of the scotoma.

Amblyopia

Amblyopia is said to exist when visual acuity is poor (less than 6/6, or 20/20) even with corrective lenses, without obvious cause. Amblyopia can be considered as either *organic* or *functional.* Schapero (1971) classified organic amblyopia as either nutritional, toxic, or congenital. Functional amblyopia includes strabismic, refractive, and hysterical (psychogenic) amblyopia. Functional amblyopia due to strabismus or refractive anomalies was formerly referred to as *suppression amblyopia* or as *amblyopia ex anopsia* (amblyopia due to nonuse).

Refractive amblyopia can occur either as a result of uncorrected anisometropia or of uncorrected astigmatism. If one eye is much more hyperopic than the other (for example, right eye +4.00D and left eye +1.00D), the more hyperopic eye will never experience a sharply focused retinal image because the less hyperopic eye will be required to accommodate a lesser amount for vision at any distance. Consequently, the more hyperopic eye routinely

suppresses, leading to amblyopia (by a process not completely understood). However, if one eye is considerably more myopic than the other (say, right eye −4.00D and the left eye −1.00D), the less myopic eye will experience a relatively sharp image for distance vision and the more myopic eye will have a sharp image for near vision; therefore, suppression will not occur, and amblyopia will not develop. It is of interest, however, that many uncorrected anisometropic hyperopes do not develop amblyopia. In any case, correction of anisometropic hyperopes at an early age should be considered.

A child having a large amount (2.00 or 3.00D or more) of uncorrected astigmatism may develop amblyopia in both eyes because neither eye experiences a perfectly sharp retinal image. This amblyopia, however, tends to be small in amount with corrected visual acuity of about 6/9 (or 20/30), and the vision often gradually improves if corrective lenses are prescribed during the early school years.

Strabismic amblyopia may occur in the deviating eye of a strabismic patient and is thought to be the result of long-continued suppression (again, by a mechanism not well understood). The visual acuity in the strabismic eye may be as poor as 6/60 (20/200) or as good as 6/7.5 (20/25). The typical response of a nonamblyope in reading the letters on the Snellen acuity chart is to read all letters in each line until a point is reached at which some (or all) of the letters in a given line cannot be distinguished. In contrast, the amblyope will often read one or two letters in each of several lines, making assessment of visual acuity difficult. This is due to a phenomenon that has been variously called *contour interaction*, the *crowding phenomenon*, or *separation difficulty*.

Due to the phenomenon of contour interaction, the visual acuity for an amblyopic eye varies with the number of stimuli present on the acuity chart. Visual acuity may be relatively poor if a chart involving several lines of letters is presented, but it tends to improve if a single line of letters is presented and improves still more if a single letter is presented. Therefore, in a routine vision screening of schoolchildren, the "whole chart" method of testing visual acuity should be used. Otherwise, cases of amblyopia may be missed.

Flom (1966) developed a visual acuity chart that takes into account the effects of contour interaction. This chart is shown in Figure 4.35. Visual acuity is determined by the patient's ability to locate the gaps in the *C*-shaped Landolt rings, while the *E*s provide contour interaction. Several charts must be used, one for each letter size.

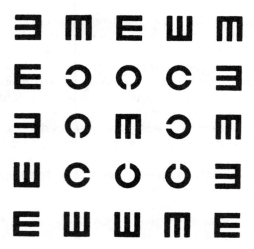

Figure 4.35 Flom's visual acuity chart for amblyopia. Acuity is determined on the basis of the Landolt rings: the tumbling *E*s are for the purpose of providing contour interaction (from M. C. Flom, 1966, pp. 63–68).

Eccentric fixation

An additional adaptation to strabismus, which occurs along with amblyopia, is *eccentric fixation*. In this condition, an off-foveal point in the retina of the deviating eye is used for fixation, both in monocular and in binocular vision. Eccentric fixation tends to occur if amblyopia persists beyond early childhood, and it is found in a large proportion of strabismic amblyopes. In esotropia, the eccentrically located retinal point used for fixation is usually in the nasal retina, whereas in exotropia it is usually in the temporal retina.

Flom (1966) has shown that the amount of eccentric fixation is closely related to the depth of the patient's amblyopia: the greater the amblyopia (i.e., the poorer the visual acuity), the larger the angle of eccentric fixation. Eccentric fixation is considered to be *parafoveal* if it is between 1 and 3 degrees; *paramacular* if between 3 and 5 degrees, and *peripheral* if greater than 5 degrees.

Most modern ophthalmoscopes are equipped with a graticule target designed for the detection and measurement of eccentric fixation. While the patient views a distant object, the examiner projects the bull's-eye of the graticule target on the patient's fovea. The patient's attention is then called to the target and instructed to look at the bull's-eye. If the position of the foveal reflex relative to the graticule target changes when the patient fixates the bull's-eye, an off-foveal point is used for fixation; the new position of the foveal reflex indicates the degree and direction of eccentric fixation. In the situation illustrated in Figure 4.36, the foveal reflex is located nasal to the center of the target, indicating that the patient is fixating with an eccentric retinal point located temporal to the fovea.

The first ophthalmoscope to become available having a graticule target for the measurement of eccentric fixation was called the Visuscope. The procedure is sometimes referred to as the Visuscope test or visuoscopy.

Anomalous retinal correspondence

As described at the beginning of this chapter, corresponding retinal points are pairs of points, one in each retina, having the same visual direction. An additional adaptation to strabismus is *anomalous retinal correspondence (ARC)*, a condition in which an off-foveal point in the retina of the deviating eye is associated, in consciousness, with the fovea of the fixing eye. In anomalous retinal correspondence the angle between the fovea and the anomalously corresponding point of the deviating eye, subtended at the nodal point, is known as the *angle of anomaly*.

Anomalous retinal correspondence is classified as either harmonious, unharmonious, or paradoxical. In *harmonious ARC*, the angle of anomaly is equal to the angle of strabismus, so the anomalous retinal correspondence serves to fully "compensate" for the strabismus; that is, the anomalously corresponding point serves to avoid both diplopia and confusion as

Figure 4.36 The use of the graticule ophthalmoscope target (Visuscope) for determining the presence of eccentric fixation.

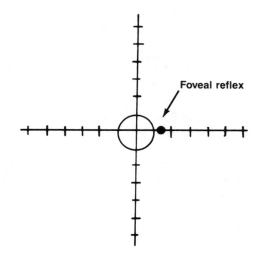

Foveal reflex

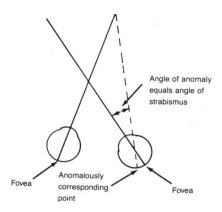

Figure 4.37 **Right esotropia with harmonious anomalous retinal correspondence.**

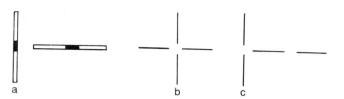

Figure 4.38 The after-image transfer test: (*a*) the stimulus; (*b*) appearance of afterimages in normal retinal correspondence; (*c*) appearance of afterimages in anomalous retinal correspondence.

shown in Figure 4.37. If the angle of anomaly is less than the angle of strabismus, the strabismus is not fully "compensated," and the ARC is referred to as *unharmonious*. If the angle of anomaly is such that the ARC not only does not "compensate" for the strabismus, but makes the situation worse, the condition is called *paradoxical ARC.*

One of the most straightforward methods of determining the presence or absence of ARC involves the use of the afterimage transfer test. Patients are first instructed to fixate, for a period of 15 or 20 seconds, the midpoint of a vertically oriented filament, using the fixing eye. This "burns" an afterimage on the retina of that eye. The patient is then instructed to fixate the midpoint of a horizontally oriented filament, using the deviating eye—again for 15 or 20 seconds—creating an after-image on the retina of that eye. The patient is then told to project the after-images of the two filaments on an unstructured surface, such as the wall at the end of the room, and to draw on a sheet of paper the two images as they appear to him or her. If the two images cross, the patient has normal retinal correspondence, but if they do not, anomalous retinal correspondence is indicated (see Figure 4.38).

It should be understood that eccentric fixation is a monocular phenomenon elicited by stimulating the deviating eye only, whereas anomalous retinal correspondence is a binocular phenomenon requiring the stimulation of both eyes.

DIAGNOSIS AND TREATMENT OF BINOCULAR VISION ANOMALIES

The procedures described in this chapter for the detection and measurement of binocular vision anomalies (phorias, fixation disparity, fusional vergence anomalies, strabismus, and the adaptations to strabismus) are intended to provide the student with a basic understanding of these anomalies. No effort is made to present a complete diagnostic regimen for any of the anomalies described. However, specific procedures for the diagnosis and treatment of anomalies of binocular vision are presented in Chapters 10 and 12. When reading those chapters, the student may find it convenient to refer to the descriptions of binocular vision anomalies given in this chapter.

Study Questions

1. Define the following terms: (a) corresponding retinal points; (b) the horopter.

2. If a subject having an interpupillary distance of 64mm fixates an object at a distance of 33cm from the spectacle plane, (a) what is the stimulus to accommodation, in diopters? (b) what is the stimulus to convergence, in prism diopters?

3. According to calculations by Ogle, what is the significance of Panum's fusional areas for fixated objects at distances of about 20m and beyond?

4. For a saccadic eye movement to the left, (a) what are the agonist muscles? (b) what are the antagonist muscles?

5. Which of the two forms of horizontal disjunctive movements—convergence or divergence—is the more highly developed function? Give evidence for your answer.

6. What are two methods that can be used clinically to stimulate a patient's accommodation?

7. List four methods that can be used clinically to dissociate the eyes.

8. What is it that prevents a latent deviation of the eyes (a phoria) from becoming a manifest deviation (a tropia)?

9. Define the following terms: (a) sensory fusion; (b) motor fusion.

10. What is the significance of Panum's fusional areas in regard to (a) the horopter? (b) physiological diplopia?

11. How do the stimulus AC/A ratio and the response AC/A ratio differ?

12. What movement or movements do the eyes make in response to (a) a large amount of prism power placed in front of one eye (e.g., 10Δ or more)? (b) a small amount of prism placed in front of one or both eyes? Give examples to illustrate your answers.

13. What characterizes stereoscopic perception of depth as an innately determined sensation, although the monocular "picture painting" clues to depth perception are thought to be acquired on the basis of experience?

14. What did Ogle mean when he talked about a fusion compulsion?

15. What term is used to designate a minute amount of underconvergence or overconvergence with respect to the plane of regard, without the occurrence of diplopia? How does this differ from strabismus?

16. If an emmetropic subject is instructed to read a row of small letters at a distance of 40cm while wearing +2.00D lenses, what is the stimulus to accommodation? For the same subject, what would be the stimulus to accommodation at 40cm while wearing −1.50D lenses?

17. Why is it more desirable for a person to have a small amount of exophoria at 40cm than to have a small amount of esophoria at the same distance?

18. What are two commonly used methods of detecting strabismus?

19. In the base-out to blur, break, and recovery test at 6m, what is happening to the visual apparatus (in terms of accommodation and convergence) when the patient reports (a) that the letters are blurred? (b) that the letters have broken into two? (c) that the letters have come back together?

20. What is the approximate speed, in degrees per second, of (a) saccadic movements? (b) following movements?

21. List and briefly describe each of the four kinds of vergence movements originally described by Maddox.

PART TWO

The Optometric Examination

The optometry student is often overwhelmed by the large number of testing procedures that must be learned in the preclinical courses. As a result, the tests tend to be performed in a "cookbook" fashion, possibly with a readily available outline of the procedures to be followed for each test. Eventually the student learns to organize the procedures in such a way that the mystery begins to disappear. One way to remove some of the mystery from the examination routine is to consider it as being made up of four parts: (1) the patient history, (2) the preliminary examination, (3) the refractive examination, and (4) the binocular vision examination.

The History

In taking the history, the chief tools used by the optometrist are his or her *ears*. On the basis of the history alone, the optometrist should be able to make a tentative diagnosis of the patient's problem or problems. This tentative diagnosis can then be reconsidered and refined on the basis of the information obtained in the preliminary examination, the refractive examination, and the binocular vision examination.

The optometric examination can be thought of as an *investigation*, in which each piece of evidence gained is used to determine the nature and then the solution of the patient's problems. This has the advantage of keeping the procedure from becoming boring, as it may well be if the practitioner looks at the examination simply as a data-collecting procedure.

The Preliminary Examination

In the preliminary examination, the optometrist uses his or her *eyes*. The purpose of the preliminary examination is to detect any gross anomaly of the visual system, such as a high refractive error, a binocular vision anomaly or disturbance in ocular motility, or an ocular or systemic disease. Many of the procedures included in the preliminary examination involve *observations* rather than measurements. These observations show the practitioner what to look for during the refractive examination and the binocular vision examination.

The Refractive Examination

During the refractive examination, the practitioner makes *measurements*. The procedures for making these measurements have changed little in the past 30 or 40 years. They involve essentially the procedures of keratometry, retinoscopy, and subjective refraction. The development of binocular refraction procedures, however, has begun to make changes in the time-honored subjective refraction routine. The development of computer-assisted refractors, both objective and subjective, is bringing about further changes.

The tentative diagnosis that was made on the basis of the history and reevaluated during the preliminary examination is further refined during the refractive examination.

The Binocular Vision Examination

Any binocular vision anomalies that may have been found or suspected during the preliminary examination are further investigated during the binocular vision examination. Although the procedures for the measurement of phorias, fusional reserves, and amplitude of accommodation have changed little in recent years, they have been supplemented by binocular refraction procedures and fixation disparity tests.

On the basis of the information obtained in the history, the preliminary examination, the refractive examination, and the binocular vision examination, the optometrist makes a diagnosis and decides on the form of treatment.

The Optometrist as a Primary Care Practitioner

It has been estimated that approximately 95 percent of the patients who seek the services of a vision care practitioner do so because of an optometric problem, whereas the other 5 percent do so because of a medical problem. Therefore, much of the optometrist's efforts during the case history and the preliminary examination must be directed toward determining whether the patient is a member of the first or the second group of patients (or perhaps both). As indicated in the Preface, optometry has placed increasing emphasis on the optometrist's role as a primary care practitioner, or as an entry point into the health care system. Although optometrists always have been primary care practitioners, this new emphasis points out an increasing understanding of the optometrist's role as a *diagnostician*. As such, the optometrist must be able to detect and diagnose not only those disease conditions affecting the eyes themselves, but also those systemic diseases that can have an effect on the visual system.

CHAPTER 5

The Patient History

PROBLEM-ORIENTED OPTOMETRIC RECORDS

The system of record keeping used in this text is based on the problem-oriented medical record system developed by Weed (1968, 1969). Weed's system had its beginnings in teaching hospitals and clinics. Although record systems used for ambulatory patients must differ in some respects from those used for hospital patients, the majority of Weed's concepts can be applied directly to optometric practice. The problem-oriented medical record system consists of four basic components: (1) the defined data base, (2) the complete problem list, (3) initial treatment plans, and (4) progress notes.

The Defined Data Base

As described by Weed (1968), the defined data base includes the patient profile, chief complaint, present illness, review of systems, physical examination, and laboratory reports. The adjective *defined* indicates that the data base is limited to those items that are deemed appropriate for an initial medical examination: with the ever-increasing number of diagnostic procedures now available, a *complete* data base would never end. However, the defined data base as described by Hurst (1972) requires a 19-page form.

For optometry, the defined data base should include a problem-oriented history, together with all of the tests of eye health, refraction, and binocular vision that are appropriate for the patient's age group. The data base would tend to vary from one practitioner to another but typically would include the following procedures:

The history: Patient profile, ocular history, and health history; family ocular and health history; and chief complaint and secondary complaints.

Preliminary examination: Uncorrected and corrected visual acuity, visual field screening tests, cover test and other ocular motility tests, tests of pupil function, tonometry, sphygmomanometry, external examination, and internal examination.

Refractive examination: Keratometry, retinoscopy, subjective refraction, and corrected visual acuity.

Binocular vision examination: Lateral and vertical phorias, fusional vergences and fixation disparities at 6m and at 40cm, gradient phoria test, binocular cross-cylinder test, amplitude of accommodation, and relative accommodation tests.

Additional procedures that may be suggested by the patient's history or symptoms include visual field examination, strabismus diagnosis, vision development tests, and low vision examination.

The Complete Problem List

The complete problem list is a sheet kept in the front of the patient's record (e.g., on the left side of a manila folder) having a numbered and titled list that includes every problem the patient has or has had. The list is constantly changed with time, as old problems are solved and new problems are identified. Weed (1972) defines a problem as "anything that requires management or diagnostic workup; this includes social and demographic problems" (p. 23). He illustrates the importance of social and psychological problems by commenting that "the management of a patient's heart failure often has more to do with his living conditions than it has to do with a urinary tract infection" (p. 54). The problem list, according to Weed, should include *all* of the patient's problems—not only the ones that can be solved by the student or practitioner who makes out the list.

Although an optometric patient's problem list would emphasize problems relating to the visual system, problems of a more general nature should be included when indicated by the patient's history or by the optometrist's findings. Particular care should be taken to include problems that tend to have ocular or visual effects, including hypertension, arteriosclerosis, diabetes, heart disease, migraine and other headache problems, multiple sclerosis, and many others. For each problem, the list includes a space for the date when the problem is entered on the list and the date when the problem is resolved. At subsequent visits the practitioner refers to the problem list, entering new problems when indicated and noting when existing problems have been resolved.

Initial Treatment Plans

Each initial treatment plan is numbered and titled on the basis of the problem (in the complete problem list) that the plan addresses. For each of the patient's problems, the initial plan should consist of the following three parts:

1. More information concerning diagnostic workup and management, including things ruled out, specific plans for each diagnostic possibility, and parameters to be followed in management of the disease.
2. Therapy, including not only drugs and other therapeutic procedures but also precise statements of goals, end points, and contingency plans.
3. Education of both the patient and family concerning the problem.

For the optometric patient, some problems will be in the province of the optometrist, but others will have to be resolved by practitioners in other disciplines. For those problems requiring the services of another health care practitioner, the initial treatment plan should indicate the type of practitioner to be consulted.

Progress Notes

As with the initial treatment plans, each progress note is concerned with a single problem and is numbered and titled accordingly. Each note is written in narrative form and should include four components:

*S*ymptomatic
*O*bjective
*A*ssessment
*P*lan

Not surprisingly, this portion of the record system is known as the SOAP system.

The progress notes are the final step in a feedback loop, often resulting in the formulation of additional plans that will be evaluated at additional progress visits. When a patient is being transferred from one practitioner to another, the final progress notes should emphasize the assessment of unresolved problems.

When applied to optometric practice, progress notes can exist only when a patient is seen by the practitioner on more than one occasion in relation to a particular problem or problems. When ophthalmic lenses are prescribed, the results are often so predictable that no follow-up visit is required. In such cases the practitioner tacitly assumes that the lenses have solved the patient's problem if the patient is not heard from within several weeks. However, for those patients whom the optometrist schedules for progress evaluation visits, the use of progress notes for each of the patient's problems will form the final step in the feedback loop.

Progress notes are of particular value to the optometrist when contact lenses are fitted. Because contact lenses tend to cause problems of their own, the careful recording of progress notes for each progress evaluation visit can give direction to the procedures performed at these visits and to the advice and instructions given to the patient. Rather than generate a separate set of progress notes for each problem, as Weed recommends, it may be preferable to use a structured form for the recording of *s*ymptomatic, *o*bjective, *a*ssessment, and *p*lan. Progress notes are also of obvious value for vision-training patients and for keeping track of low-vision patients' progress in adapting to their aids.

Recording Forms for the Problem-Oriented System

The following system of recording forms is recommended for application to optometric practice.

The original data base

This is a manila folder, which becomes the patient's permanent record and into which are bound by staples or metal clasps all subsequent record forms. The demographic and patient profile information and the results of the preliminary examination are recorded on the outer cover (side 1) of the manila folder; the refractive and binocular vision examination results, along with the initial problem list, initial treatment plans, and lens prescription are recorded on the inside right (side 3) and on the back (side 4) of the folder.

The complete problem list

This is recorded on the inside left (side 2) of the folder. This is a *permanent* list: at subsequent visits, as new problems are identified and as existing problems are resolved, this information is recorded.

Progress visit

It is convenient to have a variety of progress visit forms available for use in contact lens fitting, vision training, low-vision patient care, and other areas of optometric care. In addition, an unstructured progress visit form, for narrative recording, is often desirable.

Subsequent data base

A two-sided subsequent data base form is designed for use at annual or biannual optometric examinations. It contains the same information as is included on the form for the original data base, but it is printed on stiff paper rather than on the cardboard manila folder.

Special purpose forms

Special purpose forms may be required, depending on the practitioner, for diagnostic procedures such as strabismus diagnosis, dilated fundus examination, vision development examination, and so forth.

Whereas the original data base form and the complete problem list form are printed on the manila folder, all other forms are printed on paper and are bound by staples or metal clasps to the inside right (side 3) of the manila folder. As new forms are sequentially placed on top of the older forms, it becomes a simple matter to review the patient's previous optometric care by thumbing through the previous records. (Examples of these forms are given in Appendix A.)

DEMOGRAPHIC INFORMATION AND PATIENT PROFILE

Demographic information (name, address, telephone number, occupation, and so on) may be obtained by an aide or directly from the patient. When the latter procedure is used, the patient is given a form, usually on a clipboard, to fill out in the doctor's reception room. Such a form can also include a checklist for additional history items, including complaints, ocular history, health history, and medications taken. An example of a form used for this purpose is illustrated in Appendix A. The use of such a form does not absolve the optometrist of the responsibility of taking a history, but it can simplify the history taking by allowing him or her to concentrate on problem areas.

Weed (1972) has suggested that a new component be added to the demographic portion of the history—the *patient profile*—pointing out that the practitioner can often be more effective in providing patient care if he or she has knowledge of the patient's home life, family life, and any problems encountered in daily life. In the data base form recommended by Hurst (1972), the patient profile includes the following items: birthplace, occupation, education, marital status, religion, home situation, hobbies and special interests, average day, habits (tobacco, alcohol, and so forth), behavior during assessment, ability to communicate and understand, and other comments. The data base described by Hurst is for use with hospital patients. His patient profile, which may be more detailed than optometrists may think necessary, is taken by a member of the hospital's nursing service.

Occupation and Visual Requirements

Knowledge of the patient's occupation and visual requirements, both on and off the job, is of obvious importance to the optometrist. For the older patient, reading and working distances as well as illuminations levels are of particular importance. For patients of any age, knowledge of relative amounts of time spent at near vision as compared to distance vision pursuits is often helpful. For example, many patients who claim to have no symptoms of eyestrain accompanying reading may be found to engage in little or no reading. Knowledge of a patient's occupation and visual habits may also be helpful in determining the need for sunglasses or other protective lenses, or in advising the patient whether or not to consider wearing contact lenses.

OCULAR HISTORY

If the patient comes in wearing glasses or contact lenses, the practitioner should determine when the glasses or contact lenses were prescribed and how often (or, in the case of contact lenses, how many hours per day) they are worn. It may also be important to know when glasses or contact lenses were *first* prescribed and whether or not the patient's eyes have been examined since the present lenses were prescribed. The patient should also be questioned on any history of eye injury, disease, or operation, and appropriate details should be recorded.

The patient's present spectacle lenses or contact lenses should be neutralized and the results recorded on the record form. For spectacles, the lenses should be spotted and the distance between lens centers should be recorded, as should the presence of any vertical prism power. In addition, the lens material (glass or plastic, tint if present) and the type and size of the bifocal segment, if any, should be recorded. For contact lenses, the base curve, power, diameter, optic zone width, center thickness, tint, lens material (if known), and any other identifiable variables should be recorded. It is extremely helpful if an assistant or an optometric technician is available to determine the parameters of spectacle lenses or contact lenses. Indeed, if a practitioner has only one employee, the first procedures the employee should be taught to do (other than to act as receptionist and office manager) should be neutralizing and determining the other specifications of glasses and contact lenses.

HEALTH HISTORY AND MEDICATIONS

The patient should be questioned on the present state of health and the nature of any current or recent illness. Information concerning medications currently taken should include the name of each medication (some patients carry their medications with them) and the condition for which it is taken. The practitioner should be aware that many patients do not consider over-the-counter preparations (aspirin, antihistamines, sleeping pills, diet pills, and

so forth) as "medications." The time of the most recent medical and dental examinations should be obtained.

The patient should be questioned concerning the presence (either currently or in the past) of high blood pressure, heart disease, kidney disease, diabetes, or any other chronic disease.

FAMILY OCULAR AND HEALTH HISTORY

Questions concerning family ocular and health history should be directed mainly toward those sight-threatening conditions that are known to be inherited, including glaucoma, hypertension, and diabetes. The use of an information form filled out by the patient in the reception room is particularly helpful in providing the practitioner with information concerning the patient's health status and family ocular and health history, as these are items that otherwise may make the practitioner's history taking rather tedious and time-consuming.

THE CHIEF COMPLAINT

As a matter of convenience, the chief complaint is discussed here as the last major item in the patient history. However, many practitioners would take up the chief complaint as the first item after obtaining the demographic or patient profile information; others would place it just after questioning the patient on his or her ocular history.

The practitioner usually begins this part of the history with an open-ended question such as "How are your eyes bothering you?" or "What made you decide to have your eyes examined?" or, more directly, "What is your chief complaint?" The patient's chief complaint, as well as any secondary complaints, should be recorded in the patient's *own words* to prevent misinterpretation. For example, a patient's complaint of blurred distance vision should not be recorded as "myopia."

When the patient has responded by stating his or her chief complaint, follow-up questions should be asked to more clearly define the nature of the complaint and identify any secondary complaints. The record form should provide sufficient space for the recording of the patient's complaints and other problems in narrative form. Although checklists may be appropriate for forms completed by patients, they are not satisfactory for use by the practitioner. The great majority of patient complaints can be considered in terms of the following categories: blurred vision, eyestrain, headaches, external eye symptoms, disturbances of vision, double vision, deviating eye, protruding eye, unequal pupil size, and reading or learning problems.

Blurred Vision

In interpreting a patient's complaint of blurred vision, the practitioner should consider the many conditions that could be responsible. In most cases the patient will provide, without the need for coaxing, sufficient information to permit a tentative diagnosis. For example, a child's complaint of blurred distance vision suggests uncorrected myopia as the cause, whereas a middle-aged adult's complaint of blurred near vision suggests presbyopia. If the patient's initial statement fails to provide sufficiently detailed information, follow-up questions are necessary.

The nature of the patient's complaint often suggests rather obvious follow-up questions. In any case, the following possibilities should be kept in mind:

1. Blurred vision that occurs after prolonged close work, for a patient not of presbyopic age, may be due to uncorrected hyperopia, uncorrected astigmatism, or poor facility of accommodation.
2. Blurred vision occurring primarily in reduced illumination (as in night driving) may be due to night myopia or a receptor degeneration, such as retinitis pigmentosa.
3. Blurred vision occurring mainly in bright daylight may be due to nuclear or posterior subcapsular lens opacities.
4. Blurred vision involving a transient loss or obscuring of vision in an older adult could be due to temporal arteritis or to carotid artery occlusive disease and could therefore lead to closure of the central artery of the retina.
5. Blurred vision involving a transient loss of vision in a young adult could be due to migraine or to multiple sclerosis.
6. A possible cause of unilateral acuity loss is functional amblyopia. However, in the absence of additional testing or unless there is a definite history of strabismus, anisometropia, or high astigmatism, functional amblyopia should not be assumed to be the cause.

In many cases the practitioner's impression of the cause of the reduced vision must await the results of the refractive examination. The following possibilities should then be considered.

1. In an adult, blurred vision that accompanies a change in refraction in the direction of more myopia or less hyperopia may occur as a result of nuclear sclerosis of the lens or of increased blood sugar. Nuclear sclerosis tends to cause a unilateral change in refraction, whereas increased blood sugar causes a bilateral change.
2. In an adult, blurred vision that accompanies a change in refraction in the direction of more hyperopia or less myopia may be due to a serous detachment of the macula, if the blurred vision is unilateral, or to a decrease in blood sugar (in a diabetic patient), if bilateral.
3. In an older patient, blurred vision that is not due to a change in refraction is most likely due to lens opacities or to senile macular degeneration.

Diagnostic tests suggested by complaints of blurred vision

A complaint of blurred vision that is confirmed by a finding of reduced visual acuity but is not due to a change in refraction may often warrant additional testing. A number of diagnostic procedures are available that are designed for the purpose of determining whether the reduced visual acuity is the result of a retinal, optic nerve, or lenticular problem. Tests included in this category are the Amsler chart test, slit lamp examination with the Hruby lens, the photostress test, the swinging flashlight test, the light-brightness comparison test, color vision testing, the color saturation test, the neutral density filter test, and acuity testing with pupillary constriction. Procedures for conducting and interpreting these tests are given in Chapter 7.

Eyestrain

The term *eyestrain* is used here to describe any complaint involving a feeling of fatigue, discomfort, or pain localized in or about the eyes or thought to be associated with the use of the eyes. The term *asthenopia* is often used as a synonym for eyestrain. The term *headache* is often used by patients to describe what is discussed here as eyestrain, particularly when the ache is localized near the eyes or is thought to occur as a result of the use of the eyes.

Myopia

Complaints of eyestrain or visual fatigue are not likely to occur in myopia. As compared to uncorrected hyperopia or hyperopic astigmatism, in which distance vision can be improved by accommodating, there is little that an uncorrected myope can do to improve distance acuity. Although the myope can squint in an effort to see more clearly and may feel that his or her eyes are under a strain when doing so, the fact that vision is blurred is so obvious that most uncorrected myopes are likely to relegate any feeling of eyestrain to a secondary role.

Hyperopia

In *On the Anomalies of Accommodation and Refraction of the Eye*, Donders (1864, reprinted 1972) used the word *asthenopia* almost exclusively to designate the visual fatigue and other symptoms arising from uncorrected hyperopia. In Donders's time (the 19th century), most oculists failed to understand that convex lenses could be used for young people for distance vision; most thought they were indicated solely for presbyopia. Donders (1864) described asthenopia in the following manner:

> The eye has a perfectly normal appearance, its movements are undisturbed, the power of vision is usually acute,—and nevertheless in reading, writing and other close work, especially in artificial light, or in a gloomy place, the objects, after a short time, become indistinct and confused, and a feeling of fatigue comes on in, and especially above the eyes, necessitating a suspension of work. (p. 259)

Donders said it was generally agreed that asthenopia was due to the excessive use of accommodation, and that because asthenopia did not affect everyone, writers believed that people who were afflicted with it had a peculiar predisposition. Donders questioned the idea of a predisposition and concluded that hyperopia was the condition responsible for asthenopia.

Many of Donders's contemporaries considered asthenopia to be a form of amblyopia. Rather than prescribing convex lenses of adequate power, they prescribed weak convex lenses or no lenses at all. Children suffering from asthenopia were advised to give up their schooling, and adults were encouraged to give up their sedentary occupations and become horsecart drivers or emigrate to Australia. Donders wrote that it was a great satisfaction to be able to say that asthenopia no longer needed to be an inconvenience to anyone because it could so easily be cured by prescribing convex lenses. He also noted that opticians understood asthenopia and knew that some people required convex lenses for distance vision.

Latent hyperopia. If a patient has latent hyperopia, first attempts at refraction by means of routine fogging procedures may indicate only a small amount of hyperopia (say, 0.25 or 0.50D). However, the use of specific refraction procedures designed to fully relax accommodation may bring out the latent component of the hyperopia. (Such procedures, including the delayed subjective, "overfogging" procedures, and cycloplegic refraction are described in Chapter 9 on subjective refraction.)

Astigmatism

In uncorrected astigmatism no amount of accommodation can bring about a point focus on the retina for a point object. However, in hyperopic astigmatism one or both focal lines are located behind the retina, and accommodation can place the circle of least confusion on or near the retina. This will have the effect of improving visual acuity at the expense of a feeling of eyestrain or fatigue.

Simple or compound myopic astigmatism, in which one or both focal lines are located in front of the retina, is similar to myopia in that accommodation is not effective in clearing up distance vision. Therefore, symptoms of asthenopia would not be expected to occur. However, for near vision, accommodation may in some cases place the circle of least confusion closer to the retina and, therefore, may be accompanied by a feeling of eyestrain.

Binocular vision anomalies

Anomalies of binocular vision are often accompanied by symptoms of eyestrain. The extent of these symptoms, or the absence of symptoms, will guide the practitioner in the management of the problem.

The majority of people who have a phoria problem are relatively orthophoric at distance, but because of a relatively high or low AC/A ratio they are *esophoric* (high AC/A ratio) or *exophoric* (low AC/A ratio) at near. These two conditions are referred to respectively as *convergence excess* and *convergence insufficiency*. In the less common situations in which the patient is found to have a significant phoria at distance, the condition may or may not be accompanied by an unusually high or low AC/A ratio. If a patient is found to have a high esophoria at distance, with or without a similarly high esophoria at near, the condition is referred to as *divergence insufficiency*. If a high exophoria exists at distance, usually with a somewhat lower exophoria at near, the condition is called *divergence excess*.

Convergence excess. The patient having the syndrome of convergence excess typically complains of headaches and other signs of asthenopia accompanying close work. The asthenopia is due to the fact that negative fusional vergence must be constantly used for close work; it may be particularly severe if the patient has uncorrected hyperopia in addition to the convergence excess. Fortunately, correcting the hyperopia with plus lenses has the effect of reducing the esophoria at near, thus reducing the demand on negative fusional vergence. If the patient is not hyperopic, or if correction of the hyperopia does not fully correct the esophoria at near, additional plus lens power may be prescribed for near work only, either in the form of reading glasses or bifocal lenses.

Convergence insufficiency. The patient with convergence insufficiency, having a high exophoria at near, may complain of fatigue or even diplopia following prolonged close work. This is because constant use must be made of positive fusional vergence. The most effective treatment for convergence insufficiency usually involves visual training to build up the positive fusional vergence reserve. Many patients with apparent convergence insufficiency have what more properly is called "false convergence insufficiency." The problem is that in close work, the visual system does not respond fully to the stimulus to accommodation, and a lag of accommodation exists. For these patients, additional training to build up the facility of accommodation has been found helpful.

Divergence insufficiency. The patient having divergence insufficiency, being esophoric at both distance and near, may suffer symptoms of asthenopia, including headaches, for distance vision as well as for near vision. The treatment for this condition involves the full correction of any hyperopia, with possibly the prescription of base-out prism power for constant wear.

Divergence excess. The divergence excess patient, having a high exophoria at distance, may not suffer symptoms of eyestrain but may have occasional diplopia for distance vision tasks such as driving an automobile or viewing television. Some patients are unaware that anything is wrong until they are told that one eye occasionally turns outward. Because divergence excess is due to an abnormally high AC/A ratio, the use of minus lens power at distance (overcorrecting myopia or undercorrecting hyperopia) is often successful in reducing the exophoria. If the exophoria is also present at near, the use of base-in prism power should be considered.

Other binocular vision problems that should be considered as possible causes of asthenopia are vertical phoria, anisometropia, aniseikonia, and strabismus.

Vertical phoria. The presence of a vertical phoria, particularly if combined with inadequate vertical fusional reserves, may be responsible for headaches, diplopia, and other symptoms of eyestrain. Although visual training for the purpose of increasing the vertical fusional reserve range may be attempted, the great majority of vertical phorias respond only to the prescribing of vertical prism.

Anisometropia. Uncorrected anisometropia, even of moderate amount, may induce eyestrain by virtue of the fact that it is impossible for the accommodative mechanism to maintain clear images on both retinas at the same time. On the other hand, large amounts of anisometropia (i.e., 2.00D or more) seldom cause symptoms, as no effort is made to maintain single binocular vision.

Aniseikonia. Aniseikonia is defined as a difference in the sizes or shapes of the retinal images for the two eyes. This condition is usually the result of magnification differences brought about by corrective lenses and tends to cause symptoms of eyestrain and headache as well as perceptual distortions such as the tilting or curving of vertical objects.

Strabismus. Concomitant strabismus is an adaptation to a preexisting refractive or binocular vision problem, and if it is a successful adaptation, symptoms of eyestrain seldom occur. Paralytic strabismus occurring in early life seldom causes symptoms of eyestrain. However, paralytic strabismus occurring during adult life may cause severe asthenopia as a result of constant, intractable diplopia.

Headaches

Headaches can have numerous causes. However, when a person having a headache as a major complaint visits an optometrist, he or she usually has diagnosed the headache as being due to a visual problem. In many cases the cause of a headache problem can be determined solely on the basis of history. In other cases, well-chosen diagnostic procedures (many of which are included in a routine optometric examination) are a necessity. In *Headache: Diagnosis and Treatment*, the otolaryngologist Ryan (1954) listed 26 points to be included in a thorough headache history. The most important of these are

1. Patient's description of the headache.
2. Family history.
3. Headache's first occurrence.
4. Onset time (time of day).
5. Frequency.
6. Intensity.
7. Character.
8. Duration.
9. Cause of onset.
10. Location.

Headaches due to eyestrain

An important and obvious characteristic of eyestrain headaches is that they generally accompany prolonged use of the eyes. However, Drews (1954) has maintained that an eyestrain headache can occur the morning after prolonged use of the eyes. He calls this an "eye hangover" headache.

Most patients visiting an optometrist because of eyestrain headaches will have experienced the headache problem for a matter of weeks or months, but not for years. The pain is not so severe that the patient is driven to find the cause within a few days, but it is usually persistent enough so that the patient eventually gets around to looking into the problem. Often the origin of the problem may be traced to a change in jobs or other change in the patient's visual requirements. Eyestrain headaches tend to be of "medium" intensity, to be *dull* in character (as opposed to sharp, burning, or boring), and they tend to be located in the brow region or in the area around or behind the eyes. If prolonged use of the eyes gives rise to excessive *muscular tension*, the pain may be located in the back of the neck or in the occipital or vertical regions.

Some authors have attempted to relate headache location and severity to specific refractive and binocular vision anomalies. However, these discussions are usually not well documented by clinical data and are of limited practical importance. Once the practitioner has established the fact that the headaches occur in conjunction with the use of the eyes, the main problem will not be matching up symptoms to findings but determining whether or not the correction of the patient's refractive or binocular vision problem will also solve the headache problem.

To prescribe or not to prescribe?

One of the most difficult decisions an optometrist has to make is deciding whether or not to prescribe lenses for a patient having a previously uncorrected refractive error when the patient's only complaint is headaches. For some patients the correction of as little as 0.50D of hyperopia or hyperopic astigmatism will solve an eyestrain or headache problem. On the other hand, because the peak of the refractive error distribution curve for unselected subjects is in the neighborhood of 0.50D of hyperopia, it should be understood that not everyone who has 0.50D of hyperopia should necessarily wear correcting lenses.

The *placebo effect* of spectacle lenses was investigated by Malcolm Cholerton, a New Zealand optometrist, who prescribed plano lenses for a number of patients who complained of eyestrain but had little or no refractive error. In most cases his patients found that the lenses relieved their eyestrain for a matter of weeks or months, but the symptoms eventually returned.

Among the factors that should be taken into consideration when deciding whether to prescribe lenses for a patient who complains of an eyestrain or headache problem are the following:

1. Every effort should be made to establish whether the symptoms occur in relation to the use of the eyes. For example, if the patient is a student or a clerical worker, the practitioner should find out if the problem occurs during weekends or other times when close work is not done. Even if the answer is negative, the patient's refractive error is not necessarily the cause of the problem. Factors such as inadequate illumination, glare, and poor ventilation should be considered.

2. The patient's binocular vision status should not be ignored. High phorias at near (particularly esophoria) can be a source of eyestrain or headache, even if there is no significant refractive error.

3. The patient's age, occupation, visual habits, and other factors should be considered. For example, an accountant is more apt to require a correction for a low refractive error than is a farmer or an outdoor worker who spends little time at close work.

4. If medical and dental evaluations have found no cause for a patient's headache problem, prescribing glasses to correct the refractive error

may well be the least expensive (and certainly the least invasive) method of coming to grips with the problem. If glasses solve the problem, they may obviate the need for an extended diagnostic workup, which could include procedures such as angiograms, electroencephalograms, and CAT scans.

5. "Loaner" lenses, consisting of low-power spheres, low-power cylinders, or low-power prisms, often prove to be of great assistance in deciding whether to prescribe for low refractive errors. After a trial of several weeks, a decision often can be made whether to prescribe "permanent" lenses. The possibility of a placebo effect, however, should be kept in mind.

Nonocular Headaches

Many patients who have headaches that they believe are due to eyestrain will be found to have headaches due to other causes (Smith, tape no. 47). A large proportion of headaches are vascular in nature. Smith has pointed out that vascular headaches tend to occur on the basis of age: *migraine headaches* tend to occur in young adults; *hypertension headaches* tend to occur in the middle-aged; and headaches due to *temporal arteritis* tend to occur in older patients. Other types of headaches the optometrist should be aware of are muscular contraction headaches, cluster headaches, nasal sinusitis headaches, and headaches due to trigeminal neuralgia.

Migraine

The *classic migraine* syndrome consists of (1) a visual aura, (2) a unilateral, throbbing headache, and (3) a feeling of nausea. The visual aura has been variously described as a "scintillating scotoma," a "fortification scotoma," which expands as an everenlarging fortification, and as "heat waves." Many migraine sufferers refer to migraine headaches as "sick headaches" and find that they can abort the headache, once the visual aura occurs, by going to bed or by drinking a cup of black coffee.

The visual aura is confined to one side of the visual field and is due to the constriction of the branches of the internal carotid artery supplying the visual cortex. The headache is caused first by dilation and then by congestion of the branches of the external carotid artery and the meningeal arteries; the nausea is due to stimulation of the vagus nerve. Troost (1978) has described what he calls *common migraine*. This is a headache in which nausea is the predominant symptom, and the prodromal visual aura does not appear.

Migraine headaches must be diagnosed entirely on the basis of history and symptoms because there are no positive physical or neurological findings. The fact that migraine headaches tend to be inherited may help in the differential diagnosis. Treatment of migraine includes both prophylactic (preventive) and symptomatic medications.

Hypertension

According to Laragh (1974), hypertension is the single biggest causative factor of death and occurs in 20 percent of the adult population, half of whom have hypertensive heart disease. Smith (tape no. 47) has characterized hypertension headaches as being severe, occurring early in the morning, and usually being present on awakening and disappearing at some time during the day. He reports that many patients find that they can make the headaches go away by drinking a cup of black coffee immediately on arising, and that some patients even go to the extent of keeping a hot plate and a pot of coffee on a bedside table. Large-scale clinical trials held during the past decade have indicated that mortality resulting from hypertension can be significantly reduced by early treatment. (Further discussion of hypertension can be found in Chapter 6.)

Temporal arteritis

Temporal arteritis, also known as cranial arteritis and giant cell arteritis, has been described by Henkind and Chambers (1979) as the most frequently misdiagnosed extraocular cause of preventable visual loss, having an exceedingly high incidence of ocular involvement. The pathological process is a chronic inflammation of the cranial arteries (particularly the temporal arteries), in which giant cells are found in the inflammatory exudate. Most temporal arteritis sufferers are older people, beyond the age of 55 or 60 years.

Symptoms of temporal arteritis include headache, a general feeling of malaise and loss of appetite, scalp tenderness (noted particularly when combing the hair), and claudication of the jaw while chewing. By interfering with the blood supply to the vessels supplying the optic nerve, temporal arteritis often leads to a condition known as *ischemic optic neuropathy*. This is likely to cause a transient loss of vision, known as *amaurosis fugax*, and may lead to occlusion of the central artery of the retina.

Because the consequences of temporal arteritis are so severe, optometrists should suspect its presence whenever an older patient complains of a debilitating headache and transient loss of vision.

Diagnosis of temporal arteritis is made on the basis of an increased blood sedimentation rate and by the presence of giant cells in the inflammatory exudate as determined by temporal artery biopsy (Smith, tape no. 64). Treatment of temporal arteritis, as described by Smith, is the aggressive use of systemic steroids. Smith has emphasized that if inadequate use of steroids is made, there is an increasing chance of closure of the central artery of the retina.

Muscular contraction headache

Muscular contraction headache, also known as *tension* headache, is described by many authors as the most common form of headache. Ryan (1954) described tension headache as a vascular headache, occurring usually in the letdown phase that follows a prolonged period of stress. He described it as either a vicelike pain in the forehead, a pain located in the vertex, or a pain in the occipital area accompanied by muscular stiffness in the neck.

Many authors consider muscular contraction headache to have a psychogenic origin. Prophylactic treatment is usually directed toward altering the patient's behavior. Symptomatic treatment includes the use of analgesics, muscle relaxants, and sedatives. Because eyestrain headaches tend to occur in the same areas (frontal, vertical, and occipital) as those described for muscular contraction headache, it is likely that muscular contraction may be a contributing cause of an eyestrain headache.

Cluster headache

Cluster headache, also known as *histamine cephalalgia*, is a severe, boring, unilateral headache occurring in the temporal region and often accompanied by ipsilateral lacrimation and nasal congestion. Most sufferers of cluster headache are middle-aged men. The term *cluster* is used because of the tendency for one or more headaches to occur daily within a short period of time. Attacks typically occur at night and are more apt to occur while lying down; sometimes they can be aborted by getting up and walking around or even by sitting up in bed. Patients often describe the pain as unbearable. Treatment, particularly prophylactic, is similar to that used for migraine.

Nasal sinusitis headache

According to Ryan (1954), headache is the most predominant symptom of acute nasal sinusitis, but not of chronic nasal sinusitis. The pain is most often in the frontal region and is most pronounced when stooping down. Other symptoms include coughing due to postnasal drip, low-grade fever, and a temporary loss of the sense of smell.

Trigeminal neuralgia

Trigeminal neuralgia, also known as *tic douloureux*, is an extremely sharp, piercing, knifelike pain of sudden onset in the facial region. It can be due to inflammation of any of the three divisions of the trigeminal nerve, but it least commonly occurs in the ophthalmic division. As described by Smith (tape no. 47), trigeminal neuralgia is characterized by a *trigger zone*, and the pain can be brought about by touching a specific area of the face in washing the face, cleaning the teeth, or shaving. Many sufferers of this condition, who are usually middle-aged or older, live in a constant state of fear, dreading the occurrence of the next attack.

There is little danger of confusing trigeminal neuralgia with other headache types, in that it occurs in the facial area (usually in the areas of distribution of the maxillary and mandibular divisions) and involves a trigger zone. Anticonvulsive agents, including phenytoin (Dilantin) and carbamazepine (Tegretol), have been found to be effective forms of treatment.

External Eye Symptoms

Among the external eye symptoms most often given as patient complaints are itching and burning of the eyes, pain or foreign body sensation, sensitivity to light, excessive tearing, and a feeling of dryness. In many cases these external ocular symptoms are manifestations of asthenopia and can be relieved by the correction of the patient's refractive error or binocular vision anomaly. In other cases the symptoms are due to pathological processes involving the ocular adnexa, such as conjunctivitis, blepharitis and other lid conditions, and tear film deficiencies. In a few cases they may be due to more threatening conditions, including uveitis and glaucoma.

Itching and burning

Symptoms of mild itching and burning may accompany small amounts of hyperopia, astigmatism, or a binocular vision problem. These symptoms may occur in conjunction with hyperemia of the lid margins and conjunctiva. In many cases the correction of the refractive error or binocular vision problem will not only relieve the itching and burning but may also relieve the hyperemia. Why this occurs is not well understood: one possibility is that a part of asthenopia is a triggering of the *local axon reflex*. Efforts to compensate for the refractive error may stimulate sensory nerve endings and, therefore, be responsible for a local increase in blood supply, manifested as hyperemia of the conjunctiva and lid margins. This hyperemia is responsible for sensations of itching and burning and causes the individual to rub his or her eyes. It is thought that eye rubbing can increase the bacterial content of the tears to the point that an inflammatory process may occur (conjunctivitis or blepharitis). It has even been suggested that one of the main factors in the etiology of styes may be the rubbing of the eyes due to a small refractive error.

Blepharitis. A common cause of itching and burning of the eyelids is blepharitis, which is an inflammatory process affecting the lid margins. In the *seborrheic* form, numerous small scales, or "dandruff," may be seen clinging to the lid margins. Using the slit lamp, these scales are most easily seen by asking the patient to close his eyes and focusing the wide beam along the upper and lower lid margins. Treatment involves washing the hair and scalp with a shampoo such as Selsun and removing the scales from the lid margins with a damp cotton applicator or with half-strength Selsun or baby shampoo.

In *ulcerative* blepharitis a bacterial infection is present, the most common cause being *staphylococcus*. The ulcerated areas along the lid margin lead to loss of eyelashes. The presence of the bacterium and its toxins in the lower conjunctival sac during the night may cause symptoms of the lids sticking together on arising, and it may lead to conjunctivitis and superficial keratitis involving the lower portion of the cornea. If untreated, a chronic form of blepharitis and conjunctivitis may result and may persist for months or even years.

Allergic conjunctivitis. Intense itching is the most prominent symptom of allergic conjunctivitis. A mild, nonspecific form of conjunctivitis, known as *atopic*, or hay fever conjunctivitis, occurs in association with allergic rhinitis. Symptoms include itching, tearing, and redness of the eyes along with edema of the bulbar conjunctiva.

Vernal conjunctivitis is a form of allergic conjunctivitis occurring mainly in the spring and summer months and most commonly affecting young males. The main symptom of vernal conjunctivitis is extreme itching ("if there is no itching, it isn't vernal"). In addition, there is a stringy or ropey discharge. Vernal conjunctivitis can occur in both palpebral and limbal forms. In the palpebral form, giant cobblestone papillae are found in the upper tarsal conjunctiva, while in the limbal form, papillae occur as thickened, gelatinous opacifications in the conjunctiva surrounding the limbus.

Treatment of nonspecific allergic conjunctivitis, according to Vaughan and Asbury (1977), includes local instillation of vasoconstrictors, cold compresses to relieve the itching, and antihistamines taken orally. This form of treatment may also suffice for mild cases of vernal conjunctivitis, but for the more severe cases Allansmith (1978) recommends what she calls "pulses" of steroids: topical prednisolone is given for a period of 4 days, which usually controls symptoms sufficiently to allow the use of other forms of therapy.

Bacterial conjunctivitis. The most prominent symptoms of a bacterial conjunctivitis are irritation and redness of the eyes, a mucopurulent discharge, and complaints of the eyes sticking together in the morning. Treatment is by topical application of antimicrobial agents, the choice of agent depending on the responsible bacterium.

Pain or foreign body sensation

A patient who reports ocular pain will usually be able to state, on questioning, whether the pain is a superficial, foreign body pain or a deep-seated pain. If a foreign body is present, it will usually be embedded in the upper tarsal conjunctiva and can be removed by everting the upper lid and carefully dislodging it with a sterile cotton applicator. If a foreign body is embedded in the corneal epithelium, it sometimes may be dislodged by the use of irrigating solution. If this fails, the patient should be referred for removal of the foreign body with a foreign body spud.

A foreign body sensation in the absence of a foreign body may be due to a corneal abrasion or recurrent corneal erosion. In either case, staining of the precorneal tear film with fluorescein should make it possible to find the cause of the problem.

Deep-seated ocular pain may be caused by more severe conditions, including corneal ulcers, acute iritis, and acute glaucoma. An important indication of an internal (as opposed to an external) condition is the presence of *ciliary injection*. This is a lilac-colored injection of the deep conjunctival vessels fanning out from the limbus, as opposed to *conjunctival injection*, which is a bright red injection of superficial anastomosing vessels and is more prominent toward the fornix. Visual acuity is also an important guide. A corneal ulcer, iritis, or acute glaucoma will usually result in lowered visual acuity, whereas a foreign body or abrasion will not.

Sensitivity to light

The triad of pain, photophobia, and lacrimation is the well-known reponse to stimulation of the ophthalmic division of the fifth cranial nerve. Any condition just described, in which pain is a symptom, may be accompanied by a complaint of increased sensitivity to light. Conditions in which sensitivity to light is a predominant symptom are epidemic keratoconjunctivitis and congenital glaucoma.

Epidemic keratoconjunctivitis. This is a highly contagious form of viral conjunctivitis, beginning as an acute follicular conjunctivitis with pain, injection, and tearing. After about 7 days, raised epithelial lesions, staining with fluorescein, may be found scattered over the cornea. At this stage and in the stage to follow, photophobia may be a marked symptom. After approximately 7 more days, subepithelial opacities will be found under the epithelial lesions. In the early stages, only supportive treatment is used (astringent drops and cold compresses), but once the subepithelial opacities occur, steroid treatment may be indicated if marked acuity loss is present (Dawson, 1979).

Congenital glaucoma. Extreme sensitivity to light and excessive tearing in the first few months or years of life should cause the practitioner to suspect the presence of congenital glaucoma. These symptoms may occur prior to a noticeable enlargement in the size of the eye (buphthalmos) or glaucomatous cupping of the optic nerve head.

Excessive tearing

Apart from those conditions in which excessive tearing occurs as a result of stimulation of the ophthalmic division of the trigeminal nerve, it may be caused by any condition that interferes with the lacrimal drainage system. These conditions tend to occur at the extremes of age: in infants as stenosis of the nasolacrimal duct and in older adults as senile ectropion.

Stenosis of the nasolacrimal duct. If one of the nasolacrimal ducts fails to open in early life, dacryocystitis (inflammation of the nasolacrimal sac) may result. In addition to treatment with antimicrobial agents, probing of the nasolacrimal duct may be necessary.

Senile ectropion. In an older individual, loss of tone of the orbicularis muscle may allow the lower lid to become everted, or turned outward. When this occurs, the inferior punctum fails to make contact with the marginal tear strip, so tears overflow the lid and run down the cheek. If an older patient complains of always having to carry a handkerchief to wipe away the tears, ectropion is almost sure to be the cause. Surgery designed to shorten the tarsal portion of the lower lid is indicated.

Feeling of dryness

A complaint of a feeling of dryness of the eyes can be due to any of a number of tear film abnormalities. Lemp (1980) discussed these abnormalities in terms of aqueous deficiency, mucin deficiency, lipid abnormalities, and lid-surfacing abnormalities. More serious possible causes of a feeling of dryness are degenerations and dystrophies affecting the anterior portion of the cornea, one of the most common of which is Fuchs's dystrophy.

Aqueous deficiency. Also known as *keratoconjunctivitis sicca*, aqueous deficiency is an absolute or partial deficiency in aqueous tear production. In addition to the complaint of a feeling of dryness, the patient may complain of a sandy or gritty feeling in the eyes, a burning sensation, and sensitivity to light. Keratoconjunctivitis sicca occurs most often in older women, although it can occur in men and in younger women. If combined with dry mouth and rheumatoid arthritis, it is known as *Sjögren's syndrome*.

Clinical signs of keratoconjunctivitis sicca include (1) a deficient marginal tear strip, (2) excessive debris in the tear film, (3) mucous threads and filaments in the tear film, and (4) poor tear production when measured by means of the Schirmer tear test. The presence of mucous threads and filaments in the tear film is due not to excessive mucin production but to the lack of sufficient aqueous tear production to wash away the mucus. The main form of treatment for aqueous tear deficiency is the use of artificial tears. These can be used several times a day, if necessary, to maintain ocular comfort. In severe cases, particularly if filamentary keratitis is present, therapeutic soft contact lenses are sometimes used.

Mucin deficiency. The presence of a mucin deficiency can be determined by the use of the precorneal film breakup test, described in Chapter 7. A precorneal film breakup time of less than about 10 seconds indicates the presence of a mucin deficiency. However, before concluding that a mucin deficiency is present, the breakup test should be repeated a number of times. If the breakup occurs repeatedly in the same area, an epithelial defect rather than a mucin deficiency may be the cause (Lemp, 1980).

The most common cause of mucin deficiency is a reduced goblet cell population due to avitaminosis A. A poor breakup time may be caused by a number of other conditions, including aqueous tear deficiencies and lipid abnormalities. Treatment for mucin deficiency involves the use of artificial tears, particularly those (called *mucomimetics*) designed to have an action similar to that of mucin.

Lipid abnormalities. Chronic blepharitis may cause a qualitative change in the secretion of the Meibomian glands. This causes the release of free fatty acids and, therefore, almost instantaneous dry spot formation (Lemp, 1980).

Lid-surfacing abnormalities. Normal blinking has the effect of constantly resurfacing the tear film. If the lids do not close completely when blinking due to paralysis of the seventh nerve, dry areas may occur in the lower portion of the cornea. Other causes of lid-surfacing abnormalities are pinguecula, which can prevent the lids from resurfacing the limbal area of the cornea with mucin, and the presence of a hard contact lens, which may cause a "bridging effect." The contact lens prevents the lid from resurfacing the cornea and the conjunctiva at the nasal and temporal limbal areas, causing the well-known "3 and 9 o'clock staining."

Disturbances of Vision

Disturbances of vision that may be reported in the history include seeing "spots" before the eyes, light flashes, temporary loss of vision, a "curtain" coming down in front of the eyes, distortion in sizes and shapes of objects, and the appearance of halos and other entoptic phenomena.

Spots before the eyes

This complaint may be due to the presence of vitreous floaters occurring as a result of liquefaction of the vitreous or more serious conditions, such as pars planitis or retinal hemorrhages.

Vitreous floaters. When the vitreous has become partially liquified, which tends to occur in myopes and older people, fine vitreous opacities may cast shadows on the retina. These shadows are most commonly seen when looking at the sky or at some other unstructured background. Patients describe them as spots, strings, cobwebs, rings, or as having the appearance of strings of bacteria seen under a microscope. They move across the visual field when eye movements are made, tending to move faster than the eyes move. These floaters are called *muscae volitantes*, Latin for "flying gnats." Although these floaters are completely innocuous, other varieties of vitreous opacities have a more serious prognosis.

Pars planitis. This is a form of chronic anterior uveitis affecting the pars plana of the ciliary body and occurring usually in younger adults. The only symptom may be a complaint of floating spots due to the presence of inflammatory cells in the retro-lental space or the anterior vitreous. Vaughan and Asbury (1977) describe pars planitis as usually remaining stationary and gradually improving over a 5- to 10-year period. Complications of pars planitis include posterior subcapsular cataracts and cystoid macular edema.

Retinal hemorrhages. Hemorrhages within the retina or into the vitreous may elicit complaints of "red spots." Conditions in which retinal or vitreous hemorrhages commonly occur include diabetic retinopathy, hypertensive retinopathy, and the various blood dyscrasias. Any complaint of red spots in the visual field warrants a through examination of the retina and vitreous.

Light flashes

A complaint of light flashes, flashing lights, or light streaks lasting only a fraction of a second may indicate the presence of a vitreous detachment. The vitreous body seldom detaches anteriorly, where the vitreous base straddles the ora serrata, but posterior vitreous detachment is a relatively common occurrence in eyes in which partial vitreous liquefaction has taken place. The liquified, posterior portion of the vitreous collapses, and the ringlike posterior attachment at the optic nerve head becomes detached. Posterior vitreous detachment and collapse is a common finding in older people and occurs in the majority of aphakic eyes.

Straatsma, Foos, and Kreiger (1980) have called attention to the fact that following posterior vitreous detachment, movement of the vitreous body exerts traction on the vitreous base. This arc of vitreous traction on the anterior portion of the retina causes the characteristic *temporal arc of flashes* reported by patients who have posterior vitreous detachment, and it increases the likelihood of retinal tears. The presence of a retinal tear, particularly if it is a full-thickness tear with a flap or free operculum, may lead to a retinal detachment. When a patient complains of light flashes, a thorough peripheral retinal examination is indicated.

Light flashes due to posterior vitreous detachment must be differentiated from the *scintillating scotoma* of migraine by careful questioning. An additional cause of light flashes is an irritative lesion of the visual cortex. Harrington (1976) points out that even though these are present in just one-half of the visual field, patients often associate them with just one eye.

Temporary loss of vision

Temporary or transient loss of vision can be due to a number of causes, including migraine, multiple sclerosis, carotid artery occlusive disease, and temporal arteritis.

Migraine. The classic migraine syndrome, as already discussed, involves a visual aura followed by a "sick headache." Although some people will report this visual aura as "heat waves" or "light flashes," others will report it as a temporary loss of vision. As in all cases of migraine, the differential diagnosis depends on a thorough history.

Multiple sclerosis. Often one of the early symptoms of multiple sclerosis is a temporary loss of vision. This is due to retrobulbar neuritis and takes the form of a positive scotoma—a scotoma of which the patient is aware. The scotoma may be ameboid in shape, changing shape and disappearing, then reappearing, and usually involving the fixation area. If the patient is seen during the attack, the scotoma may be plotted on the tangent screen. In some cases of multiple sclerosis, papillitis may be present, but in others the inflammation is confined to the retrobulbar portion of the optic nerve, with the result that there are no abnormal ophthalmoscopic signs, and therefore "neither the doctor nor the patient sees anything."

Although migraine and multiple sclerosis tend to affect young or middle-aged people, carotid artery occlusive disease and temporal arteritis are most common beyond the age of 55 or 60.

Carotid artery occlusive disease. Carotid artery stenosis or occlusion occurs as a result of the deposition of atheromatous plaques within the internal carotid arteries (more often the left internal carotid) just distal to the carotid sinus. The most common ocular symptom is *amaurosis fugax*—a sudden, transient, painless loss of vision. Vision returns within seconds or minutes. The vision loss has been found to be the result of the migration of emboli consisting of platelets, fibrin, and cholesterol into the retinal arterial tree. If a patient is seen during an attack, both white and yellow emboli may be seen: the white emboli are platelets and fibrin, whereas the yellow emboli, called *Hollenhorst plaques*, are cholesterol. According to Henkind and Chambers (1979), 5–10 percent of the patients having carotid artery occlusive disease will suffer an occlusion of the central retinal artery or of a branch artery, with consequent permanent visual loss.

Temporal arteritis. Temporal arteritis, already discussed, is a relatively common cause of loss of vision in elderly people. Loss of vision may result from closure of the central artery of the retina; permanent visual loss may be preceded by one or more attacks of transient loss of vision.

Management of temporary loss of vision. Because the possible consequences of temporary loss of vision are so threatening, any patient who presents with this symptom (unless a definitive diagnosis of migraine can be made) should be referred to the appropriate practitioner for consultation. Other, less common causes of amaurosis fugax are Raynaud's disease and the aortic arch syndrome (also called "pulseless disease").

Curtain in front of the eyes

The "textbook" cause of a complaint that a curtain appears to come down in front of the eyes is a retinal detachment. The presence of a detachment should be verified by peripheral field testing and by indirect ophthalmoscopy. A *retinal detachment* is an ophthalmic emergency requiring immediate referral.

An additional cause of this complaint is *transient retinal ischemia*, due usually to either carotid artery occlusive disease or temporal arteritis. This occurs if the transient loss of vision is not complete and lasts only a few seconds.

Distortion of objects

Occasionally a patient will complain that objects appear to be distorted, either in terms of size or shape. Both of these conditions are indicated by the term *metamorphopsia*.

Distortion in size of objects may be either a perceptual or an optical phenomenon. Occasionally the patient's perception of environmental visual clues to size constancy breaks down, and the individual may be alarmed that objects such as people's faces appear to be larger or smaller than they think they should be. Optical factors that can be responsible for size distortion include newly prescribed plus or minus lenses (increasing or decreasing the sizes of familiar objects) and *accommodative micropsia*. The latter term refers to a minification of the retinal image that occurs with excessive accommodation.

If a patient reports that small objects appear to be misshappen or that a small object seems to disappear or to move when it is fixated, macular disease should be suspected. These symptoms of metamorphopsia can often be corroborated by means of the Amsler charts or by having the patient view a sheet of graph paper having a central fixation point. If macular disease such as serous detachment or macular degeneration is present, some of the lines on the chart or graph paper, near the fixation point, may appear to be wiggly, wavy, or absent. Additional testing for macular disease involves color vision testing with either the HRR test or the Farnsworth D–15 (looking for either a red-green or blue-yellow anomaly) and a careful inspection of the macular area with a slit lamp and Hruby lens.

Halos

The presence of rainbow halos around lights is one of the classic symptoms of angle closure glaucoma. These halos are often seen at night, when the pupil is at its largest. They are usually thought to be due to corneal edema, although Emsley (1963) quoted Maddox as saying that they are due to tiny hillocks raised in the corneal epithelium. Emsley described a simple procedure for differentiating glaucomatous halos from physiological halos caused by the radial structure of the crystalline lens. If a vertically oriented stenopaic slit is moved back and forth, horizontally, in front of the pupil, a halo caused by the radial structure of the crystalline lens will appear to rotate with a wheel like motion as the slit is moved. However, if the halo is caused by corneal edema in glaucoma, the halo will not rotate.

Double Vision

A patient who complains of double vision should be asked to describe (1) whether the two images are actually apart or blend into one another and (2) whether the two images are separated vertically or horizontally. Although most complaints of double

vision are the result of binocular vision problems, other possible causes of this complaint are uncorrected refractive errors and monocular diplopia.

Uncorrected refractive errors

In answer to the questions stated above, an occasional patient will report that the two images are not completely apart but tend to blend into one another. Upon refraction, the complaint may be found to be due to uncorrected astigmatism or even uncorrected hyperopia not compensated by accommodation, or to presbyopia.

Monocular diplopia

If monocular diplopia is suspected to be the cause of a complaint of double vision, the patient should be asked if it occurs when one eye is closed. The classic cause of monocular diplopia is *keratoconus*. In addition to monocular diplopia, keratoconus patients may complain of poor vision with their glasses in spite of reasonably good visual acuity. Clinical signs of keratoconus include a thinning and protrusion of the apex of the cornea seen with the slit lamp, very steep (perhaps off-the-scale) keratometer readings, and a swirling retinoscope reflex. The protrusion of the cone (Munson's sign) may also be seen as an indentation in the lower lid when the patient looks downward.

Binocular vision problems

If double vision occurs only occasionally, the patient may be found to have a large heterophoria at distance or at near (or both), with an inadequate fusional vergence range. For example, a patient who has divergence excess may experience occasional diplopia for distance visual tasks such as driving, and a patient having convergence insufficiency may complain of diplopia following prolonged reading or close work. If occasional vertical diplopia is experienced, the obvious cause would be a vertical phoria with inadequate vertical fusional reserves.

Patients with long-standing strabismus seldom complain of double vision, having long ago adapted to the condition by developing suppression, eccentric fixation, amblyopia, or anomalous retinal correspondence (or a combination of these conditions). However, if double vision has begun only recently, a recently acquired muscle paralysis or paresis should be suspected. In older patients, particular attention should be paid to the possibility of a vertical component in the diplopia: a likely cause of the diplopia is a cerebral vascular accident such as a ruptured aneurism in the Circle of Willis. In any case, any patient complaining of a recently acquired, unexplained diplopia should be referred for medical evaluation.

Deviating Eye

This complaint most often is made by a parent regarding a child. Typically, the parent complains that the eye turns *inward*. One relatively common cause of this complaint regarding a preschool child is *epicanthus*, a condition in which one or both inner canthal areas are partly covered by a fold of skin. As long as the practitioner has ascertained that the eye does not really turn in, it is only necessary to reassure the parent that the child is not cross-eyed and that the condition will almost certainly go away by about the age of 6.

If it is found that one eye does turn inward, the practitioner should complete a strabismus workup on the child. Often the esotropia will be found to be accompanied by several diopters of hyperopia. When this condition (*accommodative esotropia*) is present, correction of the hyperopia typically straightens the eyes. Because the child usually has a high AC/A ratio, a bifocal prescription may be necessary to keep the eyes straight for near work. If hyperopia is not found in the refraction, a cycloplegic refraction should be done. If hyperopia is not found by cycloplegic refraction, the child will almost surely be found to have anomalous retinal correspondence, and orthoptics and/or strabismus surgery will be required. However, surgery alone seldom provides anything more than a cosmetic cure. For a functional cure, orthoptics plus surgery is usually needed.

Protruding Eye

A parent may complain that one of the child's eyes appears to protrude or to be larger than the other. Although it is possible for one eye to actually be larger than the other (indicating congenital or infantile glaucoma in the larger eye or microphthalmos in the smaller eye), it is also possible that the eye that looks larger is a protruding (exophthalmic) eye. When this occurs, a tumor or other mass affecting the orbit or the optic nerve should be suspected.

A related complaint is that one eye appears to be partially closed or squinting. This could be congenital ptosis or congenital Horner's syndrome. The latter condition involves unilateral ptosis, miosis, and apparent enophthalmos (with the possible addition of heterochromia irides), and it is due to a lesion of the sympathetic pathway supplying the eye.

Unequal Pupil Size

It is not uncommon for a patient to discover that one pupil is noticeably larger than the other, a condition known as *essential anisocoria*. Smith ("The Pupil") has suggested that when this occurs, the patient should be requested to bring in all his old photographs so the practitioner can inspect the best of them with the indirect ophthalmoscope lens. Often these photographs show that the condition has been present for many years, with no pathological consequence.

A common cause of unequal pupil size is *Adie's tonic pupil*. This condition, occurring mainly in young women, involves the pupil of one eye constricting only very slowly in response to light. The pupil, however, does constrict in response to a near stimulus. Smith ("The Pupil") says that the "moment of truth" in the differential diagnosis of Adie's pupil is the very slow *redilation* of the pupil after a short period of near fixation. He suggests that the patient hold the reading material, to assure that the near pupillary response will occur. Adie's syndrome is caused by a lesion of the ciliary ganglion. No treatment is required. More serious causes of unequal pupil size are discussed in Chapter 6.

Reading or Learning Problems

A parent often brings a child to the optometrist with the complaint that the child is not progressing well in school. Even though the ability to read and learn is known to be dependent on a large number of factors, it is obvious that reading requires seeing, so we should not be surprised that many parents think first of the optometrist when a reading problem presents itself.

Even though many optometrists are now engaging in the diagnosis and therapy of developmental and perceptual-motor anomalies, the optometrist should not neglect the responsibility of ruling out the possibility that a refractive or binocular vision anomaly may play a part in a child's learning problem.

Refractive anomalies. The relationship between refractive state and reading ability is discussed in Chapter 3. In this discussion it is pointed out that hyperopes are more likely to have reading or learning problems than myopes. The uncorrected hyperope must use an excessive amount of accommodation for near work, whereas the uncorrected myope need use relatively little accommodation. The problem for the hyperope is not the effort involved in the greater amount of accommodation required, but in the effect this has on the relationship between accommodative convergence and accommodation.

The excessive amount of accommodation required by the hyperope brings into play an excessive amount of accommodative convergence, which may result in esophoria at near. If this occurs, negative fusional vergence must be used to avoid diplopia. Negative fusional vergence is not a well-developed function, and its constant use (along with the use of excessive accommodation) can result in symptoms of asthenopia and a distaste for reading and other close work.

Phorias. In a study by Kelly (1957) discussed in Chapter 3, it was found that myopes, whether exophoric or esophoric, tended to have above-average reading scores, whereas hyperopes having exophoria at near had good reading scores, but hyperopes who were esophoric at near had mean reading scores that were significantly low.

It must be understood, however, that relationships between reading or learning ability and refractive and binocular vision anomalies are not strong enough to have predictive value—one cannot predict whether a child will be a good reader on the basis of the child's refractive or binocular vision status.

Strabismus. Studies by Eames (1948) and Cassin (1976) have shown an association between reading failure and the presence of strabismus. However, this relationship is in all probability a result of the fact that reading failure tends to be associated with hyperopia: there is a strong relationship between strabismus and hyperopia in children. Most strabismic children have a combination of high hyperopia and strabismus.

Color vision anomalies. It is well known that the "big four" color vision anomalies—protanopia, deuteranopia, protanomaly, and deuteranomaly—occur in about 8 percent of males and in about 0.5 percent of females. Zuba (1974) has called attention to the fact that color coding is often used in progressive teaching programs and that the classroom teacher may not be aware that some children are at a disadvantage when these materials are used because of the presence of color vision anomalies. Espinda (1973), a school psychologist, found that teachers reporting on children with difficulty acquiring color discrimination skills often believed that these problems suggested intellectual inadequacy. Nearly all of these children were male and they had varying degrees of difficulty in mastering the tasks of a color-laden kindergarten and primary school curriculum.

Color vision screening should be included in the examination of all young patients, particularly if the child is found to have a reading problem. (Color vision testing and color vision counseling are discussed in Chapter 6.)

Study Questions

1. List the items of information that should be obtained in each of the following parts of the patient history: (a) ocular history; (b) health history and medications; (c) family and ocular health history; (d) chief complaint.

2. How would you describe a typical "eyestrain headache" in terms of (a) frequency? (b) intensity? (c) character? (d) duration? (e) cause of onset? (f) location?

3. How do seborrheic and ulcerative forms of blepharitis differ in terms of (a) clinical appearance? (b) cause? (c) treatment?

4. What are the possible causes for double vision? For each of these causes, what question or questions would you ask the patient to support or rule out that particular cause as a diagnosis?

5. If an adult who complains of blurred distance vision is found to have a change in refraction in the direction of increased myopia or decreased hyperopia, on what basis would you consider that a possible cause of the refractive change is diabetes as opposed to nuclear sclerosis of the lens?

6. During the history, what complaint or complaints would you expect to hear from a patient having (a) myopia? (b) hyperopia? (c) astigmatism?

7. Briefly describe the content of each of the four basic components of a problem-oriented system of optometric records: (a) the defined data base; (b) the complete problem list; (c) initial treatment plans; (d) progress notes.

8. List the patient-reported symptoms that would cause you to suspect each of the following forms of headache: (a) hypertension; (b) temporal arteritis.

9. What complaints would you expect to hear during the history if the patient has (a) convergence insufficiency? (b) convergence excess? (c) divergence insufficiency? (d) divergence excess?

10. (a) Describe the symptoms reported during the history that would lead you to make a tentative diagnosis of classic migraine headache. (b) How do the symptoms of common migraine differ from those of classic migraine?

11. Although a superficial pain in the eye is most likely due to the presence of a foreign body trapped underneath the upper eyelid or to a corneal abrasion, what conditions may be responsible for a deep-seated pain in the eye?

12. If a patient complains of a temporary loss of vision, how would the patient's age assist you in determining the cause?

13. What three parts should be included in each initial treatment plan?

14. Progress notes are intended for use with patients who will be seen by the practitioner on a number of occasions. When applied to optometric practice, on what kinds of patients is the use of progress notes most likely to be appropriate?

15. (a) What condition did Donders conclude was the cause of asthenopia? (b) What form of treatment did Donders recommend for this condition?

16. What symptoms would cause you to consider that a patient's headaches may be diagnosed as (a) cluster headaches? (b) muscular contraction headaches?

17. What complaints would you expect to hear during the history if the patient has an uncorrected vertical phoria?

18. What questions would you ask to determine whether a patient's complaint of temporary loss of vision is due to (a) migraine? (b) multiple sclerosis? (c) temporal arteritis? (d) carotid artery occlusive disease?

19. On the basis of each of the following symptoms reported during the history, what condition or conditions would you consider as a possible cause or causes? (a) itching of the eyes; (b) complaints of the eyelids sticking together in the mornings; (c) excessive tearing; (d) a feeling of dryness of the eyes.

20. What complaints would you expect to hear during the history from a patient who has strabismus?

CHAPTER 6

The Preliminary Examination

Upon completion of the history, the examiner is in a position to make a tentative diagnosis of the patient's problem or problems. During the preliminary examination, the examiner's approach should continue to be problem oriented. Problems brought to the examiner's attention during the history should be actively investigated and evaluated, and additional problems should be anticipated.

The purpose of the preliminary examination is to detect any gross anomaly such as a high refractive error, a binocular vision anomaly, a disturbance of ocular motility, or an ocular or systemic disease. Many of the procedures included in the preliminary examination are observations rather than measurements. These observations show the practitioner what to look for during the refractive examination and the binocular vision examination.

ORGANIZATION OF TESTING PROCEDURES

The procedures making up the preliminary examination should be organized so they can be done quickly, with a minimum of time lost between procedures. The practitioner should attempt to develop the skill of going quickly from one procedure to the next, working rapidly without giving the patient the impression of being rushed or of not allowing adequate time. Even while working rapidly, the practitioner will find it possible to inform the patient of the purpose of each test, making the whole experience an interesting one for the patient.

Physical Plan

The order of testing procedures to some extent depends on the type and location of instrumentation used for each test. Larger pieces of equipment should be located conveniently so the patient is not required to move from one chair to another several times during the examination. This is not only an inconvenience for the patient but wastes much of the practitioner's valuable time. Also, if an instrument is not conveniently located, the practitioner may decide not to use this instrument "unless it is really needed." This applies particularly to visual field testing equipment. If a tangent screen or other visual field testing equipment is located in a room other than the optometrist's examination room, the practitioner may tend to avoid using it on a regular basis. (However, if a trained technician or assistant does the visual field screening using an Autoplot or computerized screening instrumentation, it is desirable, of course, to have the instrument in a separate room.)

A convenient examination room arrangement is shown in Figure 6.1. The biomicroscope is located on an arm of the refracting unit, along with the

Figure 6.1 A suggested examination room arrangement.

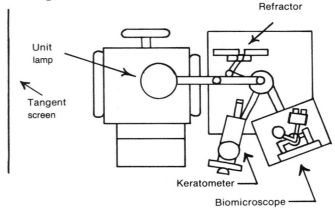

137

keratometer. The tangent screen is located to the right of the refracting unit (or it could be behind the refracting unit), so it is necessary only to swing the chair around 90 degrees (or 180 degrees), adjust the height, and begin testing. The refracting unit light is an effective source of illumination for visual field testing and can be quickly swung into place.

The location of the tonometer will depend on the type of instrumentation used. An electronic tonometer can be conveniently mounted on a shelf near the refracting unit. If an air puff tonometer is used, it will require its own table and necessitate moving the patient for this procedure. If a Goldmann tonometer is used, location will not be a problem because the instrument is attached to the biomicroscope. The only problem here is that the process of applanation may bring about some corneal distortion, so many practitioners prefer to perform this procedure *after* the refractive and binocular vision examination. Many practitioners also prefer to perform ophthalmoscopy, and perhaps biomicroscopy, at the end of the examination.

Order of Testing

The following order of testing procedures is suggested:

1. Visual acuity testing.
2. Tests of ocular motility and binocular vision.
   a. Cover tests.
   b. Corneal reflex test.
   c. Near-point of convergence testing.
   d. Near-point of accommodation testing.
   e. Motility tests.
   f. Tests of pupillary function.
   g. Tests of stereopsis.
3. Color vision testing.
4. Visual field screening.
   a. Confrontations.
   b. Tangent screen or automatic perimetry.
5. Tonometry.
6. Blood pressure measurement.
7. External examination (discussed in Chapter 7).
8. Internal examination (discussed in Chapter 7).

Visual acuity testing, the cover tests, and some of the motility tests require the use of an occluder; some of the tests for motility require the use of a penlight; the near-point of accommodation and near-point of convergence tests require the use of a millimeter ruler; and some tests (visual acuity at near, near-point of accommodation, and cover tests) require the use of a near-point acuity chart. These

small pieces of equipment can be kept in a jacket pocket or at another convenient location so the tests can be performed smoothly and rapidly. A convenient acuity chart for preliminary tests is a reduced Snellen chart glued onto a tongue depressor.

VISUAL ACUITY MEASUREMENT

The preliminary examination normally begins with the determination of visual acuity. This is a logical starting point, as any complaints of blurred vision elicited during the history can be confirmed, and patients typically expect the doctor to have them read the "eye chart." Many patients become visibly annoyed if they have to sit through a number of other tests before they are given an opportunity to read the letters on the eye chart.

Standard Testing Conditions

Visual acuity testing conditions should be as close to "standard" as possible. There are several reasons for this:

1. If testing conditions are changed from time to time due to factors such as relocating equipment, a patient's visual acuity findings may not be comparable from one visit to another.
2. In practices containing more than one examination room, a patient's visual acuity obviously should be identical in each room.
3. A patient's visual acuity findings should be identical in offices of different practitioners.
4. A patient's visual acuity may become a legal issue, such as eligibility for a driver's license, a pension, or an insurance claim.

Standard conditions for the determination of visual acuity include letter size, testing distance, chart and background illumination, and contrast.

Letter Size

As discussed in Chapter 1, "normal" visual acuity involves the ability to detect a gap subtending an angle of 1 minute of arc. For a 6m testing distance, the linear height of the gap is equal to $6(\tan 1') = 1.745$mm; for a letter 5 units high (consisting of three strokes and two gaps), the letter height is $5(1.745) = 8.725$mm or, rounding off, 8.7mm. When calibrating a visual acuity chart, the simplest procedure is to measure the height of the 6/60 (20/200) letter *E*,

Table 6.1 Height of 6/60 (20/200) *E* for various testing distances.

Distance		Height
6m	20 ft	87mm
5m	16 ft	73mm
4m	13 ft	58mm
3m	10 ft	44mm

which should be 10(8.7) = 87mm. With standard chart projectors, the projector is moved closer or farther from the screen until the correct letter size is achieved. For testing distances shorter than 6m (20 feet) the height of the 6/60 (20/200) *E* is given in Table 6.1.

Testing Distance

Because rays of light diverging from a point 6m from the eye have a vergence of 0.17D on reaching the eye, "optometric infinity" differs from real infinity by an appreciable amount. When testing distances shorter than 6m are used, what effect should we expect this to have on visual acuity?

As long as letter size is such that a 6/6 (20/20) letter subtends an angle of 5 minutes of arc at the spectacle plane, an emmetrope or an uncorrected hyperope with reasonable facility of accommodation would be expected to have no difficulty clearing up the letters at a distance less than 6m. However, an uncorrected myope would be expected to have artificially high visual acuity under these circumstances. For example, at a testing distance of 3m (10 feet), a 0.33D myope would be in perfect focus and would likely read at least one more line of letters than at the 6m distance. In the experience of the author, visual

Figure 6.2 Use of a mirror system for a short examination room.

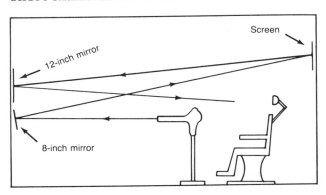

acuity for uncorrected (and corrected) myopes becomes a problem for testing distances much closer than about 5m (16 feet).

The effect of testing distance on visual acuity should not be confused with the effect of testing distance on refractive findings. For an acuity chart at 4m, the vergence of light is 0.25D for all patients, no matter what the refractive state, so myopes will tend to be underminused and hyperopes will tend to be overplussed. If the testing distance must be less than about 15 feet, the use of a mirror system should be considered.

When a mirror system is used in connection with a chart projector, the projector screen is placed on the wall behind (and above) the patient's head. A small mirror about 20cm square reflects the light from the projector onto the chart, and the patient views the chart in a larger mirror about 30cm square (see Figure 6.2).

Illumination

Illumination for visual acuity testing, as well as for other examination procedures, can be considered in terms of either illuminance or luminance. *Illuminance (E)* is the amount of luminous flux incident on a surface per unit area of the surface, and it can be specified in *footcandles. Luminance (B)* is a measure of the luminous flux emitted or reflected per unit area of a source or a reflecting surface, as measured per unit area of a light-sensitive surface. For a reflecting surface that can be considered as a perfect diffuser, luminance is equal to illuminance multiplied by the reflection factor (*r*) of the surface:

$$B = rE.$$

The use of a hand-held illuminance meter (such as the GE214 shown in Figure 6.3) for measuring clinical illumination levels has been discussed by Long and Woo (1979). To measure the illuminance of a surface with a meter of this type, place the base of the meter on or near the surface, with the head of the meter parallel to the surface, making sure not to block the light reaching the meter. Using the multiplying switch on the right side of the meter, the operator selects the scale having the appropriate sensitivity, and reads the illuminance directly from the scale. To determine the luminance reflected from the surface, hold the illuminance meter with its head parallel to and about 4 or 5cm from the surface under consideration; the illuminance reading is regarded as a luminance reading. Long and Woo pointed out that this method of measuring luminance

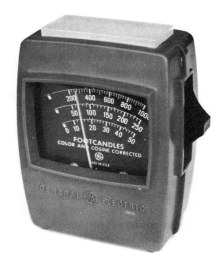

Figure 6.3   A typical hand-held illuminance meter (Woo and Long, 1979).

is strictly accurate only for perfect diffusers of unlimited extent, but it is usually an adequate approximation for the materials encountered clinically.

Woo and Long (1979) published a table listing luminance levels for use in the optometric examination (reproduced here as Table 6.2). Their recommended illuminance level of 12–20 footcandles for distance acuity charts corresponds to a luminance level of about 10–16 foot-lamberts if a reflectance

factor of 0.8 is assumed. Commercially available chart projectors provide luminance levels in excess of this amount when used with a correctly positioned screen.

It is necessary to consider not only the luminance of the acuity chart itself but also the overall room illumination. For a patient having uncorrected myopia, astigmatism, or absolute hyperopia, extremely bright room illumination may decrease pupil size to the point that acuity will be artificially high. Night myopia would be a factor to consider if there were no background illumination at all, but the high luminance level of the acuity chart itself most likely would be sufficient to minimize any effects of night myopia. Woo and Long (1979) pointed out that, because visual acuity depends on contrast as well as luminance, the room lighting in the vicinity of a projected chart should be kept low: otherwise, it will reduce the contrast of the letters on the chart. They recommend that the room lighting in the vicinity of the projector screen (with the projector turned off) should be no greater than 13 percent of the projector illuminance.

Contrast of the letters on a projected chart can also be a problem when polarized projector slides are used. To achieve maximum contrast with polarized slides, it is imperative that the line normal to the screen bisect the angle between the projector beam and the patient's line of sight (see Figure 6.4). In setting up a polarized projection system, it is a good idea to use a small mirror to determine the

Table 6.2   Illuminance levels recommended for the optometric examination (Woo and Long, 1979).

Procedure	Illuminance
External examination of the eye	100 fc (1,100 lux) at the examining chair measured in the plane parallel to and 1m from the floor
Observation of pupillary reflexes, ophthalmoscopy, slit lamp examinations, retinoscopy, keratometry	5–10 fc (55–110 lux) measured in the plane parallel to and 1m from the floor
Distance tests charts	At least 12–20 fc (130 to 215 lux), assuming a 0.8 reflecting factor
Near-point cards	Same as distance charts
Binocular crossed cylinder	1–2 fc (10–20 lux)
Addition measurements using the crossed-cylinder grid target	1 fc (10 lux)
Tangent screen	7 fc (75 lux)
Color vision testing	Macbeth or daylight lamp at 80 fc (860 lux)

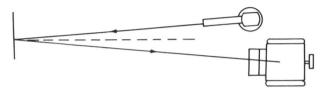

Figure 6.4   Adjustment of angle of screen for use with polarized projector slides.

correct angle for the screen. With the projector turned off, the mirror (and the angle of the screen) should be adjusted until the patient sitting in the chair can see the projector.

Testing Procedures

Distance visual acuity is determined first with no correction and then with the patient's habitual distance correction. Right eye acuity is always taken first, followed by left eye acuity and binocular acuity.

Unless there is a reason to believe that visual acuity will not be within normal limits, a recommended procedure is to present the whole chart (i.e., a block of letters from about 6/15 to 6/4.5, or 20/50 to 20/15) and ask the patient to read the smallest row of letters that can be easily seen, then to read as many letters as possible in the next row, and so forth. However, if there is reason to believe the patient is myopic, either on the basis of complaints or because of a myopic correction, the testing should begin with larger letters. In any case, the patient should be cautioned not to squint, as this will cause acuity to be erroneously high in uncorrected myopes or astigmats. Acuity is recorded in terms of the smallest complete line of letters identified (e.g., 6/6, or 20/20), or in terms of the number of letters not identified in the line in question (6/6 − 2, or 20/20 − 2), or the number of letters identified in addition to those in the line in question (6/6 + 3, or 20/20 + 3).

For measurement of visual acuity at 40cm, a reduced Snellen chart is used. This is an acuity chart printed on a stiff or plasticized card measuring about 5 × 6 inches and mounted in front of the refractor on a reading rod. The letter heights are such that a 6/6 (20/20) letter subtends an angle of 5 minutes of arc at a distance of 40cm, so acuity findings taken at 40cm are comparable to 6m findings.

Procedures for children

Because amblyopes have poorer acuity if the whole chart is presented than if a single line of letters or a single letter is presented (the phenom-

enon of contour interaction), it is important in testing children's acuity to present a block of five or six lines of letters—otherwise, amblyopia may be missed. A visual acuity chart designed by Flom (1966) to provide contour interaction is described in Chapter 4 and shown in Figure 4.35.

Most first-grade children, many kindergarten children, and even some preschool children know enough letters so acuity can be tested by means of a Snellen letter chart. Even if the child is familiar with only a limited number of letters (e.g., the letters making up the child's name), it is often possible to obtain an accurate measurement of visual acuity by having the child identify those particular letters wherever they occur in a specific line of letters.

For children between the ages of about 3 and 6 years who cannot recognize enough letters to make the use of a standard letter chart possible, *tumbling Es* can be used (see Figure 6.5). The child is given a wooden or plastic letter *E* and instructed to point the "legs" of the *E* in the same direction as those of the *E* on the chart. However, a child in this age group

Figure 6.5   The American Optical children's acuity slide.

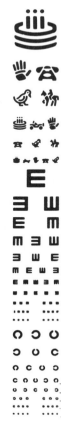

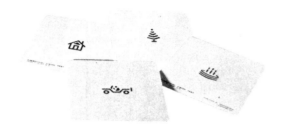

Figure 6.6   The Allen Preschool Vision test.

may not have developed the concept of laterality and, therefore, may not be capable of pointing the wooden or plastic E in the correct direction. Most children in this age group respond well if asked to state whether the legs of the E point "up, down, toward the window, or toward the door" (or whatever objects are located to the right or left of the acuity chart). It is tempting to present single lines of letters or single letters when using a tumbling E chart. This temptation can be overcome by having an assistant stand beside the chart to indicate the letter in question with a pointer.

An alternative to the tumbling E chart is the *Landolt C chart*, also shown in Figure 6.5. The child can be told that "somebody has taken a bite out of this doughnut" and asked to point to the part of the doughnut that is missing.

For the preschool child who fails to respond to the tumbling E chart or the Landolt C chart, various picture charts are available. The *Allen Preschool Vision test* (see Figure 6.6) consists of a set of seven cards, each containing a single picture, for use with children 2 years of age and older. The child is first shown the cards at close range, with both eyes open, and is asked to name each picture (the names in many cases will differ from the names an adult would be expected to use). One eye is then occluded, the examiner shuffles the cards—using the cards that appear to have the most meaning for the child—and presents them individually at increasingly greater distances. Visual acuity is recorded in terms of the maximum distance at which one or more pictures are correctly named, always using 30 as the denominator of the Snellen fraction. For example, if 15 feet is the maximum distance for the right eye and 10 feet is the maximum distance for the left eye, visual acuity will be recorded as

Right eye: 15/30 (= 20/40),

Left eye: 10/30 (= 20/60).

The *American Optical Project-o-Chart* child's acuity slide (shown in Figure 6.5) includes a series of pictures like those on the Allen cards. As with the Allen cards, the child is first asked to name each picture, and responses are then evaluated in terms of the child's names for the pictures. This can be done by having the child name the larger pictures in the first three lines of the chart while seated in the ophthalmic chair or, if necessary, by having the child walk toward the screen while the larger pictures are presented.

The *Stycar visual acuity test* consists of letter charts designed for use at 10- and 20-foot distances together with sets of miniature eating utensils and a number of toys. The child is given a large card, called a key card, and is asked to find the letter on the card that is the same as the letter on the distance chart. The eating utensil set includes a small set of utensils held by the examiner (first at 10 feet and then at 20 feet) and a large set held by the child. The child is asked to tell which utensil in the set is the same as the one held by the examiner.

The *Sheridan Gardiner visual acuity test*, like the Stycar test, provides a large key card (see Figure 6.7a) for use by the child. The child is asked to point to the letter on the key card that is the same as the letter shown on the distance chart (see Figure 6.7b). The distance chart is in the form of a spiral-bound booklet, with one letter presented on each page. The Sheridan Gardiner test also includes a reduced Snellen chart (see Figure 6.7c) for near testing.

Both the Stycar letter charts and the Sheridan Gardiner test have the advantage that letter charts rather than pictures can be used to measure the visual acuity of a preschool child, even though the child cannot name the letters.

The use of an *optokinetic nystagmus (OKN) drum* has been proposed as a method of measuring visual acuity in children. The drum presents alternating black and white stripes, and the test is based on the fact that the child cannot help but make nystagmus movements if the stripes are seen as the drum is rotated (nystagmus movements are rhythmic, conjugate movements having a slow phase in the direction of the movement and a fast, corrective movement in the opposite direction). Unfortunately, the stripes on commercially available OKN drums are so wide that when the drum is rotated at a distance close enough to attract the child's attention, nystagmus movements may be elicited when the visual acuity is no better than about 20/1000.

Another visual acuity test that has been advocated for children involves the use of sugar pellets such as those used for commercially available cake decorations. The child seated at a table is asked to name the colors of the sugar pellets placed on the table. Although this test has the advantage that the pellets

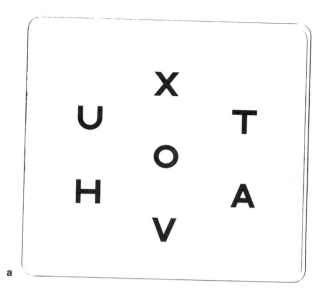

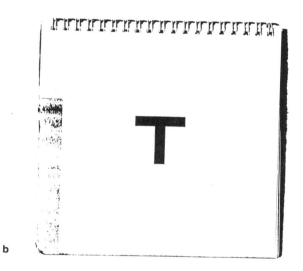

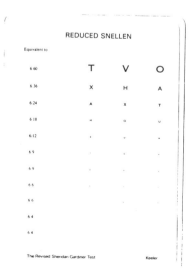

Figure 6.7 The Sheridan Gardiner visual acuity test: (*a*) child's key card; (*b*) distance chart in the form of a spiral-bound booklet; (*c*) reduced Snellen chart for near-acuity testing.

may be eaten when the test is over, only low levels of acuity are required to identify the pellets. For pellets 2mm in diameter that are identified at a distance of 25cm, the angular size of each pellet would be $\tan^{-1}(2/250)$, or 27.5 minutes of arc, corresponding (if a pellet is considered as a "gap") to a Snellen acuity of 20/550.

Contrary to many reports still in optometric literature, a 3-year-old child should be expected to have visual acuity of approximately 20/20. Failure to obtain normal acuity findings in the absence of an uncorrected refractive error, amblyopia, or ocular disease is due to communication problems rather than to a lack of development of the child's visual system.

COVER TESTS

By means of the *unilateral cover test* (also called the *cover-uncover test*), the practitioner can determine the presence or absence of a tropia. By means of the *alternating cover test*, the practitioner can determine whether a phoria or a tropia is present but cannot differentiate between the two. Thus, if the unilateral cover test results in a negative finding, a positive finding on the alternating cover test indicates the presence of a phoria. Because the alternating cover test can interfere with the manifestation of a tropia, it is customary to perform the unilateral cover test first.

Unilateral Cover Test

While wearing his or her own spectacle correction, if any, the patient's attention is called to a letter on the 6m Snellen chart. To assure that accommodation is relaxed, the letter should be no larger than one line above the patient's corrected acuity with the worse eye, and the patient should be instructed to keep the letter in sharp focus. The practitioner is seated opposite the patient, with his or her head positioned so that it does not block the patient's view of the chart. Sufficient illumination must be directed toward the patient's eyes so the practitioner can observe any eye movement.

The occluder is placed in front of the right eye, held there for about 1 second, and then removed. During this time the practitioner observes the patient's left eye for any movement. If no tropia exists, the left eye will make no movement, maintaining steady fixation both when the right eye is covered and when it is uncovered. If the right eye is strabismic (deviating either inward or outward), the left eye will maintain fixation when the right eye is covered and when it is uncovered, just as if there were no strabismus. However, if the left eye is strabismic, covering the right eye will cause it to turn outward (in esotropia) or inward (in exotropia) to take up fixation; removal of the cover will cause it to move back to its strabismic position.

Before the cover is placed in front of the left eye, a few seconds should be allowed to elapse so the eyes return to their normal (undissociated, or associated) relationship. The left eye is then covered, and the cover is held there for about 1 second and then removed. During this time the practitioner observes the patient's right eye for any movement. An absence of any movement of the right eye indicates either that there is no tropia or that the left (covered) eye may be strabismic. Whereas a movement of the right eye on covering the left eye indicates strabismus, an outward movement indicates esotropia and an inward movement indicates exotropia. The sequence of movements in right exotropia is shown in Figure 6.8. The test is repeated several times, first covering the right eye and then the left, but always allowing a few seconds for the eyes to return to their normal relationship before repeating the test.

Figure 6.8 The unilateral cover test showing right exotropia. The right eye makes no movement on being covered (*b*) or uncovered (*c*). However, when the left eye is covered (*d*), the right eye turns inward to take up fixation, and the left eye turns outward. When the left eye is uncovered (*e*), the right eye turns outward, and the left eye turns inward to take up fixation.

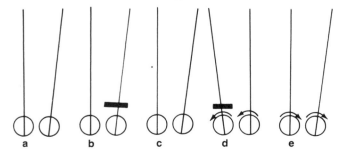

The test is repeated in a similar manner at 40cm, with the patient again instructed to fixate a letter no larger than the line above the best acuity line for the worse eye. The patient is instructed to keep the letter in sharp focus. If the patient is a child, a picture can be used as long as it includes fine detail that will serve as an accommodative stimulus. Objects such as pencil points, penlights, or visual field wands are not satisfactory for the cover test, as they do not serve as accommodative stimuli.

A reduced Snellen chart or a picture glued onto a tongue depressor is a convenient accommodative stimulus for the unilateral and alternating cover tests

Figure 6.9 Acuity chart and pictures printed on a plastic paddle made by Clement Clarke Ltd.

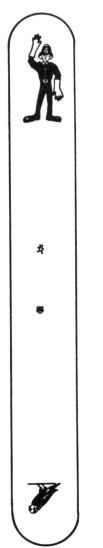
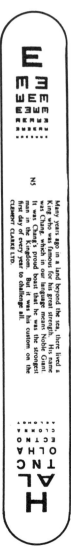

at 40cm, as is a commercially available acuity chart printed on a plastic paddle (see Figure 6.9). A good way to insure that the patient will accommodate for the distance of the chart is to have the patient hold the tongue depressor or paddle.

Strabismus may be either *unilateral*, where one eye is always the deviating eye, or *alternating*, where either eye may deviate. Unless the unilateral cover test is repeated several times, an alternating tropia may be missed, and the practitioner may conclude that the tropia is unilateral. Exotropia of relatively recent onset is particularly likely to be alternating.

A tropia may be present at some times and not at others: this is an *intermittent tropia*. For example, a patient who has intermittent exotropia may be found on one occasion to have right exotropia but on the next occasion to have only a high exophoria.

If a tropia is found at one testing distance but not at another, the condition is called a *periodic tropia*. For example, in some cases of accommodative esotropia, the patient may have no strabismus at distance but may have esotropia at near; while in divergence excess, there may be no strabismus at near but exotropia may be found on distance testing.

The following summarizes the interpretation of the unilateral cover test: the deviating (strabismic) eye makes no movement when it is covered or uncovered; when the fixing eye is covered, the strabismic eye will turn inward (if exotropic) or outward (if esotropic) to take up fixation, and it will return to its strabismic position when the occuluder is removed. It is as if the deviating eye does not fixate unless it has to, and the only time it has to is when the fixing eye is covered.

Alternating Cover Test

The conditions for the alternating cover test are the same as for the unilateral cover test. The patient wears his or her own spectacle correction, if any, and fixates a small letter (one line above best acuity for the worse eye) on the Snellen chart at 6m. The examiner sits facing the patient. The patient is instructed to keep the small letter in sharp focus.

The examiner places the occluder in front of the right eye, holds it there for about 1 second, and then quickly places it in front of the left eye. The test is repeated several times, the occluder being held in front of each eye for about 1 second before being quickly moved to the other eye. As the occluder is moved from one eye to the other, the examiner always observes the eye that has just been uncovered. If the just-uncovered eye turns inward, it

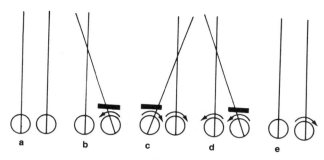

Figure 6.10   Alternating cover test showing esophoria. In the absence of the occluder (*a*), the visual axes are parallel, with each eye fixating the distant object. When the occluder is placed in front of the right eye (*b*), it turns inward; when the occluder is quickly moved to the left eye (*c*), the left eye turns inward, and the right eye turns outward to take up fixation; when the occluder is quickly moved back to the right eye (*d*), the right eye turns inward, and the left eye turns outward to take up fixation; and when the occluder is removed (*e*), the visual axes are again parallel.

indicates that while under cover it deviated outward (exophoria); if the just-uncovered eye turns outward, it obviously deviated inward (esophoria) while under cover. For the 40cm testing distance, the test is done in exactly the same manner while the patient fixates a small letter (one line larger than best acuity) on the reduced Snellen chart. The alternating cover test is summarized in Figure 6.10.

In both distance and near testing, there should be sufficient illumination on the patient's face so eye movements can be easily observed. With practice, the examiner will be able to detect a movement of 3 or 4Δ.

The examiner may wish to sharpen his or her ability to detect small amounts of movement by using a low-powered square prism. For example, if no movement is observed in the alternating cover test (indicating that the patient has no phoria for that testing distance), the examiner can repeat the alternating cover test while placing a 4Δ prism, first base-in and then base-out, in front of one eye and observing the other eye for movement. When the prism is placed in the base-in position it will create an esophoria, so the eye without the prism should be observed to turn outward on being uncovered. In the base-out position the prism will create an exophoria, so the eye should turn inward on being uncovered. Thus, if equal amounts of esophoric and exophoric movement are found (with the prism base in the two positions), the original diagnosis of ortho-phoria was correct. However, if in the base-in position little or no esophoric movement is seen, but in the base-out position a large amount of exophoric movement is seen, it indicates that the patient is esophoric rather than orthophoric.

Vertical phoria

If the patient has a vertical phoria, each eye will be seen to turn upward or downward just as the cover is removed. Because a phoria is "shared" between the two eyes, if the right eye is observed to turn downward as it is uncovered, the left eye should be observed to turn upward as it is uncovered. This indicates that the right eye, while covered, deviated upward and the left eye deviated downward. This condition could be called either *right hyperphoria* or *left hypophoria*. However, by convention, vertical phorias are always labeled in terms of the hyper-phoric eye.

In many cases a patient will be found to have both a lateral phoria and a vertical phoria. For example, if the right eye is observed to turn downward and inward as it is uncovered, the condition would be exophoria combined with right hyperphoria.

Perceived target movement

The practitioner's ability to detect a small phoria can be enhanced by asking the patient if the fixated object (the letter on the chart) appears to move as the occluder is moved from one eye to the other. If any movement is seen, the patient is asked whether the movement of the target is in the same direction or in the direction opposite to the movement of the occluder. Movement in the same direction indicates exophoria, and movement in the opposite direction indicates esophoria.

During the alternating cover test, no diplopia as such as experienced. For an exophoric patient, when the occluder is moved from the right eye (see Figure 6.11a) to the left eye (see Figure 6.11b), the image of the object that had been seen previously by the fovea of the left eye is seen by a retinal point to the right of the fovea of the right eye. Therefore, the object appears to be in the left visual field. This requires a fixation movement to the left, which is the same direction as the movement of the occluder (from the right eye to the left eye).

It should be understood that the patient does not see the fixation target while eye movement takes place. It is only perceived to move because it changes its position from "straight ahead," where it was seen

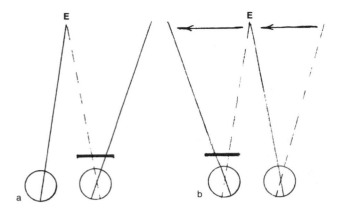

Figure 6.11 Perceived target movement in exophoria. The letter *E* appears to move in the same direction (from right to left) as the occluder.

by the left eye, to "to the left," where it was seen by the right eye. When movement is perceived rather than real (as when one traffic light blinks on while another blinks off), psychologists sometimes refer to it as *phi movement*. Thus, when a patient is asked to report the direction of movement of the fixation target during the cover test, the procedure is sometimes called the *phi movement test*.

For an esophoric patient (see Figure 6.12), the image of the object, which had previously been seen by the fovea of the left eye (see Figure 6.12a) is seen by a retinal point to the left of the fovea of the right eye (see Figure 6.12b). Therefore, the object appears to be in the right visual field. This requires a fixation movement to the right (due to the fact that the target is perceived to move to the right), which is the

Figure 6.12 Perceived target movement in esophoria. The letter *E* appears to move in the opposite direction (from left to right) as the occluder.

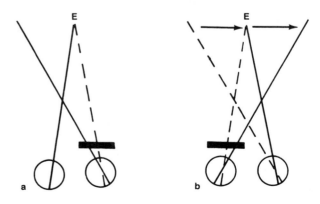

opposite of the direction of movement of the occluder (from the right eye to the left eye).

When the patient is a child, a useful procedure is to ask the child to point (using a thumb or other finger) in the direction that the letter is moving. Even preschool children, who would have difficulty with the concepts of "same" and "opposite," often have little difficulty pointing in the direction the letter is moving. If the examiner suspects a vertical phoria, the patient should be asked if the letter appears to be higher for one eye than for the other, or if it appears to move diagonally rather than horizontally.

If a strabismic patient has harmonius anomalous retinal correspondence, the letter or other fixation object will appear to be in the same position for each eye. For this reason the phi movement test should *not* be used with strabismic patients.

Measurement of the phoria or angle of squint

The alternating cover test may be used to *measure* the phoria or the angle of squint by the use of square prisms or a prism bar (see Figure 6.13). Square prisms are easier to handle than the round prisms found in trail lens sets, and they are available in sets ranging from 1–20Δ or more. Prism bars are available in horizontal form (for measuring lateral deviations) and vertical form (for measuring vertical deviations). Whichever form of prism is used, the prism is placed in front of one eye, and the

Figure 6.13 (a) Square prisms; (b) horizontal prism bar; (c) vertical prism bar.

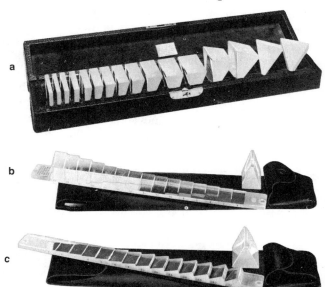

movement of the other eye is observed while the alternating cover test is performed. Prism power is increased until a reversal is noted. For example, if exo movement is observed prior to the use of prisms, base-in prism power is increased until no movement is noted, and it is then further increased until eso movement is noted. Often there will be a range from 2–4Δ of power for which no movement is noted: the prism that neutralizes the phoria or tropia will be the midpoint of the range.

CORNEAL REFLEX TEST

The corneal reflex test is a convenient test for determining the presence of strabismus at near. It is particularly useful for a child on whom results with the unilateral cover test were questionable. In this test, the patient is instructed to watch a penlight or ophthalmoscope bulb held by the examiner at a distance of about 40cm, while the examiner observes the corneal reflexes in the patient's eyes while viewing just above the light source with the dominant eye. If no tropia exists, each corneal reflex will be located approximately 0.5mm nasal to the center of the pupil. This is because the line of sight makes a small angle (about 5 degrees) with the pupillary axis. This angle, measured from the entrance pupil of the eye, is called the *angle lambda*. Whereas the corneal reflex is normally about 0.5mm nasal to the center of the pupil, it may be slightly more displaced nasally in some hyperopic eyes, and it may be near the center of the pupil or even displaced temporally in some highly myopic eyes.

Hirschberg's method

With Hirschberg's method, in esotropia, the corneal reflex for the deviating eye will be displaced temporally compared to the fixing eye, whereas in exotropia, it will be displaced nasally. The angle of strabismus can be estimated on the basis that each millimeter of displacement of the corneal reflex indicates approximately 22Δ of strabismus.

Krimsky's method

In Krimsky's method, prisms are placed in front of the deviating eye while using the alternating cover test, and the prism power is found that will place the corneal reflex in the same position for the deviating eye as for the fixing eye. This procedure presents the problem that a light source is not an adequate stimulus for accommodation. If the patient responds to the alternating cover test with square prisms or a prism bar with a test object that acts as an accommodative stimulus, the Krimsky test need not be done.

Angle lambda

In interpreting the corneal reflex test (either the Hirschberg or Krimsky methods), the practitioner should establish whether angle lambda is equal for the two eyes. To do this, each eye should be occluded alternately and the position of the corneal reflex for each eye observed. Except in unusual cases, angle lambda will be equal for the two eyes (i.e., the corneal reflexes will be in the same relative positions for the two eyes in monocular fixation). If the practitioner should find the position of the corneal reflex to be noticeably different for one eye than the other, *eccentric fixation* should be suspected. If eccentric fixation is present, visual acuity will be decreased for the strabismic eye (i.e., amblyopia).

NEAR-POINT OF CONVERGENCE

It is convenient to test for the near-point of convergence just after completing the corneal reflex test. As the penlight is slowly brought inward toward the patient's nose, the patient is asked to report when the light "breaks into two." The examiner watches the patient's eyes to determine any loss of convergence not reported by the patient. If one eye turns outward (as shown by an inward movement of the corneal reflex) without the patient reporting diplopia, it is obvious that the patient is suppressing that eye. The expected value of the near-point of convergence is approximately 8cm or less, as measured from the spectacle plane. If the near-point of convergence is found to be in the neighborhood of 12–15cm on repeated testing, the examiner should suspect the convergence insufficiency syndrome. If one eye suppresses, the fact that this occurs (and in which eye) should be recorded, as should the distance at which the eye is seen to turn outward.

Amplitude of Convergence

To determine the amplitude of convergence, the near-point of convergence must first be specified in terms of the line joining the centers of rotation of the two eyes. Although the center of rotation of the eye is thought to be about 27mm behind the spectacle plane, as a matter of convenience this distance can be assumed to be 3cm. The amplitude

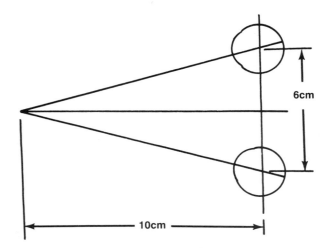

Figure 6.14   Determination of the amplitude of convergence.

of convergence (see Figure 6.14) is equal to the reciprocal (in meters) of the near point of convergence multiplied by the patient's interpupillary distance in centimeters. For a near point of convergence of 7cm, measured from the spectacle plane, and an interpupillary distance of 60mm, the amplitude of convergence would be

$$\frac{1}{0.10}\,(6) = \frac{100}{10}\,(6) = 60\Delta.$$

NEAR-POINT OF ACCOMMODATION

The near-point of accommodation can be determined monocularly for each eye as well as binocularly, while the patient wears his or her glasses or contact lenses, if any. For monocular determination of the near-point of accommodation, the left eye is occluded (it is convenient to have the patient hold the occluder) and the patient is asked to keep the 20/20 row of letters on the reduced Snellen chart in sharp focus as the card is moved closer. The patient is to report when this row of letters begins to blur and remains blurred. When a blur is reported, the near-point of accommodation is recorded as the distance (in centimeters) from the test card to the spectacle plane of the eye. The test is repeated with the right eye occluded and is then repeated binocularly.

Care should be taken to make sure the near-point card receives sufficient illumination as it approaches the patient's eyes. However, the illumination should not be so bright as to cause unnecessary constriction of the patient's pupils: this will increase the depth of focus and cause the near-point of accommodation to be erroneously low.

Amplitude of Accommodation

If the patient's refractive error is corrected while the near point of accommodation is measured, the amplitude of accommodation can be calculated simply by taking the reciprocal of the near point of accommodation, expressed in meters. For a near-point of accommodation of 8cm (as measured from the spectacle plane), the amplitude of accommodation is 12.50D.

When this test is performed while the old glasses or contact lenses are worn, the practitioner does not know whether these lenses adequately correct the patient's refractive error. Therefore, data on near-point of accommodation, taken through the old lenses, should remain in the recording form as near-point of accommodation rather than converting it to amplitude of accommodation.

MOTILITY TESTS

A number of tests have been devised to investigate the integrity of the extrinsic ocular muscles and their nerves, including the broad H test, and the diplopia field test.

Broad H Test

One of the most useful motility tests is the *broad H test*. The test is designed to test the action of the horizontal rectus muscles (the patient's eyes fixate a penlight as it is moved into the right-hand and left-hand fields) and to test the action of the vertically acting muscles, the vertical recti, and the obliques (the patient follows the penlight as it is moved to the right, then upward and downward while still turned to the right; and to the left, then upward and downward, while still turned to the left).

The broad *H* test is interpreted in terms of the *fields of action* of the six extrinsic muscles. The field of action for a given muscle refers to the field (as the patient faces it) in which that particular muscle has the greatest action. For the right lateral rectus, the field of action is the right-hand field; for the right medial rectus, the field of action is the left-hand field. The opposite applies for the left lateral rectus and left medial rectus.

The fields of action of the four vertically acting

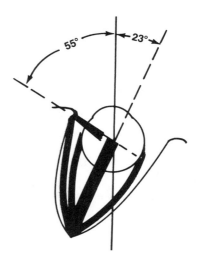

Figure 6.15   Muscle planes of the vertical rectus and oblique muscles.

muscles are based on the *muscle planes* of each of these muscles. As shown in Figure 6.15, both the superior and inferior rectus muscles lie in a plane that makes an angle of approximately 23 degrees with the straight-ahead position of the eye. This means that when the right eye is already turned outward approximately 23 degrees, the superior rectus acts as a *pure elevator* and the inferior rectus acts as a *pure depressor*. If we ask a patient to direct his or her gaze approximately 23 degrees to the right and then to look upward, any limitation in movement of the right eye is the fault of the superior rectus. Similarly, if there is a limitation in downward movement of the right eye (with gaze directed toward the right), the muscle at fault is the inferior rectus.

The superior oblique and inferior oblique muscles lie in a plane that makes an angle of approximately 55 degrees from the straight-ahead direction (see Figure 6.15). Therefore, when the eye is already turned inward approximately 55 degrees, the superior oblique acts as a pure depressor, and the inferior oblique acts as a pure elevator. Any limitation of movement when looking first inward approximately 55 degrees and then downward or upward would be due to the superior oblique (downward) or the inferior oblique (upward).

When the broad *H* test is performed, it is not necessary to have the patient direct his or her gaze *exactly* 23 degrees or 55 degrees to the right or to the left. If the gaze is directed about 30–40 degrees in each direction, any limitation of movement can be detected.

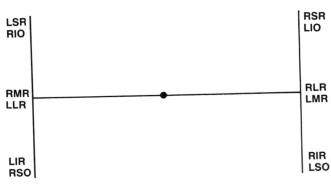

Figure 6.16   Muscles acting as elevators and depressors.

Elevators and Depressors

A muscle that turns the eye upward when it is already turned to the right is called a *right-hand elevator*, and a muscle that turns the eye downward when it is already turned to the right is called a *right-hand depressor*. Left-hand elevators and left-hand depressors are similarly defined. Figure 6.16 shows the field as seen by the patient. As shown in the figure, the muscles that act as right-hand elevators are the right superior rectus and the left inferior oblique; right-hand depressors are the right inferior rectus and the left superior oblique; and so on.

In performing the broad *H* test, the examiner faces the patient and moves the penlight in the patient's frontoparallel plane. The examiner must watch *both* eyes as the patient makes the movement: first to the right, then up, then down, and then to the left, then up, then down. Because it is difficult to watch both eyes at once, it is beneficial to perform the test twice, watching the right eye the first time and the left eye the second time.

Diplopia Field Test

If one eye appears to lag behind in any field of action in the broad *H* test, the patient can be asked to wear a pair of red/green goggles (the red lens on the right eye) while the broad *H* test is repeated. The patient is then asked to report whether *two* lights (one red and one green) are seen in each of the fields of gaze and, if so, to demonstrate how far apart the two lights appear to be. The *mnemonic of Maddox* may be used in interpreting the diplopia field test: if diplopia occurs in any field of gaze, (1) the muscle at fault is the *same-named straight muscle* or the *cross-named oblique muscle*, and (2) the most peripheral image belongs to the lagging eye.

The following example demonstrates how the mnemonic of Maddox is used. Suppose a patient reports diplopia in the left inferior field, with the green light appearing farther out (more peripheral) than the red light. The *same-named straight muscle* for the left inferior field is the *left inferior rectus*, whereas the *cross-named oblique muscle* for that field is the *right superior oblique*. Because the more peripheral image belongs to the left eye (the green image), the left inferior rectus is the muscle at fault. It should be understood that the mnemonic of Maddox applies only to underacting muscles. In this example, if a muscle were overacting, it would be the right superior oblique.

TESTS OF PUPILLARY FUNCTION

Testing a patient's pupillary function involves the use of the following tests: (1) measurement of pupil size, (2) measurement of direct, consensual, and near reflexes, and (3) the swinging flashlight test.

Pupil Size

The *size of each pupil* is measured using a millimeter ruler and estimating pupillary diameter to the nearest half millimeter. Smith (tape no. 6) recommended that measurements be made both in a lighted and a semidarkened room, as the pupils may be of equal size in one circumstance and of unequal size in another.

If the practitioner routinely uses an ultraviolet lamp (such as the *Burton lamp*) in contact lens fitting, this lamp can be used to measure pupil size in dim illumination. The fluorescence of the crystalline lens, in ultraviolet light, makes the measurement much easier.

Direct, Consensual, and Near Reflexes

To observe and evaluate *direct* and *consensual pupillary reflexes*, the patient fixates on a distant object in a semidarkened room and a penlite is used to illuminate each pupil, taking care to direct the penlite toward the macular area. The direct reflex—the constriction of the pupil of the illuminated eye—is easily seen, but it is often difficult to observe the constriction of the opposite eye, particularly if the patient has dark irides. The level of room illumination should be sufficient for the examiner to observe the constriction of the pupil of the unilluminated eye.

To observe the *near reflex*, the patient (still in semidarkened illumination) is first asked to fixate a distant object and then asked to fixate a near object such as a row of letters on a near-point card. The test should be repeated two or three times, with fixation alternating between distance and near. Again, the room illumination should be sufficient for the examiner to observe the constriction of the pupil.

Smith (tape no. 6) recommends that pupillary constriction for the direct, consensual, and near reflexes be graded on a scale from 1+ (barely noticeable) to 4+ (very strong). Another method of recording, used if all reflexes are normal, is *"PERLA,"* meaning "*P*upils *e*qual, *r*esponding to *l*ight and *a*ccommodation."

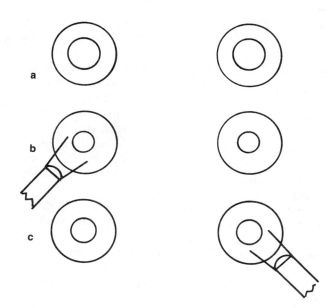

Figure 6.17 Marcus Gunn pupil: (*a*) pupil size in a semidarkened room; (*b*) both pupils constricting when the normal eye is illuminated; (*c*) both pupils dilating slightly (pupillary escape) when the light is quickly swung to the eye having an optic nerve conduction defect.

Swinging Flashlight Test

To conduct the *swinging flashlight test*, the patient fixates on a distant object in a semidarkened room. The examiner first illuminates the right eye, then the left, swinging the flashlight from one eye to the other. The procedure is repeated several times, each pupil being illuminated for about one second, so to establish a rhythm. Normally, the pupil of each eye will be seen to constrict as that eye is illuminated. However, in the presence of a Marcus Gunn pupil, the pupil of the affected eye will *dilate* slightly when that eye is illuminated. As shown in Figure 6.17, the pupils of *both* eyes will dilate when the eye with the Marcus Gunn pupil is illuminated. Because the pupil fails to constrict when illuminated, the condition is sometimes referred to as *pupillary escape.*

Interpretation of the swinging flashlight test will be discussed further in the section on pupillary anomalies.

Pupillary Abnormalities

Many people will be found to have a difference in pupil size between the two eyes sufficient to be detected when measured by a millimeter ruler (a difference of ½mm or more). This condition is known as *essential anisocoria* and is of no consequence. As noted in Chapter 5, Smith (tape no. 6) suggests that when the pupils are found to be of unequal size, the patient should be asked to supply old photographs to help the practitioner determine if the difference in pupil size is long-standing (and, therefore, likely to be essential anisocoria) or of recent origin.

In his monograph *The Pupil*, Smith describes eight pupillary abnormalities that he feels are the most important ones. Each of these are briefly discussed here, particularly in regard to their detection and diagnosis.

Adie's tonic pupil

This is a unilaterally dilated pupil with little or no reaction to light but with sluggish reaction to near stimulation. It is a relatively common clinical entity, occurring in females aged 20–30 who are otherwise healthy. It is thought to be due to a lesion of the ciliary ganglion and requires no treatment. The "moment of truth," according to Smith (tape no. 6), is the slow redilation of the affected pupil (compared to the faster redilation of the normal pupil) when the patient fixates a distant object after intently fixating his or her own finger.

Amaurotic pupil

An eye having an amaurotic pupil (an eye having no light perception) will have no direct pupillary reflex but will contract consensually when the fellow (normal) eye is stimulated by light. The fellow eye, when stimulated, will react to light but will not react consensually when the amaurotic eye is stimulated. The near reflex will be present for both eyes.

Marcus Gunn pupil

The Marcus Gunn pupil, also called the *afferent pupillary defect*, is detected by means of the swinging flashlight test. Due to a conduction defect of the optic nerve, stimulation of the affected pupil results in slightly less constriction of *both* pupils than that occurring when the normal pupil is stimulated, as shown in Figure 6.17 (Walsh, 1978). The swinging flashlight test allows comparison of the light reflex brought about by stimulating the pupil of the abnormal eye with that brought about by stimulating the pupil of the normal eye.

Among the causes of a Marcus Gunn pupil is multiple sclerosis, which may be accompanied by optic neuritis or by retrobulbar neuritis (inflammation of the optic nerve behind the globe). Smith (tape no. 6) pointed out that only a minor decrease in visual acuity may be present in an eye with a Marcus Gunn pupil.

Horner's syndrome

Horner's syndrome consists of miosis (a constricted pupil), ptosis (dropping of the upper lid), apparent enophthalmos, and a possible decrease in facial sweating on the affected side. The cause is a paralysis of the ocular sympathetic fibers responsible for pupillary dilation. The lesion can be anywhere in the long, complicated sympathetic pathway (in the midbrain, pons, upper spinal cord, middle cranial fossa, and orbit). Smith (tape no. 6) has commented that the syndrome is so subtle that it can be easily missed and that the ptosis can be detected more easily late in the day, when the patient is tired, than in the morning, when the patient is fresh.

One of the most benign forms of Horner's syndrome is that ocurring congenitally, where the lack of sympathetic innervation causes one eye to remain blue while the other turns brown (heterochromia irides). Another benign form is due to trauma involving the neck. When Horner's syndrome arises between the ages of 20 and 50 years, a malignant tumor should be suspected. Walsh has pointed out that the most common malignant tumor responsible for Horner's syndrome is a tumor of the apex of the lung. In older patients, Horner's syndrome may occur as a result of insufficiency of the basilar or vertebral arteries.

Hutchinson's pupil

Hutchinson's pupil is a fixed, dilated pupil, usually unilateral, due to a central nervous system lesion that compresses the optic nerve. Because the patient with this condition is usually very sick, an optometrist is unlikely to encounter this condition.

Light-near dissociation

Light-near dissociation is present when the pupils fail to react to light but constrict on convergence. One of the most common causes is neurosyphilis, in which case the syndrome is known as the *Argyll Robertson pupil*.

Argyll Robertson pupil

Smith (tape no. 6) states that although a true Argyll Robertson pupil is found in only 18 percent of cases of neurosyphilis, abnormal pupils are found in 80 percent of the cases. The diagnosis of neurosyphilis requires a good history, physical examination, and laboratory tests.

Aberrant regeneration of nerve III

Aberrant regeneration of nerve III may occur several months after a traumatic third-nerve palsy, and is characterized by a pseudo-Argyll Robertson pupil, a pseudo-von Graefe sign (upper lid lag when looking downward), and the presence of adduction and lid retraction on attempted vertical gaze.

TESTS OF STEREOPSIS

Stereopsis is the ability to perceive depth, or relative distance, on the basis of retinal disparity clues. The ability to perceive depth through stereopsis is considered to be innate, whereas the ability to perceive depth by monocular clues (geometrical perspective, overlay, aerial perspective, light and shadow, parallax, and height in relation to the horizon) must be learned.

One of the most commonly used tests for stereopsis is the *Titmus Stereotest* (see Figure 6.18). This test consists of a booklet containing polarized test stimuli for use at a 40cm testing distance and requires the use of cross-polarized lenses. The test includes a *stereofly*, which serves as a gross test for stereopsis, producing approximately 3,000 seconds (almost 1 degree) of retinal disparity at the 40cm testing distance. The stereofly is a particularly good test of stereopsis for preschool children. The child is asked to reach out and touch the fly's wings, which should appear to be located at some distance above the booklet. If the child's fingers touch the booklet when attempting to touch the wings, not even gross stereopsis is present.

For each of the three rows of animals on the lower

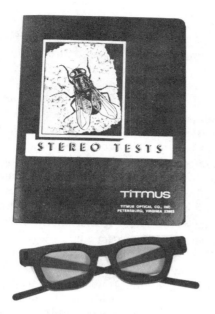

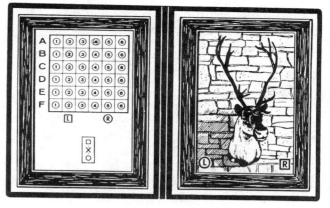

Figure 6.19   The Bernell Stereo Reindeer test.

Figure 6.18   The Titmus Stereotest.

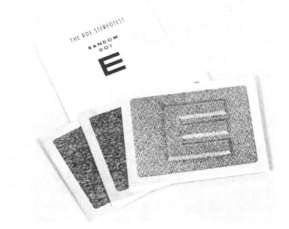

Figure 6.20   The Random Dot *E* test (demonstration plate).

left-hand side of the booklet, the child is asked which animal appears closer than the others. The retinal disparity produced in row A is 400 seconds, with the cat appearing closer; in row B the disparity is 200 seconds, with the rabbit appearing closer; and in row C the disparity is 100 seconds, with the monkey appearing closer. In each of the diamond-shaped figures on the upper left-hand side of the booklet, one of the circles (upper, lower, left, or right) should appear to be closer than the others. The angles of disparity for these figures range from 800 seconds for number 1 to 40 seconds for number 9. Griffin (1976) suggested that an interesting way to test the validity of a patient's responses is to turn the booklet upside down—the circle in each row that should appear to be above the booklet will recede into the booklet.

According to Parks (1979), patients with central fusion have 40 seconds of stereopsis or better at near, whereas patients with peripheral fusion but lacking central fusion have stereoacuity ranging from 3,000–60 seconds, averaging 200 seconds. Because stereopsis requires good visual acuity, the patient's corrective lenses should be worn along with the Polaroid filters.

The *Bernell Stereo Reindeer test* (see Figure 6.19), like the Titmus stereotest, is a polarized test providing stimuli for both gross and fine stereopsis testing. The test has the advantage that the examiner

can make the reindeer's nose wiggle by rotating the picture slightly.

The *Random Dot E test* (see Figure 6.20) consists of a demonstration plate and two test plates. The demonstration plate contains a raised letter *E* that can be seen by anyone who has reasonably good acuity, and it requires no stereopsis. Each of the test plates is printed with a polarized random dot pattern and requires the use of Polaroid glasses. A patient who has stereopsis will see a raised letter *E* in the random dot pattern of one of the test plates, whereas the other test plate will be seen as a "blank."

The examiner shows the child the demonstration plate at normal reading distance. After the child understands what is expected, the examiner shows the child both test plates, holding one in each hand at a distance of 50cm, and asks the child to point to the one containing the letter *E*. The examiner repeats the test at the 50cm distance at least four times, each time shuffling the plates before the next presentation. If the child points to the correct plate several times in a row, the two plates are presented in a similar manner at the distance of 1m. The child passes the test if he or she consistently chooses the correct plate at the 1m distance on four or five presentations. According to Reinecke and Simons (1974), the Random Dot *E* stimulates 500 seconds of disparity at 50cm and 250 seconds of disparity at 1m.

Rosner (1978) reported on a study at the University of Houston Childcare Center in which 60 children, aged 39 through 76 months, were tested by means of the Random Dot *E* at a distance of 1.5m. Each child was also given a battery of vision screening tests, including tests of ocular health, visual acuity, and near-point of convergence, as well as retinoscopy and cover tests. Ten of the 60 children failed one or more of the vision screening tests, but all 10 of these children also failed the Random Dot *E* test. Rosner concluded that when the Random Dot *E* test is given at a distance of 1.5m, it appears to be as effective in identifying children with significant refractive errors or substandard acuity as it is in identifying children with binocular anomalies.

The American Optical *Vectographic Project-o-Chart slide* provides a convenient method of testing stereopsis at 6m. This slide, described in Chapter 10, has five rows of circles. For each row of circles the patient is asked to report which circle appears to be closer than the others in the row. The retinal disparity stimulated by this test ranges from 240 seconds for the top row to 30 seconds for the bottom row.

COLOR VISION TESTING

A test of color vision should be a part of every basic optometric examination. In testing children the main concern is the detection of congenital red-green color vision anomalies, and any *pseudoisochromatic plate color test* is satisfactory. In testing adults the practitioner should be concerned with the possibility of an acquired color vision anomaly, so the patient should be screened for both red-green and blue-yellow anomalies, and each eye should be tested separately.

Red-Green Color Vision Anomalies

Normal color vision is said to be *trichromatic*, because a person having normal color vision requires

three primary colors to match any given color stimulus. The trichromatic subject will repeatedly use the same proportions of the three primary colors to match a given color sample. An *anomalous trichromat* requires three primaries just as the normal trichromat does but will match a given stimulus with different proportions of the three primaries. An anomalous trichromat may be either *protanomalous* (red-weak) or *deuteranomalous* (green-weak).

An anomalous trichromat may be differentiated from a normal trichromat by having him match a yellow stimulus with a mixture of red and green, using the Nagel anomaloscope (see Figure 6.21). When asked to make a match, the color-normal person will use the correct amount of red and green to match the yellow stimulus and in repeating the match will always return to the same proportions of red and green stimuli. However, the protanomalous trichromat requires more than the normal amount of red in the red-green combination, and the deuteranomalous trichromat requires more than the normal amount of green.

A *dichromat* is an individual who requires only two primaries to match any given color stimulus. A dichromat may be either a *protanope* (red-deficient) or a *deuteranope* (green-deficient). Rushton (1962) found that protanopes lack a red-absorbing pigment known as *erythrolabe*, and deuteranopes lack a green-absorbing pigment called *chlorolabe*. In making the Nagel anomaloscope match, the dichromat (either a protanope or a deuteranope) will accept any mixture of red and green stimuli to match the yellow, as long as he or she is able to vary the brightness of the yellow stimulus. The red and the

Figure 6.21 The Nagel anomaloscope test. The subject is asked to match the yellow stimulus by varying the luminance of the red and green stimuli.

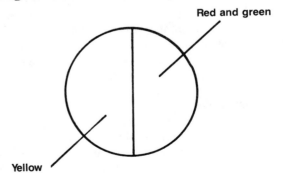

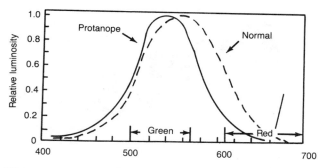

Figure 6.22 The protanope's photopic luminosity curve compared to that of the color-normal.

green stimuli appear to be the same color to the dichromat, so it does not matter which one is used.

Once it has been established that an individual is a dichromat, a differential diagnosis between protanopia and deuteranopia can be made on the basis of the protanope's insensitivity to long wavelengths. As shown in Figure 6.22, the protanope's photopic luminosity curve (the curve indicating the sensitivity of the retina to stimuli of various wavelengths) is greatly restricted in the longer wavelengths, compared to the deuteranope's or the color-normal's. Using the Nagel anomaloscope, the dichromat is asked to match a yellow stimulus first with pure red and then with pure green. (It is of interest that this presents no problem to the dichromat, because all long wavelength stimuli have the same hue.) Because of the protanope's relative insensitivity to red, less than the normal amount of yellow to match the red stimulus is required, but the normal amount of yellow to match the green stimulus is needed.

Inheritance of red-green anomalies

Red-green color vision anomalies occur so commonly that they are sometimes described as the "big four." More common in males, they are inherited as sex-linked (or x chromosome-linked) characteristics. A color-defective male receives the defective gene from his mother, who is typically color-normal. The mother, on the other hand, received the defective gene either from a color-defective father or from a color-normal mother who was a carrier. The anomaly, in effect, skips one or more generations. For a female to be color-defective, she must receive the defective gene from both her father and mother. The probability of this occurring is the square of the probability of her receiving the defective gene from only one parent. Because the

prevalence of these anomalies in males is approximately 8 percent, we would expect their prevalence in females to be about 0.64 percent (or approximately 1 in every 200 female births). For males, the breakdown for red-green anomalies is approximately as follows: protanomaly, 1 percent; deuteranomaly, 5 percent; protanopia, 1 percent; and deuteranopia, 1 percent.

Other Inherited Color Vision Anomalies

Inherited yellow-blue color vision anomalies, known as *tritanomaly* and *tritanopia*, occur much less frequently than red-green anomalies and are inherited on an autosomal rather than a sex-linked basis. As the terms indicate, tritanomaly is a form of anomalous trichromatism, whereas tritanopia is a form of dichromatism. *Monochromatism*, also called *achromatopsia*, is an extremely rare condition occurring in only one in a million people. Because all colors look the same to the monochromat, only one primary is required to match any color in the spectrum. Monochromatism may occur in either of two forms, both of which are present at birth: *typical monochromatism*, in which the retina contains no foveal cones; and *atypical monochromatism*, in which foveal cones are present. The former condition is sometimes called *rod monochromatism*, while the latter is called *cone monochromatism*. An individual with rod monochromatism will have poor visual acuity and a central scotoma due to the lack of foveal cones, whereas an individual with cone monochromatism may have normal visual acuity.

Acquired Color Vision Anomalies

Many diseases of the choroid, retina, and optic nerve can be responsible for acquired color vision anomalies. As a general rule, lesions of the choroid tend to cause yellow-blue anomalies, lesions of the retina cause either yellow-blue or red-green anomalies, and lesions of the optic nerve tend to cause red-green anomalies. Often, the presence of a unilateral color vision anomaly may enable the practitioner to detect the presence of a retinal or optic nerve disease prior to the stage when it would be detected by visual acuity testing or visual field testing (with white test objects). Conditions that may be responsible for acquired color vision anomalies include some forms of choroiditis, senile macular degeneration, other acquired maculopathies, optic neuritis, tobacco amblyopia, and other forms of optic nerve disease. As described by Glaser (1979), a conduction defect of the optic nerve acts as a high-frequency filter, serving as a barrier to conduction in the optic nerve and to which the nerve fibers associated with color vision are preferentially sensitive.

Color Vision Tests

Undoubtedly the most effective procedure for color vision testing involves the Nagel anomaloscope. With this instrument it is possible not only to detect the presence of a red-green color vision anomaly but also to make a differential diagnosis. The main problem with this instrument is its relatively high cost—not many practitioners are willing to make a major investment in an instrument designed to test for a condition that cannot be treated.

Pseudoisochromatic plates are by far the most popular of all color vision tests and are used by many optometrists. The test is in the form of a book containing a number of color plates, each plate containing a number, a figure, or in some cases an irregular winding path. Each figure is made up of dots that vary from the background in hue as well as brightness. This effect tends to camouflage the figure from patients having the color vision anomaly that the plate is designed to detect. For example, in a plate having a background of orange dots and a figure of olive green dots of the same brightness, the figure will be obvious to the color-normal but invisible to the dichromat. A typical plate is shown in Figure 6.23.

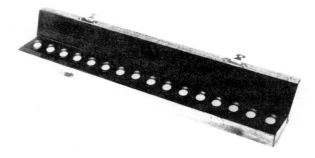

Figure 6.24   The Farnsworth D–15 color vision test.

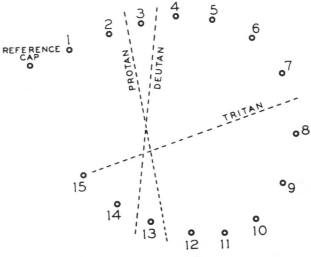

Figure 6.25 Recording form for the Farnsworth D–15 test.

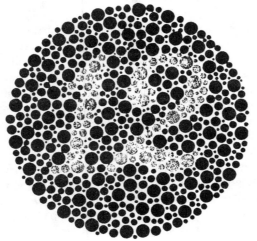

Figure 6.23   A pseudoisochromatic color plate.

Most pseudoisochromatic plates, such as those designed by Ishihara and Dvorine, are intended only for screening red-green color anomalies. However, one test—the American Optical H-R-R pseudoisochromatic plates, which unfortunately are no longer available—is designed for the detection and differential diagnosis of not only red-green anomalies but also yellow-blue anomalies. Each plate contains a triangle, a square, or a circle in any one (or more) of four locations. The subject responds, for example, by saying, "triangle in upper right and circle in lower left." This test can easily be administered to preschool children by giving the child a small watercolor paintbrush (with no paint!) and asking the child to "paint" the design he or she sees on the card.

It should be understood that the results of any pseudoisochromatic plate test are not valid unless conducted under daylight illumination. In terms of natural light, this means light from the northern sky (or from any direction if the sun is obscured by clouds). Because most optometric offices are not provided with northern light, the correct form of illumination involves the Macbeth Illuminant C—a lamp with a stand to hold the color vision booklet. It accepts an ordinary tungsten bulb, the light of which is filtered by a blue filter with specific absorption properties. If a Macbeth lamp is not available, the worst possible source of illumination is a bare tungsten bulb, since it contains too much yellow. Fortunately, a "daylight" fluorescent tube has illumination characteristics close enough to those of the Macbeth Illuminant C to make it a reasonably acceptable substitute.

The *Farnsworth D–15 test*, also known as the *dichotomous test*, is a useful, quickly performed test designed to sort people into those who are normal and those with color vision anomalies (see Figure 6.24). The test is made up of 15 color samples, and the patient's task is to line them up so they form a smooth color sequence between the two fixed samples at the ends of the tray. The results are plotted on a recording form (see Figure 6.25), and the practitioner can quickly determine whether a color vision anomaly is present. The test has the advantage of detecting not only red-green anomalies but also yellow-blue anomalies. Therefore, it is useful in screening for acquired color vision anomalies.

Color Vision Counseling

What should the color-deficient patient (or parent, in the case of a child) be told regarding the color vision defect? Most patients and parents will be interested in knowing how the condition came about. The presence of a red-green color anomaly in a child often takes the parents by surprise because the child may appear to have normal color vision.

Heath (1963) discussed the subject of color vision counseling in detail. The parents of an anomalous trichromat of preschool age should be told that the child will have only slightly greater trouble with colors than will children with normal color vision. Because all colors will appear less vivid than to the normal observer, the principal difficulties will be in the naming of pastel shades or very dark tones. Heath points out, however, that if a child has protanopia or deuteranopia, the parents should understand that many of the color names that color-normal children use to describe hues (green, yellow, orange, red, and brown) will apply to colors that all look the same to their child. When the child starts school, the parents should be encouraged to discuss their child's

problem with the teacher in sufficient detail so the teacher can understand the child's limitations and encourage him or her to perform satisfactorily within them.

Vocational counseling, although important, should be done with a certain amount of restraint. A color-defective person should not be told that certain occupational fields will remain forever closed unless the counselor is certain of the facts. For example, some of the best artists have been found to have red-green color vision anomalies. Because they see the world differently from color-normals, they often produce color combinations that the color-normal artist would not be apt to create. However, occupations in which safety hazards are involved should be stressed, of course, in any such discussion. An individual who has been diagnosed as a protanope should be told that he or she may have great difficulty seeing red taillights on cars or red traffic signals at a great distance. Even the anomalous trichromat should be told that he or she may have difficulty with traffic signals and with such things as color-coded wiring, should the patient decide to become an electrician. Once the parent and the child are aware of the kinds of problems that can occur, they are in a better position to discuss intelligently the occupational choices and other matters that may present problems.

VISUAL FIELD SCREENING

Every basic optometric examination should include some form of visual field evaluation. A detailed examination of the visual field is time-consuming and unnecessary unless there is reason to suspect the presence of a field loss. However, a visual field screening test can be done quickly and requires a minimum of equipment.

The emphasis put on glaucoma in recent years may tend to make us forget that a large number of conditions other than glaucoma can be responsible for visual field losses. Lesions of the choroid and retina, for example, often result in visual field defects. However, these lesions are usually visible with the ophthalmoscope, so their detection through visual field testing assumes a lesser degree of importance. Lesions of the visual pathway (optic nerve, optic tracts, optic radiations, and visual cortex) should be considered in any visual field screening procedure, as a visual field loss may provide the only (or the most obvious) indication that such a lesion is present.

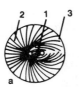

Figure 6.26 (*a*) Ganglion cell fiber distribution in the retina showing (1) papillomacular bundle, (2) radial fibers, and (3) arcuate fibers; (*b*) Seidel's sign; (*c*) partial Bjerrum scotoma; (*d*) double arcuate scotoma with nasal step.

Field Defects in Glaucoma

Visual field defects in glaucoma are the result of nerve fiber-bundle lesions. As shown in Figure 6.26a, the retinal ganglion cell fibers, traveling to the optic nerve head from the individual ganglion cells, are of three types: (1) the papillomacular bundle, made up of fibers from ganglion cells in the macular region; (2) the radial fibers, from the ganglion cells of the nasal portion of the peripheral retina; and (3) the arcuate fibers, from the ganglion cells in the temporal portion of the retina.

The arcuate fibers enter the optic nerve head at its upper and lower borders and are the first fibers adversely affected by an increase in intraocular pressure. As described by Harrington (1976), it is generally accepted that glaucomatous field defects occur as a result of diminished blood flow in the anterior optic nerve in the region of the lamina cribrosa, the arterial circle of Zinn-Haller, and the peripapillary choroidal circulation.

In the early stages of open angle glaucoma, the field defect may occur in the form of a vertical extension of the blind spot (Figure 6.26b) or a fiber-bundle scotoma extending above or below fixation to the horizontal midline in the nasal field (Bjerrum's scotoma). Only a partial Bjerrum scotoma may be present, so the practitioner may find an isolated fiber-bundle scotoma (see Figure 6.26c). In the later stages of glaucoma, a double Bjerrum scotoma may be present (one in the upper field and one in the lower field), the two coming together at the horizontal midline and forming a *nasal step* (in the nasal field, Figure 6.26d). At the same time, an overall reduction in the size of the nasal field may result in the scotoma "breaking through" the peripheral field. In terminal glaucoma, only a small temporal island of vision and/or a small central island may remain. However, even in terminal glaucoma, central vision may be relatively good when all peripheral vision has been lost.

Field Defects Due to Visual Pathway Lesions

Toxic amblyopia

Toxic amblyopia may be manifested as either a *bilateral central scotoma*, as in tobacco amblyopia, alcohol amblyopia, nutritional amblyopia, lead poisoning, or digitalis toxicity; or as *peripheral depression* or *contraction*, as in poisoning by quinine, arsenic, chloroquine, or salicylates (see Figure 6.27a). The scotoma of tobacco or alcohol amblyopia may be a *centrocecal scotoma*, involving both the fixation area and the area surrounding the blind spot (see Figure 6.27b).

Optic nerve disease

Inflammation of the optic nerve may occur in the form of *papillitis* (inflammation of the optic nerve head) or *retrobulbar optic neuritis* (inflammation of the optic nerve behind the eye). Either condition tends to cause a central scotoma with or without peripheral depression. If the inflammation is due to multiple sclerosis, there may be a transient positive scotoma (a scotoma of which the patient is aware). *Papilledema*, an elevation of the optic nerve head due to increased intracranial pressure, tends to cause visual field losses only in the later stages, and these field losses are usually permanent.

Optic chiasm

Tumors or other disease processes affecting the optic chiasm are more likely to affect the crossing fibers than the noncrossing fibers and, therefore, tend to cause temporal field loss for each eye (*bitemporal hemianopsia*). In some types of pituitary tumors, the field loss begins in the upper temporal field and progresses (clockwise for the right eye and counterclockwise for the left eye) into the lower temporal field and, finally, into the lower nasal and upper nasal fields. This progressive field loss is shown in Figure 6.28.

Postchiasmal pathway

Beyond the optic chiasm, neural fibers originating in the right half of each retina are located in the right side of the visual pathway (optic tract, lateral geniculate body, optic radiations, or visual cortex), whereas fibers originating in the left half of each retina are found in the left half of the visual pathway. Therefore, a lesion affecting the right side of the visual pathway will affect the left visual field for each eye and vice versa. Such a field loss is referred to as a *homonymous field loss*, and it can occur in the

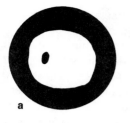 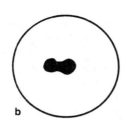

Figure 6.27   Field defects in toxic ambly-opia: (*a*) peripheral contraction; (*b*) centro-cecal scotoma.

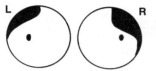 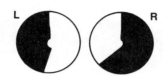

Figure 6.28   Progression of a bitemporal field loss due to a pituitary tumor affecting the optic chiasm. Note that the field defect is more severe for one eye than for the other.

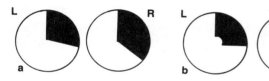

Figure 6.29   Homonymous field losses: (*a*) incongruous field defect with splitting of fixation, due to optic tract lesion; (*b*) congruous field defect with sparing of fixation, due to cortical lesion.

form of a homonymous sector defect, quadrant defect, or hemianopsia.

Homonymous field defects may be either *congruous* (the field defect having the same size and shape for each eye) or *incongruous* (the field defect differing in size and shape for the two eyes). Either *splitting of fixation* (in which half of the macular field for each eye is lost) or *sparing of fixation* (in which the macular field for each eye is intact) may occur (see Figure 6.29). In general, field defects due to lesions of the optic tracts and optic radiations tend to be incongruous and to show splitting of fixation, whereas field defects due to lesions of the visual cortex tend to be congruous and to have sparing of fixation.

Visual Field Screening Procedures

The great majority of visual field defects begin in the central visual field (i.e., within 30 degrees of fixation) or can be found in the central field at a relatively early stage. On the other hand, hemianopic field defects can be detected quickly and easily by using a peripheral field screening procedure known as *confrontations*. Therefore, the optometrist's preliminary examination should include both central and peripheral field screening procedures.

Confrontations

In the confrontation procedure, the examiner sits opposite, or "confronts," the patient and is concerned mainly with detecting restrictions in the outer limits of the visual field. Harrington (1976) recommends the following procedure:

1. The patient should have his or her back to the light and should face the examiner at a distance of about 1m.
2. A uniform dark background should be present behind the examiner.
3. The patient uses the examiner's eye as a fixation point.
4. Test objects should be 2, 5, and 10mm disks or plastic spheres attached to the end of a dull black, felt-covered wand about 2 feet in length.
5. With the patient fixating the examiner's eye, the test object is moved inward from the periphery in an arc simulating the curve of an imaginary perimeter. The patient is instructed to report when he or she first sees the object. The test is usually done in 8 half-meridians (0, 45, 90, 135, 180, 225, 270, and 315 degrees).
6. With a suitable test object, the examiner can outline the patient's blind spot, demonstrating what is meant by the disappearance of the test object.
7. Two test objects can be used simultaneously, one in the temporal field and one in the nasal field. This technique is valuable in detecting hemianopic field defects that might otherwise be easily missed. Harrington refers to this procedure as the *extinction phenomenon*: the presence of the stimulus in the seeing field gives the impression of "extinguishing" the test object in the nonseeing field.

Smith (tape no. 3) described a method of confrontations in which the examiner uses his or her own hand rather than test objects. The examiner presents one finger, two fingers, five fingers, or a fist in the patient's peripheral field and asks the patient to report what he or she sees.

Central field screening

Even though a great many instruments are now available for central visual field screening, the tangent screen remains the simplest and certainly the least expensive instrument for this procedure. As already stated, it is convenient to mount the tangent screen on a wall beside the ophthalmic chair. To do field screening it is then necessary only to swing the ophthalmic chair 90 degrees, raise or lower the chair so the patient's eyes are at the level of the fixation point, and adjust the headrest for the standard 1m testing distance. The refracting unit light can serve as a good illumination source for the tangent screen.

Flat test objects are superior to spherical ones, as the object (white on the front and black on the back) can be quickly flipped over to test the patient's response. The target should be mounted on a handle long enough so it is unnecessary for the examiner to stand in front of the tangent screen.

A good way to begin the testing procedure is to map out the patient's blind spot, going from nonseeing to seeing, using a large, white test object (5 or even 10mm). This procedure is interesting to the patient, and it provides an opportunity to check the speed and accuracy of responses. Once the blind spot has been grossly mapped out, a smaller test object (2 or 3mm) is used to more accurately determine the limits of the blind spot and to check for any vertical extensions of the blind spot. During the testing procedure the patient should be instructed to fixate intently on the central fixation point, and the examiner should be positioned so that constant checking can be made to be sure the patient is fixating.

To detect scotomas within the central field (like the fiber-bundle defects of glaucoma), the test object should be moved in a radial direction at intervals of about 5 degrees. This can be done most easily by forming a rosette pattern. The speed of movement should be carefully controlled—it should not be so fast that the patient does not have the opportunity to inform the examiner that the test object disappears, but it should not be so slow that the patient loses interest in the procedure. From time to time the test object should be flipped over, to make sure the patient reports its disappearance. In addition to moving the target in the radial direction, particular attention should be paid to the midlines: vertical for the detection of hemianopic defects and horizontal for the detection of a nasal step.

If the patient wears glasses, they should be worn for the tangent screen examination (unless they are of very low power). If the patient's glasses are bifocals, the practitioner can substitute a trial lens or uncut lens held by the patient. When this is done, correction for as much as 1.00D of astigmatism can be neglected.

The Amsler charts

The Amsler charts, designed by Marc Amsler of Zurich and published by Hamblin Instruments Ltd., consist of a series of seven grid-like charts designed for evaluating the central visual field, mounted on stiff cardboard in a ring binder. Although the use of these charts is not necessarily recommended as a screening procedure for all patients, the charts are inexpensive, easy to administer, and effective for confirming the presence of macular lesions. They should, therefore, be available in all optometric offices.

Indications. The Amsler chart test should be done whenever macular disease is suspected as a result of (1) an unexplained visual acuity loss, (2) a report of a visual disturbance in or near the fixation area (metamorphopsia), or (3) a questionable appearance of the macular area in ophthalmoscopy or biomicroscopy.

Procedure. Each chart has an overall size of 10cm vertically and horizontally, and each small square measures 5mm in each direction. When viewed at a distance of 28–30cm, the entire chart subtends an angle of 20 degrees, and each square subtends an angle of 1 degree. As shown in Figure 6.30, when the patient fixates the spot at the center of the chart, the chart image covers an area of the nasal retina extending about two-thirds of the way to the optic nerve head. The seven Amsler charts can be described as follows:

Chart 1. The standard chart, consisting of a white grid on a black background with a central fixation point. It is used in every case and in many cases is sufficient. (See Figure 6.30.)

Chart 2. Similar to the first chart, with the addition of two diagonal lines extending from the fixation point. It is for use with patients having a central scotoma, and the patient is asked to "look where the two lines would cross."

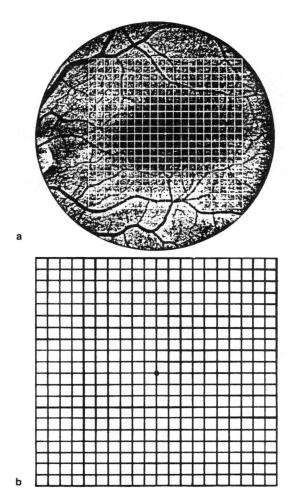

a

b

Figure 6.30 (a) Portion of the retina involved when visual field is investigated by means of the Amsler charts; (b) Amsler recording chart. A replica of chart 1, printed in black on white background (from M. Amsler, *Amsler Charts Manual*, Hamblin Instruments, 1949).

Chart 3. A red grid on a black background for use when investigating scotomas for color.

Chart 4. Has white dots (but no lines) on a black background and is designed to detect scotomas only.

Chart 5. Has white parallel lines on a black background, and it is oriented both horizontally and vertically to detect metamorphopsia.

Chart 6. Has black parallel lines on a white background; also is designed for detecting metamorphopsia.

Chart 7. Similar to chart 1 but contains smaller squares in the central 8 degrees.

The manual that accompanies the Amsler charts provides the examiner with a series of questions that should be asked when chart 1 is presented. Some of these questions are as follows:

1. "Do you see the white spot in the center of the squared chart?"
2. "Keeping the gaze fixed on the white spot in the center, can you see the four corners of the big square? Can you also see the four sides of the square? In other words, can you see the whole square?"
3. "While keeping the gaze fixed on the central fixation point, do you see, in the whole square, the network intact? Or are there interruptions in the network of squares, like holes or spots? Is it blurred in any place? If so, where?"

The answers to these questions will often suggest that additional charts be used. For example, if the patient is unable to see the central fixation point, the second chart (having the diagonal lines) should be presented. A patient often will be able to map out a scotoma, an area of metamorphopsia, or other field loss with great precision. A pocket in the back of the binder contains a pad of recording charts (black lines on white background). Either the practitioner or the patient can do the recording.

Visual Field Screening Devices

Visual field screening by the use of confrontations and the tangent screen, although not requiring expensive equipment, has the disadvantage (if done with care) of occupying a disproportionate amount of a busy practitioner's time. With the use of a visual screening device, a standardized procedure can be carried out in just a few minutes—because no interpretation of the findings is required while the test is being done, most practioners are pleased to turn the procedure over to a well-trained assistant or technician.

Harrington-Flocks multiple pattern screener

The first visual field screening device to be introduced was the Harrington-Flocks Multiple Pattern screener. This instrument consists of a booklet containing 20 pages; each page has a central fixation spot and three or more stimuli in the peripheral field. The central fixation spot is illuminated by ambient room illumination, but the peripheral stimuli are printed in fluorescent ink and are visible only when illuminated by ultraviolet light. The device is equipped with a chinrest; alignment for the patient's eyes is accomplished by making sure that for each eye, a large cross disappears within the blind spot. For each eye, each of ten pages is presented sequentially, and the ultraviolet light source is turned on to expose the fluorescent spots for only a fraction of a second. The patient is asked to report how many dots are seen each time the ultraviolet light is turned on. As described by Harrington, the 33 stimuli used (for all ten pages for each eye) cover most of the visual field within a 25-degree radius and encompass the majority of visual field defects.

An important advantage of this instrument is that stimuli are presented simultaneously in the left and right halves of the visual field. This makes it possible to detect hemianopic field defects that can escape detection in ordinary field testing as a result of the *extinction phenomenon*—the stimulus on the intact side of the visual field will "extinguish" the stimulus in the defective side of the field. According to Harrington, the extinction phenomenon is particularly likely to be present in lesions affecting the parietal lobe of the cortex.

Friedman field analyzer

The Friedman field analyzer is a screening device for the central field that utilizes a total of 15 stimulus patterns, each consisting of two, three, or four spots of light (see Figure 6.31). It consists of a black mat screen, 40cm in diameter, designed for testing at a 33cm distance. Holes in the screen are illuminated by a xenon flash tube. The flash can be triggered either by the examiner or by the patient and has a duration of one-third second. Neutral density filters, in 0.2 log unit steps, control the luminance level, which is selected on the basis of the patient's age.

Figure 6.31   The Friedman field analyzer.

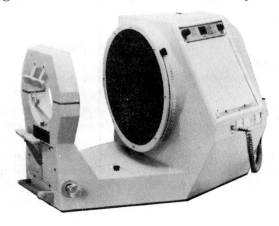

Similar to the Harrington-Flocks instrument, each time a new group of stimuli is presented, the patient is asked to report how many spots are seen. To compensate for the fact that the more peripheral retina has poorer resolving power than the central retina, spots toward the periphery are larger than central spots.

The Friedman Field Analyzer can be used either as a screening instrument or, by increasing the illumination for each target in a stepwise manner, for the performance of static perimetry. Yellen and Sherman (1979) reported on a study in which 66 eyes previously diagnosed as glaucomatous were tested by means of both the Friedman Field Analyzer and the Bausch and Lomb Autoplot. Forty-two of the 66 eyes were found to have field defects by the field analyzer, but only 23 were found to have field defects when examined by the Autoplot with 1/1000 or 2/1000 stimuli.

Automated field screening instruments

In recent years a large number of automated visual field testing instruments have been introduced, most of which are intended for use as screening instruments and for the performance of a complete visual field examination. These instruments, like the Harrington-Flocks and Friedman instruments, make use of *static perimetry*, which involves the use of multiple stimuli, rather than the conventional *kinetic perimetry*, as used with the tangent screen.

One of the first automatic field screening instruments to be introduced was the *Synemed Fieldmaster* (see Figure 6.32), which has been described by Johnson and Keltner (1980a, 1980b). This instrument has a uniformly illuminated white hemispherical field having 99 holes, each of which can be illuminated by a fiber-optic element. Each spot is illuminated in a programmed, randomized sequence, using a method referred to as *supra-threshold static perimetry*. The patient presses a button each time a stimulus is seen, and each response is recorded on heat-sensitive paper. The accuracy of fixation is monitored by light reflected from the patient's cornea; if the patient fails to fixate the central fixation spot, a warning tone is emitted, and the testing is discontinued until fixation is resumed. Keltner and Johnson (1985) have reported that the time required to run the screening program is 2-½ minutes per eye, whereas the time required to run a full visual field is 4 minutes per eye.

The *Automatic Tangent Screen* (see Figure 6.33), marketed by Computation Company, is a tangent screen, approximately 1m square, mounted on a wall and used at a 1m testing distance. There are 114 stimuli in the form of light emitting diodes (LEDs), and the stimulus pattern makes a "bow-tie" arrangement. A device resembling an electronic calculator, located at the left side of the instrument, allows the intensity, number of stimuli, and speed of presentation to be programmed. The fixation target is a red LED located at the end of a 2mm tube. Fixation is monitored by a stimulus in the blind spot area. When a patient responds to a blind spot stimulus, the instrument retests the last several spots to verify the results. Missed stimuli are automatically repeated; separate LED indicators representing the missed stimuli can be presented on the upper-left corner of the instrument and can be recorded manually. Keltner and Johnson (1985) reported the time for running the screening program as 2-½ minutes per eye. (Other automated visual field testing instruments are described in Chapter 7.)

Figure 6.32 The Synemed Fieldmaster.

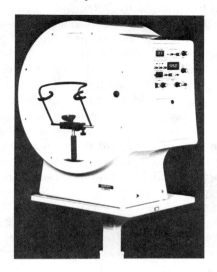

Figure 6.33 The Computation Company's Automatic Tangent Screen.

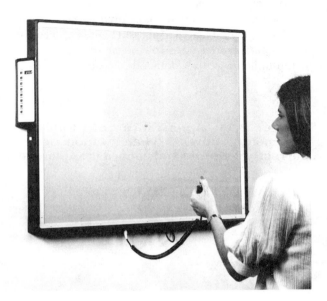

TONOMETRY

Although a definitive diagnosis of open angle glaucoma is made on the basis of changes in the appearance of the optic nerve head and the accompanying nerve fiber-bundle field defects, these changes may be preceded for many years by an elevation in intraocular pressure. A measurement of intraocular pressure (IOP), therefore, should be included in any routine optometric examination.

What Is the "Normal" IOP?

Schwartz (1980) has proposed several models for frequency distributions of intraocular pressure. In the distribution curves shown in Figure 6.34, the large curve to the left indicates the population of nonglaucomatous eyes with a mean of approximately 15mmHg, whereas the small curve indicates the population of glaucomatous eyes. For the normal (nonglaucomatous) population, a pressure of 21mmHg would fall approximately 2 standard deviations to the right of the mean; therefore, 97.5 percent of nonglaucomatous eyes would be expected

Figure 6.34 Intraocular pressure distribution curves for normal and glaucomatous eyes (Schwartz, 1980).

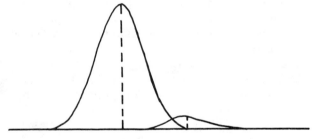

to have pressure values of 21mmHg or less. Thus, if a patient's pressure is found to be above 21mmHg, there is a good chance that the patient belongs to the glaucomatous group rather than the nonglaucomatous group; and the greater the pressure value (above 21mmHg), the greater the chance that glaucoma is present.

Indentation and Applanation Tonometry

Indentation tonometry, as performed by the *Schiötz tonometer*, is a convenient and easily performed method of tonometry, but in recent years it has been superseded to a great extent by applanation tonometry. A weight-loaded instrument, it is applied to the anesthetized cornea as the patient lies in a supine position looking upward, and the IOP is determined on the basis of the amount of indentation of the cornea produced by the standard 5.5g weight. Indentation tonometry suffers from the fact that the measurement is not a pure IOP measurement but is contaminated by the effects of the rigidity of the cornea and sclera and, to a lesser extent, by the curvature of the cornea. Myopic eyes tend to be relatively less rigid than emmetropic or hyperopic eyes, so Schiötz readings tend to be erroneously low in myopia and erroneously high in hyperopia.

The object of *applanation tonometry* is to merely flatten (applanate) the cornea; the IOP is determined on the basis of the amount of pressure that must be applied by the tonometer probe to applanate a corneal area of a predetermined size. The effects of the rigidity of the ocular coats and the corneal curvature are negligible in applanation tonometry, so an accurate measurement of intraocular pressure can be obtained.

Methods of applanation tonometry

Presently available instrumentation for applanation tonometry includes the Goldmann applanation tonometer, the MacKay-Marg electronic tonometer, the American Optical Noncontact tonometer, and the Tonomat tonometer. The Goldmann tonometer was the first instrument developed for applanation tonometry and it is still the standard to which all other methods of tonometry are compared. It was designed for use with the Haag-Streit slit lamp but is also available for use with other slit lamps. The MacKay-Marg and the AO Noncontact tonometers have the advantage of not requiring a corneal anesthetic, but they are relatively expensive instruments. The Tonomat is inexpensive but, like the Goldmann, requires the use of an anesthetic. However, the use of the Goldmann tonometer is recommended. The practitioner will certainly make regular use of the slit lamp during routine examinations, and both the additional cost and the additional time required for Goldmann tonometry as a part of the slit lamp examination are minimal.

Goldmann tonometer. The Goldmann tonometer probe is 3.06mm in diameter—a diameter selected to minimize the effects of corneal bending and the pressure exerted by the tear fluid—and is in the form of a biprism. In performing Goldmann tonometry, the cornea is first anesthetized with proparacaine (0.5 percent) and fluorescein is instilled. The cobalt blue filter is used and the slit lamp source is used to illuminate the tonometer probe. The tonometer scale is set at a value of 1 (indicating a pressure of 10mmHg), and the probe is carefully advanced toward the patient's cornea by moving the joystick forward as the patient fixates straight ahead and slightly upward. Initially, the probe is placed slightly below the patient's visual axis to avoid contact with the eyelashes; when the probe reaches a point 2–3mm in front of the cornea, the instrument is raised (by raising the slit lamp) until it is centered on the cornea. Just prior to contact, the examiner will see a pair of faint purple semicircles that will indicate whether or not the alignment is correct. When the probe contacts the cornea, two green semicircles will be seen, and the spring control knob should be adjusted until the inner edges of the two semicircles coincide (as shown in Figure 6.35). To determine intraocular pressure, the scale reading at which the inner edges of the semicircles coincide is multiplied by 10. A detailed procedure for use of

Figure 6.35 Appearance of Goldmann tonometer mires when tonometer is correctly centered and cornea is applanated.

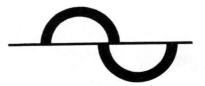

the Goldmann tonometer has been given by Spaeth (1980).

MacKay-Marg tonometer. The MacKay-Marg electronic tonometer can be kept on a shelf or table near the ophthalmic chair, and tonometry is performed while the patient sits upright in the chair. The probe, somewhat smaller than a fountain pen, is placed momentarily on the cornea while the patient fixates straight ahead. Although the instrument was designed to be used without a corneal anesthetic, obtaining readings on some patients without an anesthetic is difficult or impossible. The probe applanates an area considerably larger than the area contacted by the plunger to minimize the effects of corneal bending. The plunger displacement is very small, but it is magnified electronically and recorded by a penwriter on moving tape. Pressure readings with the MacKay-Marg tonometer tend to be about 2mmHg higher than readings with the Goldmann tonometer.

Noncontact tonometer. Using the American Optical Noncontact tonometer, a puff of air flattens a circular area of the cornea. Applanation is detected when a segment of the cornea behaves optically as if it were a plane mirror. The optical system of the instrument insures that a reading is taken when the nozzle is at a specific distance from the cornea. As the stream of air flattens the cornea, the intraocular pressure is inferred from the force of the airstream against the cornea at the instant of flattening (by the position of a piston within a cylinder). The instrument, mounted on a table, has a chinrest and a forehead rest. No anesthetic is required. The examiner first demonstrates how the instrument works by having the patient place a finger in front of the nozzle and actuating the puff of air by pushing the control button. With the patient seated at the instrument, the examiner centers the nozzle a few millimeters in front of the patient's cornea and then, looking through the telescope, further adjusts the position of the nozzle until a small red target is in sharp focus in the center of a circle. The patient is instructed to watch the red target and not to move; the examiner then pushes the button, actuating the puff of air. Usually two or three readings are taken for each eye. A number of comparative studies have shown that results with the noncontact tonometer compare favorably with those of the Goldmann tonometer.

Tonomat tonometer. The Tonomat tonometer consists of two cylindrical metal probes—one for each eye—and comes in a box that also contains a supply of paper Tono-caps, a supply of brown dye, and a measuring magnifier. The patient is placed in a supine position looking upward, and a drop of anesthetic is instilled into each eye. For each eye, a Tono-cap is placed on one of the probes and is covered with dye. While the patient fixates a finger, the examiner applanates each cornea with one of the probes, using the paper-covered end. For each probe, the dye will have been removed by the precorneal film from the area of applanation. The area of applanation, thus, is measured as the diameter of the area where the dye has been removed. If the eye is astigmatic, the nondyed area will be elliptical in shape and an estimate of the average diameter of the area must be made. The Tonomat has the advantage of being inexpensive, having no moving parts and therefore requiring no calibration.

Referral on the Basis of Tonometry Findings

Any patient having intraocular pressure of 21mmHg or more should either be referred for ophthalmological consultation or should be closely monitored by the optometrist. Whereas changes in the optic nerve head (high cup/disk ratio, thinning or notching of the rim of the cup, or pallor) or the presence of fiber-bundle field defects would confirm a clinical impression of glaucoma, an elevated pressure in the absence of optic nerve head or visual field changes may simply mean that the pressure elevation has been present for too short a time for these changes to occur. Because pressures may vary by several millimeters, depending on the time of day the readings are taken, repeated readings at different times of day should be considered for borderline readings. Also, a higher pressure in one eye than in the other, by 3mmHg or more, should indicate referral or monitoring. (Ophthalmoscopic findings in glaucoma are discussed in Chapter 7.)

To judge the accuracy of pressure readings, at least two readings should be taken for each eye on each occasion the pressure is checked. Factors such as apprehension and co-contraction of the ocular muscles may result in erroneously high readings, so when multiple readings are taken it is usually fair to assume that the *lowest* reading is the correct one.

BLOOD PRESSURE MEASUREMENT

In recent years optometrists have become increasingly aware of the importance of measuring blood pressure as a part of every routine optometric examination. Although it is true that with the ophthalmoscope the optometrist can detect generalized hypertension and arteriolar sclerosis, these conditions can be found at much earlier stages by measuring the patient's blood pressure.

There would be little advantage in the early detection of hypertension unless effective forms of treatment were available. Freis (1974) called attention to the fact that studies conducted beginning in 1964 have shown that antihypertensive therapy can control blood-pressure elevation in the great majority of cases and can significantly reduce both morbidity and mortality from cardiovascular complications of hypertension.

Epidemiology of Hypertension

Hypertension is not only mankind's most common disease, but according to Laragh (1974), it is the biggest single causative factor of death. Laragh estimated that on the basis of a criterion of blood pressure of 160/95mmHg or higher, 20 percent of the adult population has hypertension. Unfortunately, only about one-half of the hypertensive population is aware of the disease, and only about one-half of those who know they have the disease are under treatment. Further, treatment is successful in only about one-half of the cases being treated, so only about one in eight people who have hypertension is receiving adequate treatment. It has been established that hypertension is more common in men than in women and is much more prevalent in blacks than in whites.

Risk factors in hypertension, as discussed by Hutchinson ("Hypertension"), include social and economic status (apparently more highly educated people are more likely to take advantage of medical facilities), inheritance, salt intake, weight, cigarette smoking, and stress. Although nothing can be done about one's race, sex, or inheritance and little can be done about social or economic status, risk factors over which a patient can exert some degree of control are salt intake, weight, smoking, and stress.

Hypertension has been characterized as the "silent disease," because the symptoms are so minimal that the patient may not be aware of the presence of the disease. When symptoms do occur, the most prominent is headache. Smith (tape no. 47) described the hypertensive headache as occurring early in the morning and being relieved by drinking a cup of black coffee.

Complications of Hypertension

Untreated hypertension can be responsible for a large number of potentially fatal complications involving the heart, blood vessels, brain, and kidneys.

Congestive heart failure. Because of the increased arteriolar resistance in hypertension, the heart has to work harder to pump the blood through the vascular system. The heart begins to enlarge, both because of the inability to expel the blood coming into it and because of ventricular hypertrophy, and this leads to eventual failure.

Coronary artery disease. It has been found that both diastolic and systolic hypertension substantially increase the risk of coronary artery disease as well as ischemic heart disease. Antihypertensive therapy for patients having ischemic heart disease can significantly improve their survival rate.

Aortic aneurysm. The increased vascular resistance in hypertension causes dilation of the aorta and pressure on the blood vessels in the aorta's wall. This leads to necrosis of the medial aortic wall, which is followed by a splitting, or dissection, of the wall known as *dissecting aneurism*.

Cerebral vascular conditions. Cerebral hemorrhages, thrombosis, and ruptured aneurysms are much more likely to occur in individuals with elevated blood pressure.

Renal disease. Renal failure is a common cause of death in individuals with hypertension, particularly in malignant hypertension.

Hypertension Screening

It is undoubtedly true that a large proportion of the population visits a medical practitioner only rarely. Many of these same people, however, visit an eye practitioner on a regular basis. The optometrist, therefore, can play a valuable role in the community by screening for hypertension—the role is appropriate for the optometrist because hypertension can result in significant visual morbidity.

Screening for hypertension can easily become a part of the optometrist's routine examination procedure. A good time to perform sphygmomanometry is just after taking the case history, when the patient is relaxed. If visual acuity and other preliminary tests are done by an assistant or a technician, he or she may be the ideal person to measure blood pressure. Many types of sphygmomanometers are now available. Both the mercury and aneroid instruments require a stethoscope to listen to the Korotkoff sounds, whereas the electronic instruments convert these sounds to visual signals. The American Heart Association (AHA) has published a good pamphlet describing blood pressure measurement (Kirkendall, Burton, Epstein, and Freis, 1967) from which the following description is abstracted.

The rubber cuff is wrapped around the arm (in the initial examination, the pressure in each arm should be checked and recorded), and the arm is placed on a desk or tabletop so it will be in roughly the same horizontal plane as the heart. The cuff is then inflated with air to a pressure greater than the systolic pressure, causing the brachial artery to collapse. The brachial artery is located (on the inner side of the arm, at the elbow), and the stethoscope is placed over it.

As the pressure of the air in the cuff is released, the first sounds to be heard will be soft, tapping sounds. These are phase I of the Korotkoff sounds, and they are heard when the pressure in the cuff has fallen to a level just below the systolic pressure, allowing blood to flow through the artery. As the pressure in the cuff is lowered, the amount of time the blood flows through the artery is increased, causing first a swishing sound (phase II), followed by a louder, crisper sound (phase III). As the pressure is further decreased, a soft, muffled, "blowing" sound is heard (phase IV), and with further decrease in pressure all sound disappears (phase V).

The *systolic pressure* is the point at which the initial tapping sound is heard for at least two consecutive beats (phase I). According to the AHA pamphlet, the best index of *diastolic pressure* is the onset of the muffled sound of phase IV. However, some authors state that the criterion for diastolic pressure is phase V, the cessation of all sound.

Referral Criteria

Although many physicians believed that elevated blood pressure is a "normal" condition for older people, it was shown by Kannel, Gordon, and Schwartz (1971) in the Framingham study that higher arterial pressures are potentially more damaging for older people than for younger people. The Framingham study also showed that high systolic pressure was more strongly associated with coronary heart disease than high diastolic pressure, and that systolic pressure alone was a good predictor of stroke and congestive heart failure.

In the Framingham study, blood pressure was considered normal if systolic pressure was below 140mmHg and diastolic below 90mmHg. Hypertension was indicated for systolic pressure of 160mmHg or greater and diastolic pressure of 95mmHg or greater; pressures between these values were considered borderline. A recommended referral procedure is to refer for further evaluation all patients who have systolic readings of 160mmHg or above, or diastolic readings of 95mmHg or above; and to reschedule patients having borderline readings (between 140 and 160mmHg and between 90 and 95mmHg) for a second screening. If a patient is found to have borderline pressures on the second screening, the practitioner must decide whether to refer the patient or to schedule additional screening visits. These referral criteria are summarized in Table 6.3.

Table 6.3   Blood pressure referral criteria.

Visit	Systolic	Diastolic	Disposition
First	Below 140	Below 90	Normal: do not refer
	140–160	90–95	Borderline: rescreen
	160 or above	95 or above	Elevated: refer
Second	Below 140	Below 90	Normal: do not refer
	140–160	90–95	Monitor or refer
	160 or above	95 or above	Elevated: refer

Treatment of Hypertension

According to Freis (1974), the two main problems in hypertension therapy are (1) getting the patient to the physician and (2) persuading the patient to continue treatment once it has begun. For a patient who had no symptoms before the treatment was begun, the "symptoms" that can be caused by the medication may persuade the patient to discontinue treatment even though it is keeping blood pressure under control. Patient education, therefore, is an important aspect of treatment.

Antihypertensive therapy involves the use of three classes of pharmaceutical agents: (1) *diuretics*, which reduce blood volume by increasing the excretion of sodium and water; (2) *direct-acting vasodilators*, which reduce peripheral vascular resistance by acting directly on vascular smooth muscle; and (3) *sympathetic blockers*, which act centrally by reducing sympathetic activity. Treatment usually begins with one of the thiazide diuretics, which have the advantage of a slight vasodilator action in addition to their diuretic action. If a second drug is used, it is selected from either the second or third category. In some cases, three drugs (one from each category) are used.

Unfortunately, none of the drugs used in antihypertensive therapy are without adverse effects. Perhaps the most pronounced adverse effect of the thiazide diuretics is potassium depletion, which causes a feeling of fatigue and weakness (often making the patient feel worse than before the treatment). Physicians avoid this problem by prescribing potassium replacement therapy, either in the form of medication or fruits, such as bananas and oranges, which are high in potassium. Other possible adverse effects of the thiazide diuretics are increased blood glucose, nausea, and cardiac arrhythmia.

The effective treatment of hypertension requires good doctor-patient communication. Wilbur and Barrow (1974) suggest the physician provide every patient with the following information:

1. Hypertension is a major cause of stroke, heart failure, and kidney failure.
2. Hypertension is the "silent killer": you cannot tell by the way you feel whether or not you need your medication.
3. Hypertension is usually a lifelong condition, and you will have to have your blood pressure monitored for the rest of your life once it has been found to be elevated.
4. Taking antihypertensive medication daily has been proved beneficial.

TESTS PERFORMED BY AN OPTOMETRIC TECHNICIAN

Optometric technicians trained in the two-year associate degree programs given at many schools of optometry and community colleges are taught to perform most, if not all, of the procedures described in this chapter. However, practicing optometrists vary greatly in their willingness to delegate these procedures to a technician.

As a general principal, it is desirable to delegate a procedure to an optometric technician as long as the procedure requires no interpretation or decision making on the part of the examiner *while the test is being done*. Using this criterion, procedures that could be delegated to a trained technician would include visual acuity measurement, stereopsis testing, color vision screening, visual field screening, tonometry, and blood pressure measurement. Some practitioners would be reluctant to delegate visual field screening and tonometry to a technician, saying these tests require interpretation by the examiner. However, according to the author's experience in the Optometric Technician Program at Indiana University, a well-trained technician is completely capable of performing these tests. It is imperative, however, that the practitioner work closely with the technician when a "new" procedure is being performed, monitoring the technician's work for several weeks. The practitioner must also routinely recheck any abnormal or borderline findings.

Although a trained optometric technician can adequately perform the cover test, corneal reflex test, near-points of accommodation and convergence tests, and broad *H* motility test, for most of these tests practitioners can pick up many nonquantifiable clues if they do these tests themselves. This series of tests can be done in just a few minutes' time by the experienced practitioner, so little time would be saved by having the procedures performed by a technician.

Because the pupillary reflex tests require interpretation on the part of the examiner while the tests are being done, they should be done by the practitioner rather than a technician. This applies also to the external and internal examination (discussed in Chapter 7).

Finally, in any discussion of the use of optometric technicians, state optometry laws and regulations must be taken into consideration. In some states the optometry law stipulates that certain specific tests must be performed by the optometrist in every optometric examination.

Study Questions

1. What are the stimuli to accommodation (expressed in diopters) and convergence (expressed in prism diopters) for a patient having an interpupillary distance of 64mm (a) for a distance of 6m? (b) for a distance of 40cm?

2. When performing the alternating cover test, why should the phi movement test not be used for a patient who may be strabismic?

3. A clinical impression (diagnosis) of glaucoma would be confirmed not by a high intraocular pressure reading, but by one or both of what two findings?

4. What problems may a child have in seeing and interpreting colors if he or she is (a) an anomalous trichromat? (b) a deuteranope or a protanope?

5. When the near-point of accommodation is taken while the patient wears old glasses, why is it *not* appropriate to record the reciprocal of the near-point of accommodation as the amplitude of accommodation?

6. When a projected chart is used for measuring visual acuity, what are two problems that may result if an excessive amount of overall room illumination is used?

7. In measuring the visual acuity of a child, why should a block of five or six rows of letters be used rather than a single row of letters or a single letter?

8. In the unilateral cover test, when the right eye is covered the left eye turns inward to take up fixation, but when the left eye is covered the right eye makes no movement. What is the diagnosis?

9. Describe the sound heard in the stethoscope indicating (a) the systolic pressure; (b) the diastolic pressure.

10. If you take three tonometer readings on a patient's eye (all with the same tonometer) and all three readings have different values, which of the three readings is most likely to be the correct one? Why?

11. In the Framingham study, what ranges of systolic and diastolic pressures were considered to be borderline?

12. What are two commercially available visual acuity tests that have the advantage that letters rather than pictures are used to measure a preschool child's visual acuity, even though the child is unable to read?

13. In the diplopia field test, the patient reports the greatest vertical diplopia in the upper right field. (a) Either of which two muscles may be at fault? (b) If the most peripheral image belongs to the left eye, which of the two muscles is underacting?

14. What pupillary anomaly may be caused by each of the following conditions? (a) basilar or vertebral artery insufficiency; (b) a lesion of the ciliary ganglion; (c) multiple sclerosis.

15. Where would you expect a lesion to be for each of the following visual field defects? (a) a homonymous hemianoptic field defect with macular splitting; (b) a congruous homonymous hemianoptic defect; (c) a field defect involving the superior temporal quadrant of the visual field for each eye.

16. In the alternating cover test, when the right eye is covered the left eye is observed to turn outward, and when the left eye is covered the right eye is seen to turn outward. What is the diagnosis?

17. How should a patient's visual acuity be recorded, using English notation, if the patient can see the 20/400 *E* at a distance no farther than (a) 10 feet? (b) 5 feet? (c) 2 feet?

18. Why is it important for the examiner to watch the patient's eyes during the near-point of convergence test?

19. When a patient is instructed to fixate a source of light while one eye is occluded, (a) where is the corneal reflex normally located in relation to the center of the pupil? (b) what would be your tentative diagnosis if the position of the corneal reflex (with monocular fixation) differed considerably for the two eyes?

20. List the ocular muscles (for both eyes) that act as (1) right-hand elevators; (b) right-hand depressors; (c) left-hand elevators; (d) left-hand depressors.

CHAPTER 7

The Ocular Health Examination

Historically, the procedures making up the ocular health examination (the external and internal examinations) have been completed as a part of the preliminary examination. However, with indirect ophthalmoscopy under dilation now a routine optometric procedure, the internal examination is normally postponed until after the completion of the refraction and the binocular vision examination. Additional procedures (performed only when indicated), including gonioscopy, biomicroscopic examination of the posterior segment under dilation, and photodocumentation, are also done at the completion of the examination. But because of the importance of establishing the clarity of the lens and the macular area before beginning objective and subjective refraction, it is strongly recommended that biomicroscopy and direct ophthalmoscopy (without dilation) be done in the latter part of the preliminary examination.

THE USE OF DIAGNOSTIC PHARMACEUTICAL AGENTS

When U.S. laws regulating the practice of optometry were passed in the 48 states early in the 20th century, without exception the phrase "without the use of drugs" appeared in the definition of optometry. This qualification was the result of pressure from the medical profession—the optometrists of the day clearly preferred to have a "drugless" profession rather than no profession at all. In recent years, one by one, the state laws have been changed. Diagnostic pharmaceutical agents can now be used legally in all but a few of the 50 states, and laws permitting their use are under consideration in the others. Nothing in the following discussion should be interpreted as recommending or suggesting that optometrists make use of diagnostic pharmaceutical agents in states where the law forbids their use.

Diagnostic Agents Used in Optometric Practice

Three classes of diagnostic pharmaceutical agents are useful in the everyday practice of optometry. First, *topical anesthetics* are useful in anesthetizing the cornea prior to tonometry or gonioscopy. Second, *mydriatics* are used for dilating the pupil prior to such procedures as binocular indirect ophthalmoscopy, biomicroscopy involving the structures of the posterior segment of the eye (with the aid of a Goldmann fundus lens or a 60D or 90D condensing lens), and fundus photography. The third class of agents, *cycloplegics*, are useful in both objective and subjective refraction of patients having (or suspected of having) latent hyperopia or ciliary spasm. (Readers are referred to Chapter 9 for a discussion of cycloplegic agents and cycloplegic refraction.)

Instillation of drugs

Mitchell (1959) has given precise instructions for instilling drops into the conjunctival sac. He makes the following points:

1. The patient's head should be tilted back far enough so the face is almost horizontal. When this is done, the liquid can be dropped into the lower conjunctival sac without being splashed on the upper lashes or on the cornea.

2. The patient's head should be tilted slightly toward the side of the eye in which the drop is to be instilled. The drop will then be contained in the lateral portion of the conjunctival sac, minimizing the tendency for it to drain through the puncta into the canaliculi.

3. The practitioner should use the little finger of the left hand to pull down the patient's lower lid, hold the dropper bottle in the right hand so it is no more than 1 inch above (and immediately over) the lower fornix, and instill the drop.

4. The patient will be less likely to blink at the wrong moment if warned when the drop is about to fall.

5. It is useless to instill more than one drop at a time, because the conjunctival sac will only hold one drop. If a second drop is needed, the practitioner should wait about 1 minute for the first drop to be absorbed.

6. After instillation of the drop, the patient should be told to look straight ahead so the lower conjunctival sac is deepened. The patient is then told to close the lids slightly, and any overflow is wiped away.

Haine (1981) recommends what he calls the "lid-pinch" method. As the patient looks upward, the practitioner pulls the lower lid outward, making a pocket of the lower conjunctival sac, and then instills the drop. The lid is held in this position for several seconds, allowing the solution to penetrate into the mucosa of the conjunctival sac.

Topical anesthetics

The corneal and conjunctival epithelium is richly supplied with sensory nerve endings. It is thought that topical anesthetics act by reducing the permeability of the nerve cell membranes to sodium ions. This blocks nerve conduction by interfering with depolarization, so the threshold potential level is not reached and the nerve action potential does not occur.

The first agent to be used as a local anesthetic in ophthalmology was *cocaine*. As described by Ellis (1977), cocaine is a naturally occurring alkaloid derived from the leaves of *Erythroxylon coca*, a plant growing in the high altitudes of the Andes. The Indians in the region ground the leaves and packed them into wounds to relieve pain. The active agent, cocaine, was isolated in 1860 and was first used as an ocular anesthetic in 1884. Cocaine is no longer used in routine procedures such as anesthesia for tonometry and gonioscopy because of side effects that include drying and even desquamation of the corneal epithelium.

The most commonly used topical anesthetics in ophthalmology and optometry are *proparacaine*, *benoxinate*, and *tetracaine*. All three of these agents have a rapid onset of anesthesia and a duration of about 20 minutes. For tonometry or gonioscopy, only one drop (or two at most) is required. Before the anesthetic is instilled, the patient should be warned not to rub the eyes until sensation has returned, to avoid causing an abrasion.

Proparacaine (Ophthaine, Ophthetic, Alcaine), used in 0.5 percent ophthalmic solution, is considered by many practitioners to be the agent of choice, as the possibility of adverse effects with the preparation is very small. *Benoxinate* (Dorsacaine), used in 0.4 percent ophthalmic solution, should be used with caution if the patient has cardiac disease, thyroid disease, or allergies. *Tetracaine* (Pontocaine), used in 0.5 percent ophthalmic solution, can cause central nervous system stimulation bringing on convulsive activity and depression if accidentally introduced into the bloodstream (Ellis, 1977).

An important effect of topical anesthetics is to increase the permeability of the corneal epithelium to other preparations (Davies, 1972). For this reason, a mydriatic or cycloplegic drug may have a greater effect than would otherwise be anticipated if applied soon after the application of a topical anesthetic.

Mydriatics

Two classes of drugs produce a mydriatic effect when instilled into the eye. *Sympathomimetic agents* directly or indirectly stimulate the dilator pupillae muscle of the iris, mimicking the action of the sympathetic division of the autonomic nervous system, and bring about dilation of the pupil. The sympathomimetic agents most often used as mydriatics are *phenylephrine* (Neosynephrine) and *hydroxyamphetamine* (Paradrine). Phenylephrine is available in either a 10 percent or a 2.5 percent ophthalmic solution. Although in the past the use of the 10 percent solution was thought necessary, Jauregui and Polse (1974) found that when phenylephrine is used in conjunction with the anesthetic proparacaine, 0.5 percent, a solution of only 2.5 percent is necessary; maximum mydriasis occurs in 35–45 minutes and lasts 3–6 hours.

Antimuscarinic (Atropine-like agents) antagonize the muscarinic action of acetylcholine by blocking its action on structures innervated by postganglionic parasympathetic nerve fibers, paralyzing both the constrictor pupillae and the ciliary muscle. The antimuscarinic agents most often used for mydriasis are *cyclopentolate* (Cyclogyl) and *tropicamide* (Mydriacyl). In view of the possible side effects of *cyclopentolate* (to be discussed), its use should be avoided when only a mydriatic (as opposed to a cycloplegic) effect is desired. Tropicamide (Mydriacyl) is available in 0.5 percent and 1.0 percent ophthalmic solutions. Using the 0.5 percent solution, two drops instilled into the conjunctival sac will usually produce a full mydriasis in about 15 minutes, and the pupil returns to normal in 8–9 hours (Davies, 1972).

Adverse effects of mydriatic agents. In a survey of the literature concerning adverse effects of diagnostic pharmaceutical agents, Hopkins and Lyle (1977) reported three instances of adverse cardiovascular effects associated with the use of phenylephrine. However, in all cases an excessive dose of 10 percent phenylephrine was used. The recommended dosage of phenylephine is now one drop of the 2.5 percent solution, and no adverse effects have been reported with this solution.

An additional problem with phenylephrine is that if mydriasis should be followed by an attack of acute glaucoma, the use of pilocarpine to bring about miosis may cause pupillary-block glaucoma. Because of this possibility, Chang (1977) recommends that for an eye with an intact iris, tropicamide is a safer mydriatic than phenylephrine.

A number of reports of side effects due to the use of cyclopentolate have been reported by Ellis (1977) and Hopkins and Lyle (1977). These side effects included confusion, ataxia, hallucinations, speech difficulties, and convulsions. All of these cases involved children, all but one involved a higher-than-recommended dose of cyclopentolate or the use of cyclopentolate in combination with other antimuscarinic agents, and none of the reactions appeared to be life threatening. Hopkins and Lyle stated that adverse reactions to tropicamide in the literature are conspicuous by their rarity.

In summary, the agent of choice for mydriasis is tropicamide. Some practitioners recommend the use of phenylephrine in combination with tropicamide to achieve a greater (and faster) dilation. However, only one drop of the 2.5 percent solution of phenylephrine should be used. In any case, the mydriatic effect can be enhanced by prior instillation of one drop of 0.5 percent proparacaine. The use of cyclopentolate should be reserved for the cycloplegic refraction of young children suspected of having latent hyperopia (see Chapter 9).

Risk of Angle Closure

The possibility that an attack of angle closure glaucoma could occur as a result of the instillation of a cycloplegic agent must be considered. Parasym-pathetic blocking agents (including atropine, cyclopentolate, and tropicamide) can cause an attack of angle closure glaucoma by increasing the laxness of the peripheral iris, whereas sympathomimetic agents such as *phenylephrine hydrochloride* (Neosyne-phrine) can cause an attack of angle closure glaucoma by tightening up the dilator of the iris, causing pupillary block.

As described by Simmons and Dallow (1976), in eyes with a convex iris and relative pupillary block (which causes an exaggerated pressure differential between the posterior and anterior chambers), the laxness of the iris brought about by the use of a parasympathetic blocking agent makes it possible for the iris to be pushed into the trabecular meshwork, causing closure of the angle. The possibility of angle closure is greatest at the position of middilation of the pupil, according to Simmons and Dallow, probably because both the relative pupillary block and the peripheral laxness of the iris are at a maximum in this position.

The risk of angle closure can be reduced to an absolute minimum if the examiner makes use of the slit lamp to estimate the anterior chamber angle prior to the instillation of a cycloplegic agent.

Estimation of Anterior Chamber Angle

Observation of the anterior chamber angle requires the use of an instrument called a *gonioscope*. However, the width of the anterior chamber angle can be estimated quite accurately using the biomicroscope. Using a narrow slit, the examiner illuminates the cornea and the iris from an angle of approximately 60 degrees and views the illuminated area from the straight-ahead position. While viewing an optic section of the cornea at the very edge of the temporal limbus, the practitioner estimates the width of the shadow formed between the slit lamp beam illuminating the cornea and the beam on the surface of the iris. As shown in Figure 7.1, the angle can then be graded on a scale from 4 (wide open) to 0 (closed angle).

If the width of the shadow on the iris is equal to or greater than one-half the width of the corneal

Figure 7.1   Estimation of anterior chamber angle.

Grade 4   Grade 3   Grade 2   Grade 1

optic section, a *grade 4 angle* exists, whereas a shadow between one-fourth and one-half of the width of the corneal optic section indicates a *grade 3 angle*. According to Lichter (1976), for a grade 3 or grade 4 angle, the angle formed by the front surface of the iris and the peripheral portion of the cornea is from 30–45 degrees, and the angle is incapable of closure. If the width of the shadow is one-fourth the width of the beam on the cornea, a *grade 2 angle* exists. Lichter defines a grade 2 angle as one that may occlude under certain circumstances. Such circumstances, although not specified by Lichter, might include dilation of the pupil due to darkness or instillation of a cycloplegic or mydriatic agent. If the width of the shadow is less than one-fourth the width of the beam on the cornea, the angle is a *grade 1 angle* and is susceptible to closure. If no shadow is present, the angle is closed (the patient is undergoing an attack of angle-closure glaucoma!), and the angle is defined as *grade 0 angle*.

The practitioner can freely dilate a grade 3 or grade 4 angle without fear of angle closure. Grade 2 angles should be dilated only with very good reason and when prior arrangements for treatment of a possible emergency have been made; grade 1 angles should never be dilated. Before making a decision on dilation, the angle for each eye should be estimated in both the nasal and temporal quadrants.

Van Herick, Shaffer, and Schwartz (1969) examined 400 eyes both by gonioscopy and the slit-lamp technique and found that the drainage angle width correlated well for the two procedures. As for the frequency of occurrence of dangerously narrow angles, these investigators published data concerning angle widths as determined by the slit lamp on 2,185 unselected patients examined over a 5-year period. As shown here, they found that only 37 patients (1.64 percent) had grade 1 or grade 2 angles; 2,148 (98.36 percent) had grade 3 and grade 4 angles:

Grade	Number	Percentage
1	14	0.64
2	23	1.0
3	1,321	60.0
4	827	38.36

Gonioscopic evaluation of the angle

Although few optometrists include gonioscopy in their normal examination routines, the report of Cockburn (1981), an Australian optometrist, is of interest. Cockburn performed gonioscopy on the left eyes of 300 successive patients ranging in age from 5–87 years. He used a Zeiss four-mirror goniolens and confined his observations to the superior aspect of the angle, as this is where appositional closure and formation of synechiae tend to occur first. He found that 6 percent of his patients had some or all of the trabeculae obscured from gonioscopic view and, therefore, the angles were considered to be significantly narrowed; 2 percent had only the anterior half (or less) of the trabeculae in view and thus were considered to be critically narrowed.

Cockburn (1981) compared these results to those of a study he had previously performed using the Van Herick slit-lamp technique on 509 successive patients. In this study, 7.5 percent of the patients were found to have a shadow width of 0.3 or less as compared to the width of the corneal beam. He also compared his results to those of Van Herick, Shaffer, and Schwartz (1969), who reported that only 1.64 percent of 2,185 unselected patients were found to have angles of grade 2 or less (shadow width of 0.25 or less than that of the width of the corneal beam), and to a previous study by Van Herick, Shaffer, and Schwartz (1969) in which the prevalence of narrow angles, using the same criterion, was found to be 4.6 percent.

Cockburn concluded that, because it is unlikely that optometrists will perform gonioscopy on all patients to identify the 6 percent who will have significant narrowed angles, the Van Herick test should be used, and those eyes having angle width assessments of *0.3 corneal units or less* should be considered as having significantly narrow angles.

Reversal of angle closure

Because reversal of angle closure is a therapeutic procedure rather than a diagnostic procedure, practitioners who are permitted by law to use diagnostic but not therapeutic pharmaceutical agents should make preparations (in advance) for emergency treatment of angle closure, should it occur. This usually can be done by working out an arrangement with a local ophthalmologist or, if there is no ophthalmologist in the vicinity, a general medical practitioner or a hospital emergency treatment center. For example, the arrangement may call for the optometrist to instill pilocarpine or timolol on an emergency basis and get the patient as quickly as possible to the ophthalmologist, general physician, or emergency room for continuation of the treatment.

An angle-closure attack due to the instillation of a mydriatic or cycloplegic agent would probably occur several hours after the patient left the practitioner's office. Symptoms of such an attack include pain in and around the eye, blurred vision, and, in some cases, gastrointestinal symptoms such as nausea and vomiting, which tend to mask the nature of the disease (Gombos, 1977). Examination of the patient will indicate an edematous cornea, partially dilated, poorly reactive pupil, and markedly elevated intraocular pressure.

In the past, some authors have advocated the routine use of a miotic agent after mydriasis or cycloplegia to insure that an attack of angle-closure glaucoma does not occur. However, Garston (1975) warned against the routine use of a miotic agent after dilation. Not only does pilocarpine constriction tend to last longer than the mydriasis, but there is evidence that pupillary block can be brought about by the use of a miotic. This is due to the fact that in middilation (as may occur when a miotic is used for an already dilated pupil), the border of the iris tends to press firmly against the lens capsule.

Gombos (1977), discussing hospital emergency room treatment of angle-closure glaucoma, described both topical and systemic forms of treatment. For topical treatment he recommended the instillation of the pilocarpine, 2 percent, every 10 minutes, or eserine, 0.75 percent, at the same time intervals. For systemic treatment he recommended the intravenous route (because the patient is usually nauseous) using acetazolamide (Diamox), an intravenous dose of 500mg being administered initially and followed by a dose of 250mg every 4 hours by mouth after the nausea has subsided. Gombos also discussed the use of the hyperosmotic agents mannitol, urea, and glycerol (the latter administered by mouth) in systemic treatment. Terry (1977) warned that, because glycerol can raise the blood sugar level, it should be used with care (if at all) for elderly diabetic patients, whereas isosorbide has no caloric value and can be safely given to diabetic patients.

As noted by Gombos (1977), an acute attack of angle-closure glaucoma will almost certainly recur if the eye is not operated on. Therefore, after successful medical treatment of the patient's first angle-closure attack, the patient should be examined by an ophthalmologist (using tonometry and gonioscopy), and a peripheral iridectomy should be done as soon as the condition of the eye is suitable for surgery.

THE EXTERNAL EXAMINATION

The examiner's approach during the external and internal examination, like the history taking and the preliminary examination, should be problem oriented. Problems identified during the history and the preliminary examination should be further evaluated, when appropriate, and additional problems should be anticipated. A problem-oriented mental set on the part of the practitioner not only insures better patient care but has the advantage of keeping the procedure from becoming tiresome. The external examination includes a gross inspection of the external structures of the eye using oblique illumination, and examination by means of the biomicroscope.

Use of Oblique Illumination

Most of the external examination is done by *oblique illumination*: the optometrist illuminates a given structure from an oblique angle and inspects it with or without magnification. The least sophisticated method of oblique illumination involves the use of the refracting unit light and the practitioner's naked eye. A better method involves the use of a penlight and a binocular loupe. The best method involves the use of the slit-lamp biomicroscope. For the part of the examination that can be performed by direct rather than oblique illumination, *distance magnification* can be easily provided by the ophthalmoscope with its auxiliary lenses. A +10.00D lens will enable the optometrist to have a clear, magnified view of ocular structures seen at a distance of 10cm.

In one of the first textbooks describing the use of the slit-lamp biomicroscope, Doggart (1948) emphasized that the ocular structures should not be studied under the high magnification of the biomicroscope until they first have been studied under low magnification or with no magnification at all, using oblique illumination. However, many practitioners today spend a minimum of time (or none at all) examining the patient under lower magnification before beginning biomicroscopy.

Biomicroscopy

The biomicroscope derives its name from the fact that it enables the practitioner to observe, under magnification, the living tissues of the eye. At the risk of stating the obvious, it may be remarked that due to the transparency of its media, the eye is the only structure of the body that is available for noninvasive histological examination during life.

The biomicroscope consists of an illumination system, an observation system, and the necessary mechanical apparatus for their support and coordi-

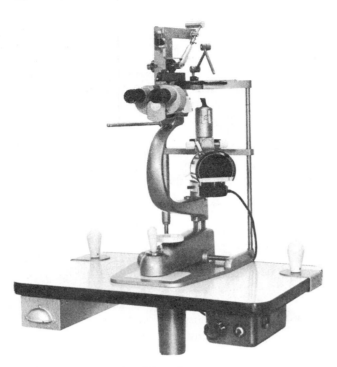

Figure 7.2   Zeiss biomicroscope.

nation. The illumination system is in the form of a bright, focal source of light with a slit mechanism and circular apertures of various sizes. The observation system is a binocular microscope capable of a wide range of magnification. When using the biomicroscope, the examiner typically illuminates an ocular structure with a beam of the desired width and observes the structure at an oblique angle.

In terms of design, there are two major types of biomicroscopes. In the design typified by the Zeiss and the American Optical instruments, the light source is located below the level of the slit, near the base of the instrument (see Figure 7.2). In the other design, typified by the Haag-Streit and other instruments, the light source is located at the top of the instrument (see Figure 7.3). The latter form of instrumentation has the advantage of having a very intense source of light, but the disadvantage of having fewer choices of magnification.

Adjustment of the instrument

All modern slit-lamp biomicroscopes have the following controls:

1. A joystick, by means of which the illumination and observation systems (which are linked together) can be moved backward and forward and from side to side.

2. A screw arrangement, incorporated into the joystick in some instruments, for moving the illumination and observation systems, upward and downward.

3. An adjustable headrest and chinrest, with a line or other marker to indicate the desired level of the patient's eyes. If the chinrest is adjusted so the patient's eyes are at this level, the examiner will find that a sufficient range of movement will be available in both the upward and downward directions.

4. Controls for the adjustment of slit width and slit height and for the rotation of the slit; and controls for the interposition of a cobalt blue filter and (for some instruments) a green, or red-free, filter.

5. Magnification controls, including two or more pairs of readily changeable objective lenses and two sets of eyepieces. One instrument, the Nikon slit lamp, is equipped with a continuously variable "zoom" magnification system.

6. An on/off switch and an illumination control, usually provided with three levels of illumination. To keep from dazzling the patient and to avoid premature burning out of the bulb, low or moderate illumination should be used for the majority of routine slit-lamp procedures.

7. A focusing rod, which is mounted in place of the chinrest. Following the instructions provided with the instrument, the slit source and the

Figure 7.3   Haag-Streit biomicroscope.

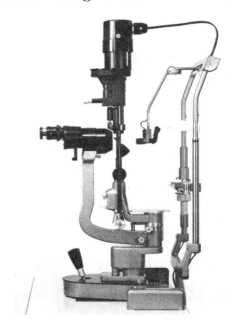

microscope are adjusted, using the focusing rod, so they are parfocal (i.e., focus in the same plane).
8. A fixation object for the patient.

Seating and aligning the patient

Before the slit-lamp examination is begun, the patient should be seated comfortably at the instrument, with the chair or stool positioned high enough so he or she is leaning slightly forward into the instrument's headrest. Some slit lamps are provided with hand grips, which are useful to help the patient maintain a steady position throughout the examination. The examiner's position is also important: the stool should be adjusted so the microscope is at eye level without the need to hunch forward. Before seating the patient, the slit source and the microscope should already have been adjusted for parfocality, and the microscope should have been adjusted for the examiner's interpupillary distance.

The Haag-Streit 900 slit lamp has a monocular fixation target with an adjustable-focus optical system, which makes it possible for the patient to fixate the target without the necessity for accommodation or convergence. Most other slit lamps have a simple illuminated target that requires accommodation and convergence on the part of the patient. With these instruments, some practitioners instruct the patient to look at the practitioner's ear or at an object across the room.

In making preliminary adjustments of the light source, the examiner should take care not to unnecessarily expose the patient's eyes to the slit-lamp beam. Preliminary adjustments can be made on the patient's sclera near the limbus or on the closed eyelid.

For the novice, the first problem in the use of the slit lamp is finding the patient's cornea. This can be most easily done by focusing the slit on the patient's closed eyelid, using low magnification and a slit of medium width, and then instructing the patient to open his or her eyes. By moving the joystick forward very slightly, the oily appearance of the tear layer will be noted. If the patient is asked to blink two or three times, the presence of the tear layer can be appreciated by the appearance of debris moving upward and downward in the tear film with each blink. The slit can then be narrowed down, and an optic section of the cornea can be seen.

Methods of illumination

It is convenient to discuss the use of the biomicroscope in terms of methods of illumination. As Doggart (1948) pointed out, in actual practice we do not solemnly proceed from one method of illumination to the other. Rather, methods overlap and swiftly alternate with one another. Nevertheless, the practitioner must become thoroughly familiar with each method of illumination and know on what occasions each should be used.

Direct illumination. In making use of direct illumination, the slit-lamp beam and the microscope are both focused sharply on the structure to be observed. As shown in the top diagram in Figure 7.4, the beam and the microscope are arranged so they are at an oblique angle to one another. In direct illumination, either a wide or a narrow slit can be used.

When the *wide slit* is used, the practitioner can concentrate on viewing the surface itself (e.g., the surface of the precorneal film or the surface of the cornea), or observe a transparent structure (such as the cornea) as a three-dimensional figure known as a *parallelepiped* (shown in Figure 7.5). Using the

Figure 7.4 Methods of illumination (Grosvenor, 1963).

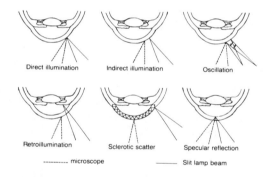

Figure 7.5 Parallelopiped and optic section (Grosvenor, 1963).

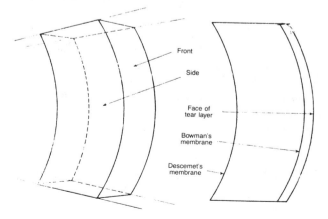

parallelepiped, the corneal stroma (which makes up 90 percent of the thickness of the cornea) will appear to be optically empty in the absence of any opacities. The normal corneal stroma contains sensory nerve fibers, which are fine and silky in appearance, splitting into branches at acute angles.

With the *narrow slit*, an optic section of the cornea, anterior chamber, or crystalline lens can be observed (see Figure 7.5). It is the optic section that gives rise to the term *biomicroscope:* a section of the living eye can be observed much the same as if a slice of it were placed on a microscope slide. When the cornea is observed in an optic section, three bright bands will be seen: two closely spaced anterior bands and a posterior band. The most anterior of the bands is formed by the precorneal film and appears to be yellow-green in color if fluorescein has been instilled. The second bright band is formed by *Bowman's membrane*, and the epithelium occupies the space between the two anterior bright bands. The posterior band is formed by *Descemet's membrane*, and the wide space between the second and third bright bands is occupied by the corneal stroma. The optic section is useful in localizing opacities or other lesions within the cornea, anterior chamber, or lens, as well as estimating the depth of a lesion within one of these structures.

Indirect illumination. In using indirect illumination, the beam is focused on an opaque or translucent structure located to one side of the area to be observed by the microscope, and this area is observed somewhat in shadow by virtue of scattered light.

Oscillation. Oscillation is a variation of indirect illumination in which the microscope is kept in focus on the structure to be observed and the beam is oscillated back and forth, alternately resulting in direct illumination and indirect illumination. Fine corneal scars, opacities, and other lesions are often isolated more readily by using oscillation than either direct or indirect illumination.

Retroillumination. Also referred to as *transillumination*, retroillumination involves focusing the beam on a surface beyond (or behind) the area to be observed. For example, the cornea can be observed in retroillumination by illuminating the iris and focusing the microscope on the cornea, observing the cornea in the light reflected back from the iris. It is sometimes difficult to know whether one is using, at a given moment, retroillumination or indirect illumination. During inspection of the cornea, it may be illuminated partly by retroillumination and partly by indirect illumination. In fact, these two methods (with the addition of direct illumination and oscillation) can be employed almost simultaneously as different areas of the cornea are observed.

Sclerotic scatter. If a slit of medium width is directed toward the limbus from a wide angle, the scattering of light by the cornea will cause the appearance of a halo all the way around the cornea at the limbus. The light traverses the cornea by total internal reflection. Therefore, if the cornea is free of opacities, the light will pass through the cornea unhindered, but if an opacity, abrasion, or foreign body is present, it will be visible due to the local scattering of the light. Sclerotic scatter is useful in detecting corneal abrasions, embedded foreign bodies, edema, and other conditions that may occur in connection with contact lens wear.

The *split-limbal method*, a variation of sclerotic scatter, has been described by Korb and Exford (1968). It is used for the detection of *round edema*, or *central corneal clouding* resulting from contact lens wear. Korb and Exford (1968) described this method of illumination as a combination of sclerotic scatter and retroillumination. The width of the beam should be about 1.5mm for a blue iris or 3.0mm for a brown iris; the angle of incidence should be between 45 and 60 degrees; and observation should be made in complete darkness, just after removal of the lens. The practitioner should become partially dark adapted before using the procedure, and the observation should be made with the naked eye rather than with the aid of the binocular microscope. Central corneal clouding appears as a circular patch of clouding, off-white in color, against the dark background of the pupil. Its position corresponds to the centering of the contact lens.

Specular reflection. Using a slit of medium width, if the source and the microscope are placed at equal angles from the normal to the corneal surface, the image of the source will be observed. This image of the slit lamp source is referred to as the *zone of specular reflection*. This method is particularly useful in observing both the corneal epithelium and the endothelium. The corneal epithelium forms a bright image of the source (Purkinje's image no. 1), while the endothelium forms a relatively dim image (Purkinje's image no. 2) seen just to one side of the image formed by the epithelium. To observe the endothelium, high magnification (from 30× to 40×) must be used.

Precorneal Film Breakup Test

The precorneal film breakup test is valuable not only in predicting which patients are likely to be unsuccessful contact lens wearers, but also in determining the likelihood of a dry eye problem due to a mucin deficiency. Fluorescein is applied to the bulbar conjunctiva by means of a moistened fluorescein strip, and the patient is instructed to blink several times and then stare straight ahead (but not looking into the light source) without blinking. Using the wide beam and the cobalt blue filter, the examiner begins to count while watching for the appearance of one or more amoebalike black patches in the precorneal film. The appearance of these black patches indicates that the tear film has "broken up." Using normal subjects, Holly (1973) found that the majority of breakup times fell in the 15-through-34-second range and that in no instance was the breakup time less than 10 seconds.

Lemp (1973) pointed out that in the presence of an inadequate mucin layer, the evaporation of tears when blinking is prevented can allow lipids from the superficial oily layer to migrate to the corneal surface. When the mucin layer has become sufficiently contaminated by lipids, the tear film ruptures and dry spots begin to form. A breakup time of less than 10 seconds is usually considered a negative factor in patient selection for contact lens fitting, particularly in the case of hydrogel lenses. Lemp (1980) emphasized that the practitioner should be looking for randomly distributed dry spots when performing the breakup test. Dry spots that repeatedly occur in the same area could be due to an epithelial defect and, therefore, should not be considered as a true indication of tear film breakup time.

Applanation Tonometry

It is convenient to perform Goldmann applanation tonometry as a part of the routine slit-lamp examination, since the Goldmann tonometer is mounted on the slit lamp. Due to the possibility of abrading the cornea while performing Goldmann tonometry, some practitioners prefer to put off both the slit-lamp examination and tonometry until after completing the refraction and binocular vision

examination. (The procedure for performing Goldmann applanation tonometry is described in Chapter 6.)

A PROBLEM-ORIENTED SLIT-LAMP ROUTINE

The examiner should develop a problem-oriented slit-lamp examination routine so that all structures of the anterior segment of the eye can be examined quickly and efficiently. Although the order in which the ocular structures are examined tends to vary from one practitioner to another, the following routine is recommended:

1. *The precorneal film.* Fluorescein is instilled, and the examiner performs the precorneal film breakup test, notes the width of the lower marginal tear strip, inspects the tear film for the presence of mucus or other debris, and inspects the epithelium for staining.
2. *The cornea.* The cornea is examined in optic section using the narrow beam, following which the beam is widened and directed toward the iris so the cornea can be inspected by retroillumination. Specular reflection is next used to examine the endothelium, and the beam is then focused on the limbal area so the cornea can be evaluated by sclerotic scatter.
3. *Anterior chamber angle.* The beam is narrowed down and the anterior chamber angle width estimated, first in the temporal and then in the nasal quadrant.
4. *Eyelids and conjunctiva.* The beam is swept across the upper and lower lids while the lid margins are inspected. The lower lid is everted and the lower tarsal conjunctiva inspected, following which the upper lid is inverted and the upper tarsal conjunctiva inspected. The bulbar conjunctiva is then examined.
5. *The anterior chamber, iris, and lens.* The anterior chamber angle is examined for the presence of flare and cells using the conical beam, after which the iris is examined with a moderately narrow slit. The slit is then narrowed down for examination of the lens in optic section at as oblique an angle as possible. The slit lamp is then directed toward the other eye, and the examination routine is repeated.

Precorneal film

A practitioner who emphasizes the fitting of contact lenses should conduct a thorough examination of the precorneal film, including the breakup test, on every patient. If the patient later inquires about contact lenses, the important information concerning the tear film will already have been obtained.

Following the breakup test, the width of the marginal tear strip (the cylindrical-shaped strip of tears formed where the upper and lower lid margins meet the bulbar conjunctiva) should be mentally noted, and the tear film should be carefully inspected for excess debris, mucous threads, and corneal filaments. While inspecting the precorneal film, any superficial fluorescein staining of the cornea or the bulbar conjunctiva should be noted.

Problems that the practitioner should anticipate while inspecting the tear film are mucin deficiency, aqueous tear deficiency, lipid abnormalities, and lid-surfacing abnormalities. (These conditions are discussed in Chapter 5 and are only briefly summarized here.)

Mucin deficiency. As indicated earlier, a precorneal film breakup time of less than 10 seconds indicates the presence of a mucin deficiency. Holly and Lemp (1971) found that patients with such short breakup times, although having adequate aqueous tears, have abnormally low or nonexistent goblet cell populations. The most obvious cause of a deficient goblet cell population is vitamin A deficiency.

Aqueous deficiency. The term *keratoconjunctivitis sicca* is often used synonymously with *aqueous deficiency*, which is defined as an absolute or partial deficiency in aqueous tear production. The main symptom of aqueous tear deficiency is a foreign body sensation, usually bilateral, progressing to a constant burning sensation. Clinical findings observed with the slit lamp include a scanty marginal tear strip, excess debris in the tear film, mucous threads, and corneal filaments (Lemp, 1980).

Lipid abnormalities. Lemp (1980) pointed out that in chronic marginal blepharitis, qualitative changes in the Meibomian gland secretion may result in the release of fatty acids. This may lead to almost instantaneous dry spot formation and punctate epithelial erosions.

Lid surfacing abnormalities. The precorneal film is able to maintain the corneal epithelium in a hydrated state only if the lids can continually resurface the epithelium with hydrated mucus. This resurfacing may be deficient when a pinguecula is present, when the lids fail to close completely because of a seventh nerve paralysis, or because of inadequate blinking.

Lid surfacing abnormalities lead to localized areas of epithelial desiccation (drying) due to the deficient mucin layer in the affected areas. When fluorescein has been instilled, these areas of desiccation appear as punctate staining.

The cornea

Once the examination of the precorneal film has been completed, the cornea is examined. An optic section of the cornea is observed using a narrow beam with both direct and indirect illumination. The beam is swept horizontally across the cornea. Abrasions, scars, and other opacities can be seen with this procedure, and their depth within the cornea can be estimated. If the beam is widened and focused on the iris while the microscope is focused on the cornea, using retroillumination, opacities not seen under direct or indirect illumination may become visible.

To obtain a magnified view of the corneal endothelium, specular reflection is used. With high magnification and good illumination the endothelial mosaic can be visualized, as shown in Figure 7.6. Following this, the slit-lamp source is rotated temporally so the limbal area can be illuminated using sclerotic scatter. This is the last step in the examination of the cornea, after which the examiner can proceed with estimation of the anterior chamber depth.

Problems that should be anticipated when examining the cornea include epithelial staining,

Figure 7.6 The corneal endothelium *(left)* seen in specular reflection. The reflection of the light source *(right)* is from the corneal epithelium.

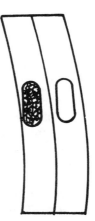

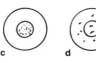

a   b   c   d   e

Figure 7.7 Patterns of corneal staining: (a) 3 and 9 o'clock staining due to a hard contact lens; (b) foreign body stain; (c) apical stippling due to a tight contact lens; (d) staining due to viral conjunctivitis; (e) staining due to staphylococcus.

scars, active inflammatory conditions, degenerations, dystrophies, and pigment deposition.

Epithelial staining. Epithelial staining occurs as a result of localized destruction of epithelial cells and may have a great variety of causes. The staining that can occur as a result of drying of the cornea due to a deficient mucin layer has already been described. Another common cause of epithelial staining is mechanical abrasion of the cornea, which may be due to an injury (such as a fingernail scratch) or a loosely fitting contact lens. Punctate staining can occur as a result of corneal anoxia, caused by a tightly fitting contact lens or by contact lens overwearing. Punctate staining can occur as a result of superficial keratitus due to a bacterial or viral infection of the cornea. One of the more common causes of superficial keratitus is *epidemic keratoconjunctivitis (EKC)*, caused by an adenovirus. Patterns of epithelial staining due to various conditions are shown in Figure 7.7.

Corneal scars. Many patients will be found to have small corneal scars due to old injuries, corneal ulcers, or other infections. One of the most common corneal ulcers is a *marginal ulcer*, which occurs near the limbus and often appears in conjunction with an attack of acute conjunctivitis, or *pink eye*. These small ulcers have no effect on vision but leave a permanent scar. Scars due to larger, central corneal ulcers like a serpiginous ulcer usually interfere markedly with vision.

Corneal scars are classified as *maculae* (very small, barely visible spots), *nebulae* (diffuse scarring), and *leukomae* (large, dense white scars). If a corneal scar is seen, its presence should be indicated on the patient's record, both in writing and in the form of a diagram. Such drawings and even photodocumentation are important when a patient is to be fitted with contact lenses. If a patient notices a previously existing corneal scar after the lenses have been fitted, he or she may blame the lenses (and the practitioner) for the scar.

Active inflammatory conditions. These conditions include superficial keratitis, deep keratitis, and anterior uveitis. As already described, superficial keratitis is characterized by epithelial staining. Other signs of superficial keratitis, including circumcorneal injection and conjunctival follicles, are described later in the chapter in the section on conditions of the lids and conjunctiva. Because the cornea has no blood supply, the consequences of infection of the deeper corneal layers are evident not only in the cornea but in the conjunctiva, anterior chamber, and iris. Deep keratitis in the active stage may be accompanied by circumcorneal injection, corneal infiltrates (large, whitish areas underneath the epithelium), keratic precipitates, hypopyon, and anterior chamber flare and cells. Keratic precipitates are aggregations of leukocytes and infective material appearing gray-white in color and deposited on the posterior surface of the cornea. Hypopyon is an accumulation of similar material at the bottom of the anterior chamber, and anterior chamber flare and cells are the result of this material being dispersed within the aqueous.

Corneal degenerations. Textbooks on ocular disease describe a large number of types of corneal degeneration. The most common, occurring mainly in older people, is *arcus senilis*. This is a whitish or yellowish opacity occurring in the form of an arc or even a complete circle just inside the limbus, with a clear area between the opacity and the limbus. It is due to the deposition of cholesterol esters and other material in the corneal stroma, and it is of no consequence other than a possible indication of a high serum cholesterol level.

Corneal dystrophies. The most common corneal dystrophy is *Fuchs's endothelial-epithelial dystrophy*. It begins in the form of *corneal guttata*, which are small, wartlike prominences on the endothelium occurring in the axial portion of the cornea of middle-aged and older people. Guttata are most easily seen with the slit lamp by retroillumination or specular reflection. In the areas where the guttata exist, large numbers of endothelial cells are either absent or nonfunctional, so the barrier function of the endothelium is eventually compromised. Fluid from the aqueous enters the cornea under the intraocular pressure, diffuses to the epithelium, and causes pronounced epithelial edema.

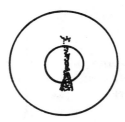

Figure 7.8   Kruckenberg's spindle.

Pigment deposition. The most obvious form of pigment deposition is *Kruckenberg's spindle*, a vertically elongated, spindle-shaped deposition of iris pigment on the corneal endothelium (see Figure 7.8). In more obvious cases it can be seen by direct illumination, but otherwise its detection may require retroillumination. The presence of a Kruckenberg spindle indicates the loss of a large amount of iris pigment, some of which may clog the spaces in the trabecular meshwork and cause *pigmentary glaucoma.* Another form of pigmentation is *pigment dusting* of the endothelium, a deposition of fine pigment granules that can be seen only with retroillumination. Pigment dusting should also alert the practitioner to the possibility of pigmentary glaucoma.

Estimation of the anterior chamber angle

Recall that the final step in the examination of the cornea involves sclerotic scatter. On completion of this procedure, the anterior chamber angle is estimated, first in the temporal and then in the nasal quadrant, and a mental note is made of the angle (grade 4, 3, 2, 1, or 0) for later recording. Anterior chamber angle width is known to vary with a number of factors, including the following.

Age. As the eyeball grows, the anterior chamber tends to increase in depth in spite of the gradual increase in thickness of the crystalline lens as new lens fibers are formed. However, at about the age of 20 (Spooner, 1957) the eyeball no longer increases in size, so the continual increase in thickness of the crystalline lens tends to cause the anterior chamber depth to decrease gradually with age (rather than increase). Clinical experience indicates that the great majority of children and teenagers have grade 3 or 4 angles.

Refractive error. Myopic eyes, being large, tend to have deep anterior chambers and thus wide angles; hyperopic eyes, which tend to be small, tend to have shallow anterior chambers and thus narrow angles. Aphakics (people who have undergone surgery for removal of the crystalline lens) tend to have deep anterior chambers and wide angles. On the basis of variation of the anterior chamber angle with age and refractive error (and with some oversimplification), one may expect the following: aphakics and young myopes tend to have grade 4 angles, young hyperopes and older myopes tend to have grade 3 or 4 angles, and older hyperopes (or even, occasionally, myopes) may have grade 2 or even grade 1 angles.

Swelling of the crystalline lens. In the early stages of a senile cataract, the lens tends to swell, bringing about a narrowing of the anterior chamber angle. Even a myope, who would be expected to have a relatively wide angle, may be found to have a grade 2 or 1 angle in the presence of an early senile cataract. A narrow angle in combination with a senile cataract should suggest referral for ophthalmological evaluation.

Eyelids and conjunctiva

After estimating the anterior chamber angle, the practitioner's attention is turned to the eyelids and conjunctiva. The positions of the lids are noted, particularly whether the lower lid tends to turn inward or outward. The slit beam is swept first across the upper lid and then across the lower lid, during which the skin of the lids is inspected for signs of inflammation, growths, or lumps, and the lid margins and lashes are inspected.

The tarsal conjunctiva lining the lower lid is easily inspected for inflammation or follicles by everting the lower lid. The upper lid, however, has a much stiffer tarsal plate, so eversion requires some practice. The least sophisticated method of everting the upper lid requires the use of a cotton swab as a fulcrum. The patient is instructed to look downward and to press his or her head firmly into the headrest while the practitioner presses the cotton swab (oriented horizontally) against the upper lid at the sulcus just above the lid margin. Using the thumb and forefinger of the other hand, the practitioner everts the lid while using the cotton swab as a fulcrum. With practice, it will be possible (for the majority of patients) to use the index finger of one hand rather than the cotton swab as the fulcrum. Even better is the one-handed method of upper lid eversion. The practitioner uses the index finger of the preferred hand as the fulcrum and, grasping the lid margin with the thumb of the same hand, quickly twists the hand and everts the lid. The tarsal conjunctiva of the upper lid is then inspected for the presence of inflammation, follicles, or papillae.

The bulbar conjunctiva is then inspected for any signs of vascular injection or engorgement and for surface irregularities such as pingueculae or pterygia. Particular attention should be paid to the limbal conjunctiva. At the limbus, the conjunctival vessels end in a series of marginal loops, known as *peripheral arcades*. Normally the cornea is devoid of blood vessels, but in some pathological conditions small vessels from the limbal arcades will be seen to extend across the limbus into the cornea.

Problems the practitioner should be aware of in the examination of the eyelids and conjunctiva are considered here in terms of the positions of the eyelids and puncta, the skin of the eyelids, the lid margins, the tarsal conjunctiva, and the bulbar conjunctiva.

Positions of the eyelids and puncta. The eyelids should be grossly inspected for signs of *entropion* (turning inward) or *ectropion* (turning outward) of the lid margins. Both of these conditions are more likely to involve the lower than the upper lid, and both tend to occur mainly in elderly patients. A complication of entropion is the fact that the lashes tend to turn inward (*trichiasis*) and rub against the cornea, causing pain and eventual scarring. A complication of ectropion is the fact that the puncta may be constantly everted, allowing tears to spill out of the lower conjunctival sac onto the cheek (*epiphora*). Both the upper and lower puncta should be inspected to make sure that they press inward against the bulbar conjunctiva and are therefore able to drain away the tears.

Skin of the eyelids. Among the abnormalities that may involve the skin of the eyelids are inflammatory conditions such as *dermatitis* and the presence of one or more yellowish, raised areas known as *xanthelasma*. The latter condition tends to occur in older people near the inner canthus (even on the side of the nose), and it requires no treatment other than possible removal for cosmetic reasons.

Lid margins. The lid margins should be inspected for signs of blepharitis and for styes and other localized lesions. Blepharitis, an inflammation of the lid margins, occurs in the form of either seborrheic or ulcerative blepharitis. In *seborrheic blepharitis*, flakes of "dandruff" can be seen at the lid margins at the base of the lashes. The most effective method of inspecting the lid margins for

dandruff flakes is to ask the patient to close his or her eyes and to sweep the slit lamp beam across the margins of the closed lids. Seborrheic blepharitis usually accompanies dandruff of the scalp, causes mild itching, and tends to contraindicate successful contact lens wear. *Ulcerative blepharitis* is caused by a bacterial infection and is a more serious condition than seborrheic blepharitis. The lids are reddened, and tiny ulcerated areas are found along the lid margin, tending to cause the lashes to fall out. While seborrheic blepharitis can be treated with selenium sulphate (a dandruff-removing shampoo), ulcerative blepharitis requires antibiotic treatment.

A stye, or *hordeolum*, is an infection of a lash follicle, whereas an *internal stye*, which presents itself at the lid margin just behind the lashes, is an infection of a Meibomian gland. Either condition is an inflammatory lesion causing the cardinal symptoms of redness, swelling, heat, and pain. On the other hand, a *chalazion* is a chronic granulomatous infection of a Meibomain gland and does not usually cause inflammation.

Many varieties of neoplasms, malignant as well as benign, may be found on the skin of the lids or at the lid margins. The most common malignant tumor of the lid is the *basal cell carcinoma*, which most commonly occurs on the lower lid as a pearly elevation or even as a notch in the lid margin. It gradually erodes the lid and, if not removed, may even erode the orbit.

Tarsal conjunctiva. In many viral and allergic forms of conjunctivitis, *follicles* will be seen in the tarsal conjunctiva. These are localized areas of lymphoid hyperplasia appearing as white or gray elevations in the upper or lower tarsal conjunctiva. In children, conjunctival follicles may occur in the absence of any signs of inflammation, a condition known as *folliculosis*. In some forms of allergic conjunctivitis, *papillae* can be seen in the upper tarsal conjunctiva. These contain tufts of blood vessels and differ in appearance from follicles; they are flat-topped and have a smooth, velvety appearance. Wearers of contact lenses sometimes develop follicles or papillae in the upper tarsal conjunctiva, apparently due to either the mechanical trauma caused by the contact lens or to an allergic reaction to protein materials contaminating the lens surface.

Bulbar conjunctiva. In the presence of an external source of inflammation such as conjunctivitis or a foreign body, the superficial conjunctival vessels will be *injected*, or overly full of blood. In

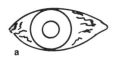 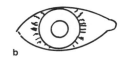

Figure 7.9 *(a)* **Superficial and *(b)* deep injection of the bulbar conjunctiva.**

superficial conjunctival injection, the vessels are bright red in color, the injection is more prominent toward the fornix than toward the limbus, and the injected vessels move freely when the lower lid is moved. However, in the presence of an internal disease such as keratitis or iritis, the deep vessels surrounding the limbus are injected. In *deep* injection, the affected vessels are purple or lilac in color, extend outward from the limbus in a radial manner, and do not move when the lower lid is moved. However, both types of injection can occur together, so a diagnosis of a condition as external or internal should be made only with the consideration of additional signs and symptoms. (See Figure 7.9.)

Anterior chamber

Following the examination of the lids and the conjunctiva, the anterior chamber is examined by means of the *conical beam* obtained by selecting the smallest aperture available (both vertically and horizontally), using high magnification. The purpose of the conical beam is to inspect the anterior chamber for the appearance of flare and cells, either of which indicate the presence of either a keratitis or a uveitis. The visualization of anterior chamber flare and cells takes advantage of the Tyndall phenomenon: in an optically empty medium such as the aqueous humor, any opaque object will appear as white or gray in an otherwise dark field.

Other more obvious conditions affecting the anterior chamber are hypopyon and hyphema. As already noted, *hypopyon* is a collection of leucocytes and other material at the bottom of the anterior chamber accompanying a corneal ulcer. *Hyphema* is a pool of blood at the bottom of the anterior chamber, occurring usually as a result of blunt trauma to the eye.

Iris and lens

After examination of the anterior chamber, the conical beam is replaced by the slit beam, and the iris and lens are examined. The iris is subject to a number of abnormalities and disease processes, but most of these are rather gross and do not require for their discovery the high level of magnification of

which the slit lamp biomicroscope is capable. One of the most commonly found anomalies of the iris is the presence of *nevi:* clusters of pigment cells that are found in the majority of irides. Congenital anomalies having to do with the pupil include corectopia, coloboma, and aniridia. *Corectopia* is an off-center pupil. *Coloboma* is a sector-shaped absence of iris tissue resulting in a keyhole-shaped pupil. It is due to premature closure of the fetal fissure of the eye. *Aniridia* is a somewhat less than complete lack of an iris, occurring as an autosomal dominant inherited condition and accompanied by glaucoma and other abnormalities that make for a poor prognosis. As for some of the more threatening, acquired conditions, in *acute iritis* the pupil is constricted, whereas in *acute angle-closure glaucoma* it is dilated and misshapen.

The crystalline lens is examined with the narrow slit, the light source entering the eye at as large an angle as the diameter of the pupil will allow. To obtain as large a pupil as possible, it may be necessary to reduce the illumination of the slit to the lowest possible level. An optic section of the lens, as shown in Figure 7.10, will reveal the anterior upright Y-suture and the posterior inverted Y-suture, along with the zones of discontinuity separating the embryonic, fetal, and adult nuclei. The lens is subject to opacities of many kinds, including congenital, senile, traumatic, and toxic cataracts as well as those that occur secondary to other disease processes. By far the most prevalent of these are *senile cataracts*. Unfortunately, most older people have such small pupils that, unless the pupil is dilated, the practitioner may find that less can be learned about a patient's cataract by means of the slit lamp than can be learned with the ophthalmoscope. Figure 7.11 shows the appearance of each of the three major types of senile cataracts with dilation of the pupil. The cortical cataract is shown with the wide beam of the slit lamp, while the nuclear and posterior subcapsular cataracts are shown with the narrow beam in optic section.

Recording of findings

The slit-lamp examination for the right eye being completed, the left eye is examined and the findings are then recorded. The completeness of recording slit-lamp findings varies greatly from one practitioner to another. The briefest method of recording findings involves a notation of the anterior chamber angle for each eye and a brief comment such as "everything within normal limits" or, more briefly, "WNL" (assuming, of course, that all findings *are*

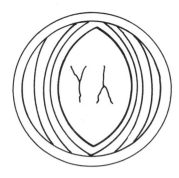

Figure 7.10   The lens in optic section. The beam of light is striking the eye from the left side.

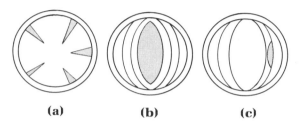

(a)   (b)   (c)

Figure 7.11   Senile cataracts: *(a)* Cortical, with wide beam; *(b)* Nuclear, with narrow beam; and *(c)* Posterior subcapsular, with narrow beam coming from the left. Because dark field illumination is used with the slit lamp, opacities in the media appear to be white or gray.

within normal limits). The most complete form of recording would involve notation of the chamber angle width followed by a list of all the structures of the anterior segment of the eye, with brief comments concerning such characteristics as the clarity of each structure.

The practitioner must somehow strike a balance between a too-brief and sketchy recording of findings and a voluminous, time-consuming procedure. What is important in the recording process is to make note of the presence of any variation from normal, even if it is a nonthreatening condition, so on future examinations there will be no doubt whether a given variation from normal existed previously. A recommended procedure, which has the advantage of enabling the examiner to record findings fully and in a minimum of time, is to use a record form that lists each of the anterior segment structures, followed by sufficient space for notes concerning any variations from normal and any drawing the practitioner may wish to make. A

suggested recording format for the slit lamp examination is shown in Appendix A.

Examination of the vitreous and retina

Without the use of special lenses, only the most anterior portion of the vitreous body can be examined with the slit lamp. For examination of the more posterior portions of the vitreous and the retina, a dilated pupil and the use of the Hruby lens or the Goldmann contact lens are necessities. (Examination of the vitreous and retina with the slit lamp are discussed later in this chapter.)

THE INTERNAL EXAMINATION

The first ophthalmoscope, invented by Babbage in 1847, was simply a mirror that reflected light into the patient's eye. A hole in the silvering served as a peephole for the examiner, and the light source was a candle or a gas lamp located beside and somewhat behind the patient's head. In 1851, Helmholtz developed the first ophthalmoscope to receive the attention of the medical profession. This instrument made use of multiple thin plates of glass that served the function of a semisilvered mirror and required no peephole. Improvements in the ophthalmoscope were made rapidly, the candle or gas lamp eventually being replaced by an electric light bulb mounted in the instrument.

The self-luminous ophthalmoscope, like all instruments designed for examining the human eye, consists of an illumination system and an observation system. The illumination system is made up of the light source, condensing lenses, a reflecting prism, and a series of apertures. The observation system consists of a peephole and a bank of spherical lenses that are used to compensate for the patient's refractive error and to bring structures in the anterior segment of the eye into view.

The instrument just described is the *direct ophthalmoscope* (see Figure 7.12). With it the examiner views an upright, virtual image of the patient's fundus magnified by the optical system of the patient's eye. By interposing a strong convex lens in the path of the light leaving the patient's eye, the examiner can observe an inverted, real image of the fundus, a procedure known as *indirect ophthalmoscopy*. In addition to the fact that the image is upright in one case and inverted in the other, direct and indirect ophthalmoscopy differ in that the image size is larger and the field of view smaller in direct than in indirect ophthalmoscopy.

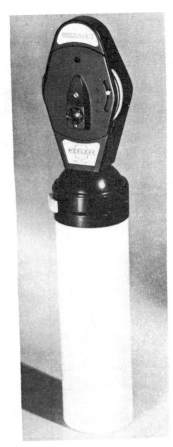

Figure 7.12   The direct ophthalmoscope.

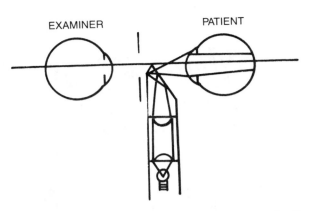

Figure 7.13 Illumination system of the direct ophthalmoscope.

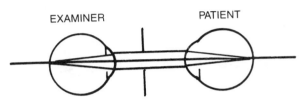

Figure 7.14 Observation system of the direct ophthalmoscope.

The Direct Ophthalmoscope

When the light from the ophthalmoscope strikes the patient's retina, it is reflected diffusely in all directions so each illuminated point serves as a source of light (see Figure 7.13). As shown in Figure 7.14, if the patient is emmetropic and is completely relaxing accommodation, a point of light on the retina will leave the eye as a bundle of parallel rays; if the examiner is emmetropic with accommodation relaxed, these parallel rays of light will focus sharply on the retina, so the examiner will clearly see the patient's fundus. However, if either the patient or the examiner is not emmetropic or if either is not completely relaxing accommodation, the examiner will see the patient's fundus clearly only by interposing lenses behind the peephole. For example, if the examiner is emmetropic, the patient is a 3.00D hyperope, and both completely relax their accommodation, the examiner will require a +3.00D lens to see the patient's fundus clearly.

It is tempting to imagine that the direct ophthal-

moscope can be used to measure the patient's refractive error. To some extent this is true, but there are two problems: (1) one can never be sure that both the examiner and the patient are fully relaxing accommodation; and (2) a correct measurement of the refraction must involve illumination of the patient's macular area, and the resultant pupillary constriction usually prevents the practitioner from viewing the macular area sufficiently long to do a "refraction." Whereas the optic nerve head or the retinal vessels may serve as good targets for ophthalmoscopic refraction, the length of the eye is not necessarily the same at these locations as it is when the macular area is considered.

Magnification

In performing direct ophthalmoscopy, the patient's eye can be considered a simple magnifier having a focal length of 16.67mm (the distance between the principal plane of the eye and the primary focal plane). The magnification of a simple magnifier is calculated on the basis that the object of regard (the patient's fundus, in this case) would ordinarily be placed at a distance of 25cm from the viewer's eye (the "least distance of distinct vision").

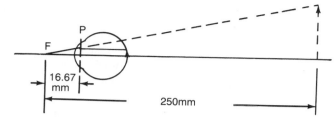

Figure 7.15 Magnification of the direct ophthalmoscope.

Referring to Figure 7.15, the magnification (M), therefore, would be calculated as follows:

$$M = \frac{250mm}{16.67mm} = 15\times.$$

This relationship is for an emmetropic eye. For a myopic eye the magnification is greater, and for a hyperopic eye it is less than $15\times$. Emsley (1963) has shown that when the patient's ametropia is corrected with the appropriate lens in the peephole, the magnification is $19\times$ for a 10.00D myope and $13\times$ for a 10.00D hyperope.

Field of view

Emsley has shown that the field of view for an emmetropic eye having a 4mm pupil—assuming that the peephole of the ophthalmoscope is 3mm in diameter and is located 35mm from the reduced surface of the patient's eye—is 6.5 degrees, which is close to the angular size of the optic nerve head. The field of view is somewhat smaller in myopia and larger in hyperopia.

Procedure for direct ophthalmoscopy

The patient is seated in the ophthalmic chair at a height that is comfortable for the examiner. The headrest should be adjusted so the patient's head, although held erect, will have support during the examination. The patient is asked to look at a fixation target high on the opposite wall or on the ceiling, and is told that the examiner's head may occasionally block the view of the fixation target but to "look through my head" in the direction of the target if this occurs. The examiner uses the right eye to examine the patient's right eye and the left eye to examine the patient's left eye.

If the examiner wears glasses for the correction of a refractive error, he or she may find it convenient to remove them for ophthalmoscopy, putting the "best sphere" correction in the peephole of the ophthalmoscope. However, if the correction involves more than 1.00D or so of cylindrical power, clear vision for ophthalmoscopy may be impossible with a spherical lens. While viewing the patient's fundus, the examiner should consciously attempt to relax accommodation. This can be aided by imagining that, when looking into the patient's pupil, he or she is looking at an outdoor scene through an open window.

Direct ophthalmoscopy involves three procedures: (1) inspection of the ocular media at a distance, (2) examination of the anterior segment of the eye, and (3) examination of the posterior segment.

With the patient fixating the distant fixation target and with no lenses in the peephole, the examiner begins by inspecting the ocular media from a distance of about 20–25 inches. At this distance, opacities in the media (particularly cortical cataracts) can be seen that could be easily missed during "close in" ophthalmoscopy. Following this, the examiner places a +8.00 or +10.00D lens in the peephole and moves in to a distance of 4 or 5 inches to inspect the anterior structures of the eye. Little time is required here, in that the lids, conjunctiva, cornea, anterior chamber, and iris will have already been examined by means of the slit lamp.

After the anterior structures have been examined, the examiner gradually reduces the amount of lens power in the instrument while focusing on the internal structures of the eye—the lens, vitreous, and finally the retina. When the retina has been reached, the optic nerve head, retinal vessels, and the macula should be clearly visible with no lens in the peephole if the patient is emmetropic. For patients having ametropia of 1.00D or more, appropriate lenses must be placed in the ophthalmoscope peephole, or the fundus details will not be clearly seen. After inspection of the optic nerve head, the retinal vessels, the fundus background, and the macular area, the examiner next evaluates the peripheral fundus. This is done by instructing the patient to look in the direction corresponding to the portion of the fundus to be examined. To examine the superior fundus, the patient is instructed to look upward; for examination of the nasal fundus, the patient is told to look inward; and so forth. The evaluation of the peripheral fundus completes the process of direct ophthalmoscopy.

The Indirect Ophthalmoscope

In the simplest form of indirect ophthalmoscopy, the direct ophthalmoscope is held at arm's length from

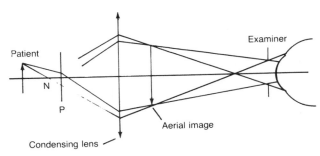

Figure 7.16   Observation system in indirect ophthalmoscopy (not to scale: redrawn from Emsley, 1963). The examiner views a magnified, inverted, aerial image located between his or her own eye and the condensing lens.

the patient's eye (approximately 40cm), and a condensing lens is placed in the light path in front of the patient's eye. The examiner holds the ophthalmoscope in the dominant hand and the condensing lens in the nondominant hand, and steadies this hand by placing the fingertips against the patient's forehead. As shown in Figure 7.16, the condensing lens forms a real, inverted, aerial image between the condensing lens and the ophthalmoscope, and it is this aerial image that the examiner views through the ophthalmoscope peephole. If the eye is emmetropic the light leaving the eye forms a parallel beam, so the aerial image is formed at the focal plane of the condensing lens.

Magnification and field of view

The magnification due to the condensing lens is determined by dividing the refracting power of the patient's eye by the power of the condensing lens (Emsley, 1963). For a +13.00D condensing lens, assuming the eye is emmetropic and has a refracting power of 60.00D, the magnification due to the lens would be

$$M = \frac{60}{13} = 4.5\times.$$

The magnification is also affected by the distance at which the aerial image is viewed by the examiner. If it is viewed at the 25cm "least distance of distinct vision," the magnification is simply that due to the condensing lens, or, in this case, 4.5×. However, the actual viewing distance is approximately 40cm, so the resulting magnification is equal to

$$\frac{25}{40}(4.5\times) = 2.8\times.$$

The magnification would be greater for a hyperopic eye and less for a myopic eye.

The field of view, using the +13.00D condensing lens, has been given by Emsley (1963) as 25 degrees for an emmetropic eye (four times that of direct ophthalmoscopy) and somewhat smaller for a hyperopic eye and larger for a myopic eye.

Some examiners prefer to use a stronger condensing lens to have a larger field of view but with lower magnification. For a +20.00D condensing lens, the magnification due to the lens would be

$$\frac{60}{20} = 3\times.$$

For a 40cm viewing distance, the resulting magnification would be

$$\frac{25}{40}(3\times) = 1.9\times.$$

American Optical monocular indirect ophthalmoscope

The American Optical Corporation offers a compact 5× monocular indirect ophthalmoscope that incorporates an inverting lens system so the examiner views an upright, rather than an inverted, image (see Figure 7.17). This instrument makes indirect ophthalmoscopy much more convenient than it is with the previously described system in

Figure 7.17   The monocular indirect ophthalmoscope.

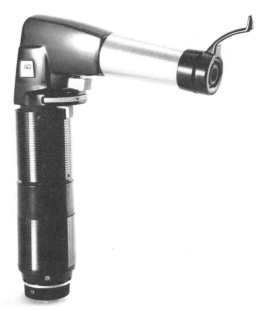

which a direct ophthalmoscope and a hand-held condensing lens are used. An important advantage of this instrument is that the peripheral fundus can be viewed through the nondilated pupil. The instrument is gaining favor, particularly in those states where the use of diagnostic drugs is not allowed.

Procedure for monocular indirect ophthalmoscopy

Practitioners who regularly make use of the monocular indirect ophthalmoscope usually depend on it for the major part of the ophthalmoscopic examination, performing indirect ophthalmoscopy prior to direct ophthalmoscopy. By doing so, the examiner "sees the forest before looking at the trees" and uses the direct ophthalmoscope only for a more highly magnified inspection of the optic nerve head, the blood vessels, the macula, and any suspicious area of the posterior portion of the fundus already identified by use of the indirect ophthalmoscope.

The indirect ophthalmoscope not only has the advantage of providing a better overall picture of the fundus due to the greatly expanded field of view, but it is surprisingly effective in the examination of the peripheral fundus. Even with a pupil as small as 3 or 4mm, it is usually possible to examine the fundus far enough in the periphery to see the vortex vein ampules, which are just behind the equator and are seldom seen in direct ophthalmoscopy. Like indirect ophthalmoscopy, the peripheral fundus is examined while the patient looks in the direction corresponding to that portion of the fundus the examiner wishes to inspect.

The binocular indirect ophthalmoscope

In the late 1940s, Schepens designed a headborne binocular indirect ophthalmoscope that provides the examiner with a brightly illuminated, stereoscopic view of the patient's fundus (see Figure 7.18). Using this instrument, the examiner works at arms' length from the patient and views the aerial image of the patient's fundus by means of a hand-held condensing lens. The condensing lens is held at a distance from the patient's eye equal to the focal length of the lens. The most commonly used condensing lens powers are +14.00 and +20.00D.

Magnification decreases with increasing power of the condensing lens, being approximately 2.7× for the +14.00D lens and 1.9× for the +20.00D lens. The field of view increases with increasing condensing lens power. In spite of the fact that the magnification is much lower than the 15× provided by direct ophthalmoscopy, image resolution is surprisingly good as a result of both the high level of illumination and the presence of stereoscopic depth perception.

When the binocular indirect ophthalmoscope is used for general examination, the patient may either be seated upright in the ophthalmic chair or the chair may be adjusted to the reclining position so the patient is supine, looking toward the ceiling. The examiner is positioned above the patient's head (with respect to the patient), thus viewing the patient's fundus upside down and backward.

Binocular indirect ophthalmoscopy

Binocular indirect ophthalmoscopes based on Schepens's original design are available from a number of manufacturers. Binocular indirect ophthalmoscopy requires the use of a mydriatic agent. Optometrists who make use of this procedure on a routine basis defer the instillation of mydriatic drops until after completion of the refractive and binocular vision examinations, since these procedures should be done while the physiological functions of the visual system are operating normally.

For routine examination with the binocular indirect ophthalmoscope, the patient is seated upright and is directed to look in extreme positions of gaze as the peripheral fundus is evaluated. The examiner then scans the central area of the posterior pole while the patient's eyes are in the primary position. Because of the intense radiation generated by the indirect ophthalmoscope source, care should be taken not to direct the light in any one area of the retina for an extended period of time.

For fundus drawing, the ophthalmic chair is adjusted in the reclining position so the patient is

Figure 7.18 The binocular indirect ophthalmoscope.

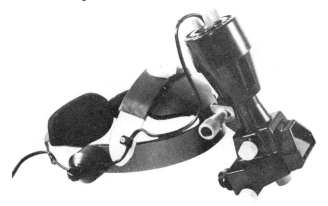

supine, facing the ceiling. The examiner is positioned above the patient's head, viewing the patient's fundus upside down and backward. Because the binocular indirect ophthalmoscope produces an image that is upside down and backward, a fundus drawing made by the examiner (when turned upside down) will have the correct up-down and right-left relationships.

Indications for binocular indirect ophthalmoscopy. With the current general use of diagnostic pharmaceutical agents, the first decision the practitioner must make is whether to routinely dilate every patient or to use dilation only on the basis of predetermined criteria such as those listed below. If the practitioner *does* elect to dilate every patient, the next decision is whether to routinely use binocular or monocular indirect ophthalmoscopy. Those practitioners who are relatively recent graduates will, in most cases, have become accustomed to using binocular indirect ophthalmoscopy on a routine basis, and will likely continue to do so in practice. Many of those older practitioners, however, who began practice when only direct and/or monocular indirect ophthalmoscopy were used, will be likely to continue to use these procedures.

If the practitioner elects *not* to dilate each patient, using direct and monocular indirect ophthalmoscopy on a routine basis, the use of dilation and binocular indirect ophthalmoscopy should be considered in the following circumstances:

1. The undilated pupil may be too small to obtain an adequate view of the fundus.
2. Even with a relatively large pupil, the presence of crystalline lens opacities may prevent observation of fundus details. However, the greater illumination of the binocular indirect ophthalmoscope, together with the stereoscopic depth perception, will usually provide improved visibility of the fundus.
3. Due to the increased prevalence of posterior vitreous detachment and, therefore, the increased chance of retinal tears that may lead to retinal detachment, high myopes (about 5.00D or more) should have a dilated fundus examination on a routine basis.
4. Patients who have undergone cataract surgery are particularly at risk for retinal detachment, since approximately two-thirds of aphakic patients have posterior vitreous detachment.
5. Diabetic patients, particularly those having retinopathy in the posterior fundus, should have a dilated fundus examination.
6. Any patient complaining of flashing lights or other unexplainable entoptic phenomena should have a dilated fundus examination.

Procedure. Due to the extreme brightness of the binocular indirect ophthalmoscopy source, a maximum amount of dilation is necessary. This can be accomplished by first instilling one drop of proparacaine, 0.5 percent, followed in 1 minute by one drop of tropicamide, 1 percent. If there are no contraindicating factors, 1 drop of 2.5 percent phenylephrine may also be instilled. For patients with dark irides, a second drop of tropicamide, 1 percent, may be necessary if dilation is not under way within 10 minutes after instillation of the first drop. Maximum dilation is usually present by the end of 25 or 30 minutes.

The examiner should place the instrument on his or her head as comfortably as possible, hold one thumb straight ahead at a distance of about 50cm, and adjust the interpupillary distance. The condensing lens should be held so the convex surface faces the examiner. Before examining a patient, the examiner should practice with a schematic eye. The + 20.00D condensing lens is held at a distance of 50cm from the eye, and an aerial image is formed between the condensing lens and the examiner (about 5cm in front of the condensing lens). The examiner should practice moving his or her head and the condensing lens in such a manner that the head, the condensing lens, and the patient's pupil are all on a common axis (see Figure 7–19).

Figure 7.19   The common axis principle in binocular indirect ophthalmoscopy (Garston and Cavallerano, 1980).

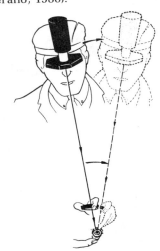

When examining a patient, the examiner is positioned above the patient's head, the ophthalmic chair being adjusted in a sufficiently low position so the condensing lens can be held at approximately arm's length. Because the patient must have a minute or two to become light adapted, Brockhurst (1956) has suggested that the examiner should first inspect the cornea, lens, and vitreous, using low illumination and without using the condensing lens.

Following this, the fundus examination is begun. The examiner tilts the condensing lens slightly to displace reflections from its surface toward the edge of the lens. Starting with the lens close to the patient's eye, the examiner brings the condensing lens away from the patient until the patient's pupil entirely fills the lens. Using the +20.00D lens, the examiner should be about 14–16 inches from the condensing lens (the ophthalmoscope incorporates a +2.00D lens, in order to make little accommodation necessary at this distance). Standing directly over the patient and moving the condensing lens forward and backward slightly if necessary, the examiner should have no trouble getting the central portion of the patient's fundus into view. Once this is done, the examiner instructs the patient to look upward while viewing the superior fundus and downward while viewing the inferior fundus, exactly as would be done in direct or monocular indirect ophthalmoscopy. The only difference is that the portion of the fundus seen is reversed and inverted.

Standing above the patient's head, the examiner is free to move to the position necessary to observe the desired quadrant of the fundus. For example, to view the inferior fundus, the examiner stands at the patient's forehead; to examine the nasal fundus, the examiner stands temporal to the patient. In all cases, the examiner views the quadrant of the patient's fundus 180 degrees from where he or she is standing. To cope with the inverted and reversed image, Garston and Cavallerano (1980) suggest the examiner completely forget that the image is inverted rather than attempt to reverse and invert the image in his or her mind. These authors make the point that when viewing the inferior fundus (or any quadrant for that matter), one is actually seeing the inferior fundus, but seeing it in reverse. In drawing the fundus, the fundus chart is placed upside down on the patient's chest. When the completed drawing is viewed right side up, it is a true representation (in terms of up-down and right-left) of the patient's fundus.

In examining the fundus with the binocular indirect ophthalmoscope, the examiner should get into the habit of estimating distances in *disk diameters*. The examiner should be able to identify and draw not only the optic disk, retinal vessels, and macular area but also the following structures (shown in Figure 7.25): the vortex vein ampullae, near the equator; the long ciliary nerves and arteries, located in the horizontal meridian at the 3 and 9 o'clock positions; short ciliary nerves and arteries, located usually near the vertical meridian; and the nasal and temporal ora serrata.

Fundus abnormalities that the examiner should look for during binocular indirect ophthalmoscopy include pigment abnormalities, paving stone degeneration, retinoschisis, lattice degeneration, and retinal breaks or holes. [Detailed discussion of these abnormalities is beyond the scope of this text. However they are very well described by Straatsma, Foos, and Feman (1980), and Straatsma, Foos, and Kreiger (1980) (in volume 3, chap. 26 and 27 of Duane *Clinical Ophthalmology*, 1980).]

A PROBLEM-ORIENTED OPHTHALMOSCOPY ROUTINE

As with biomicroscopy, the practitioner should develop a problem-oriented examination routine; one that constantly and actively looks for evidence of specific, predictable problems. As with biomicroscopy, the examination routine should be thorough but should flow smoothly and efficiently from one procedure to another. (Because the examination routine for the anterior segment structures is discussed in an earlier section on biomicroscopy, it is not repeated here.) A problem-oriented examination of the following structures is discussed: the crystalline lens, vitreous body, optic nerve head, retinal vessels, macular area, fundus background, and peripheral fundus.

Crystalline lens

With the direct ophthalmoscope, it is often possible to detect lens changes at an earlier stage than would be possible in biomicroscopy with the undilated pupil. This is due partly to the fact that the lower levels of illumination used in ophthalmoscopy allow a larger pupil, and partly because the ophthalmoscope allows the examiner more freedom of movement than is available in biomicroscopy. A procedure that is helpful in the early detection of *nuclear cataracts* is *oblique illumination*: if the ophthalmoscope is directed toward the patient's eye at an angle of 60 degrees or more and the examiner observes the patient's pupil with the naked eye, a milky appearance of the relatively large pupil indicates that a nuclear cataract is present.

While examining the patient's lens with the +8.00 or +10.00D lens in the peephole of the direct ophthalmoscope, the examiner should rotate his or her head (and the ophthalmoscope) to view the lens periphery from various angles. Using this procedure it is possible to identify cortical lens opacities at an earlier stage than would be possible with the slit lamp. Particular attention should be paid to the inferior nasal quadrant of the anterior cortex, in that cortical water clefts, spoking, wedges, and lamellar separation are most apt to occur in this portion of the lens (Phelps, 1976). These and any other lens opacities will appear to be black, due to the bright-field background illumination of the fundus, as contrasted with their gray or white appearance in the dark-field illumination used in biomicroscopy.

The appearance of a dark, grainy shadow at or near the center of the posterior portion of the lens may indicate the presence of a *posterior subcapsular cataract*. This form of cataract can occur either as a senile cataract or as a result of the systemic administration of steroids or other drugs.

Vitreous body

As the plus lens power in the direct ophthalmoscope is gradually reduced, increasingly more posterior portions of the vitreous body come into view. Although the vitreous body contains large numbers of fibrils, these cannot be seen with the ophthalmoscope but require the use of the slit lamp with the Hruby lens or the Goldmann fundus lens. With the ophthalmoscope, the normal vitreous appears to be optically empty.

In an active case of *choroiditis*, the posterior vitreous may contain fine, dustlike opacities. These can be seen best with the optic nerve head as a background.

Ocular fundus

The examination of the ocular fundus includes an evaluation of the appearance of the optic nerve head, the retinal vessels, the macular area, the fundus background, and the peripheral fundus. A schematic diagram of the normal ocular fundus is shown in Figure 7.20, and the appearance of the normal fundus is summarized in Tables 7.1 and 7.2.

Optic nerve head

The optic nerve head is the most prominent landmark of the fundus and is ordinarily the first

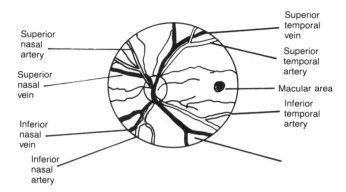

Figure 7.20   Schematic drawing of normal ocular fundus (redrawn from Nover, 1974).

structure to be inspected in the fundus examination. To locate the optic nerve head, the examiner should direct the beam parallel to the patient's line of sight; for example, if the patient is looking upward at a fixation target on the ceiling, the examiner should be looking downward at a similar angle. The beam should also be directed somewhat nasal to the patient's line of sight because the optic nerve head is located some 15 degrees nasal to the center of the fovea. The optic nerve head should be evaluated for color, elevation, appearance of the border, and type of cupping. Cupping can be evaluated by either (or both) of two systems: the Elschnig system and the cup/disk ratio system.

Color. The presence of tiny blood vessels within the optic nerve (the circle of Zinn-Haller) gives the optic nerve head a slightly pinkish tinge, although less pink than the fundus background. If physiological cupping exists, the central portion of the optic disk appears to be relatively whitish in color, and the crisscross appearance of the lamina cribrosa may be seen. A dead white or a porcelain white appearance of the optic disk is evidence of *optic atrophy*, which would be accompanied by a marked loss of central vision and a Marcus Gunn pupil. In a disk having a large amount of cupping, a grayish white pallor of the rim of the disk or of a portion of the rim suggests the possibility of glaucoma.

Elevation. If the optic nerve head is found to be elevated, as compared with the surrounding fundus, papillitis or papilledema should be suspected. The amount of elevation can be determined by focusing the ophthalmoscope on a blood vessel at or near the center of the disk and then focusing on a vessel just

Table 7.1   Appearance of a normal ocular fundus (Nover, 1974).

Disk	Color	Red-yellow; more pronounced on the nasal side. The temporal half may appear pale.
	Form and size	Round to oval; diameter, 1.5–1.7mm.
	Margins	Sharp; occasionally a pigment ring or conus.
	Vessels	Originate within a physiologic excavation.
Retina	Periphery	Lighter than central area. Occasional irregularities of pigmentation and lighter areas visible.
	Fovea	Appears darker than surrounding retina. Marginal reflex at the border of the macula. The yellow color visible only in red-free illumination.
	Vessels	Arteries: light red, straight, white reflex stripes. Veins: dark red, tortuous, pulsation. Caliber: vein to artery = 3:2.
	Choroid vessels	White, pink, yellow-white background; no reflex stripes; very tortuous; numerous anastomoses (only visible if there is dense pigmentation of the intervascular spaces, tessellated fundus, or sparse pigmentation of retinal pigment epithelium, albinotic fundus).

Table 7.2   Physiologic color variations in the normal ocular fundus (Nover, 1974).

	Even red fundus	Tessellated fundus	Blond fundus (albinotic)
Retinal pigment epithelium	Dense and even pigmentation	Little pigmentation	Sparse or no pigmentation
Choroidal melanocytes	Obscured	Marked pigmentation	Sparse or no pigmentation
Choroidal vessels	Obscured	Visible as red, anastomosing net; intervascular spaces are black-brown	Visible as a red net on the yellow-white scleral background

outside the disk. A difference of 3.00D (between the optic nerve head and the retina) represents approximately 1mm of elevation. In *papillitis*, an inflammation of the optic nerve, the elevation seldom exceeds 3.00D; however, in *papilledema*, edema of the optic nerve as a result of increased intracranial pressure, the elevation may be as much as 9.00D. In either case, the retinal arteries and veins may be badly congested, possibly with flame-shaped hemorrhages near the disk. Occasionally, the optic nerve head of a perfectly normal eye will appear to be elevated. This condition is called *pseudopapilledema* and is most likely to occur in hyperopic eyes. If an elevated optic nerve head has a scalloped border,

drusen of the optic nerve should be suspected. These are small elevations of the optic nerve head, and may be accompanied by a visual field loss.

Border of the optic disk. The optic nerve head sometimes has a narrow ring of pigmentation at the border, particularly the temporal border. This is a perfectly normal condition and is choroidal pigment showing through where the retinal tissue has pulled away from the optic nerve. It is called a *choroidal crescent*. A *scleral crescent* is a white, crescent-shaped area temporal to the disk, occurring in myopia as a result of both the retina and choroid pulling away from the optic nerve.

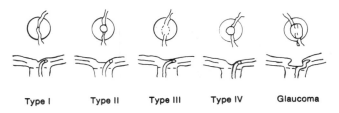

Type I   Type II   Type III   Type IV   Glaucoma

Figure 7.21 Elschnig's disk types (redrawn from Shlaifer, 1959).

Cupping. Shortly after the turn of the century, Elschnig proposed a method of optic disk typing. On the basis of descriptions by Kronfeld (1951) and Shlaifer (1959), Elschnig's disk typings may be characterized as follows (see Figure 7.21).

Type I. Elschnig's Type I disk has no physiological cup, the surface of the nerve head being essentially flat and in the same plane as the retinal surface.

Type II. In Type II, a physiological cup is present and is cylindrical in shape, as shown in both the surface and cross-section diagrams.

Type III. Type III is a saucer-shaped cup, usually present in the portion of the disk temporal to the location of the central retinal artery and vein.

Type IV. This is the typical myopic cupping. In this type, the retinal arteries and veins are pushed toward the nasal border of the disk, and a rather wide and deep cup is present, having its greatest depth nasally and becoming increasingly shallow temporally.

Type V. This disk type includes a number of miscellaneous categories, including myelinated nerve fibers, edematous or atrophied disks, and glaucomatous atrophy.

Glaucomotous cup. In a fully developed glaucomatous cup, the margin of the cup extends almost to the disk margin itself, and the vessels seem to disappear under the lip of the "bean pot" excavation. While such an advanced glaucomatous cup is easy to identify, an early glaucomatous cup easily may be confused with Elschnig's Type II, Type III, or Type IV disk. Kronfeld suggested that the practitioner make a simple drawing of the patient's cupping as it relates to the optic nerve head, so when the patient returns (presumably after an absence of a few years) the cupping can be compared to that in the diagram, and a new diagram can be made.

Cup/disk ratio. A convenient way of characterizing the cup is to record what has become known as the cup/disk ratio. Actually recorded as a decimal fraction rather than as a ratio (see Figure 7.22), the cup/disk ratio is an estimate of the diameter of the cup as related to the diameter of the disk and usually refers to the horizontal meridian. For example, a cup/disk ratio of 0.5 indicates that the diameter of the cup is half the diameter of the disk. Armaly and Sayegh (1969) have reported that only about 6 percent of their group of subjects had cup/disk ratios of 0.6 or greater, so a cup/disk ratio of this magnitude should arouse suspicion of the presence of glaucoma.

Congenital anomalies. A relatively common and sometimes alarming congenital anomaly of the optic nerve is the presence of *myelinated nerve fibers.* Myelination of the optic nerve fibers normally stops at the lamina cribrosa, but if it does not, an appearance like Figure 7.23 may result. This is a harmless condition but it may cause a visual field defect (an extension of the physiological blind spot) if the condition is extreme. Another common congenital anomaly is the presence of remnants of embryonic tissue covering a part of the disk or surrounding the blood vessels as they enter (or exit) the disk.

Retinal vessels

In examining the retinal vessels, the practitioner should note the relative caliber of the arteries and

Figure 7.22 Cup/disk ratios.

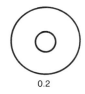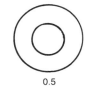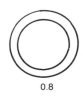

0.2   0.5   0.8

Figure 7.23 Myelinated nerve fibers.

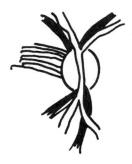

veins (the V/A ratio) The practitioner should look for irregularities in the caliber of arteries and veins, evaluate the condition of the arteriovenous crossings, evaluate the light streak of the arteries, and look for venous and arterial pulsation.

Vein/artery ratio. For arteries and veins beyond the first bifurcation, a retinal artery normally has a caliber slightly less than the corresponding vein. This is usually expressed as a V/A ratio of 3/2. In *hypertensive retinopathy* the arteries are attenuated, with the result that the V/A ratio may be reduced to 2/1 or even 3/1. Along with this attenuation, localized irregularities in the caliber of the arteries may occur along with focal constrictions.

Irregularities in caliber of veins. Dilation, tortuosity, and beading of the retinal veins may occur in *sickle-cell anemia* and in other blood dyscrasias.

Arteriovenous crossings. Where an artery and a vein cross, they share the same outer layer (tunica adventitia). Therefore, if an artery becomes sclerosed (as in *arteriolar sclerosis*, which accompanies hypertension), traction is exerted on the wall of the vein. As shown in Figure 7.24, this traction causes the arteriovenous (A/V) crossing changes of compression, deviation, humping, tapering, and banking. In general, the more pronounced the crossing changes, the more serious is the patient's arteriolar sclerosis.

Figure 7.24 Arteriovenous crossing changes: *(a)* normal crossing; *(b)* early arteriovenous compression; *(c)* deviation of vein; *(d)* humping of vein; *(e)* tapering of vein; *(f)* banking of vein (from Scheie and Albert, 1977).

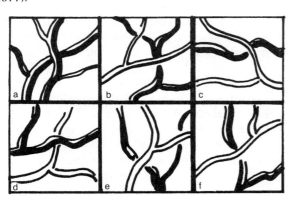

Arterial light streak. When we look at a normal retinal artery with an ophthalmoscope, we do not see the arterial wall. All that is seen is a column of blood with a cylindrical surface, and as the ophthalmoscope is moved, the reflection of this blood column, or light streak, may be seen to move. If the arterial wall becomes sclerotic as a result of hypertension, the light streak may appear at first to be accentuated and widened. However, in the later stages this may lead to a "copper wire" or "silver wire" artery appearance. As described by Scheie and Albert (1977), grades 1 and 2 of arteriolar sclerosis are indicated by an increase in the width of the light streak and the presence of arteriovenous compression; grade 3 is indicated by the presence of "copper wire" arteries and further advanced A/V compression; and grade 4 is indicated by the presence of "silver wire" arteries and even more severe A/V compression. In this classification, *compression* is used to indicate all of the crossing changes shown in Figure 7.24.

Arterial and venous pulsation. The central artery and central vein of the retina should be evaluated for the presence of pulsation where they exit (or enter) the optic nerve. Pulsation of the central retinal artery is definitely abnormal. It occurs only when the intraocular pressure exceeds the diastolic pressure of the retinal artery (which is normally about one-half that of the brachial diastolic pressure) and, therefore, indicates that the patient is experiencing an attack of glaucoma. Spontaneous pulsation of the central vein, on the other hand, is a normal condition in about 80 percent of all people. The presence of spontaneous venous pulse should be recorded so that if at any time in the future it is found not to be present, either papilledema or impending closure of the central retinal vein may be suspected.

Macular area

Inspection of the macular area involves the problem that once the light from the ophthalmoscope strikes the macular region, the pupil constricts, and, in many cases, the examiner loses sight of the macula. This problem can be solved to some extent by using the narrow macular beam and by dimming the light source so the pupillary constriction will not be as extreme. With some patients a request to "look at my light" will result in an opportunity to visualize the macular area for a brief moment. For other patients a request to "look at the top edge of my light" or to "look at the bottom edge of my light" will be accompanied by less pupillary constriction than if the patient were to look directly at the light. The examiner should evaluate the macular area in terms of the presence or absence of the foveal reflex, as well as look for any pigmentation, depigmentation, or other unusual appearance.

Foveal reflex. The foveal reflex occurs as a result of the reflection of the light from the ophthalmoscope in the foveal pit. It appears as a bright pinpoint of light that moves sideways or up and down in response to movement of the ophthalmoscope. The foveal reflex is usually brighter and more easily seen in children than adults, probably due to the greater transparency of the retinal tissue and the larger pupil. For each eye the examiner should record whether the foveal reflex is present and, if it is, whether it is bright, dull, barely present, and so forth. Absence of the foveal reflex may indicate the presence of *central serous retinopathy, macular edema,* a *macular dystrophy,* or other macular abnormality. However, in older patients, the foveal reflex is often absent, even when no disease is present.

Macular pigmentation. Because the retinal pigment epithelium is more dense in the macular area than in the surrounding retina, the macular area normally appears somewhat darker than the surrounding retina. Indeed, this hyperpigmentation of the macular area is what allows the examiner to identify it and determine where to look for the foveal reflex. In senile macular degeneration there tends to be pigment clumping in the macular area, along with areas of depigmentation. This has been variously referred to as a "salt-and-pepper" appearance or as a "moth-eaten" appearance. There are also a number of conditions in which a heavily pigmented ring is present in the periphery of the macular area and has a "bull's-eye" or "beaten-bronze" appearance. The "bull's eye" is horizontally oval and is often somewhat larger in extent than the optic disk. This type of pigmentation is characteristic of a form of juvenile macular dystrophy known as *Stargardt's disease* and is also seen in *chloroquine retinopathy.*

Drusen. The presence of drusen is a relatively common finding in or near the macular area. Drusen appear as white or yellow, round, oval, or otherwise-shaped elevations in the retina. They usually occur in both eyes. They have been described as deposits of amorphous material in the inner portion of Bruch's membrane, just underneath the pigment epithelium, and they involve some destruction of the pigment epithelium. They occur in senile macular degeneration and other degenerative conditions and also occur occasionally in younger people as an inherited condition. They have no effect on vision unless occurring in the foveal area, and they are not amenable to treatment.

Fundus background

The fundus background has a mottled appearance due to the presence of the retinal pigment epithelium. There is usually a thinning of the pigment epithelium toward the periphery of the retina, so the choroidal vessels can be seen. Rather than being end arteries like the retinal vessels, the choroidal vessels freely intertwine and have a basket-weave appearance.

In *albinism* and *albinoidism* there is a marked thinning of the retinal pigment epithelium throughout the retina—the choroidal vessels are clearly visible, giving rise to the terms *tigroid fundus* and *tesselated fundus.* There is a thinning of the retinal pigment epithelium in high and moderate myopia due to the stretching of the eyeball, and the pigment epithelium tends to become thinner with age, regardless of refractive error.

Abnormalities that may occur in the fundus background include areas of hyperpigmentation, hemorrhages (round, flame-shaped, and preretinal), microaneurisms, cotton-wool exudates, and hard exudates.

Hyperpigmentation. The most common cause of hyperpigmentation in the fundus background is *retinal pigment epithelium hyperplasia,* which occurs in the form of single or multiple patches of black pigment with well-defined borders, varying in size from the width of a retinal vessel to the size of the optic disk or larger. There is no visual loss and no treatment is required.

Hyperpigmentation of the choroid is less common than hyperpigmentation of the pigment epithelium and may occur either in the form of a choroidal nevus or a choroidal melanoma. A *choroidal nevus* is slate gray or even blue gray in appearance (because of the presence of the overlying retinal pigment epithelium) and usually has indefinite borders. Nevi are benign and require no treatment. A *choroidal melanoma* may look little different than a nevus, but at some stage it will be raised above the level of the surrounding retina, forming a mass within the globe. Choroidal melanomas are malignant tumors that may eventually metastasize, causing death. The treatment is *enucleation* (surgical removal of the eye).

Hemorrhages. *Round* or *dot hemorrhages* are those located in the deeper layers of the retina. One common cause of round hemorrhages is the rupture of microaneurisms in *diabetic retinopathy. Flame-shaped hemorrhages* occur in the nerve fiber layer of the retina, and their shape is due to the nerve fiber distribution in the affected area. They occur in the later stages of hypertensive retinopathy, in papilledema, and in a large number of other conditions. *Preretinal hemorrhages* occur as a result of the bleeding of small, newly formed vessels on the surface of the retina or the optic nerve. They are usually large hemorrhages and tend to be "boat shaped" due to the infiltration of blood, by gravity, between the retina and the vitreous. Preretinal hemorrhages occur in the proliferative forms of diabetic retinopathy, sickle-cell anemia, and other retinopathies. The treatment for a preretinal hemorrhage is light or laser coagulation.

Microaneurisms. Microaneurisms are so small that many of them are beyond the resolving power of the direct ophthalmoscope. The first indication that anything is wrong may be when they rupture, resulting in small dot hemorrhages. Many retinal surgeons treat microaneurisms and small hemorrhages in diabetes with light or laser coagulation.

Cotton-wool exudates. Cotton-wool exudates are white, cottony-appearing deposits in the retina that are somewhat smaller than the optic disk. They were formerly thought to be inflammatory exudates but are now known to be infarcted areas in the nerve fiber layer occurring as a result of local retinal ischemia. They occur in diabetic retinopathy and in the later stages of hypertensive retinopathy.

Hard exudates. Hard exudates are yellowish, waxy-appearing deposits in the retina resulting from localized retinal edema. They are part of the clinical picture of diabetic retinopathy and result from changes in the capillary walls.

Peripheral fundus

As noted earlier, to view the peripheral fundus the examiner instructs the patient to look in the direction corresponding to the portion of the fundus to be examined—the patient is instructed to look upward if the examiner wishes to examine the

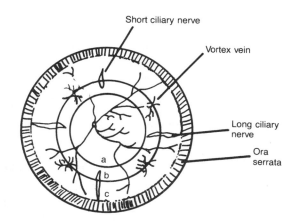

Figure 7.25 Approximate area of fundus seen: (a) direct ophthalmoscope and undilated pupil; (b) monocular indirect ophthalmoscope and undilated pupil; (c) binocular indirect ophthalmoscope and fully dilated pupil (fundus record form from University of Alabama form OPT 102).

superior fundus, and so on. The extent of the peripheral fundus that can be examined depends on the instrumentation used. The inner circle in Figure 7.25a indicates the approximate area of the fundus that can be seen with the direct ophthalmoscope with an undilated pupil (the actual area would depend on the patient's pupil size, refractive error, and other variables); the outer circle in Figure 7.25b indicates the approximate area that would be seen with the monocular indirect ophthalmoscope and an undilated pupil. With the binocular indirect ophthalmoscope and a fully dilated pupil, it is possible to view the fundus all the way to the ora serrata, as indicated in Figure 7.25c.

Landmarks. Peripheral fundus landmarks that can be seen with the monocular indirect ophthalmoscope include the vortex vein ampules and the long and short ciliary nerves (see Figure 7.25). The four vortex vein ampules are located in the oblique meridians of the fundus, just anterior to the equator, and close to the outer limit of the field of view as seen by the monocular indirect ophthalmoscope. They are easily seen in lightly pigmented fundi, appearing to be reddish or pink in color against the pale peripheral fundus background. However, in darkly pigmented fundi they are usually hidden by the retinal pigment epithelium. The long and short ciliary nerves are radially oriented and are a glistening white in appearance.

Peripheral fundus lesions. The peripheral fundus lesions that are of major interest in the examination of the peripheral fundus are those that may lead to retinal detachment. This detachment occurs not between the retina and the choroid, but between the retinal rods and cones and the pigment epithelium, with the pigment epithelium remaining attached to Bruch's membrane of the choroid. As described by Straatsma, Foos, and Kreiger (1980), the retinal pigment epithelial cells are joined firmly to each other by a continuous belt of tight intercellular junctions known as the *zonula occludens*. The inner surfaces of the pigment epithelial cells have irregular processes extending into the spaces between the outer segments of the rods and cones, and these spaces are filled with a mucopolysaccharide material that forms a relatively weak bond. This bond can be broken by fluid passing from the vitreous through a break in the sensory retina, particularly if traction is exerted on the retina by the vitreous.

Conditions that are apt to lead to retinal detachment include retinal tears, lattice degeneration, and retinal holes (see Figure 7.26). Retinal tears are usually *U*-shaped or *V*-shaped, with the "top" of the *U* or *V* directed anteriorly, toward the ora serrata, and with a tapered flap (operculum) extending into the vitreous. Lattice degeneration involves one or more sharply demarcated, circumferentially oriented lesions in the anterior retina, criss-crossed with fine white lines and with pigment accumulations in the areas of the white lines (which are atrophic blood vessels). Retinal holes are round holes with smooth, rounded margins, located near the ora serrata.

Recording of findings

As with the slit-lamp examination, one must strike a balance between a sketchy, incomplete recording of findings and a recording procedure that is laborious and time-consuming. A recommended format that enables the examiner to record the findings in a minimum of time as well as include sufficient blank space for any drawings is shown in Appendix A.

ADDITIONAL OCULAR HEALTH EXAMINATION PROCEDURES

The armamentarium of the optometrist include a large number of additional procedures, normally used only when indicated by the patient's history or by the results of the preliminary or ocular health examination. These procedures include gonioscopy; slit-lamp examination with the Hruby lens, the Goldmann fundus lens, or the 60D or 90D condensing lens; ocular photodocumentation; visual field testing; neurodiagnostic tests; exophthalmometry; ophthalmodynamometry; and ocular ultrasonography.

Gonioscopy

Without special instrumentation it is impossible to observe the anterior chamber angle because, as shown in Figure 7.27a, rays of light reflected from structures in the angle strike the air-tear interface at an angle greater than the critical angle and, therefore, are totally internally reflected. The first method of gonioscopy to be developed made use of a very thick contact lens (see Figure 7.27b), which allows the rays of light from the anterior chamber angle to be transmitted directly into the eye of the examiner. This procedure is called *direct gonioscopy*, and the lens is called the *Koeppe lens*. A method developed later by Goldmann makes use of a contact lens fitted with one or more mirrors designed for reflecting the light from the anterior chamber angle into the examiner's eye (see Figure 7.27c). This procedure is called *indirect gonioscopy*, and the lenses available for performing indirect gonioscopy include several versions of the Goldmann lens as well as the Zeiss goniolens.

To make use of the Koeppe lens, the patient must recline in a supine position; the examiner makes use

Figure 7.26 Peripheral retinal lesions that may lead to retinal detachment (fundus record form from University of Alabama form OPT 102).

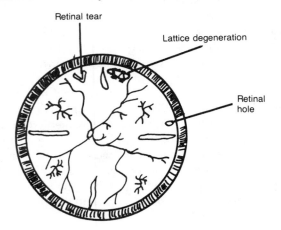

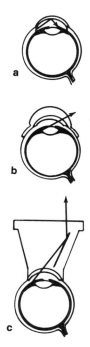

Figure 7.27 *(a)* **Rays of light coming from the anterior chamber angle are totally internally reflected;** *(b)* **direct gonioscopy with the Koeppe lens;** *(c)* **indirect gonioscopy with the Goldmann lens.**

of a small, portable binocular microscope and a focal illuminator. As compared with indirect gonioscopy, direct gonioscopy with the Koeppe lens has several advantages: (1) minimal patient cooperation is necessary and (2) the examiner can easily visualize any quadrant of the anterior chamber angle. Further, the angles for the two eyes can be compared by placing a Koeppe lens on each eye.

To perform indirect gonioscopy with the Goldmann or Zeiss goniolens, the patient is seated at the slit lamp, and both the illumination and observation systems of the slit lamp are used. The indirect method, therefore, has the advantage that a bright, narrow beam can be used to view an optical section of the anterior chamber angle.

Indications for gonioscopy. Although the method described by Van Herick, Shaffer, and Schwartz (1969) enables the practitioner to make a reasonably accurate estimation of the anterior chamber angle, the only way to actually visualize the angle is by means of gonioscopy. Additional indications for gonioscopy include a number of situations in which information concerning the angle (apart from the estimation of its width) is desirable. For example, gonioscopy should be performed on a patient found to have a *Kruckenberg spindle* (deposition of pigment cells on the corneal endothelium) to see if pigment has been deposited in the trabecular meshwork. If *rubeosis iridis* (new blood vessels on the surface of the iris) is found to be present, gonioscopy should be done to rule out the presence of new blood vessels in the anterior chamber angle. A third indication for gonioscopy is to rule out the presence of *angle recession* following an injury in which an eye has been submitted to blunt trauma. Gray (1977, 1978) listed the following indications for gonioscopy: shallow anterior chambers; open or narrow angle glaucoma; anterior or posterior uveitis; iris or ciliary body masses; intumescence of the crystalline lens; dislocation or subluxation of the lens; rubeosis iridis; central artery or central vein occlusions; ocular contusion; intraocular foreign bodies; essential iris atrophy; and any symptomatology suggestive of acute, subacute, or chronic angle closure.

Procedure. The procedure for performing gonioscopy with the Goldmann lens has been described in some detail by Gray (1977, 1978). The first step in the procedure involves placing on the clean gonioscopy lens (washed with soap and water) two drops of 1.6 percent *hydroxyethyl cellulose* solution, being careful not to introduce air bubbles into the solution. Following this, the patient's cornea is anesthetized with one drop of 0.5 percent proparacaine hydrochloride. While the patient is seated at the slit lamp with his or her chin in the chinrest and forehead firmly against the forehead rest, the examiner instructs the patient to look upward and everts the lower lid with the thumb (right thumb for the patient's right eye, and left thumb for the left eye). The examiner then grasps the goniolens with the thumb and first finger of the other hand and tilts the goniolens so one edge is positioned at the inferior cul-de-sac. Placing the thumb of the free hand gently against the patient's upper lid, the examiner instructs the patient to look straight ahead, and then pivots the lens onto the patient's cornea.

After releasing the thumb from the upper lid, the examiner continues to hold the lens between the thumb and the index finger, while supporting the lens underneath by the second or middle finger. The last two fingers are rested on the patient's cheek to prevent excessive pressure against the patient's cornea. The goniolens is then rotated, using the thumb and the index finger, to view the various quadrants of the anterior chamber angle. Using a broad beam of 2mm or more, the slit lamp and microscope are aligned at 0 degrees to each other, with 10× magnification; the beam is directed toward the center of the gonioscope mirror. Using this procedure, the portion of the anterior chamber angle facing the gonioscope mirror will come into view as the microscope is focused, and the magnification can be increased to view the angle.

To remove the goniolens, the examiner gently rocks it back and forth. If the lens does not loosen with this procedure, the seal can be broken by exerting a small amount of pressure on the sclera or by irrigating the eye with saline solution. Once the goniolens has been removed, the eye should be rinsed with irrigating solution and the goniolens washed with soap and water. The cornea should be inspected with fluorescein and the cobalt blue filter for signs of epithelial staining.

Interpretation. In interpreting what is seen in gonioscopy, the examiner becomes something like a "little man standing on the lens capsule" (see Figure 7.28). Using this analogy, the surface of the iris constitutes the "terrain," and Schwalbe's line (the termination of Descemet's membrane) constitutes the "horizon." The structures in the anterior chamber angle are all located between the most peripheral portion of the iris and Schwalbe's line.

In a completely open angle (grade 4), the "little man standing on the lens capsule" will see the following structures, from the "horizon" downward: (1) Schwalbe's line, (2) the trabecular meshwork, (3) the scleral spur, and (4) the ciliary body. In general, all four of these structures will be seen in a grade-4

angle. The first three structures will be seen in a grade-3 angle, only the first two will be seen in a grade-2 angle, and only Schwalbe's line will be seen in a grade-1 angle.

Schwalbe's line is opaque and white in appearance. According to Licther (1976), it is thought to be made up of trabecular fibers that turn to run circumferentially around the angle. It may be raised slightly and may appear to glisten.

The trabecular meshwork, located just below Schwalbe's line, is normally dull gray in appearance but in many eyes is identified by the presence of faint pigmentation. If the pigmentation is particularly prominent, the possibility of pigmentary glaucoma should be considered.

The scleral spur is seen as a thin white line below the translucent (or pigmented) trabeculum. It represents the most anterior aspect of the sclera. (Recall that the longitudinal muscle fibers of the ciliary muscle insert into the scleral spur.)

The ciliary body band, located just below the scleral spur, varies in appearance from dull brown to pale gray. In about one third of normal eyes, *iris processes* will be seen to bridge across the ciliary body band, extending anteriorly over the scleral spur and terminating just behind the trabeculum. [For additional information on the interpretation of gonioscopic findings, readers are referred to Licther (1976) and Gray (1978).]

Examination with the Hruby Lens

The Hruby lens is a −60.00D lens mounted on the slit lamp in such a way that it can be placed very close to the patient's cornea without touching it (see Figure 7.29a). With the slit lamp it is ordinarily possible to examine ocular structures only as far back as the most anterior portion of the vitreous humor. However, by neutralizing the refractive power of the eye, the Hruby lens makes it possible to examine the posterior vitreous and the retina. As described by Colenbrander (1979), when the Hruby lens is used close to the cornea, the fundus image will be close to the fundus itself and of approximately actual size. Therefore, the magnification is essentially that of the microscope: at 16× it will be approximately that of direct ophthalmoscopy, but at higher magnification settings it will be correspondingly greater than that of direct ophthalmoscopy. Use of the Hruby lens has the advantage over direct ophthalmoscopy of binocular vision and the consequent perception of stereoscopic depth. However, viewing is limited to the posterior portion of the

Figure 7.28 Examiner's view of the anterior chamber angle in gonioscopy. The surface of the iris is the "terrain," and Schwalbe's line is the "horizon."

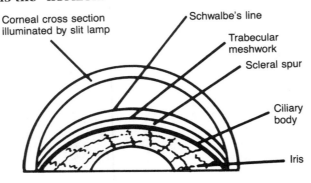

Corneal cross section illuminated by slit lamp

Schwalbe's line

Trabecular meshwork

Scleral spur

Ciliary body

Iris

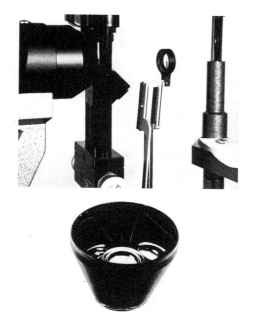

Figure 7.29 *(a)* **The Hruby lens;** *(b)* **the Goldmann fundus lens.**

fundus. Another disadvantage is that the pupil must be dilated.

Indications. By using the narrow slit with the Hruby lens, it is possible to determine the presence of areas of elevation above or depressions below the retinal surface. Therefore, examination with the Hruby lens is particularly indicated when macular detachment, macular degeneration, or other macular conditions are suspected on the basis of ophthalmoscopy. Hruby lens examination is also indicated when papilledema, drusen of the optic disk, or other optic nerve pathology is suspected on the basis of ophthalmoscopy. A third indication for Hruby lens examination is vitreous liquefaction, posterior vitreous detachment, or other degenerative changes in the vitreous when a patient complains of floaters, flashing lights, or other entoptic phenomena.

Procedure. To use the Hruby lens, the slit lamp source and microscope are both oriented in the zero position. While the patient watches the fixation object provided with the instrument, the Hruby lens is gradually moved forward until the narrow slit is focused on the retina. The focusable fixation object provided with the Haag-Streit 900 slit lamp is particularly useful for this procedure, as it can be moved to whatever position is necessary without requiring

the patient to accommodate. The examiner will soon develop skill in bringing the desired area of the retina into view by moving the fixation object, thus controlling the retinal position viewed not by moving the slit lamp beam but by controlling the patient's fixation. If examination of the posterior vitreous is desired, the retina (i.e., the optic nerve head or a large retinal vessel) can first be brought into focus; the joystick can then be moved backward, causing the posterior vitreous to come into focus.

Examination with the Goldmann Three-Mirror Fundus Lens

The Goldmann three-mirror lens is designed for use in the examination of the retina and vitreous as well as the anterior chamber angle (see Figure 7.29b). Indications for its use in examining the retina and vitreous are to some extent similar to those for the Hruby lens, with the important exception that its use is not confined to the examination of the posterior pole. The three mirrors of the Goldmann fundus lens are inclined at angles of 73, 67, and 59 degrees.

Procedure. Prior to beginning the procedure, the anterior chamber angle is estimated, using the biomicroscope, to make sure that the angle is open. As when performing gonioscopy, two drops of 1.6 percent hydroxyethyl cellulose solution are placed in the lens, being careful not to introduce air bubbles into the solution. The patient's cornea is then anesthetized with one drop of 0.5 percent proparacaine hydrochloride. The lens is then placed on the eye, using the same procedure as that described earlier for the Goldmann goniolens.

As described by Tasman (1976), the examination is begun by using the flat central portion of the lens to examine the central 30 degrees of the fundus as well as the cornea, the lens, the anterior chamber, and the anterior and posterior vitreous. The slit-lamp beam is oriented both horizontally and vertically in traversing the vitreous cavity from side to side and from top to bottom. The 73-degree mirror is then used to examine the fundus from the posterior 30-degree area to the equator; the 67-degree mirror is used to examine the fundus from the equator to the pars plana; and the 59-degree mirror (designed for gonioscopy) is used for viewing the extreme fundus periphery. The areas that may be viewed through each portion of the three-mirror lens are shown in Figure 7.30. Detailed instructions for examination of the vitreous with the three-mirror lens are given by Tasman (1976) and Jaffe (1969).

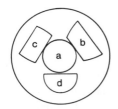 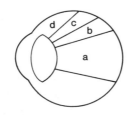

Figure 7.30   The areas that may be observed through each portion of the Goldmann 3-mirror lens: *(a)* **Flat anterior surface;** *(b)* **73-degree mirror, for viewing posterior to the equator;** *(c)* **57-degree mirror, for viewing from the equator to the ora serrata;** *(d)* **59-degree mirror, for viewing from ora serrata to ciliary body and for use in gonioscopy.**

Biomicroscopic Examination with +60D and +90D Condensing Lenses

Biomicroscopic examination of the retina and vitreous with the aid of a +60D condensing lens was first described by El Bayadi (1953). The early form of the technique was not widely accepted because it required a relatively long working distance and resulted in poor image quality. However, with the recent availability of Volk +60D and +90D biaspheric lenses, image quality is as good as or better than that obtained with the Hruby lens. Further, the technique has the advantage, as compared to the Goldmann three-mirror lens, of being noninvasive.

Indications. Indications for the examination with the +60D and +90D lenses are similar to those for examination with the Hruby lens and the Goldmann three-mirror lens. Cavallerano, Gutner, and Garsten (1986) have noted that the fundus can be observed almost to the equator, and that the vitreous can be examined by moving the slit lamp back slightly. They have suggested the use of the +90D lens for examining the optic disc of a patient with ocular hypertension or glaucoma, as well as for observing subtle changes in the macular area in early diabetic retinopathy, macular edema, and age-related maculopathy.

Procedure. The procedure for the use of the +60D or +90D lens has been described by Cavallerano et al. (1986) and Quintero (1986). Cavallerano et al. prefer the +90D lens rather than the +60D lens because the former is held closer to the patient's eye, permitting the examiner to rest his or her hand on the forehead rest of the slit lamp. They also prefer

the +90D lens because its aerial image is closer to the patient and does not require the slit lamp to be racked as far back as for the +60D lens.

After estimation of the anterior chamber angles, dilation is carried out as described earlier. The patient is seated at the biomicroscope, and the observation system is adjusted so that a stereoscopic view of the anterior segment of the eye is obtained. The illumination system should be directed at an angle of about 5 degrees from the direction of motion of the microscope, taking care that the light source does not occlude one of the microscope oculars. The patient is instructed to look straight ahead, and the slit lamp is adjusted so that a beam about 2–3mm wide is centered on the patient's pupil. The condensing lens is held between the thumb and index fingers of the left hand while examining the patient's right eye, and in a similar manner with the right hand while examining the patient's left eye. The index finger should project about 1cm behind the lens, allowing the tip of the finger to rest gently on the patient's brow. While looking outside the microscope oculars, the slit-lamp beam is focused sharply on the surface of the condensing lens closest to the examiner. The examiner then looks through the oculars and begins slowly to move the biomicroscope away from the patient's eye until the aerial image of the fundus is in focus—this image is located at a point in space between the anterior surface of the condensing lens and the microscope oculars, approximately 1 inch in front of the condensing lens. Once the aerial image is in focus, any magnification level of which the slit lamp is capable may be used.

While the condensing lens is held steadily before the patient's eye, the posterior fundus is scanned by moving only the joystick. Due to the large amount of prism power induced by the condensing lens, moving the joystick laterally decenters the slit-lamp beam sufficiently to make it possible to examine a large area of the posterior fundus. The peripheral fundus may also be examined by instructing the patient to look upward, downward, to the left, and to the right, and readjusting the slit-lamp beam for each new direction of fixation. The vitreous may then be examined by racking the slit lamp backward slightly.

OCULAR PHOTODOCUMENTATION

A variety of methods of ocular photodocumentation are available to the optometrist. These include external ocular photography by means of a standard single-lens-reflex (SLR) camera with the necessary auxiliary equipment, anterior segment photography by means of the photo slit lamp, fundus photography, fundus fluorescein angiography, and specular microscopy.

Why use photodocumentation?

The main reason for using ocular photodocumentation is to provide the practitioner with a permanent record of the appearance of a lesion or other abnormality to serve as a basis for future comparison. This is particularly important for lesions that are apt to progress or for benign tumors that may at some future time increase in size or show signs of becoming malignant. However, photodocumentation also allows the practitioner to send photographs to ophthalmologists, dermatologists, or other practitioners to whom patients may be referred. Further, photodocumentation is patient education: some patients appreciate having a photograph of an abnormal condition and being able to observe its progress or lack of progress. Still another reason for using photodocumentation, applying particularly to fundus fluorescein angiography and specular microscopy, is to confirm a diagnosis of a suspected condition. In fundus fluorescein angiography the events change so rapidly that photodocumentation is a necessary part of the procedure, whereas in specular microscopy the diagnosis of a corneal endothelial abnormality or disease can be made only after enlargement of the photographic record. Finally, by photographing unusual conditions, the practitioner can communicate with other practitioners by giving lectures and writing articles, as well as contribute information that may increase the understanding of ocular disease processes.

External photography with a single-lens-reflex (SLR) camera

An ordinary SLR camera can be adapted easily and inexpensively for external ocular photography. Long (1979) described a system of external photography making use of an SLR camera with a 50 or 55mm lens. Additional required equipment includes (1) a close-up attachment; (2) a telextender, also called a teleconverter; (3) an electronic flash unit; and (4) a straight flash bracket and bounce shoe for mounting the flash unit on the camera.

The close-up attachment makes the camera myopic and can be in the form of either positive lenses mounted in front of the camera lens—which produce refractive myopia—or extension tubes (hollow tubes mounted between the lens and the camera body)—which produce axial myopia.

The teleconverter is a negative-power optical system mounted between the camera lens and the camera body that has the effect of magnifying the image with a corresponding restriction of the field of view. Long recommends a 2× teleconverter, which increases the focal length of the 50mm normal lens to an effective focal length of 100mm. This is much less expensive than a prime telephoto lens and has the advantage of permitting a closer approach to the subject than would be possible with a telephoto lens of the same focal length. It also has a smaller entrance pupil than is possible with most telephoto lenses, permitting a greater depth of field. The smaller entrance pupil, however, makes the system "slower" than a prime telephoto lens, requiring more light for exposure.

Long (1979) recommends an inexpensive strobe flash unit having a guide number of about 45 ASA-ft for film of ASA 64 or ASA 25. A strobe unit fires at 1/1,000 second or less, effectively stopping any motion of the subject or the subject's eyes. The straight flash bracket screws into the camera's tripod mount to mount the strobe unit to one side of the camera, and the bounce shoe is a small device that fits between the strobe and its mount. Long recommends the following equipment and exposures:

1. *Full-face portrait.* Lens-to-subject distance: approximately 1m; normal lens with 2× teleconverter; strobe mounted on flash shoe of camera; f/4.8.
2. *Half face or both eyes.* Lens-to-subject distance: about 50cm; normal lens with 2× teleconverter; strobe mounted on flash shoe of camera; f/11.
3. *Single eye with adnexa.* Lens-to-subject distance: approximately 20cm; normal lens with 2× teleconverter and +4.00D close-up lens or 16mm extension tube mounted between lens and teleconverter; strobe mounted on flash bracket through bounce shoe, usually temporal to patient and aimed by adjustment of bounce shoe; f/11.
4. *Single eye isolated.* Lens-to-subject distance: approximately 15cm; normal lens with 2× teleconverter and +6.00D close-up lens or 26mm extension tube mounted between lens and teleconverter; strobe mounted as for single eye with adnexa; f/11.

Several shots should be taken of the subject at both the optimal f/number and at greater and lesser f/numbers. [Readers interested in the various systems for external ocular photography are referred to Olsen (1979a), who describes the following systems: (1) Nikon Micro-Nikkor Auto 55mm, f/3.5 lens; (2) Nikon Micro-Nikkor Auto 105mm, f/4 lens; (3) Kodak Instatech X; (4) Photoeaze external camera; (5) Nikon Medical-Nikkor Auto 200mm, f/5.6 lens; (6) SLR camera with supplementary plus lenses; (7) SX–70 Polaroid camera; and (8) Polaroid CU–5 close-up Land camera.]

Slit-lamp photography

As discussed by Mann (1970), the first successful system of slit-lamp photography was developed by Goldmann in 1940. Since that time, several photo slit lamps have been introduced, but unfortunately many are so expensive that their cost can be justified only for hospitals and clinics.

The first reasonably priced photo slit lamp to be made available was the Nikon photo slit lamp. The instrument incorporates the basic Nikon slit lamp having a zoom-lens system, and it has the advantage that the photographic attachment (including the camera body, mounting brackets, and flash mechanism) can be added to the preexisting slit lamp. It has the disadvantage, as pointed out by Gutner (1979) and Perrigin (1980), of having a mirror that is mechanically moved into position and that completely blocks the view of the eye composing the photograph for a significant period of time. The examiner's other eye, which sees the patient's eye from a different angle of observation than that which the film will record, must be used in composing the photograph. A slight eye movement can cause the examiner to miss what he or she is trying to document.

Perrigin (1980) reviewed the available equipment for slit-lamp photography. The three most expensive photo slit lamps described by Perrigin are the Jena model 210, the Rodenstock 2001, and the Zeiss. The Jena has the same disadvantage described for the Nikon: the examiner has to shoot "blind." However, both the Rodenstock and the Zeiss have the choice of either 50/50 or 70/30 beam splitters rather than having a mechanically moved mirror. Less expensive photo slit lamps are the Marco IIB and V models, the Topcon SL–5D, and the Nikon. The Marco instruments are equipped with 50/50 beam splitters, whereas the Topcon SL–5D (see Figure 7.31) is equipped with a 70/30 beam splitter. Perrigin commented that the Topcon instrument is well designed and, in his experience, is the most desirable of the photo slit lamps available for combined use in both routine biomicroscopy and slit-lamp photography. An additional advantage of the SL–5D

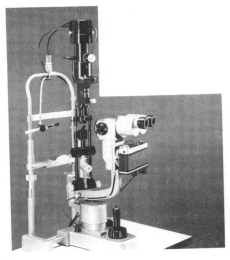

Figure 7.31   The Topcon SL–5D photo slit lamp.

is that the instrument is provided with a switch for moving the beam splitter out of the optical path for routine (nonphotographic) use.

With the photo slit lamp, the practitioner should be able to photographically document anything seen during a routine slit-lamp examination (although possibly at lower magnification).

Goniophotography. Olsen (1979b) describes a method of goniophotography making use of the Nikon photo slit lamp and the Goldmann single-mirror goniolens. For optimum results, Olsen suggests magnifications of 16 or 25× (since the 10× eyepiece is not included in the optical system when the camera is used, the actual magnification is 1.6 or 2.5×). He also recommends flash-intensity (I) setting 2 and aperture (A) setting 3 with a 2mm slit at 25× without filters. The microscope is placed perpendicular to the plane of the face and back surface of the goniolens, and the goniolens mirror is placed opposite the section of the angle to be photographed. For photographing the superior and inferior angles, the illumination system is swung 10–20 degrees to the side opposite the side where the photographic system is mounted. For photographing the medial and temporal angles, the microscope and illumination system are made coaxial, and the horizontal slit beam is inclined at an angle of 10–20 degrees. Olsen also describes the use of the Kowa RC–2 fundus camera (described here in the section on fundus photography) in combination with the Goldmann single-mirror goniolens, as well as the

Nikon slit lamp and the Kowa fundus camera in combination with the Koeppe direct goniolens. Olsen concludes that the Nikon photo slit lamp/Goldmann goniolens combination produces the best overall results for the typical optometric practice.

Photography with the +90D lens

Cavallerano et al. (1986) describe the use of the slit lamp and +90D lens for photographic documentation. They report that their best results were obtained by shooting at a magnification of 25× (ISO 400) using a flash output of 20 watt-seconds; and that polaroid prints can also be taken at 25× magnification using a Polaroid type 779 film (ISO 600) at a flash output of 80 watt-seconds. Background illumination is not recommended in either situation because it would increase the number of reflections in the photograph. Cavallerano et al. suggest that the examiner look monocularly through the eyepiece that shows the photographic image to insure accurate focus and consistent results. They further point out that the maximum width of the beam may not exceed one-half the diameter of the condensing lens to obtain useful photographic documentation.

Fluorescein photography

With the appropriate exciter and barrier filters, fluorescein is used to photograph staining of the corneal or conjunctival epithelium and in contact-lens fluorescein photography. Long (1979) recommends a Wratten 47A blue filter over the strobe head for the exciter filter and a Y2 yellow filter over the camera objective for the barrier filter. These filters require an increase in exposure of about four f-stops.

Fundus photography

Although the first successful instrumentation for fundus photography, as described by Hurtes (1976), was developed in 1886, fundus photography has been used on a regular basis in ophthalmological departments in hospitals and clinics only since the 1940s, and by optometry schools and clinics only during the past two decades. The availability of mydriatic agents in the majority of the 50 states today is bringing fundus photography to the attention of increasing numbers of practicing optometrists. Practitioners who have given little thought to fundus photography may not be aware that a hand-held fundus camera can be purchased for only a few thousand dollars and that a very good table-mounted instrument can be purchased for about the price of a subcompact automobile. They may also not be aware that a fundus camera can be used to take photographs of the conjunctiva, cornea, iris, and crystalline lens.

Field of view. In terms of the available field of view, three categories of fundus cameras are available. For some years the "standard" fundus camera has required the use of a mydriatic agent and has had a 30-degree field of view, which is large enough to include the optic nerve head, the macular area, and a bit more on either side. With these instruments the magnification of 2.5× (similar to that of an indirect ophthalmoscope) can be doubled by the use of a 2× lens to show greater fundus detail, but with a consequent reduction in the field of view to 15 degrees.

Recently, a number of "nonmydriatic" fundus cameras having a 45-degree field of view have been introduced. With these instruments the patient is seated in a dimly illuminated room to allow the pupils to dilate, and the fundus is then illuminated with a low-intensity, infrared light.

In a third category of fundus camera, allowing a field of view of 148 degrees, the camera objective must make contact with the cornea. Although this camera is able to show much more in the periphery than the standard 30-degree camera and has the further advantage of requiring only one picture rather than a montage of pictures to illustrate an extensive fundus lesion, the image is so minified that there is a much poorer image resolution than is available with the 30-degree camera. Gutner (1979) has pointed out that these large-field cameras were designed not to supplant but to supplement ordinary fundus cameras. Mainly because of the greater cost of the instruments in the second and third categories (but also because of the specialized uses for which they are designed), the great majority of optometric practitioners and clinics having fundus cameras have the standard 30-degree instrument.

Instrumentation. The various instruments available for fundus photography have been reviewed by Perrigin (1980). The least expensive fundus cameras available are two hand-held models, the Kowa RC–2 (see Figure 7.32) and RC–3. The RC–3 provides both 2.6× and 5.3× magnification, with corresponding fields of view of 30 and 15 degrees. The optical system of the Kowa camera is that of an indirect ophthalmoscope (as are the optical systems of all fundus cameras), and the instrument is used in much the same way as an ophthalmoscope is used. With a 20.00 or 30.00D condensing lens, it can be used as an indirect ophthalmoscope. Perrigin

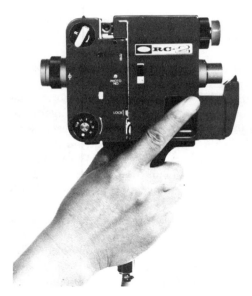

Figure 7.33   The Topcon TRC–JE fundus camera.

reports that this instrument takes good photographs and has the advantage that it also can be used for external ocular photography. As compared with table-mounted instruments, the Kowa's maneuverability makes it possible to photograph lesions in the far periphery with a sufficiently dilated pupil. An additional advantage is that due to its portability, it can be easily used for procedures such as screening programs and examinations in patient's homes.

The least expensive table-mounted fundus cameras are the Topcon TRC–JE, TRC–FE, and TRC–FET. Perrigin (1980) recommends the lowest priced,

Figure 7.32   The Kowa RC–2 hand-held fundus camera.

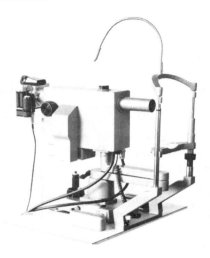

the TRC–JE, as a good choice for the average practitioner (see Figure 7.33). This camera has the standard 30-degree field of view with 2.5× magnification and comes with a standard 35mm camera back. With this camera it is possible to take pictures at the rate of one frame every 10 seconds, and satisfactory external ocular photographs can be taken. The TRC–FE and TRC–FET are the same basic camera as the TRC–JE but have a second camera back (for fundus fluorescein angiography) and the capability of taking photographs at the rate of one frame per second. In addition, they can double the magnification to 5×. The TRC–FE camera is used at the University of Houston College of Optometry, and it has been found to be completely satisfactory and unusually durable. As an option, a Polaroid camera back is also available. Even though this has the obvious advantage of immediate reinforcement for the photographer, it has the disadvantage of relatively poor image quality. In addition, Polaroid prints are of little value for use in lectures or seminars. If the practitioner would like to supply a patient with a print but ordinarily uses slides rather than prints, Perrigin (1980) has suggested that the slide be projected on a screen and a picture of it be taken with a Polaroid camera.

The more expensive, standard 30-degree-field fundus cameras include the Zeiss fundus camera and the Jena model 211 Retinophot. Several 45-degree-field, nonmydriatic fundus cameras are now available, the least expensive of which is the Topcon TRC–NW2. In a slightly higher price range are cameras having a variable field of view (usually from 20 degrees to 45 or 60 degrees) and, consequently, variable magnification: the Topcon TRC–W, TRC–WT, and TRC–W3, and the Canon CF–607. The Pomerantzeff Equator Plus camera, which provides a 148-degree field and requires contact between the objective lens and the cornea, is the most expensive fundus camera, at a cost of approximately $20,000.

Indications. When a fundus camera is available, the practitioner will find it useful to take fundus photographs not only for the documentation of progressive or possibly progressive conditions (macular changes, suspicious cup/disk ratios, retinal or choroidal pigmentation, hypertensive or diabetic retinopathy, and so on), but also when a patient is dilated for binocular indirect ophthalmoscopy or for examination with the Hruby lens or the Goldmann fundus lens. Once the patient has been dilated, the small amount of additional time for fundus photography is negligible.

Procedure. Dilation for fundus photography, like for binocular indirect ophthalmoscopy, can usually be accomplished by the instillation of one drop of proparacaine, 0.5 percent, followed after about 1 minute with one drop of tropicamide, 1 percent, and possibly one drop of 2.5 percent phenylephrine. For patients with dark irides, a second drop of tropicamide may be necessary if dilation has not begun by about 10 minutes after the first drop. Dilation is usually complete in 25–30 minutes.

The various specifications, including film speed and flash settings, tend to vary from one fundus camera to another, so the instruction manual should be consulted. Every fundus camera is provided with a movable fixation target and will require some practice for the examiner to be able to predict where the fixation target should be placed to take a picture of a given area of the retina (the fixation target is for the eye not being photographed). In extreme cases, such as lesions in the periphery, the patient's head may have to be tilted in the headrest. A running record should be kept of all shots, including the date, patient's name, eye (R or L), and tentative diagnosis.

Survey of photographic instrumentation

Scott (1979) sent questionnaires to more than 100 practitioners and clinics that were assumed to be involved in ocular photodocumentation on a regular basis to determine their preferences in photographic instrumentation. Sixty-one responses were received. The following are responses for optometrists in private practice (in order of preference):

External eye and adnexa
1. 35mm camera, 55mm macrolens, external mounted flash, K–25 film.
2. 35mm camera, 100mm macrolens, external mounted flash, E–200 film.
3. 35mm camera, medical Nikkor lens, internal flash, E–64 film.
4. 35mm camera, normal lens with extension tubes, ring flash, E–64 film.
5. Fundus camera.
6. Modified Polaroid SX–70.

Slit-lamp photography
1. Nikon, E–200 film.
2. Topcon SL–5D.

Fundus photography
1. Topcon TRC–FE.
2. Topcon TRC–FET.
3. Kowa RC–2.

Fundus fluorescein angiography

As noted by Cullen (1979), the original paper describing fundus fluorescein angiography was published in 1961 by Novotny and Alvis. Since that time, fundus fluorescein angiography has become an important diagnostic tool in ophthalmology. However, for several reasons it is unlikely that this procedure will soon become a routine part of optometric practice: (1) it requires the injection of sodium fluorescein into the antecubital vein (in front of the elbow), whereas most if not all diagnostic drug laws allow only for drugs instilled into the conjunctival sac; (2) although reactions to intravenous fluorescein are rare, they can occur and, according to Scheie and Albert (1977), can include vertigo, bronchospasm, myocardial arrhythmia, myocardial infarction, shock, and cardiac arrest; and (3) emergency resuscitation equipment, 1:1000 epinephrine hydrochloride, parenteral corticosteroids, benadryl, aminophylline, and aramine should always be instantly available. Nevertheless, ophthalmologists (particularly retinal surgeons) with whom optometrists consult are making increasing use of fundus fluorescein angiography, so optometrists should be well informed of the procedure and its interpretation.

Instrumentation. Instrumentation for fundus fluorescein angiography includes a fundus camera capable of taking pictures at the rate of one per second. Black and white film is used. A suitable exciter filter (blue, over the strobe source) and a barrier filter (yellow, over the camera objective) must be used.

Indications. Conditions or suspected conditions in which fundus fluorescein angiography can aid in diagnosis or management include diabetic retinopathy (in any stage); macular changes such as central serous retinopathy, cystoid macular edema, dystrophies, or degenerations; choroidal nevi or melanoma; retinal hemorrhages for any reason; papilledema, papillitis, or other optic nerve changes; and closure of a retinal artery or vein. This list is not intended to be complete, but it illustrates the wide range of conditions in which fluorescein angiography is employed.

Procedure. The procedure for fundus fluorescein angiography described here is based to a great extent on the discussion of Scheie and Albert (1977). The patient's pupils must be maximally dilated using tropicamide, 1 percent, and phenylephrine, 10 percent. Prior to the injection of fluorescein, a complete clinical examination of the fundus is done using direct and indirect ophthalmoscopy and the Goldmann fundus lens. Color fundus photography also is done along with a preinjection black and white photograph. The patient is instructed concerning the procedure, including the reason for performing the procedure and the expected side effects (including the fact that the patient will feel a "flush" when the dye enters his or her system, will see a series of flashing lights, and may feel faint or nauseated. The skin will appear to be yellow for a few hours after the procedure, and the dye will pass out in the urine, making it appear greenish-yellow).

From 5–10cc of sodium fluorescein is rapidly injected into the antecubital vein, and photographs are taken at 1-second intervals from 5 to 25 seconds after the injection, followed by photographs at 2, 5, and 10 minutes. Within 12 to 15 seconds after injection, the filling of the choriocapillaris provides an evenly mottled, choroidal flush, or background fluorescence. About 1 second after the choroidal fluorescence appears, first the retinal arteries and then the veins can be seen to fill.

Due to the zonula occludens, which binds the retinal pigment epithelial cells to Bruch's membrane and to each other, the retinal pigment epithelium acts as a *physical* barrier for the passage of fluorescein into the retina. Due to the presence of a large amount of pigment, it also acts as an *optical* barrier to the choroidal fluorescence. For example, where the retinal pigment epithelium is thin (at the location of one or more drusen), the choroidal fluorescence will be brighter than usual; where it is thick (at the macula), the choroidal fluorescence will be diminished.

Interpretation. Blocking of fluorescein, or *hypofluorescence*, can occur due to zones of hyperpigmentation, hemorrhage, or decreased vascularity (such as zones of capillary nonperfusion). *Hyperfluorescence* is seen where the pigment epithelium is atrophic or rarified, where drusen are present, or where abnormal deposits are present. In making a diagnosis, the timing of the events taking place is important. For example, in cystoid macular edema, a petal-shaped area of hyperfluorescence may persist surrounding the macular area after the choroidal fluorescence and the fluorescence of the retinal arteries and veins has ceased. For angiograms depicting specific entities, readers are referred to Chapter 9 of Scheie and Albert (1977), or Behrendt's discussion in Volume 3, Chapter 4, of Duane (1976).

Readers interested in more detailed information on ocular photodocumentation are referred to Long (1984).

Specular microscopy

With the advent of extended-wear contact lenses, contact lens practitioners have become aware that a prolonged embarrassment of the oxygen supply to the cornea can result in adverse changes in the corneal endothelium. With the use of ultrasound in cataract surgery and the widespread fitting of intraocular lenses, ophthalmic surgeons also have reason to be concerned about the corneal endothelium. To permit examination of the endothelium in much greater detail than is possible with the routine use of the slit lamp and specular reflection, an instrument known as the *specular microscope* has been developed. The specular microscope applanates an area of the cornea approximately 1mm by 1mm (requiring a corneal anesthetic), an area containing approximately 2,000 endothelial cells. It is a highly specialized, expensive instrument and is available largely in hospitals and teaching clinics.

Holden, Zantos, and Jacobs (1978) developed a system for photographing endothelial cells with a magnification of 60–70× and without the necessity for contacting the cornea. Their system makes use of an SLR camera mounted behind one of the eyepieces of a Nikon slit lamp. Zantos and Holden (1977) used this system for photographing the endothelium of unadapted soft contact lens wearers. They found that small, black spots, or "blebs," appeared in the endothelial mosaic approximately 10 minutes after insertion of the lenses (see Figure 7.34). The number and size of the blebs increased with lens wear until a maximum was reached, but continued lens wear was accompanied by apparent adaptation and a decrease in the number of blebs. Removal of the lenses resulted in rapid return of the endothelial mosaic to a normal appearance.

In describing their technique, Zantos and Holden (1977) made the point that the conventional method of slit lamp photography involves the use of a beamsplitter or a mirror, either of which fails to provide sufficient magnification to record endothelial detail. The necessary magnification was achieved by mounting the camera behind one of the eyepieces, using a coupling device. If higher magnification is needed (than that provided by the slit lamp and camera), the slides can be rephotographed with a magnifying slide copier.

Barr and Schoessler (1980) used the technique developed by Zantos and Holden (1977), modifying

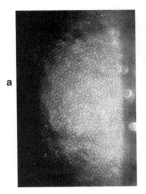 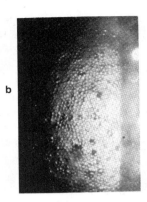

Figure 7.34 *(a)* **Normal corneal endothelium;** *(b)* **the appearance of "blebs" in the endothelium after 10 minutes of contact lens wear** (Zantos and Holden, 1977).

the system by providing the Nikon slit lamp with a protractor and pointer assembly that made it possible to set the fixation lamp at a constant angle, both horizontally and vertically. They fitted 12 subjects with one hard (PMMA) contact lens—using the opposite eye as a control—and took endothelial photographs prior to lens insertion and at various times thereafter up to 4 hours of wear. The 12 subjects were found to have an average number of 8 endothelial blebs after 30 minutes of lens wear, which was reduced to an average of 3 blebs after 6 hours of wear. Barr and Schoessler concluded that the presence of the blebs was not due to edema, and they speculated that they were the result of a build-up of carbon dioxide in the corneal tissue due to the physical barrier presented by the contact lens.

It appears that the Zantos-Holden technique of viewing endothelial cells is firmly established as a research procedure. Recently, Nikon developed an endothelial camera not requiring contact with the cornea and providing magnifications during observation of 30 and 60×. The instrument also can be used for gross photography and slit-lamp photography, but it is provided only with a monocular (rather than a binocular) microscope, and has the disadvantage that the maximum magnification that can be provided in a photograph is 5 or 10×.

VISUAL FIELD TESTING

Central and peripheral visual field screening procedures were introduced in Chapter 6. As noted there, if visual field screening results in the detection of a visual field loss, the practitioner may wish to reschedule the patient for a more complete visual field examination. However, if the patient is to be referred for ophthalmological or neurological consultation, the findings of the screening procedures may be considered adequate. Whether the optometrist reschedules the patient for a complete visual field examination depends to some extent on his or her relationship with consulting practitioners. In some cases, the consultant may prefer to do a complete visual field workup, thus making the optometrist's field examination redundant; in other cases, the consultant may prefer to have the optometrist do the field workup. Availability of local consultants is also an important consideration: if no ophthalmologist or neurologist is available locally, the optometrist may find it advantageous to do a more complete evaluation than would be done otherwise.

Central Field Testing

Tangent screen

The procedure for central field screening using the tangent screen is described in Chapter 6. When the tangent screen is used only as a screening device, it is not necessary to record the findings on a chart unless a field loss is found (however, the examiner should record on the patient's record that central fields were found to be within normal limits). When a patient is rescheduled for a tangent screen examination on the basis of a positive screening result, the findings should be recorded on a standard recording chart. A convenient way to record the findings is to use black-headed pins (which are invisible to the patient) to record the blind spot, the peripheral limits of the central field, and any scotomas. At the completion of the procedure, the positions of the pins can be recorded on the chart, and any scotomas or other field defects can be indicated.

As discussed in Chapter 6, if the patient normally wears glasses, they should be worn for the tangent screen examination. Bifocal wearers may hold a loose trial lens or uncut lens blank in front of the eye being tested (up to 1.00D of cylinder can be neglected). Smith (tape no. 3) recommends that central field testing not be done on aphakic patients unless contact lenses are worn, due to the extreme magnification effects caused by aphakic spectacles.

Once the blind spot has been plotted (preferably with a large test object), a 3mm test object should be used for most routine tangent screen testing; it should be moved in a rosette pattern over the central visual field. The speed of movement should be slow enough so the patient will have time to respond if the test object disappears, but not so slow that the patient's attention will not be maintained. The test object (black on the back side) should be flipped over occasionally to test the patient's responses: if the test object does not "disappear" when flipped over, the patient cannot be expected to report the presence of a visual field defect if one exists.

Smith (tape no. 3) has made the point that targets no smaller than 3mm in diameter should be used for tangent screen testing. For 1 and 2mm targets, the wand is likely to be a stronger stimulus than the target itself, causing the patient to respond to the fact that the wand rather than the target is seen. If the patient shows a constriction in the upper field or upper temporal field, the most likely cause is a drooping upper lid. In such a case, the patient should be asked to open the eyes wide or to hold up the upper lid of the eye being tested with a finger.

If space is available, a 2m tangent screen is much superior to a 1m screen. A 2m tangent screen is 2m square, and testing is done at a distance of 2m. A convenient and effective way to construct a 2m tangent screen is to use two 4 × 8 pieces of wallboard covered with black felt. Such a tangent screen extends from the floor to the ceiling and can be conveniently placed at the end of the examining room. With a 2m tangent screen, for a field defect of a given angular size, the linear size will be double that for a 1m tangent screen. This greatly increases the probability that the field defect will be found.

Whether a 1 or 2m tangent screen is used, illumination over the surface of the screen should be as even as possible. However, illumination need not (and should not) be high: the standard illumination for tangent screen testing is usually specified as 7 footcandles.

Projecto-light pointer

Smith (tape no. 3) highly recommends the use of a *projecto-light pointer* for tangent screen examination. This is a flashlight pointer operated either by batteries or by a 110-volt circuit; it is often used by lecturers when presenting slides. Smith instructs the practitioner to remove the diaphragm from the flashlight (usually in the form of an arrow) and to stand behind the patient while the patient fixates the fixation point in the center of the tangent screen. The examiner repeatedly turns on the flashlight—only for an instant—in different areas of the visual field and asks the patient to report the position of the light. To control fixation, every other stimulus

goes into the blind spot. If the patient reports seeing the stimulus in the blind spot, it is obvious that accurate fixation is not being maintained. Smith is enthusiastic about the use of the projecto-light pointer in tangent screen testing, calling it "the best thing since sliced bread."

Bausch & Lomb Autoplot

The Bausch & Lomb Autoplot is a 1m tangent screen made of gray vinyl (see Figure 7.35). It has a central, cross-shaped fixation point, and the examiner projects an illuminated test object varying in diameter from 0.5 to 15mm in either white, red, green, or blue light. A pantograph arrangement is used to move the stimulus and to record the findings. Because only the test object is illuminated, the screen must be illuminated externally. A level of illumination of only 1 footcandle is required.

The examination procedure is similar to that used with the tangent screen. The examiner faces the patient and is thus able to monitor the patient's fixation closely. To test the patient's responses, the examiner may extinguish the test object by obstructing the optical system or by moving the aperture slightly to one side. Although the Autoplot is much more expensive than a tangent screen, both the examination and recording of the visual field are greatly simplified.

Jenkel-Davidson Lumiwand

The Jenkel-Davidson Lumiwand is a self-luminous test object mounted on the end of a 1m-long black

Figure 7.35   The Bausch & Lomb Autoplot: *(a)* the projection and plotting mechanism; *(b)* the instrument and screen mounted on a table for use.

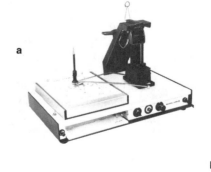
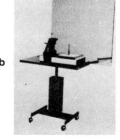

wand. The size of stimuli can be varied from 1 to 10mm, and illumination levels of 1, 3, and 9 millilamberts are available. The Lumiwand is designed for use with a black felt tangent screen and an illuminated fixation light. When the Lumiwand is used, the level of illumination must be sufficient so the examiner is able to monitor the patient's fixation, but low enough so the patient is not able to see the handle of the Lumiwand. Harrington (1976) suggested that a small nightlight be mounted on the wall above the tangent screen to enable the examiner to monitor the patient's fixation. Because the Lumiwand is illuminated only while the examiner presses a button on the handle, extinguishing the stimulus to test the patient's response can be done simply.

Peripheral Field Testing

Equipment available for peripheral field testing include the arc perimeter, the Aimark projection perimeter, and the Goldmann and other hemispherical projection perimeters.

Arc perimeter

Arc perimeters are distributed by Bausch & Lomb, American Optical, and other companies. These instruments employ a 333mm testing distance (one-third that of the tangent screen) and make use of hand-held or mechanically activated test objects. They are designed for determining the peripheral limits of the field of vision in horizontal, vertical, and oblique meridians. By turning the perimeter arc sequentially into each of six positions for each eye, the peripheral limits of the field can be plotted for 0 and 180 degrees, 30 and 210 degrees, 60 and 240 degrees, 90 and 270 degrees, 120 and 300 degrees, and 150 and 330 degrees. Test objects varying from 1–12mm or more in diameter are available. In determining the peripheral limits of the visual field, the examiner begins testing each half-meridian by holding the test object at the extreme limit of the perimeter arm and moving it inward, thus moving it from "nonseeing to seeing," while monitoring the patient's fixation. For each half-meridian, more than one test object can be used, each test object plotting (for all half-meridians) an *isopter* of the peripheral field (see Figure 7.36). Commonly used test objects are 1, 3, and 6mm (corresponding to ⅙, ½, and 1 degree of arc at the 333mm distance). As shown in Figure 7.36, the extent of the peripheral field, with a 3mm test object, is approximately 90 degrees temporally, 70 degrees inferiorly, 60 degrees

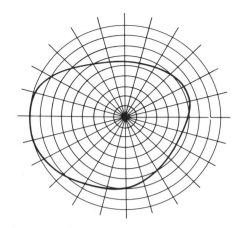

Figure 7.36   Visual field isopter as plotted by means of an arc perimeter (3/330 white test object).

nasally, and 55 degrees superiorly. The actual extent of the normal peripheral field for an object of a given size and a given level of illumination (7 footcandles) will depend on such anatomical features as the patient's nose, overhang of the superior orbital ridge, or a tendency for the upper lid to droop.

Aimark projection perimeter

The Aimark projection perimeter, made by Curry and Paxton, is an arc perimeter having a projected test object rather than a hand-held or mechanically actuated test object (see Figure 7.37). The lack of a

Figure 7.37   The Aimark projection perimeter.

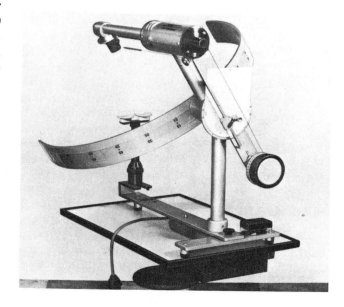

physical test object avoids any noise that would otherwise occur, and eliminates the clues that are unavoidable when a physical rather than an optical test object is used (e.g., moving of the examiner's arm). Peripheral field isopters are determined in the same manner as with the mechanical arc perimeter, moving the projected spot inward along the perimeter arm from nonseeing to seeing. Smith (tape no. 3) prefers the Aimark perimeter to the Goldmann hemispherical perimeter (see the following section) because it is possible to reach around and hold the patient's eyelid up, thus avoiding the upper field artifact that can otherwise occur. (However, the patient's lid can be taped up to overcome this problem.)

Goldmann hemispherical projection perimeter

The Goldmann perimeter is a hemispherical projection perimeter having a radius of curvature of 300mm (see Figure 7.38). The advantages of the Goldmann perimeter are that the illumination of the patient's entire visual field is controlled (whereas with an arc perimeter the illumination on the wall behind the perimeter is an unknown quantity), and both the test object and the background illumination are subject to accurate calibration so that exact conditions of illumination can be recreated on repeated testing. Another advantage is that not only the plotting of peripheral isopters but also central and midperipheral field testing are possible.

The inside surface of the hemisphere is painted a mat white, and the projector arm is moved by means of a pantograph arrangement that also is used for

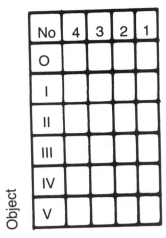

Figure 7.39   Standard test stimuli used with the Goldmann perimeter.

recording the findings. Each position of the pantograph handle corresponds exactly to the position of the spot of light on the surface of the hemisphere. The examiner observes the patient's eye (to monitor fixation) through a telescope in the back of the instrument. To test the patient's responses, the test object can be noiselessly extinguished by moving a slide. The projected targets vary in size from $\frac{1}{16}$mm^2 to 64mm^2, and neutral density filters allow for target luminosities ranging from 3.16 to 100 millilamberts. The size and intensity of the target are designated using the grid shown in Figure 7.39, in which intensity decreases from right to left and size increases from top to bottom. Tate (1970) recommends that the zero target sizes not be used (the ones represented by the top row in Figure 7.39). In using the Goldmann perimeter, three isopters are usually plotted, using stimuli such as, for example, I–4, II–4, and III–4. With these stimuli the illumination is 100 millilamberts in each case, and the stimulus sizes are 0.5, 1, and 2mm, respectively.

Static Perimetry

The method of perimetry discussed thus far—in which a test object of a given size and intensity is moved to determine the extent of the field of view or to determine the presence of a scotoma within the visual field—is called *kinetic perimetry*. *Static perimetry*, on the other hand, involves the use of multiple stimuli in various predetermined positions that can be varied in illumination. A given stimulus

Figure 7.38 The Haag-Streit Goldmann hemispherical perimeter, front and back views.

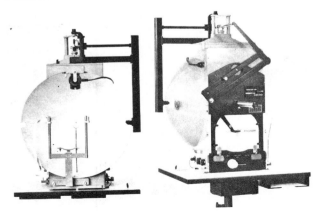

can be presented at several illumination levels in a stepwise fashion (starting with the lowest illumination), or the illumination can be increased gradually in a continuous fashion until the patient reports that the test object is seen. The Goldmann perimeter can be adapted for static perimetry, and the automated instruments to be described, operate on the basis of static rather than kinetic perimetry.

Harrington (1976) described the procedure of static perimetry used with the Tubinger perimeter. Stationary stimuli (spots of light) are presented, and luminance is increased, stepwise, until the patient signals that the stimulus is seen. The stimulus is then moved to a new location in the meridian, and the luminance is again increased until the patient reports that it is seen. This is repeated usually at 1-degree intervals within the central 15 degrees of the field, and at 5-degree intervals in the peripheral field. Approximately 50 stimulus exposures are made along a single meridian. The examination usually is made along four meridians (90, 180, 135, and 45 degrees). If depressions are found, they can be explored along new meridians or in a circular fashion. This procedure can be followed by kinetic perimetry, using the same instrument.

Automated static perimeters

As a result of the availability of computerization technology, a large number of automated static perimeters have been introduced in recent years. Although these instruments were originally developed mainly for use in visual field screening, many of them have now been perfected to the point that they can be used for detailed field evaluation, with the result that they are rapidly replacing not only the conventional perimeter and tangent screen but even the Goldmann perimeter.

Two of these automated instruments, the Synemed *Fieldmaster* and the Computation Company's *Automatic Tangent Screen*, are described in Chapter 6 and illustrated in Figures 6.32 and 6.33. Currently available automated and semiautomated perimeters have been described by Keltner and Johnson (1985). Of the 22 instruments described by these authors, only three (the Digilab 350 and two models of the Automatic Tangent Screen) are tangent screens; all others are bowl perimeters. Methods of presenting stimuli include the use of fiber-optic elements (as with the Fieldmaster), light-emitting diodes (as with the Automatic Tangent Screen), and projection systems. Most of these instruments are designed for visual field screening and complete visual field examination, using suprathreshold static

perimetry. The time necessary for a visual field screening varies from about 2–9 minutes per eye, whereas the time necessary for a complete visual field evaluation varies from about 4–20 minutes per eye. Most of the instruments capable of a complete evaluation, described by Keltner and Johnson, are in the $12,000–$15,000 price range.

In a review of automated perimeters, Walters (1986) discusses screening perimetry versus full-threshold perimetry, making the point that whether an instrument does a screening or a full-threshold procedure is largely determined by the software and not by the hardware. Walters strongly recommends that the optometrist have an instrument that is capable of *full-threshold testing*. His rationale for this recommendation is as follows: when visual field screening is done routinely, the practitioner can be confident of any results that are found to be within the normal range; but if abnormal results are obtained, it is not always clear if a real visual difficulty exists. If patients having abnormal screening fields are routinely referred for ophthalmological evaluation, false positive referrals will undoubtedly be made; but if the optometrist can follow through with full-threshold testing for those patients who fail the screening, the over-referral rate will not only be lower but the practitioner will be able to monitor the results of any subsequent therapy.

Walters (1986) evaluated two screening instruments, the *Topcon SPB–1000* and the *Kowa AP–340*, and four instruments capable of a complete threshold evaluation, the *Humphrey Field Analyser 620*, the *Digilab 750*, the *Dicon AP–2520*, and the *Quantum 412*. The salient features of these instruments, as described by Walters, are summarized in Table 7.3 (screening instruments) and Table 7.4 (full-threshold instruments).

The two screening instruments described by Walters (1986), as shown in Table 7.3, are similar in that they (1) are hemispherical perimeters having a background illumination of 31.5 apostilbs (equal to that provided by the Goldmann perimeter), (2) make use of light-emitting diodes, (3) provide data input by means of a video screen and a light pen, (4) do not provide for the storage of data, and (5) are not capable of being upgraded for full-threshold testing. The Topcon instrument has the disadvantage of low-stimulus intensity (435 apostilbs, less than half that available in the Goldmann perimeter), whereas the Kowa instrument's fixation control, which operates by sensing the patient's eye movements, is unnecessarily sensitive and tends to respond to head movements and eye blinks. An additional problem

Table 7.3   Comparison of automated field screening instruments.

	Topcon SBP–1000	Kowa AP–340
Cost	$11,000.	$9,900.
Stimuli	235 LEDs	340 LEDs
Size	2mm	1mm
Intensity	Max. 425asb[a]	4–3, 400asb[a]
Color	585nm (Orange)	570nm (Y–G)
Background	31.5asb[a]	31.5asb[a]
Fixation control	Blind spot monitoring and TV monitor	Automatic sensing of eye movement; telescope
Data input	Video screen and light pen	Video screen and light pen
Output	No data storage; immediate printout on 11 × 23.5cm paper	No data storage; immediate printout on 11cm-wide paper strip
Advantages	No "black hole" effect[b] (LEDs are illuminated at 31.5 apostilbs)	Central 25-degree full-threshold test; good gray scale; fast printout
Disadvantages and problems	Screening instrument;[c] can do limited threshold testing, represented on a line graph that cuts through the visual field; LEDs are too dim	Fixation monitor is too sensitive; has the "black-hole" effect;[b] no adequate check for false positives or false negatives; not a full-fledged threshold instrument[c]

[a]Apostilbs (background intensity of Goldmann perimeter is 31.5 apostilbs).
[b]See text for explanation of "black-hole" effect.
[c]Incapable of being upgraded for full-threshold testing.

with the Kowa AP–340 is that each LED is presented inside a "black hole" in the white perimeter background, with the result that all potential stimuli locations are obvious to the patient during the entire procedure, and the patient's task is therefore to determine when a yellow-green light appears inside a black hole rather than to determine when a stimulus appears as an increment on an unstructured white background. The "black-hole" effect does not occur with the Topcon SBP–1000 because all of the LEDs are constantly illuminated at a level equivalent to the 31.5 apostilb background.

As shown in Table 7.4, all of the full-threshold instruments make use of light-emitting diodes with the exception of the Humphrey 620, which is a projection perimeter. The Humphrey instrument is also unique in having a variable stimulus size (which can be as large as 64mm^2, the equivalent of the Goldmann V), and in having red, blue, and green filters available for color-field testing. All four of the instruments have blind-spot monitoring of fixation, and two (the Humphrey 620 and the Dicon AP–2530) also have a telescope for this purpose. For these two instruments, input is by means of a video screen and a light pen, whereas input for the Digilab 750 and

the Quantum 412 is by means of a dedicated IBM personal computer. All four instruments provide floppy-disc storage of data, make use of a dot-matrix printer for data output, and are provided with a "gray scale" in addition to numeric scales.

The only full-threshold instrument that suffers the "black-hole" effect is the Dicon, which also has the disadvantage of a long delay in obtaining a gray-scale printout. Both the Digilab and the Quantum instruments have eliminated the "black-hole" effect by covering the hole with a translucent plastic sheet, which is "transilluminated" by the LED when it is lit. But both of the instruments have a maximum stimulus intensity of 1,000 apostilbs as compared to the maximum of 10,000 apostilbs available for the Humphrey and Dicon instruments. An advantage of the Quantum 412 not shared by the other instruments is the capability of running a "pseudokinetic" program, in which stimuli are serially illuminated, giving the appearance of motion. In summing up his evaluation, Walters (1986) could unequivocally recommend only the Humphrey 620 Field Analyser, noting that this instrument is versatile and easy to use, and has avoided many of the major problems from which the other machines suffer. He suggests

Table 7.4 Comparison of automated full-threshold visual field instruments. (Walters, 1986)

	Humphrey 620	Digilab 750	Dicon AP–2520	Quantum 412
Cost	$14,950.	$14,000.	$14,495.	$12,095.
Stimuli	Projection	256 LEDs	520 LEDs	412 LEDs
Size	1–64mm^2	2mm	1mm	2.5mm
Intensity	0.08–10,000[a]	0.08–1,000[a]	0.12–10,000[a]	Max. 1,000[a]
Color	W (and R, B, G)	570nm (Y–G)	570nm (Y–G)	570nm (Y–G)
Background	31.5asb[a]	3.15 or 31.5asb[a]	31.5asb[a]	4 or 31.5asb[a]
Fixation control	Blind-spot monitoring and telescope	Blind-spot monitoring	Blind-spot monitoring and telescope	Blind-spot monitoring
Data input	Video screen and light pen	IBM PC keyboard	Video screen and light pen	IBM PC keyboard
Output	Disc storage (2 drives); DM printer	Disc storage (1 drive); DM printer	Disc storage (1 drive); DM printer	Disc storage (1 drive); DM printer
Scales	Gray scale; db scale; deficit scale	Gray scale; numeric scales	Gray scale; db scale	Gray scale; db scale
Advantages	Versatile; excellent gray scale; can do foveal thresholds	Versatile; keyboard input; no "black-hole" effect[b]	Sufficient intensity; sufficient number of LEDs	Sufficient intensity and number of LEDs; no "black-hole" effect;[b] has pseudokinetic program
Disadvantages and problems	Evaluates only the central 60 degrees	Insufficient stimulus intensity; too few LEDs; poor gray scale; no telescope to monitor fixation	Black-hole effect;[b] delay in obtaining gray-scale printout	Long delay in obtaining gray-scale printout; poor gray scale

[a]Apostilbs (background intensity of Goldmann perimeter is 31.5 apostilbs).
[b]See text for explanation of "black-hole" effect.

that, if the practitioner cannot afford the cost of the 620, the next best option is the Humphrey 605 (a screening instrument) or the 610 (which lacks the disc storage), either of which can be upgraded to the level of the 620 at a later date, if desired.

NEURODIAGNOSTIC TESTS

When a patient has reduced visual acuity in one eye or an ocular motility problem, and when the cause of the problem is not obvious, the practitioner can make use of one or more of a large number of *neurodiagnostic tests*.

Objective neurodiagnostic tests

Objective neurodiagnostic tests available to the optometrist include tests of pupillary function, tests of ocular motility, and electrodiagnostic procedures. The first two of these procedures are discussed in Chapter 6, and readers are referred to these discussions of testing procedures and their interpretation. Electrodiagnostic procedures are discussed in a later section in this chapter.

Subjective neurodiagnostic tests

Subjective neurodiagnostic tests include the photostress test, the brightness comparison test, diagnostic color-vision tests, the color saturation test, the neutral density filter test, acuity testing with pupillary constriction, and acuity testing through opaque media.

Photostress test. The photostress test is designed to differentiate between a retinal problem and an optic nerve problem in a patient who has reduced visual acuity in one eye. A penlight is directed into the patient's "good" eye for 10 seconds, after which the patient's attention is directed to the line of letters on the distance Snellen chart just above the best visual acuity line for that eye. The time necessary for the patient's acuity to recover to the point that the line in question can be read is recorded as the recovery time for that eye. The same procedure is then repeated for the "bad" eye. If the recovery time is about the same for each eye, the cause of the lowered visual acuity is an optic nerve lesion. However, if the recovery time is considerably longer for the "bad" eye (say, 100 seconds or longer versus 40 or 50 seconds for the "good" eye), the cause of the lowered visual acuity is in the retina. As discussed by Glaser (1979), the prolonged recovery time can be considered as caused by a delay in the regeneration of visual pigments after being bleached with bright light.

Brightness comparison test. The brightness comparison test is also designed to differentiate between a retinal problem and an optic nerve problem in a patient who has reduced visual acuity in one eye. The examiner briefly directs a penlight into each of the patient's eyes—beginning with the "good" eye—and asks the patient if there is a difference in the brightness of the light for the two eyes. If there is a difference, Glaser (1979) suggests the patient be asked, "If the light is worth a dollar in this eye [light in the intact eye], what is it worth in this eye [light in the abnormal eye]?" If the light in the abnormal eye seems to be dimmer than that in the intact eye, the cause of the problem is an optic nerve lesion; otherwise, it is a retinal lesion. Glaser describes this test as the subjective counterpart to the swinging flashlight test. This test should *not* be done just after tests such as the photostress test or indirect ophthalmoscopy.

Diagnostic color-vision tests. Color vision should be tested for each eye separately for any patient having unexplained lowered visual acuity. Optic nerve conduction defects tend to cause red-green color-vision anomalies, whereas retinal disease can cause either red-green or yellow-blue color-vision anomalies. Many of the color-vision tests described in Chapter 6 are designed only for the purpose of color-vision screening and are unable to differentiate between red-green and yellow-blue color-vision anomalies.

The American Optical HRR pseudoisochromatic plate test, which unfortunately is no longer avail-able, differs from other pseudoisochromatic plate tests in that it is designed to differentiate between red-green and yellow-blue anomalies. The least expensive and most quickly performed diagnostic color-vision test available is the Farnsworth D–15 test described in Chapter 6. On the basis of the way the patient sorts the 15 color samples, he or she can be categorized as a color-normal, a protan (red anomaly), deutan (green anomaly), or a tritan (yel-low-blue anomaly). (See Figure 5.24 in Chapter 5.)

The standard for comparison in the field of diagnostic color-vision testing is the Nagel anomalo-scope. However, due to its high cost, this instrument is available in few, if any, optometric offices. A less expensive and highly effective diagnostic test is the Farnsworth-Munsell 100–Hue test (see Figure 7.40). This is an expanded version of the D–15 test, consisting of four trays containing a total of 88 (not 100) color samples. The patient sorts the color samples in each of the four trays in what appears to be a logical color sequence, and the results are plotted on a polar coordinate plot (see Figure 7.41). When the graph has been plotted, a diagnosis of the specific color-vision anomaly (if any) can be made.

Color saturation test. Glaser (1979) described a simple test designed to differentiate between retinal and optic nerve problems. The patient is asked to look at the red top of a mydriatic bottle first with one eye and then with the other, and then is asked if there is a difference in the color of the two caps. If there is an optic nerve conduction defect, the patient will report that the cap seems to be faded or desaturated for the defective eye.

Neutral density filter test. When a patient is found to have lowered visual acuity in one eye, the practitioner may be tempted to assume that it is due to a long-standing functional amblyopia. However, in such cases a diagnosis of functional amblyopia is tenable only if (1) there is a definite history of poor visual acuity; (2) the patient is strabismic, anisome-tropic, or has high astigmatism that was not corrected at an early age; or (3) a diagnosis of ambly-opia is indicated by the results of the neutral density filter test. As described by Glaser (1979), a 2-log unit neutral density filter (which reduces incident illumi-nation by a factor of 100) will cause little or no reduction in visual acuity in an eye with functional amblyopia. However, in the presence of an optic nerve conduction defect such as retrobulbar neuritis, visual acuity will be drastically reduced

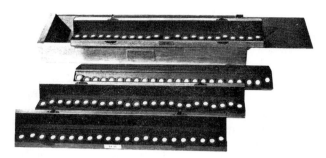

Figure 7.40 The Farnsworth-Munsell 100–Hue test.

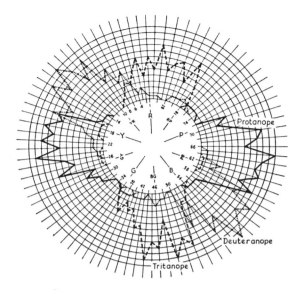

(e.g., from 20/60 normally to 20/200 or 20/400 through the neutral density filter).

Acuity testing with pupillary constriction. If a patient has a nuclear or a posterior subcapsular cataract affecting mainly the axial light rays, he or she may complain of blurred vision in bright daylight in spite of normal or near-normal visual acuity when tested under the usual clinical conditions. If visual acuity is reduced substantially when a penlight is directed toward the eye to constrict the pupil, the patient's complaint of blurred vision in bright daylight can be better understood. One solution to this problem may be the use of dark-green or gray sunglasses for driving and other daytime, outdoor activities. If this does not solve the problem, cataract surgery may be considered even though reading vision is still adequate.

Acuity tests through opaque media. When a patient has a mature cataract, assessment of the visual acuity must be made prior to cataract surgery. Otherwise, in spite of a successful operation, the patient may have reduced vision due to macular degeneration or other forms of retinal disease. A number of tests of retinal function can be employed, and retinal function is deemed to be adequate if the following criteria are met: (1) the patient can see the light of a penlight in any portion of the peripheral visual field and can report its direction; (2) the patient can perceive two penlights as two, when they are held about 2 inches apart at a distance of 2 feet; and (3) the patient can identify colors produced by holding red and green filters in front of a penlight.

A number of instruments making use of interference fringes recently have been introduced to assess a patient's visual acuity through a cloudy lens. One of these instruments is the Retinometer, made by Rodenstock for use with the Haag-Streit slit lamp.

Figure 7.41 Recording form for the Farnsworth-Munsell 100–Hue test. Typical plottings for a protanope, deuteranope, and tritanope are shown. If all color samples were placed in the proper sequence (normal color vision), all points would be plotted along the inner circle.

Using a coherent source of laser light, two laser beams are directed through an area of the lens where the opacity is the least dense, and interference fringes are formed on the retina. The fringes can be oriented in vertical, horizontal, or oblique meridians, and the spatial frequency can be varied, corresponding to visual acuity ranging from 6/120 (20/400) to 6/6 (20/20). By this means the patient's acuity after cataract surgery can be predicted. If acuity with the laser fringes is poor, the patient probably has macular degeneration or other macular disease. Richter and Sherman (1979) stated that in their clinic, attempts to assess a patient's visual acuity with the Retinometer in the presence of a very dense cataract have not always been fruitful. An additional interferometer, the Visometer, is made by Haag-Streit.

CONTRAST SENSITIVITY TESTING

In the routine measurement of visual acuity, charts are designed so that *contrast* is as high as possible—very black letters are shown on a very white background—and the object of the test is to determine the smallest row of letters (specified in terms of the angular subtense of a stroke or a gap) that the patient can correctly identify. However, many visual tasks in real life require not the identification of small, high-contrast objects but the identification of relatively large, low-contrast objects. Although low-contrast visual acuity charts have been available for many years, the development of effective clinical methods for testing vision at different levels of contrast has occurred mainly during the past decade.

Contrast may be defined as the ratio of the difference between the maximum and minimum luminance of a test stimulus divided by the sum of the maximum and minimum luminance, or

$$\frac{L_{max} - L_{min}}{L_{max} + L_{min}}.$$

To express contrast as a percentage, the ratio is multiplied by 100. Although the contrast of black print on a white background is quite close to 100 percent, the contrast involved in many daily visual tasks, such as viewing an airplane in a cloudy sky or the recognition of a human face, may be close to zero.

In contrast sensitivity testing, the patient is presented with repetitive stimuli in the form of vertically oriented *gratings* at various contrast levels. These may be *square-wave gratings* or *sine-wave gratings*, and are designed so that the average luminance (half the sum of the luminance of the bright and dark bars) is constant for all gratings. The spacing between any two bars in a grating is specified in terms of *spatial frequency*, which is analogous to the width of a stroke or gap in a letter on a visual-acuity chart. For example, a spatial frequency of 30 cycles per degree (30 bars and 30 gaps per degree) would indicate a stroke or gap width of one minute of arc, and, therefore, would be the equivalent of 6/6 (20/20) visual acuity.

The gratings may be presented to the patient in a variety of ways. For example, they may be electronically generated and displayed on an oscilloscope screen or a computer monitor, printed on paper and presented on cards or in a booklet, or projected onto a screen. The range of spatial frequencies used in such tests typically extends from 0.5 cycles per degree (the equivalent of 6/320, or 20/1200 visual acuity) to 30 cycles per degree (the equivalent of 6/6, or 20/20 acuity). The angular width of the grating is usually about 3–5 degrees, with the result that a 0.5 cycle-per-degree grating would present only 2–3 bars, whereas a 30 cycle-per-degree grating would present 90–150 bars.

Contrast is varied for a grating of a given spatial frequency using any of a number of psychophysical methods. When electronically generated gratings are utilized, the grating may first be presented at a low contrast, the contrast then being increased until the grating is seen. On the other hand, the grating may be presented at a high contrast, the contrast being decreased until the grating is no longer seen. Another method involves the randomized presentation of gratings of varying contrast (method of constant stimuli). Although this method is psychophysically sound, the time required for its use may not be justified in a clinical setting. As with visual-acuity testing, testing is normally done monocularly.

Plotting contrast sensitivity data

The method used for plotting contrast sensitivity data is illustrated in Figure 7.42. Spatial frequency is plotted along the x-axis and contrast sensitivity (the reciprocal of contrast threshold) is plotted along the y-axis. As shown in Figure 7.42, the curve has the shape of an inverted *U*, contrast sensitivity reaching a peak at about 3–6 cycles per degree and gradually decreasing at both lower and higher spatial frequencies. The subject's visual acuity can be estimated by extrapolating the upper end of the curve to the x-axis. For the data plotted in Figure 7.42, the dashed line intersects the x-axis at approximately 45 cycles per degree, indicating a visual acuity of 6/4.5 (20/15).

Figure 7.42 Contrast sensitivity plot, showing spatial frequency along the x-axis and contrast sensitivity (the reciprocal of contrast threshold) along the y-axis. Snellen acuity can be estimated by extrapolating the upper end of the curve to the x-axis (Loshin and White, 1984).

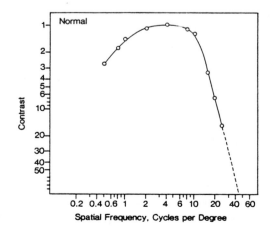

Changes in contrast sensitivity with age

Although the corrected visual acuity of a healthy eye remains relatively stable with increasing age, it is of interest that contrast sensitivity has been found to decrease with increasing age. An understanding of age changes in contrast sensitivity for the healthy eye is of importance, because there is abundant evidence that pathological changes such as cataracts and macular degeneration can cause significant losses in sensitivity for certain spatial frequencies. Contrast sensitivity for 70 subjects in their 60s, 70s, and 80s, free of significant ocular disease, was compared to that for 33 subjects in their 20s–50s, also free of ocular disease (Sekuler et al., 1982). The results, shown in Figure 7.43, indicated that, although subjects of all ages had approximately equal sensitivity for lower spatial frequencies (0.5 and 1 cycles per degree), there was a decrease in sensitivity for the higher frequencies with each decade of life. Reduced contrast sensitivity at higher spatial frequencies for older subjects was also found by Owsley et al. (1983). Noting that the average retinal illuminance of a 60-year-old eye has been estimated by Weale (1963) as being only about one-third of that of a 20-year-old eye (due to a smaller pupil diameter and increased optical density of the crystalline lens), Owsley et al. performed contrast sensitivity testing on a group of 20-year-old subjects while wearing a

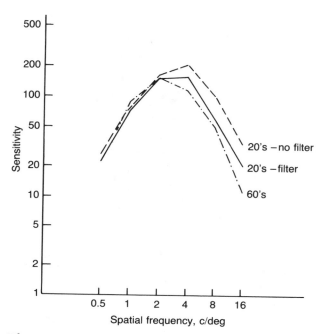

Figure 7.44 For 20-year-old subjects wearing a neutral density filter, contrast sensitivity decreased at higher frequencies (Owsley et al., 1983).

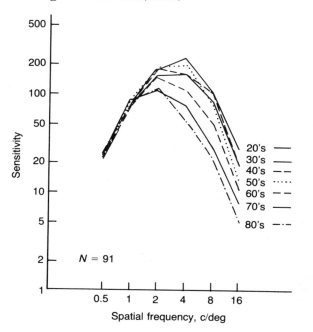

Figure 7.43 Change in contrast sensitivity with age (Sekular et al., 1982).

neutral density filter that decreased the retinal illuminance by a factor of approximately three. Contrast sensitivity for these subjects through the filter was found to decrease for the higher spatial frequencies (see Figure 7.44), but not to the extent of the decrease found for the older subjects. Owsley et al. concluded that a part of the decrease in contrast sensitivity for older subjects may be due to neural rather than optical factors.

Clinical methods of contrast sensitivity testing

In recent years a number of clinical contrast sensitivity tests have been introduced, including electronically generated sine-wave gratings with video-monitor displays, the Arden plate test, and the Vistech Vision Contrast Test System.

Currently available electronically generated gratings include the Caldwell CTS–5000 and the Nicolet Optronix CS–2000. Using these gratings, the patient can signal when the pattern is first detected (with increasing contrast) or when the pattern can no longer be seen (with decreasing contrast), or the examiner may choose to adjust the contrast. An advantage of electronically generated gratings is that

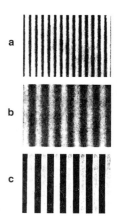

Figure 7.45 The Arden grating test. Gratings (a) and (b) differ in spatial frequency, whereas gratings (b) and (c) differ in contrast (Arden, 1978).

they may be presented not only as stationary patterns but also as *flickering* or *moving* patterns.

The Arden plate test, introduced in 1978 and available from American Optical Corporation, consists of a booklet containing several sine-wave grating patterns. Each grating is oriented vertically, but the contrast varies from the top to the bottom of the grating, being lowest at the top of the page

and highest at the bottom (see Figure 7.45). For each grating, the examiner or the patient gradually moves a card (which masks the grating) downward over the page until the point is reached at which the grating is seen. At that point, the examiner records the contrast from a scale provided with the grating. After a practice trial, the procedure is repeated for each of six plates.

The Vistech contrast sensitivity chart, developed by Ginsburg (1984), consists of a chart made up of six rows of 3-inch-diameter sine-wave gratings (see Figure 7.46). Each row consists of a sample grating and a series of test gratings of a given spatial frequency but differing in contrast. Spatial frequencies utilized (from the top to bottom row) are 1, 2, 4, 8, 16, and 24 cycles per degree. Each grating is oriented in one of three directions: vertical, slanted 15 degrees to the right, or slanted 15 degrees to the left. The task of the patient is to report the orientation for each grating in each row. When the testing is completed, the data are plotted and compared to the "normal" contrast sensitivity curve. Two separate Vistech charts are available: the VCTS–6500 for distance testing, and the VCTS–6000 for near testing. A projector slide, the VCTS–500S, is also available.

Results obtained using the Vistech chart and the Optronix CS–2000 were compared by Ginsberg (1984) for a group of 83 volunteer subjects. Ages of

Figure 7.46   The Vistech contrast sensitivity test.

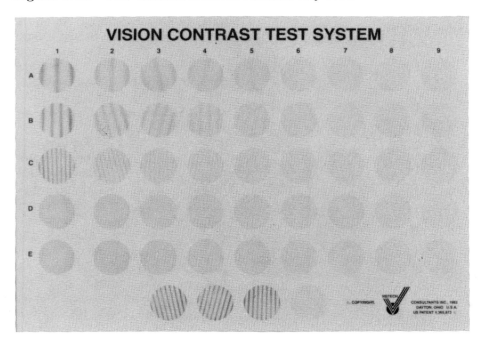

the subjects ranged from 9–75 years, and subjects reporting any ocular pathology were excluded. Although the population means of contrast sensitivity correlated highly for the two tests, Ginsberg reported "a small, nonsignificant but systematic difference" in the results of the two tests. Results for the Vistech chart indicated slightly lower sensitivities at the higher spatial frequencies and slightly higher sensitivities at the lower spatial frequencies. In addition, the high spatial frequency cut-off for the Vistech chart was found to be 46 cycles per degree (an approximate equivalent of 6/4.5 or 20/15 visual acuity) as compared to 57 cycles per degree (an approximate equivalent of 6/3 or 20/10 visual acuity) for the Optronix test.

Diagnosis by means of contrast sensitivity testing

Contrast sensitivity testing has been shown to be useful in the diagnostic work-up of a number of conditions, including glaucoma, optic nerve disease, macular degeneration, albinism, and amblyopia. Using the Arden plates, Arden and Jacobson (1978) reported that contrast sensitivity for 50 glaucomatous eyes was found to be significantly reduced as compared with contrast sensitivity of eyes of normal subjects. Arden and Gucukoglu (1978) tested retrobulbar neuritis patients with both the visually evoked response and the Arden gratings. They found that the possibility of making a positive diagnosis with the visually evoked response alone was 0.54, whereas the possibility of making a positive diagnosis with the Arden gratings alone was 0.71.

The contrast sensitivity of six patients having senile macular degeneration with moderate acuity reduction was investigated by Brown and Garner (1983). They found that the contrast sensitivity was depressed for both high and low frequencies when compared to age-matched controls, and that the peak sensitivity was shifted toward lower frequencies. Contrast sensitivity of patients with more advanced macular degeneration was studied by Loshin and White (1984), who measured contrast sensitivity for 40 patients selected from the University of Houston Low Vision Clinic, each of whom had senile macular degeneration with reduced visual acuity and a central visual field loss. Curves for eight representative subjects indicated results similar to those of Brown and Garner (1983): decreased sensitivity at all spatial frequencies when compared to normal subjects, with a shifting of the peak sensitivity toward lower spatial frequencies. It is of interest, however, that four of the eight subjects were found

to have consistently higher contrast sensitivity for one eye than for the other at all spatial frequencies, the preferred eye being the one with the higher Snellen visual acuity; whereas for the other four subjects the eye having the higher peak sensitivity was found to have the lower sensitivity for the higher frequencies (the curves for the two eyes crossing over at the higher frequencies) and consequently the lower Snellen acuity. Loshin and White (1984) made the point that these latter subjects preferred to use the eye having the higher peak sensitivity rather than the eye having the higher Snellen acuity.

The possibility that contrast sensitivity testing can differentiate between optical and neural causes of a visual loss was suggested by Woo (1985). Contrast sensitivity, measured on a 70-year-old man having bilateral cataracts and senile macular degeneration, indicated high frequency losses for both eyes. One year after the original testing, the patient returned to report a reduction in vision and increased discomfort due to glare. Although Snellen visual acuity and acuity for retinal interference fringes were unchanged, a further reduction in contrast sensitivity was found for both eyes. On the assumption that retinal interference fringe acuity is influenced only by neural limitations whereas contrast sensitivity is influenced by both neural and optical limitations, Woo concluded that the further loss of vision was due to progression of the cataracts rather than to the senile macular degeneration. This conclusion was of importance, because it pointed to possible treatment options.

Contrast sensitivity was measured in albinotic patients by Loshin and Browning (1983), using both vertically oriented and horizontally oriented gratings. Subjects for the study included eight patients aged 15–31 years, each having pendular nystagmus and strabismus. Testing was done for the nonstrabismic eye of each subject. For four of the patients, contrast sensitivity was higher for horizontal gratings than for vertical gratings, for all spatial frequencies. For the other four patients, contrast sensitivity was higher for horizontal than for vertical gratings for high and medium spatial frequencies, but lower for frequencies below 2 cycles per degree. Loshin and Browning concluded that, although a number of factors may be responsible for the superior contrast sensitivity for horizontal gratings (including high astigmatic error, nystagmus, and possible neural modifications), the meridional differences for these patients were highly related to the direction of the nystagmus.

The use of contrast sensitivity testing in amblyopia has been explored by a number of researchers. Electronically generated sine-wave gratings were used to measure contrast sensitivity for both the amblyopic and nonamblyopic eyes of ten strabismic amblyopes by Hess and Howell (1977). For five of the subjects, contrast sensitivity of the amblyopic eye was depressed only at the lower spatial frequencies (labeled by the authors as "type 1"), whereas for the other five subjects, contrast sensitivity for the amblyopic eye was depressed for all frequencies (labeled "type 2"). Although Hess and Howell were unable to account for the two types of responses, their data indicated that with one exception the amblyopic eyes of the type 2 subjects had poorer visual acuity than those of the type 1 subjects. Anisometropia was not a determining factor, one of the type 1 subjects and two of the type 2 subjects being anisometropic.

Although the contrast sensitivity data of Hess and Howell (1977) did not differentiate between strabismic and anisometropic amblyopia, contrary results were reported by Lundh and Lennerstrand (1983), who tested contrast sensitivity by means of computer-generated stimuli. They found that eleven children having strabismic amblyopia had major high-frequency losses but only minor losses in the low and middle frequencies, whereas ten children having combined strabismic and anisometropic amblyopia were found to have losses of about the same degree for all frequencies. After treatment, patients in both groups were found to have significantly improved contrast sensitivity for the high frequencies but not for the medium and low frequencies.

Contrast sensitivity testing was used to evaluate the improvement in three amblyopic patients by Woo and Dalziel (1981). Each of the three patients was given a form of treatment for amblyopia (known as CAM treatment) in which the nonamblyopic eye was occluded for each 7-minute session, during which the patient viewed a series of rotating square-wave gratings underneath a clear plastic plate on which the patient played games to ensure cooperation. After the treatment, there was no improvement in visual acuity but substantial improvement was noted in contrast sensitivity in all cases. This improvement was still present 16 months later for one patient, but was not present after 12 months for the second patient and after 18 months for the third. Woo and Dalziel concluded that the CAM therapy appeared to bring about an improvement in contrast sensitivity. In an earlier paper, Lennerstrand and Lundh (1980) reported no improvement in visual acuity of 8 of 24 amblyopic children who had been given the CAM treatment, but contrast sensitivity was found to improve for 4 of the 8 children.

The effect of contact lenses on contrast sensitivity

Contact lens wearers sometimes complain of unsatisfactory vision, in spite of Snellen visual acuity of 6/6 (20/20) or better. This phenomenon has served as a stimulus for studies of contrast sensitivity of contact lens wearers, most of which have found a tendency for contrast sensitivity to be poorer with contact lenses than with spectacles. The following causes for this reduced contrast sensitivity have been proposed: (1) uncorrected or residual astigmatism; (2) corneal edema occurring with contact lens wear; (3) spherical aberration; and (4) contact lens coatings, deposits, or discolorations.

Applegate and Massof (1975) found that contrast sensitivity was lower with contact lenses than with an equivalent spectacle correction, and that the decrease in contrast sensitivity was more severe for three subjects fitted with soft contact lenses than for three subjects fitted with hard contact lenses. They found the differences in contrast sensitivity to be minimal at the higher spatial frequencies but to be more pronounced at intermediate spatial frequencies of 2–4 cycles per degree. They suggested that uncorrected astigmatism may have been partially responsible for their findings. In a study involving nine soft contact lens wearers, Bernstein and Brodrick (1981) found no systematic differences between contrast sensitivity with soft contact lenses and spectacles, nor did they find any systematic changes during an 18-hour period of testing. They attributed these results (as compared to those of Applegate and Massof) to the fact that none of their subjects had more than 0.12D of uncorrected astigmatism. Decreased contrast sensitivity of contact lens wearers was found by Mitra and Lamberts (1981) who, finding that the decrement was more pronounced after two weeks of lens wear, suggested that lens deposits or spherical aberration may have been responsible.

Using soft contact lenses having center thicknesses of 0.12mm, 0.07mm, and 0.03mm (Bausch & Lomb B3, U3, and O3 lenses, respectively), Grey (1986) found a gradual loss of contrast sensitivity during the first hour of wear, the severity of the losses increasing with lens thickness. Because it was found that corneal thickness increased while wearing the lenses and that the thickness increase was greater the thicker the lenses, it was concluded that the decrement in contrast sensitivity was due to corneal edema.

Contrast sensitivity for edges

Making the observation that contrast sensitivity for a *single edge* appears to be a reliable indicator of the peak contrast sensitivity function, Verbaken and Johnston (1986a, 1986b) have reported the development of a contrast sensitivity test making use of a boundary between light and dark backgrounds, rather than a bar grating. The new test (shown in Figure 7.47), called the Melbourne Edge Test, consists of 20 circular stimuli, each 25mm (1 inch) in diameter. The test consists of a series of edges, separating light and dark backgrounds, of reducing contrast, with variable orientation as the identifying feature. The subject is shown a key card that presents four circles having vertically, horizontally, and obliquely oriented lines. Using the key card, a four-alternative-choice method is used, the patient being asked to identify the orientation of each of the test edges. The test was administered to 497 consecutively presenting clinical patients. In analyzing their results, subjects were split into three groups on the basis of visual acuity and media haze, and it was found that the edge contrast sensitivity test provided diagnostic data that would not have been available from the testing of visual acuity alone.

Evaluation of contrast sensitivity testing as a clinical technique

The Arden plate test, the first contrast sensitivity test designed for clinical use, has been evaluated by Owsley et al. (1983) who have made the following points: (1) the threshold can be crucially affected by the rate at which the grating is uncovered; (2) the illumination level significantly affects the threshold, yet there is no standard procedure for controlling illumination for the test; (3) it has been found that older observers give a large number of false positive responses; and (4) at recommended viewing distances the Arden plates test for spatial frequencies no higher than 6.4 cycles per degree, whereas losses of sensitivity in older patients have been found (using other tests) in frequencies as high as 16 cycles per degree.

Although the inexpensive and easily administered tests of contrast sensitivity were designed for clinical use, Glover, Bird, and Yap (1987) found that these tests are of little value when used with young amblyopic children. These researchers used Arden plates and Vistech charts to measure the contrast

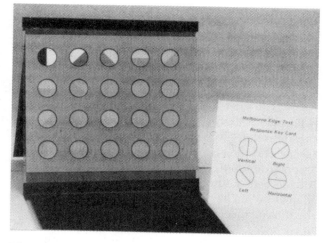

Figure 7.47 The Melbourne Edge Test (Verbaken and Johnston, 1986).

sensitivity of 40 unselected amblyopic patients from 3–12 years old, and found that only 16 of the 40 children were able to provide reliable results on the Arden plates, whereas only 8 of 20 children provided reliable results on the Vistech near charts, and 8 of the 20 children provided reliable results on the Vistech distance charts. In general, the children who failed to provide reliable results were the younger children. Glover et al. noted that many of the children could not understand the tests sufficiently to produce reliable results, and that others had difficulty concentrating on the tests, leading to a high incidence of false positive and false negative results. They concluded that the Arden and Vistech tests were of limited value in routine assessment of amblyopia in young children.

An interesting observation of the utility of contrast sensitivity testing was made by Yates et al. (1987), who determined contrast sensitivity norms for 103 subjects free of ocular disease and between the ages of 21 and 40 years. Finding (as would be expected) that the subjects who had the highest sensitivity at the higher spatial frequencies were those who had the highest Snellen visual acuity, Yates et al. asked if there are advantages to contrast sensitivity testing above and beyond conventional acuity measurements. They answered this question by relating an anecdote involving two clients at a state agency for the blind who had equal Snellen acuity, one of whom could operate a machine for stamping metal parts and one who could not: had it not been for contrast sensitivity testing, showing poor contrast for low spatial frequencies for the second client, the client would have been accused of malingering.

ELECTRODIAGNOSTIC PROCEDURES

Clinically useful electrodiagnostic procedures include the electroretinogram, the electro-oculogram, and the visually evoked response. An *electroretinogram (ERG)* is the record of the mass response of the retina to an intense flash of light, and in a duplex retina like the human being's it is dominated by the rod mechanism. The *electro-oculogram (EOG)* is recorded in response to movements of the eye and arises mainly from the retinal pigment epithelium. The *visually evoked response (VER)* is an electrical response of the visual cortex that can be evoked by having the patient view an oscillating checkerboard or striped stimulus pattern.

Electroretinogram

When the whole retina is subjected to an intense flash of light, the mass response of the retina can be recorded if a suitable electrode is placed on the anesthetized cornea with the aid of a contact lens, and a second electrode is placed on the face or forehead. The ERG, shown in Figure 7.48, is made up of the initial negative *a*-wave; a positive *b*-wave; a slowly rising, positive *c*-wave; and a *d*-wave, or off-effect. It is thought that the *a*-wave originates from the inner segments of the rods and cones, the *b*-wave originates from the bipolar cells, and the *c*-wave originates from the retinal pigment epithelium.

The *b*-wave is not only the most prominent feature of the ERG, it also has received the most attention from the point of view of diagnosis. The height of the *b*-wave (i.e., the distance from the trough of the *a*-wave to the peak of the *b*-wave) has been found to be greater in the dark-adapted, or rod, retina than in the light-adapted, or cone, retina, and it is diminished or lacking in conditions in which the rods are abnormal. To elicit the photopic ERG response (which requires suppression of the activity of the rods), a highly light-adapted eye is stimulated by a flickering red light: rods are not only insensitive to red light but are insensitive to a high-speed flicker. To elicit the scotopic ERG response, the dark-adapted eye is stimulated by a flash of blue light (see Figure 7.49a). For both the photopic and the scotopic ERG response, the entire retina is stimulated by means of a mat white sphere called a *Ganzfeld*, which distributes the light evenly over the retina.

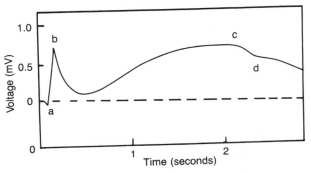

Figure 7.48 Schematic representation of the electroretinogram.

Because the ERG response is dominated by rods, it is typically found to be normal in the presence of macular dystrophies. However, it is found to be either abnormal or flat in retinitis pigmentosa and other diseases affecting the rods, so it is an important diagnostic procedure whenever a rod abnormality is suspected. Walters (1981) has found that the ERG response may be abnormal in a large variety of rod dystrophies in which the typical bone corpuscle pigmentation of retinitis pigmentosa is absent. Conversely, even when bone corpuscle pigmentation is present, the ERG response may be normal, confirming a diagnosis of pseudoretinitis pigmentosa. There is one variety of retinitis pigmentosa in which electroretinography can be particularly helpful: a lipid abnormality known as *a-beta-lipoproteinemia*, it is the only type of retinitis pigmentosa for which effective treatment has been found. Its diagnosis is confirmed on the basis of blood tests in which acanthocytosis (malformed erythrocytes) and lowered levels of fat-soluble vitamins, including vitamin A, are found. Treatment by large doses of vitamin A leads to a more nearly normal ERG response and, presumably, to an arrest or reversal of the loss of vision.

Most cases of retinitis pigmentosa are the result of either autosomal dominant, autosomal recessive, or sex-linked recessive inheritance. The most common (as well as the most severe) is the autosomal recessive form, which is most likely to occur in families involving the marriage of first cousins. Because an abnormal ERG response can be found prior to retinal pigmentation or any other sign of retinitis pigmentosa, the presence of an abnormal ERG response provides the opportunity for parent counseling concerning such matters as a child's educational and vocational choices.

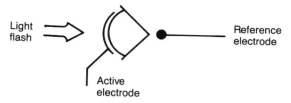

Electroretinography

a

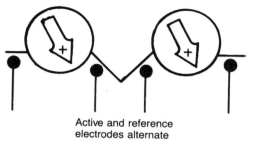

Active and reference
electrodes alternate

Electro-oculography

b

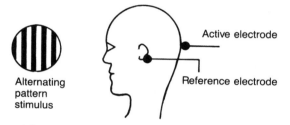

Alternating
pattern
stimulus

Active electrode

Reference electrode

Visually evoked response testing

c

Figure 7.49 Clinical electrodiagnostic procedures. (a) A deep-blue light is used to produce a rod ERG, a red light on a dark field produces a rod-plus-cone ERG, and a fast red light or a red light on a light field produces a cone ERG. (b) Because the eye is like a small battery (cornea positive), eye movements produce a voltage change across the two electrodes, and because eye movements are held constant in EOG testing, any change in the voltage measured can be attributed to changes in the activity of the pigment epithelium. (c) In recording the VEP, patterned stimuli are used to assess the visual system's response to changes in spatial frequency. (From Walters, 1981.)

Electro-oculogram

There exists a potential difference of about 6 mV between the cornea and the back of the eyeball, so movement of the eye will cause changes in potential

if one electrode is placed near the inner canthus of the eye and another is placed near the outer canthus (see Figure 7.49b). To record the EOG response, the patient is instructed to fixate back and forth between two fixation points 40 degrees apart. The potential is measured under conditions of dark adaptation and again under light adaptation, and the potential difference for a normal subject is found to be more than twice as great for light adaptation as for dark adaptation. The result is expressed as the EOG ratio, which is defined as the light peak amplitude divided by the dark trough amplitude, multiplied by 100.

As described by Afanador (1977), the apparatus has a green fixation light in the center and peripheral red fixation lights on each side. The green fixation light is turned on for 45 seconds, after which it is turned off, and the red lights are alternately illuminated for 1 second each for a period of 15 seconds. The patient is instructed to look at whatever light is on and is told that he or she will be in the dark for 12 minutes followed by 12 more minutes during which the patient must continue watching the lights.

Afanador reported that for 38 normal subjects, EOG ratios averaged 2.33/1 with a standard deviation of ±0.33. An EOG ratio of 1.75/1 is considered to be abnormal. Abnormal EOG ratios have been reported in Best's disease (vitelliform degeneration) and in other pigment epithelium abnormalities. In Best's disease the ERG is found to be normal, in spite of the abnormally low EOG ratio. Abnormally low EOG ratios have also been reported in malignant melanoma of the choroid.

Visually evoked response

If an electrode is placed on the scalp near the inion and the patient is instructed to view an oscillating checkerboard or striped pattern, a potential that is indicative of cortical activity can be recorded (see Figure 7.49c). Because the VER amplitude is depressed by defocus, the recording of the VER while the patient looks through lenses of different powers has been advocated as a method to measure refractive error (see Chapter 10). Other possible uses of the VER, listed by Siegfried (1977), include the ruling out of optic nerve disease, objective assessment of amblyopia, examination for macular dystrophies, and detection of suspected malingerers.

Present status of electrodiagnostic procedures

Although many claims have been made for the diagnostic efficacy of electrodiagnostic procedures (and in particular, the VER), the state of the art at the present time is such that we can say with confidence only that:

1. The ERG is an extremely useful tool in detecting the presence of retinitis pigmentosa, even in the absence of the typical bone corpuscle pigmentation of the retina. This is particularly true for children afflicted with Usher's syndrome, a condition in which a deaf child will ultimately become legally blind due to a recessive form of retinitis pigmentosa.
2. The EOG is useful in the differential diagnosis of abnormalities of the retinal pigment epithelium such as Best's disease.
3. The VER should still be considered to be in the experimental stage, as few—if any—claims for its usefulness have been substantiated by controlled clinical studies.

Electrodiagnostic equipment is so specialized and its use indicated so infrequently by the typical private practitioner that it is available only at the larger optometric and ophthalmologic centers. For example, all schools of optometry in the United States and Canada now have electrodiagnostic clinics. However, the practitioner should be aware of the existence of electrodiagnostic procedures and should consider making use of electrodiagnostic services in selected cases.

ADDITIONAL DIAGNOSTIC PROCEDURES

Exophthalmometry

There are a number of abnormalities in which one or both eyes will appear to protrude more than the normal amount. If just one eye appears to protrude, the examiner should suspect the presence of an orbital tumor, pseudotumor, abscess, or other space-taking mass. If both eyes appear to protrude, the most likely cause is Grave's disease (exophthalmic goiter). However, in the early stages of Grave's disease, the eyes may not actually protrude but may appear to protrude because of retraction of the upper eyelids.

An *exophthalmometer* is an instrument designed to measure the amount of protrusion, or exophthalmia, of each eye relative to the outer orbital margin. The Hertel exophthalmometer uses a mirror system that allows the examiner to measure the protrusion of each eye while facing the patient (see Figure 7.50a). The normal range of readings is from 12–20mm, and readings in excess of 20mm are considered abnormal. Vaughan and Asbury (1977) make the point that the exophthalmometer is particularly useful in following the progress of a patient having exophthalmia.

Greenberg (1977) has described the Luedde exophthalmometer, which is a clear plastic stick ruled in millimeters, one end of which is tapered. The tapered end is placed firmly against the lateral orbital margin, and the instrument is oriented perpendicular to the plane of the face. The examiner views the eye from the temporal side and notes the position of the corneal apex relative to the exophthalmometer scale. This instrument suffers from the same problem encountered if the examiner attempts to measure the position of the cornea with a millimeter ruler—there is no way to make sure that the ruler is held perpendicular to the facial plane and that the examiner's line of sight is parallel to the facial plane. The resulting parallax can be responsible for sizable errors. Also, as pointed out by Greenberg, it is not possible to simultaneously compare readings for the two eyes, as it is with the Hertel instrument.

Ophthalmodynamometry

Carotid artery insufficiency, also called carotid artery occlusive disease, is a major cause not only of

Figure 7.50 *(a)* **The Hertel exophthalmometer;** *(b)* **footplate of the ophthalmodynamometer** (from Pence, 1980).

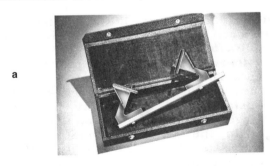

a

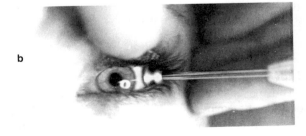

b

cerebral vascular accident (stroke) but also of blindness due to closure of the central artery of the retina in older patients. Patients suffering from carotid artery insufficiency may complain of transient loss of vision (amaurosis fugax), and the examiner may find one or more yellowish, shiny cholesterol plaques, called *Hollenhorst plaques*, at or near a bifurcation in one of the retinal arterioles.

The presence of carotid artery insufficiency can be detected by *ophthalmodynamometry*. In this procedure, pressure is exerted on the sclera to increase the intraocular pressure to the point where the central artery of the retina begins to pulsate and then collapses. Pence (1980) notes that as the central artery of the retina begins to close, it is supplied a greater blood flow by the ophthalmic artery; therefore, ophthalmodynamometry is actually a measurement of the relative ophthalmic artery pressure. The term *relative* is used here because the pressure reading is affected by the intraocular pressure, the ocular rigidity, and other factors. More than 90 percent of internal carotid artery obstructions occur below the origin of the ophthalmic artery, just distal to the point where the common carotid artery divides into the internal and external carotids, therefore, adversely affecting the blood flow into the ophthalmic artery and into the retinal arteries.

The ophthalmodynamometer exerts pressure on the sclera in much the same way a blood pressure cuff exerts pressure on the arm. When the central artery of the retina collapses, the intraocular pressure equals or slightly exceeds the pressure within the artery. Ophthalmodynamometry can be done by either the *compression method*, in which a spring-loaded cylinder is used to apply pressure on the sclera, or the *suction method*, in which a suction cup is placed on the sclera, and a vacuum is created by pulling out a syringelike plunger, raising the pressure within the eye. The compression method is described here and is shown in Figure 7.50b.

Procedure. The patient's pupil is first dilated by means of a mydriatic, and a local anesthetic is instilled into the eye. The patient is instructed to fixate upward and nasally, and the footplate of the ophthalmodynamometer is placed on the sclera temporal to the limbus. The footplate must be tangential to the sclera and the shaft of the ophthalmodynamometer must be kept perpendicular to the sclera as the pressure is applied. The examiner views the optic nerve head with an ophthalmoscope while the pressure is increased. With increasing pressure, the veins will pulsate and then collapse, following

which the arteries at the edge of the disk will begin to pulsate (indicating the systolic pressure) and then will collapse (indicating the diastolic pressure). It is advisable that the examiner work with an assistant, who can read the pressure dial when the examiner reports arterial pulsation beginning and arterial collapse occurring.

For patients with normal internal carotid artery circulation, the difference in pressure readings for the two eyes should be less than 15 percent; differences greater than 20 percent between the two eyes represent a definite reduction in internal carotid blood flow on the side with the lower pressure. Ophthalmic artery pressure can also be evaluated as it relates to brachial artery pressure as determined in routine sphygmomanometry. Normally, systolic ophthalmic artery pressure (relative ophthalmic artery pressure, as measured by ophthalmodynamometry) should be about three-fourths the systolic brachial artery pressure; diastolic ophthalmic artery pressure should be about two-thirds the diastolic brachial artery pressure. However, for patients with high blood pressure these fractions will be somewhat higher. When the ophthalmodynamometry pressure value is less than 50 percent of the corresponding brachial artery pressure, internal carotid artery disease should be suspected.

In routine practice it is necessary to assess only diastolic pressure to evaluate the patency of the ophthalmic artery. This negates the possible adverse effects of shutting off the arterial flow. [For additional information on ophthalmodynamometry, readers are referred to the excellent review by Pence (1980).]

Ophthalmic Ultrasonography

As described by Scheie and Albert (1977), ophthalmic ultrasonography utilizes high-frequency ultrasound waves emitted by a probe placed directly on the eye or near the eye by means of a waterbath. Echos from ocular tissues are viewed on the screen of an oscilloscope. Two forms of ultrasound examination are available: *time-amplitude*, or *A-scan*, which provides a linear-dimensional picture; and *intensity modulation*, or *B-scan*, which provides a two-dimensional cross section of the eye and orbit.

A-scan ultrasonography measures the time delay and echo-wave form. The time delay is converted to distance, in millimeters, by multiplying the time by a velocity constant. For several years it has been used for measuring the axial dimensions of the eye (anterior chamber depth, lens thickness, vitreous chamber depth, and the axial length of the eye). Instrumentation, procedures, and results obtained with A-scan ultrasonography are discussed in Chapter 11.

In B-scan ultrasonography, echos are seen as aggregations of white dots on a black background, providing an acoustic cross section of the eye and orbit. In a normal eye these aggregations of white dots indicate the locations of the cornea, iris, anterior chamber, posterior wall of the globe, and retrobulbar orbital fat. Echos are not obtained for the lens substance nor for the vitreous unless opacities are present. Because it is used as an aid in the diagnosis of specific ocular and orbital diseases and abnormalities, B-scan ultrasonography is considered as a secondary or tertiary care procedure and would not normally be done on a primary-care basis. Indications for its use include the diagnosis of intraocular tumors, detachments and other lesions of the retina, lesions of the vitreous, orbital tumors, and other orbital lesions.

Study Questions

1. Using the slit lamp, which method of illumination is used for (a) observing the corneal endothelium? (b) looking for central corneal clouding due to contact lens wear? (c) inspecting the anterior chamber for flare and cells? (d) observing a cross section of the crystalline lens? (e) looking for pigment dusting of the endothelium or a Kruckenberg spindle?

2. What anterior chamber angle grading would you expect to find for a patient who is (a) a 12-year-old myope? (b) a 60-year-old hyperope? (c) an aphakic patient?

3. How does the indirect ophthalmoscope differ from the direct ophthalmoscope in regard to (a) magnification? (b) field of view?

4. In what direction should the examiner tell the patient to look (a) when wishing to view the inferior fundus? (b) when wishing to view the temporal fundus of the right eye?

5. What term is used to designate infarcted areas in the nerve fiber layer of the retina occurring as a result of local retinal ischemia?

6. What condition would you expect if a patient was found to have a scanty marginal tear strip, excess debris in the tear film, and mucous threads?

7. What term is used to indicate the presence of leucocytes and infective material deposited on the posterior surface of the cornea? What term is used to indicate the presence of similar material at the bottom of the anterior chamber?

8. A tear film breakup time of how many seconds (or less) would cause you to conclude that a patient may not be a successful contact lens wearer?

9. What are deposits of amorphous material in the inner portion of Bruch's membrane, just underneath the retinal pigment epithelium, appearing as white or yellow elevations in the retina? What is the prognosis when this condition is present?

10. In chronic marginal blepharitis, a qualitative change in the Meibomian gland secretion can cause what tear film problem? Why?

11. What term is used to designate each of the following conditions? (a) a turning inward of the lower eyelid, which may cause (b) the lashes to turn inward, rubbing against the cornea; (c) a turning outward of the lower eyelid, which may cause (d) tears to spill out of the lower conjunctival sac onto the cheek.

12. What would be the magnification of an indirect ophthalmoscope using a 15.00D condensing lens (a) for a working distance of 25cm? (b) for a working distance of 40cm?

13. Give the Elschnig disk cupping (I, II, III, or IV) for each of the following: (a) a wide and deep cup, with the vessels pushed nasally, typical of myopia; (b) a flat disk with no cupping; (c) a saucer-shaped cup, usually located in the portion of the disk temporal to the location of the central artery and vein; (d) a cylindrically shaped cup.

14. What peripheral fundus condition involves one or more sharply demarcated, circumferentially oriented lesions crisscrossed with fine, white lines and with an accumulation of pigment?

15. Pigment clumping and a "moth-eaten" appearance in the macular area indicate the possible presence of what condition?

16. It has been found that a cup/disk ratio of what value is present in only 6 percent of normal subjects?

17. What term is used to designate small, wartlike prominences in the endothelium in the axial portion of the cornea of a middle-aged or older person? What corneal dystrophy can this condition lead to?

18. What generalized vascular condition is indicated by the presence of (a) compression occurring at retinal arteriovenous crossings? (b) attenuation of arteries, resulting in an altered vein/artery ratio?

19. When using the Van Herick technique for estimation of the anterior chamber angle width, what is the width of the shadow on the iris compared with the width of the corneal beam for an angle of (a) grade 1? (b) grade 2? (c) grade 3? (d) grade 4?

20. What term is used to designate (a) flat-topped elevations of the tarsal conjunctiva, smooth and

velvety in appearance and associated with some forms of allergic conjunctivitis? (b) gray or white elevations of the tarsal conjunctiva, which are localized areas of lymphoid hypertrophy occurring in some forms of viral, bacterial, and allergic conjunctivitis?

21. What risks, if any, are involved in the use of each of the following topical anesthetics: (a) cocaine; (b) proparacaine; (c) benoxinate; (d) tetracaine.

22. List the possible indications for the performance of gonioscopy.

23. What advantage does a 2-meter tangent screen have as compared to a 1-meter tangent screen?

24. How does static perimetry differ from kinetic perimetry?

25. What neurodiagnostic test can be described as "the subjective counterpart of the swinging flashlight test?"

26. The diagnosis of what condition or conditions can be confirmed (a) if there is an abnormal electroretinogram? (b) if there is an abnormal electro-oculogram?

27. What adverse effects have been reported with the use of (a) 10-percent phenylephrine? (b) cyclopentolate? (c) tropicamide?

28. List a number of possible diagnoses that would suggest the use of the slit lamp and Hruby lens.

29. (a) Using a nonmydriatic fundus camera with a 45-degree field, how is it possible to obtain a fundus picture with an undilated pupil? (b) How does the procedure for the use of a 148-degree fundus camera differ from that of the ordinary fundus camera having a 30-degree field?

30. According to Smith, (a) why should targets no smaller than 3mm be used for tangent screen testing? (b) what is the most likely cause of a constriction in the upper or upper-temporal field?

31. If a patient with reduced acuity in one eye responds that the red top of a mydriatic bottle appears to be desaturated with one eye as compared to the other eye, what is the cause of the reduced acuity?

32. After successful treatment of an angle-closure attack, what should be done to ensure that a further attack does not occur?

33. In using a project-o-light pointer for tangent screen testing, how can the optometrist make sure that the patient is fixating accurately?

34. If a patient has a prolonged recovery time on the light-stress test, is the patient's poor acuity caused by a retinal problem or by an optic nerve problem?

35. What are the advantages of the Goldmann hemispherical perimeter as compared to an arc perimeter?

36. In using the binocular indirect ophthalmoscope, when directing the light beam toward the superior fundus, is the practitioner (a) seeing the superior fundus or the inferior fundus? (b) seeing it upright or inverted?

37. What is the advantage of using double stimulation in visual field testing (test objects presented simultaneously in both the left and right visual fields)?

38. If a patient having a nuclear or posterior subcapsular cataract complains of poor vision in bright daylight in spite of normal or near-normal Snellen acuity, how can the optometrist confirm this complaint in the examining room?

39. Why is it not advisable to routinely use a miotic agent after mydriasis or cycloplegia?

40. In routine tangent screen testing, how can the optometrist test the validity of the patient's responses?

41. (a) What symptoms reported by a patient or what clinical findings would indicate the need for ophthalmodynamometry? (b) This test is designed to confirm the diagnosis of what condition? (c) What are the criteria for a positive finding?

42. What is the "black-hole" effect? How can it be avoided?

43. What information is provided by contrast sensitivity testing that is not provided by visual acuity testing with a Snellen chart?

44. Does contrast sensitivity vary with age in normal subjects (those free of ocular disease)?

45. In what pathological conditions can contrast sensitivity testing provide diagnostic information that is not provided by visual acuity testing or other routine optometric procedures?

CHAPTER 8

Objective Refraction

The determination of the refractive state of the eye involves both objective and subjective refraction. In *objective refraction*, the examiner determines the refractive state of the eye on the basis of the optical principles of refraction without the need for subjective responses on the part of the patient. In *subjective refraction*, the examiner determines the refractive state entirely on the basis of the patient's subjective responses.

The classical methods of objective refraction are keratometry and retinoscopy. In *keratometry*, the refracting power of the cornea is determined in each of the two principal corneal meridians. Keratometry, therefore, provides the practitioner with information about the astigmatism of the eye but no information about spherical ametropia (myopia or hyperopia). *Retinoscopy* provides the practitioner with information concerning both spherical ametropia and astigmatism; it includes *static retinoscopy*, in which the patient fixates a distant target, and *dynamic retinoscopy*, in which the patient fixates a near object.

During the past decade, many methods of automated objective refraction have been developed. These, together with methods for automated subjective refraction, are discussed in Chapter 11.

KERATOMETRY

Optical Principles

The cornea is both a convex refracting surface and a convex mirror. If information about the refracting power of the cornea is desired, it should be necessary only to reflect an object of known size and at a known distance off the corneal surface, determine the size of the reflected image with a measuring telescope, and calculate the refracting power on the basis of an assumed index of refraction. Unfortunately, the small nystagmoid movements of the eye make such measurement impossible.

Doubling principle

Suppose the object to be reflected from the cornea is an illuminated circle with a small cross on either side. If one attempts to measure the size of the reflected image of this object, or *mire*, with a telescope reticle, the zero position of the reticle scale would first be lined up with the left-hand cross (see Figure 8.1a). However, by the time the scale reading could be made at the position of the right-hand cross, the eye would have moved enough so an accurate reading would be impossible.

However if the illuminated object is doubled—by a prism, for example (see Figure 8.1b)—it will be necessary only to superimpose the right-hand cross belonging to one image with the left-hand cross belonging to the other to obtain an accurate measurement of the image size.

The *doubling principle* was first used by Helmholtz. He used two small glass plates with plane parallel faces, placed at an angle, to cause a doubling of the reflected image seen through the telescope. Using this arrangement, the amount of doubling

Figure 8.1 Measurement of the size of a reflected image (a) by means of a telescope reticle scale and (b) by means of a doubling system.

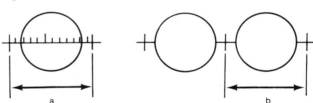

231

could be varied by varying the angle between the two glass plates.

Helmholtz's original instrument was not sufficiently accurate for clinical use. The first clinically useful instrument, known as the Javal-Shiötz keratometer (later manufactured as the Universal ophthalmometer and currently available as the Haag-Streit keratometer), used a *Wollaston prism* as a doubling device. The original American Optical ophthalmometer (also known as the Chambers-Inskeep ophthalmometer) used a *biprism* as a doubling device.

The Bausch & Lomb keratometer makes use of two prisms, one oriented horizontally and the other oriented vertically, so that horizontal and vertical doubling occur simultaneously. This method of doubling is also used in the newer American Optical instrument (the CLC ophthalmometer) and in many of the Japanese keratometers.

Keratometric formula

In Figure 8.2, PQ represents an illuminated object (a portion of the keratometer mire) and P′Q′ represents the image of this object formed by the cornea. The magnification of the image can be expressed by the Newtonian formula:

$$\frac{h'}{h} = -\frac{f}{x} = -\frac{r}{2x}$$

and

$$r = -2x\frac{h'}{h},$$

where

x = the distance from the object PQ to the focal plane of the cornea.

When the instrument is used, the mire image (P′Q′) is viewed through a telescope, the objective of which is brought to a constant distance from the image when it is in focus. Because the position of the

mire PQ is fixed in relation to the telescope, the distance d (distance between object and image) is also a fixed quantity. Because the object distance is large with respect to the focal length of the cornea, we can substitute d for x in the above equation. Thus,

$$r = -2d\frac{h'}{h}.$$

Because the distance d and the mire object size (h) are both constants, it is obvious that the radius of curvature is proportional to the size of the mire image, or

$$r = kh'.$$

The instrument can be calibrated to give a reading in terms of the radius of curvature (r) expressed in millimeters, or in terms of the refracting power (F) expressed in diopters. In the latter case an index of refraction must be assumed. When he designed the original instrument, Helmholtz used the value 1.3375 as the index of refraction to account not only for the air-to-cornea refraction but also for the cornea-to-aqueous refraction. This value is used in the calibration of most modern keratometers.

Instrumentation

In the Bausch & Lomb keratometer (see Figure 8.3), the light beam reflected from the patient's cornea passes through four apertures, as shown in Figure 8.4. In this figure, the left and right apertures contain a horizontally placed and a vertically placed prism, respectively, whereas the upper and lower apertures contain no prism.

The upper and lower apertures constitute a *Scheiner's disk* mechanism, enabling the operator to keep the instrument in sharp focus. If the instrument is not in focus, the image formed by these apertures will be double, as shown in Figure 8.5a; if it is in focus, the image will be single, as shown in Figure 8.5b.

Because horizontal and vertical doubling can be accomplished simultaneously, the instrument is referred to as a *one-position keratometer*. In contrast, instruments equipped with a Wollaston prism or a biprism, which enable doubling only in one direction, must be rotated 90 degrees between the horizontal and vertical measurements. Therefore, they are referred to as *two-position keratometers*. When the meridians of greatest refraction and least refraction are found, the difference in refracting power between the two meridians represents the corneal astigmatism.

Figure 8.2 The cornea as a spherical mirror.

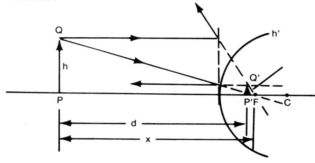

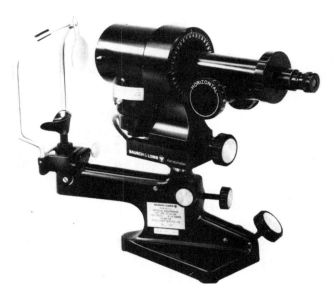

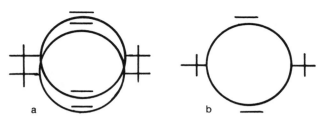

Figure 8.5 The Scheiner's disk focusing mechanism *(a)* out of focus and *(b)* in focus.

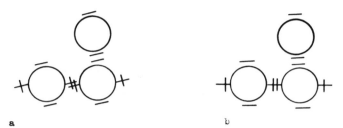

Figure 8.6 Locating the principal meridians of the cornea; *(a)* incorrect meridians; *(b)* correct meridians.

Figure 8.3 The Bausch & Lomb keratometer.

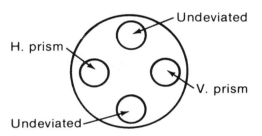

Figure 8.4 Apertures in the keratometer optical system.

Once the telescope has been clearly focused on the mire images, it is necessary to rotate the barrel of the instrument to locate one of the two principal meridians. As the barrel is rotated, a position will be found where the horizontal limbs of the two crosses will appear to be continuous with one another (see Figure 8.6b) rather than obliquely oriented (see Figure 8.6a). When this occurs, the base-apex lines of the two doubling prisms will be parallel to the two principal meridians of the cornea.

A cross-sectional diagram of the Bausch & Lomb keratometer is shown in Figure 8.7. Two measuring drums (M and N) are placed one on each side of the telescope; the left drum controls the travel of the horizontal prism (parallel to the axis of the instrument) and the right drum controls the travel of the vertical prism. The measuring drums are calibrated in terms of refractive power, in diopters, reading to the nearest 0.12D. The instrument is provided with

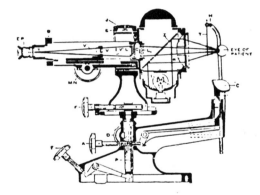

Figure 8.7 Cross-sectional diagram of Bausch & Lomb keratometer.

a meridional scale (S) for use in determining the locations of the principal meridians.

The whole instrument can be moved toward or away from the patient's cornea by turning the knurled knob (F). This is the knob that monitors focusing of the instrument via the Scheiner's disk. When the instrument is used, one hand is needed to control the measuring drum (M or N), but the other hand should always be placed on the focusing knob (F) to make sure the undeviated (lower right) image is kept single.

The eyepiece (EP) of the telescope includes a cross hair reticle, which is focused before the patient is seated in front of the instrument. Once this has been done, the images of the mires will be viewed in the plane of the reticle.

Calibration

The instrument should be calibrated on a regular basis using as a "cornea," a ⅝-inch, bright steel ball bearing. The bearing can be mounted on the back of the occluder, using modeling clay, or on a commercially available attachment called a *contactometer*. The ⅝-inch ball has a radius of 0.794mm (⁵⁄₁₆ inch), which converts (using the keratometer's index of refraction of 1.3375) to 42.50D.

After focusing the eyepiece, the examiner should take a series of three readings on the steel ball, just as would be done with a patient's eye. However, because the ball is spherical, no astigmatism should be found. If the instrument is correctly calibrated and if the examiner's readings are accurate, all three readings should be 42.50D, or within ±0.12D of 42.50D. If the three readings are all within ±0.12D of a value other than 42.50D (e.g., a series of readings such as 43.00, 43.12, and 42.87D), it indicates that the instrument is not correctly calibrated. However, if the three readings are widely scattered (e.g., 43.00, 41.87, and 42.50D), this is an indication that the operator's accuracy is poor.

Procedure

The procedure for determining the refracting power of a patient's cornea in the two principal meridians involves the following steps.

1. *Focusing the eyepiece.* The occluder (T) is placed in front of the patient's end of the keratometer (before the patient is seated at the instrument), and the light switch is turned on. Starting with the eyepiece turned all the way out, it is turned inward slowly until the cross hairs are in sharp focus. The reason for starting with the eyepiece all the way out is to relax the operator's accommodation.

2. *Adjusting the instrument to the patient.* The patient's chair or stool should be adjusted so he or she will have to lean forward slightly to place the chin in the chinrest. The patient is asked to place the chin firmly in the chinrest and the forehead against the forehead rest, and to grasp the base of the instrument with both hands.

3. *Aligning the instrument.* The body of the instrument has two horizontally placed "spears," which are useful in adjusting the instrument to approximately the correct height. While looking outside the instrument, the knurled knob (E) is adjusted until the right "spear" is at the level of the outer canthus of the patient's right eye.

If the instrument is then aimed at the bridge of the patient's nose, a shadow will be seen (still looking outside the instrument) on the bridge of the nose. The focusing knob (F) should then be turned back and forth until the shadow appears at its darkest. The instrument is then swung over to the right eye, and the three mire images will be seen in relatively clear focus. The instrument then should be aligned so the cross hairs are in the center of the undeviated (lower right) mire image.

4. *Instructing the patient.* The patient is instructed to keep his or her eyes open wide (but told it is all right to *blink*), and to watch the image of the eye in the center of the instrument. However, a patient with a large refractive error may not see the eye's reflection and should be told to look into the center of the instrument.

5. *Finding the primary meridian.* The *primary meridian* is defined as the meridian closest to 180 degrees, as measured by the plus signs of the mire image; the *secondary meridian* is 90 degrees from the primary meridian and is measured by the minus signs of the mire image. Holding one hand on the focusing knob and making sure that the two lower right mire images coincide, the operator rotates the barrel of the instrument approximately 30 degrees in each direction, finding the position at which the crosses are continuous (as shown in Figure 8.6).

6. *Taking the readings.* In taking the horizontal reading, the right hand is kept on the focusing knob to make sure that the undeviated mire image remains single, while the left hand is used to bring the two crosses into superimposition. When this has been completed, the reading in the vertical meridian is taken while the left hand is kept on the focusing knob and the right hand is used to bring the two minus signs into superimposition. The instrument is then aligned for the patient's left eye, and the left eye readings are taken.

7. *Recording the findings.* By convention, the power in the horizontal meridian is recorded first, followed by the power in the vertical meridian. Typical findings would be recorded as follows:

R: 42.00 at 180; 43.00 at 90.

L: 42.25 at 170; 43.50 at 80.

The finding for the right eye indicates that the refracting power in (or along) the 180-degree meridian is 42.00D, and the refracting power in the 90-degree meridian is 43.00D.

Interpreting the Findings

The difference in power between the two principal meridians indicates the power of the cylindrical lens necessary to correct the patient's corneal astigmatism, and the meridian of least refracting power indicates the position of the minus axis of the correcting cylinder. For the patient whose findings are given above, the cylindrical lenses necessary to correct the corneal astigmatism would be R: − 1.00 × 180; L: − 1.25 × 170.

We refer to corneal astigmatism as *with-the-rule* when the weakest corneal meridian is at or near 180 degrees (and, therefore, the minus axis of the correcting cylinder is at or near 180 degrees) and as *against-the-rule* when the weakest corneal meridian is at or near 90 degrees (and the minus axis of the correcting cylinder is also at or near 90 degrees). If the principal meridians are between 30 and 60 degrees or between 120 and 150 degrees, the corneal astigmatism is said to be *oblique*. In the great majority of eyes, the weakest meridian of the cornea is at or near 180 degrees, and corneal astigmatism is with-the-rule.

Corneal Versus Refractive Astigmatism

Refractive astigmatism, also called *total astigmatism*, as determined by retinoscopy or by subjective refraction, is made up of both *corneal* and *internal astigmatism*. Internal astigmatism is due to such factors as the toricity of the back surface of the cornea and the tilting of the crystalline lens with respect to the optic axis of the cornea.

Javal's rule, an empirically determined relationship between corneal and refractive astigmatism, states:

$$A_t = p(A_c) + k,$$

where

A_t = Total (refractive) astigmatism.

A_c = Corneal astigmatism.

p = Approximately 1.25.

k = 0.50D against-the-rule astigmatism.

Substituting the values of p and k, the relationship becomes

$$A_t = 1.25(A_c) -0.50 \text{ axis } 90.$$

This relationship has been found to hold true on a statistical basis but is of limited use in predicting refractive astigmatism in individual cases on the basis of corneal astigmatism. However, experience shows that it is an extremely useful guide.

Using the above examples, Javal's rule would indicate that we should expect the following amounts of refractive astigmatism (findings for the patient whose corneal astigmatism was found to be −1.00 axis 180 for the right eye and −1.25 axis 170 for the left eye):

R: 1.25 (−1.00 axis 180) −0.50 axis 90

= − 1.25 axis 180 −0.50 axis 90

= − 0.75 axis 180.

L: 1.25 (−1.25) −0.50 axis 90

= − 1.56 axis 170 −0.50 axis 90

= − 1.06 axis (approx.) 170

= (approx.) −1.00 axis 170.

Although the obliquely crossed cylinders for the left eye, with axes of 170 and 90 degrees could be resolved mathematically, in the clinical situation this is not justified.

The relationship between keratometric and refractive astigmatism (for amounts of corneal astigmatism up to 3.00D with-the-rule and 2.00D against-the-rule), as calculated using Javal's rule, is shown in Table 8.1 and Figure 8.8. Inspection of Figure 8.8 indicates the following:

1. In the absence of corneal astigmatism, the expected amount of refractive astigmatism is −0.50D against-the-rule.
2. If the corneal astigmatism is −0.50D with-the-rule, virtually no refractive astigmatism is expected.
3. If the corneal astigmatism is −2.00D with-the-rule, the expected refractive astigmatism is also −2.00D with-the-rule.
4. If the corneal astigmatism is −2.00D against-the-rule, the expected refractive astigmatism is −3.00D against-the-rule.

If keratometry is done routinely, estimated refractive astigmatism can be quickly calculated mentally prior to performing retinoscopy. In most cases the astigmatism found in retinoscopy will be in the same direction as and within approximately 0.50D of the amount determined by Javal's rule.

A simplified form of Javal's rule

Grosvenor, Quintero, and Perrigin (1988) compared keratometric and refractive astigmatism

Table 8.1 Total (refractive) astigmatism predicted on the basis of Javal's rule.

Corneal astigmatism	Predicted total astigmatism
−2.00 × 90	−3.00 × 90
−1.00 × 90	−1.75 × 90
0	−0.50 × 90
−1.00 × 180	−0.75 × 180
−2.00 × 180	−2.00 × 180
−3.00 × 180	−3.25 × 180

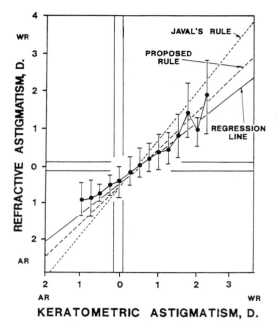

KERATOMETRIC ASTIGMATISM, D.

Figure 8.9 Comparison of keratometric and refractive astigmatism for a group of optometric patients. A close approximation to the regression line is the dashed line indicating that refractive astigmatism is predicted by combining keratometric astigmatism with −0.50D × 90 (from Grosvenor, Quintero, and Perrigin, 1988).

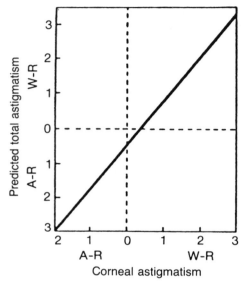

Figure 8.8 The relationship between keratometric astigmatism and refractive astigmatism, as predicted by Javal's rule.

for three subject populations—myopic children, clinic patients, and patients examined in an optometric practice—totaling 1,058 eyes. For each subject population the data were plotted on a graph, as shown in Figure 8.9, and the regression line representing the relationship between keratometric and refractive astigmatism was determined as follows.

For the myopic children:

Refractive astig.

$\quad$ = 0.76(keratometric astig.) −0.40 × 90.

For the clinic patients:

Refractive astig.

$\quad$ = 0.84(keratometric astig.) −0.32 × 90.

For the optometric practice patients:

Refractive astig.

$\quad$ = 0.87(keratometric astig.) −0.43 × 90.

For all three subject groups it was found that the straight line having the equation,

refractive astig.

$\quad$ = 1(keratometric astig.) −0.50 × 90,

provided a better fit for the mean data than did Javal's original rule. Therefore, Grosvenor et al. recommended the use of the simplified version of Javal's rule—requiring only that the keratometric astigmatism be combined with −0.50 × 90—pointing out that if a simplified form of a rule provides a more accurate result than a more complicated form, there's little reason not to use the simplified form.

The relationship between keratometric astigmatism and refractive astigmatism, on the basis of the rule recommended by Grosvenor et al., is illustrated in Table 8.2 and Figure 8.10. Using this relationship:

1. In the absence of corneal astigmatism, the expected amount of refractive astigmatism is $-0.50D$ against-the-rule.

2. If the corneal astigmatism is $-0.50D$ with-the-rule, no refractive astigmatism is expected.

3. For any given amount of corneal astigmatism, the expected refractive astigmatism is determined by combining the corneal astigmatism with -0.50×90.

Improving Keratometer Accuracy

Brungardt (1969) pointed out that keratometer findings tend to be less accurate in the vertical

Table 8.2 Total (refractive) astigmatism predicted on the basis of the Grosvenor et al. (1987) simplification of Javal's rule.

Corneal astigmatism	Predicted total astigmatism
-2.00×90	-2.50×90
-1.00×90	-1.50×90
0	-0.50×90
-1.00×180	-0.50×180
-2.00×180	-1.50×180
-3.00×180	-2.50×180

Figure 8.10 Graphical comparison of keratometric and refractive astigmatism based on the rule recommended by Grosvenor, Quintero, and Perrigin (1987).

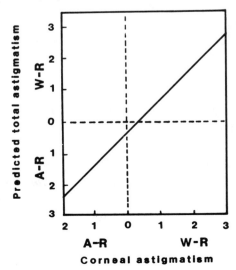

meridian than in the horizontal meridian. Using a Bausch & Lomb keratometer for daily readings on the same subject, he found the total range of findings to be 0.37D in the horizontal meridian but 0.75D in the vertical meridian. In terms of the variation around the midpoint of the range in each meridian, this would amount to a variation of $\pm 0.19D$ for the horizontal meridian and $\pm 0.37D$ for the vertical meridian.

One possible cause of inaccuracy in the vertical meridian is the vertical doubling of the minus sign of the main mire image when the instrument is out of focus. If the operator allows even a slight amount of doubling of the Scheiner's disk mechanism while superimposing the minus signs, the findings will be inaccurate. Another source of inaccuracy is that, if the patient fails to keep his or her eyes open wide enough, drooping of the eyelid may cause one of the minus signs to disappear. In this case, the operator will think the two minus signs are superimposed when, in fact, only one minus sign is seen.

There are two possible methods of improving keratometer accuracy, particularly in the vertical meridian. The first method is rotating the barrel of the keratometer through an angle of 90 degrees after taking the reading in the horizontal meridian, thus using the plus signs of the mire image for taking the vertical as well as the horizontal reading. The second method, proposed by Shick (1962), is the modification of the plus and minus signs of the keratometer mires so findings can be taken by vernier alignment rather than by superimposition. Shick's method of mire modification is illustrated in Figure 8.11.

Figure 8.11 Schick's keratometer mire modification (redrawn from Shick, 1952).

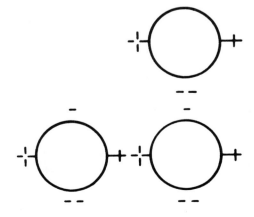

Peripheral Keratometry

The cornea is known to be flatter in the periphery than at the apex. The extent of this peripheral flattening can be investigated by the use of a plastic disk provided with appropriate fixation points and mounted on the front of the keratometer. The disk shown in Figure 8.12 has fixation points located approximately 2, 3, 4, and 5mm outward from the keratometric axial point (the point on the surface of the cornea intersected by the optic axis of the keratometer). A typical plot of corneal refracting power as related to direction of fixation is shown in Figure 8.13. In this graph, *fixation upward* indicates that the refracting power of the *lower* part of the cornea is being determined, and so forth. The graph

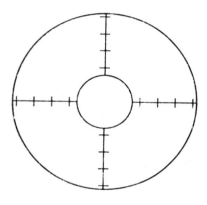

Figure 8.12 Plastic disk with fixation points for use in peripheral keratometry (Grosvenor, 1961).

Figure 8.13 A typical plot of peripheral keratometry data (Grosvenor, 1961).

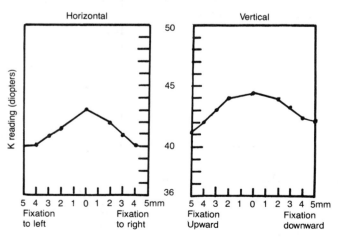

indicates that for this subject, the corneal refracting power decreases from 3.00 to 5.00D in each of the four semimeridians.

Because hard contact lenses are designed on the basis of the peripheral flattening of the cornea, practitioners who fit these lenses may find that peripheral keratometry data are useful. For example, peripheral keratometry data for a patient with keratoconus (as shown in Figure 8.14) may indicate that the cornea flattens as much as 9.00 or 10.00D in the periphery.

A commercially available instrument that attaches to the Bausch & Lomb keratometer for the purpose of performing peripheral keratometry, the Topogometer, is shown in Figure 8.15.

Should Keratometer Findings Be Taken on All Patients?

Although some vision care practitioners feel that keratometry is an optional or even an unnecessary procedure, there are many reasons for including a keratometer finding in every data base optometric examination:

1. Keratometer findings require only a few minutes' time, and the result of Javal's rule (calculated mentally) can be used to speed up both retinoscopy and subjective testing.
2. The keratometer findings can be referred to at a later date, should any corneal injury or disease occur.
3. One of the most obvious signs of keratoconus is distortion of the keratometer mire images, along with a marked corneal steepening (as high as 48.00 or 50.00D, or off the scale). In the absence of routine keratometry, cases of keratoconus can be easily missed.
4. Many patients will ask about the possibility of wearing contact lenses, and advice cannot intelligently be given in the absence of keratometer findings.

Corneal Astigmatism and Contact Lenses

Hard contact lenses typically are rigid enough to maintain their curvature while being worn. Therefore, when spherical hard contact lenses are fitted, corneal astigmatism is for all practical purposes eliminated but internal astigmatism remains. Internal astigmatism averages about −0.50D against-the-rule, and patients who have no more than this amount of (uncorrected) internal astigmatism while wearing

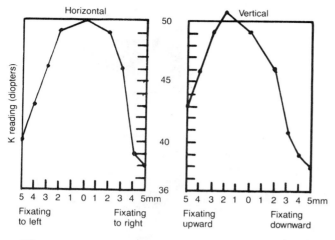

Figure 8.14 Plot of peripheral keratometry data for an eye with keratoconus (Grosvenor, 1961).

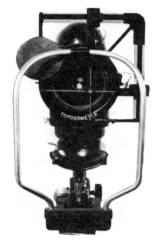

Figure 8.15 Topogometer, attached to a Bausch & Lomb keratometer.

hard contact lenses usually have acceptably clear and comfortable vision with the lenses. However, a few people have as much as 1.00 or 1.50D of internal astigmatism, and this is usually sufficient to cause blurred vision, symptoms of eyestrain, or both. The amount of astigmatism that will remain uncorrected can be predicted by comparing the patient's refractive astigmatism to his or her corneal astigmatism. If this difference is greater than 0.50D, vision with hard contact lenses may be poor. The best way to predict the amount of astigmatism that will remain uncorrected is to refract the patient while wearing trial contact lenses. Harris and Chu (1972) found that for corneas having with-the-rule astigmatism, a

contact lens having a center thickness of 0.13mm or less can flex, or bend, on the cornea enough to reduce or eliminate the uncorrected astigmatism that would be predicted. Although most hard contact lenses have spherical front and back surfaces, lenses with toric front surfaces are available for patients having so much internal astigmatism that clear, comfortable vision cannot be obtained with spherical lenses.

Soft contact lenses are usually flexible enough that they conform to the corneal surface while being worn. Therefore, spherical soft contact lenses correct neither corneal nor internal astigmatism. Hence, the predicted amount of uncorrected astigmatism with spherical soft contact lenses will be the refractive, or total, astigmatism of the eye. It has been found that soft contact lens wearers have unsatisfactory vision if refractive astigmatism is greater than -0.75 or $-1.00D$ with-the-rule, or greater than -0.25 or $-0.50D$ against-the-rule or oblique. However, soft contact lenses are now available with toric front surfaces, so astigmatism can now be corrected for wearers of these lenses.

INSTRUMENTATION FOR CLINICAL REFRACTION

The trial lens set and trial frame (see Figures 8.16 and 8.17) constitute the simplest form of instrumentation for use in clinical refraction. The typical trial lens set incorporates pairs of plus and minus spherical lenses ranging from ±0.12 to $\pm20.00D$, pairs of minus cylinders ranging from -0.12 to $-6.00D$, and pairs of prisms ranging from 1 to 15Δ or more. Also included are such items as occluders, pinholes, and Maddox rods.

The trial frame contains cells for four lenses in front of each eye. The strongest lens is placed in the back cell, with increasingly weaker lenses, as required, placed in the forward cells. All three of the front cells (one of which will usually contain a cylindrical lens) can be rotated by turning the knurled knob located temporal to the lens cell, and a cylinder axis scale is provided for each eye. Interpupillary distance can be adjusted by turning the knurled knobs at the top of the frame (one for each eye). Additional knurled knobs allow adjustment of temple length, pantoscopic tilt (the angle of each lens with respect to the vertical plane), and the vertex distance (distance from the cornea to the back surface of the lens in the back cell).

Retinoscopy, subjective refraction, and binocular

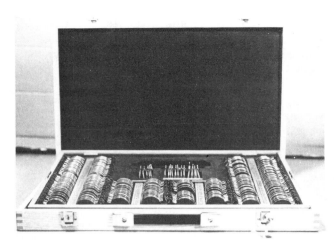

Figure 8.16   Trial lens set.

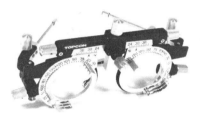

Figure 8.17   Trial frame.

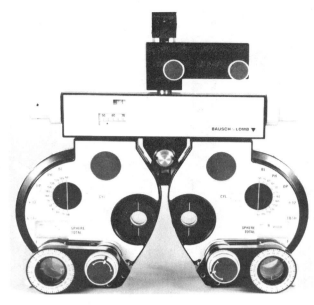

Figure 8.18   The Bausch & Lomb refractor.

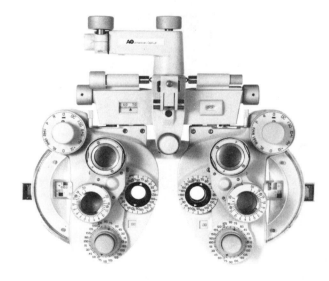

Figure 8.19 The American Optical Rx-Master phoroptor.

vision testing were done by means of the trial frame and trial lenses before modern refracting instrumentation became available, and some refractionists still prefer the trial frame and trial lenses.

Refractors or Phoroptors

The terms *refractor* and *phoroptor* are generic terms used more or less interchangeably to describe instruments designed for refraction and phorometry. The most widely used instruments in the United States are the Bausch & Lomb refractor (see Figure 8.18) and the American Optical Rx-Master phoroptor (see Figure 8.19). Each of these instruments is mounted on a floor stand or wall bracket and is equipped with a wide range of spherical and cylindrical lenses and a variety of auxiliary lenses and prisms. Each is equipped also with Jackson crossed cylinders for use in refining cylinder axis and power (described in Chapter 9), and Risley rotating prisms designed for measurement of phorias and fusional vergences (described in Chapter 10). Each instrument has a calibrated reading rod for the presentation of reduced Snellen charts and

other charts for near-point testing, as well as the necessary adjustments for setting the instrument for the patient's interpupillary distance, for leveling the instrument, and for determining vertex distance.

Although trial lenses and a trial frame can be used for retinoscopy and subjective refraction as effectively (if not as quickly) as a refractor or phoropter, these instruments are capable of a number of testing procedures that cannot be done with a trial frame. For example, tests requiring the Risley rotating prisms—namely, lateral and vertical phorias and fusional vergence findings—cannot be done with a trial frame because of the weight of the rotating prisms (although phorias can be done with a trial frame by using a Maddox rod). Near-point findings requiring small changes in lens power, such as the relative accommodation tests (described in Chapter 10), cannot be done easily with a trial frame.

Even though the additional time required to manipulate trial lenses and their limitations in regard to binocular vision testing makes their routine use impractical in a busy practice, they are useful in a number of circumstances:

1. Children below the age of 5 or 6 years can seldom sit still long enough behind a refractor to make its use feasible.
2. Trial lenses are much larger in diameter than refractor or phoroptor lenses, so the examiner can monitor the patient's eye position during the refraction and can perform the cover test through the correcting lenses.
3. When trial lenses are used, the subjective end point can be easily verified by having the patient look at an object through an open window while the examiner makes appropriate lens changes.
4. Near-vision testing can be done with the patient's head tilted forward in the usual reading position.
5. For the presbyopic patient, the power of the bifocal addition can be verified while the patient holds reading material at an accustomed reading distance or sits at a desk or a table.
6. With trial lenses and a trial frame, refractions can be done in patients' homes or in hospitals and convalescent homes.

Practitioners who use refractors for routine examinations often make use of trial lenses for many of these procedures.

MEASUREMENT OF INTERPUPILLARY DISTANCE

The practitioner must know the patient's *interpupillary distance* (distance between the centers of the pupils of the two eyes, commonly called *PD*) to center the refractor or phoroptor lenses in front of the eyes. On completion of the examination, the PD will again be of importance if ophthalmic lenses are to be prescribed, because it is used to specify the positions of the optical centers of the lenses.

The traditional method of measuring the interpupillary distance has been to measure the distance from the temporal edge of the right pupil to the nasal edge of the left pupil (which is equal to the distance between the centers of the two pupils) using a millimeter ruler. However, a more accurate method is to measure the distance between the *corneal reflexes* of the two eyes. When the patient fixates a light source, the corneal reflex denotes the point where the visual axis, or line of sight, passes through the cornea. For most people, the corneal reflex is located about ½mm nasal to the center of the pupil, with the result that measurement of the distance between the centers of the pupils will usually result in a PD measurement that is in error by being 1mm too great.

Procedure. To measure the patient's distance PD, the examiner faces the patient at a distance of approximately 40cm and holds a millimeter ruler in the patient's spectacle plane. The examiner holds a penlight underneath his or her left eye (aimed toward the patient's right eye), and the patient is instructed to look at the examiner's left eye while the examiner aligns the corneal reflex of the right eye with the zero point on the millimeter ruler scale (see Figure 8.20a). The examiner then holds the penlight underneath his or her right eye (aimed toward the patient's left eye), instructs the patient to look at the examiner's right eye, and notes the reading on the scale corresponding to the position of the corneal reflex of the left eye.

To measure the patient's near PD, the examiner faces the patient at a distance of 40cm, holding the

Figure 8.20 (*a*) **Measurement of distance PD; (*b*) measurement of near PD.**

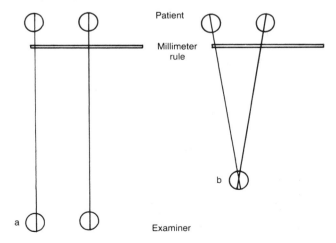

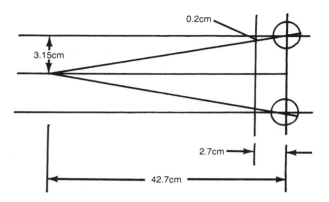

Figure 8.21   Calculation of near PD on the basis of distance PD, for a distance PD of 63 mm (6.3 cm).

penlight underneath his or her right eye (which is aligned with the patient's midline), and aims the penlight toward the bridge of the patient's nose. The patient is instructed to look at the examiner's right eye, and the examiner first aligns the corneal reflex of the right eye with the zero point on the millimeter ruler scale. The examiner then notes the reading on the scale corresponding to the position of the left corneal reflex (see Figure 8.20b). For the 40 cm distance, the near PD will usually be about 4 mm less than the distance PD. By means of simple calculations involving similar triangles it can be shown that the difference between the distance and near PDs is 3.5 mm for a distance PD of 55 mm, 4.0 mm for a distance PD of 63 mm, and 4.5 mm for a distance PD of 71 mm (see Figure 8.21). If the examiner is amblyopic in one eye, the patient's near PD can be measured using the normal eye and the appropriate amount (usually 4 mm) can be added to obtain the distance PD.

STATIC RETINOSCOPY

Optical Principles

The purpose of retinoscopy is to obtain an objective measurement of the patient's refractive state. In *static retinoscopy*, the refractive state is determined while the patient fixates an object at a distance of 6 m. In *dynamic retinoscopy*, the refractive state is determined while the subject fixates an object at some closer distance, usually at or near the plane of the retinoscope itself.

The development of retinoscopy occurred serendipitously when it was found that the plane mirror used in ophthalmoscopy, when moved back and forth, would result in the movement of light and shadow within the patient's pupil. As noted by Millodot (1973), Sir William Bowman reported the movement of this light and shadow effect in 1859. French ophthalmologist Cuignet reported, in 1873, that movement of the ophthalmoscope mirror resulted in the presence of a kaleidoscopic array of light within the patient's pupil. However, Cuignet mistakenly attributed this phenomenon to the cornea. Parent (1880) attributed the lights and shadows to the retina and suggested first the term *retinoscopie* and, later, the term *skiascopie*.

As with any optical instrument, the retinoscope is made up of an illumination system and an observation system. The simplest form of modern retinoscope is the spot retinoscope having a plane mirror. The initial explanation of the optical principles involved in retinoscopy will be in terms of this relatively simple instrument.

Illumination system

The illumination system of the spot retinoscope consists of a bright focal source of light and a semi-silvered mirror that reflects light from the source into the patient's eye, as shown in Figure 8.22a. Because the effective source (S') is located just behind the mirror, when the examiner rotates the mirror, the spot of light will move across the patient's face in the same direction as that of the mirror. For example, if the mirror is tilted upward, the spot of light on the patient's face (or on the front of the refractor) will move upward; if the mirror is tilted

Figure 8.22   Illumination system of a plane-mirror retinoscope: *(a)* mirror is directed toward patient's pupil; *(b)* mirror is tilted upward, causing spot of light on retina to move upward.

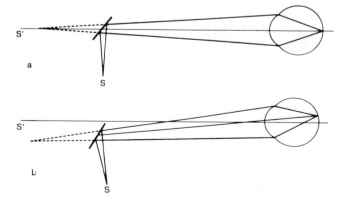

to the right, the spot of light will move on the patient's face toward the right (from the point of view of the examiner).

Our concern here, however, is the spot of light on the patient's retina in relation to the tilting of the mirror. As shown in Figure 8.22b, when the mirror is rotated upward, the spot of light moves upward on the patient's retina, or in the same direction as the spot of light moving across the patient's face. This may be explained on the basis of the relationship between the visual field and the retina. An object that is below the foveal line of sight (the effective source, located behind the mirror in this case) will be imaged above the fovea, whereas an object in the visual field located above the foveal line of sight will be imaged below the fovea. Likewise, an object in the visual field located temporal to the foveal line of sight will be imaged on the nasal retina. The spot of light on the patient's retina moves in the same direction as that of the light moving across the patient's face, regardless of whether the patient is myopic, emmetropic, or hyperopic.

Observation system

It should be understood that, contrary to ophthalmoscopy, the state of refraction of the examiner's eye is not involved in the process of retinoscopy. As Emsley (1963) pointed out, it is only necessary that the examiner see clearly what is happening in the patient's pupil. Hallak (1976) calculated that, on the basis of a 15mm distance between the retinoscope peephole and the first principle plane of the examiner's eye, the examiner's refractive error would have to be at least 35.00D of myopia for the effect on the patient's retinoscopy finding to be as much as 0.12D.

The basic principle involved in the observation system is that if the patient's accommodation is relaxed, *neutral motion* of the reflex seen within the patient's pupil (defined below) occurs when the peephole of the retinoscope is conjugate to the patient's retina. For a myopic eye, neutral motion will be observed, with no lenses in front of the eye, when the retinoscope's peephole is placed at the far-point of accommodation of the eye. For a 2.00D myope, neutral motion will be observed when the peephole is 50cm from the primary focal plane of the patient's eye; and for a 1.50D myope, neutral motion will be observed when the peephole is 67cm from the eye's primary focal plane.

Recall that only a myopic eye has its far-point of accommodation located at a finite distance in front of the eye. An emmetropic eye's far-point of accom-

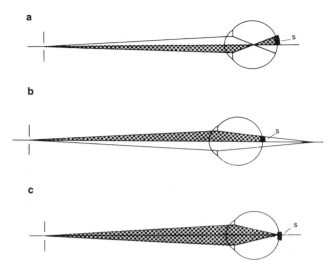

Figure 8.23   Observation system of a plane-mirror retinoscope: (a) myope, showing "against" motion; (b) hyperope, showing "with" motion; (c) emmetrope, showing "neutral" motion. S designates the spot of light on the patient's retina.

modation is located at infinity, and a hyperope's far-point of accommodation is located at some point behind the primary focal plane of the eye. Therefore, although any myopic eye could be "scoped" by simply finding the required position of the retinoscope peephole for neutral motion of the reflex, to scope an emmetrope or a hyperope it is necessary to use convex lenses.

In practice, the retinoscope is positioned either 50 or 67cm from the primary focal plane of the patient's eye. The point of neutrality is determined for each principal meridian of the eye by placing appropriate lenses in the refractor. Before the finding is recorded, a "working distance" lens power (+2.00 or +1.50D) is subtracted from the total lens power in the refractor.

In the discussion that follows, we are not concerned with working distance lenses but with whether the patient is myopic, emmetropic, or hyperopic *with respect to the peephole of the retinoscope*. In the three diagrams in Figure 8.23, the spot of light (S) on the retina can be thought of as a source of light emitting rays of light in all directions. However, only that bundle of rays corresponding to the observation system of the retinoscope is of interest in our discussion.

Figure 8.23a shows what occurs when the patient is myopic with respect to the plane of the retinoscope's peephole. When the spot of light is in the upper part of the patient's retina, the reflex in the plane of the pupil will be seen in the lower part of the pupil (and, of course, when the spot of light is on the lower part of the retina, the reflex will be seen in the upper part of the pupil). With a myope, therefore, "against" motion is observed as the mirror (actually, the whole instrument) is tilted upward and downward or sideways.

Figure 8.23b shows what occurs when the patient is hyperopic with respect to the plane of the peephole. When the spot of light is on the upper part of the retina, the reflex is seen in the upper part of the pupil (and when the spot is on the lower part of the retina, the reflex is seen in the lower part of the pupil). Thus, "with" motion is observed as the instrument is tilted upward and downward.

Figure 8.23c shows that, when the patient is emmetropic with respect to the plane of the peephole, the pupil is illuminated only when the spot on the retina is on the optic axis of the eye. When this occurs, the whole pupil is illuminated instantaneously. There is no motion of the reflex observed in the pupil. Therefore, this is known as *neutral motion* and is also sometimes referred to as *complete flashing*.

In performing retinoscopy, the examiner will find that the motion of the reflex is slow if there is a large amount of uncorrected myopia or hyperopia. As neutrality is approached (as appropriate lenses are placed in front of the patient's eyes), the movement of the reflex increases in speed. At neutrality, the movement of the reflex is infinitely fast—with the result that, as already stated, the whole pupil is illuminated simultaneously.

Instrumentation

The modern retinoscope differs from the simple instrument described above in two respects: (1) it incorporates a concave mirror in addition to the plane mirror, and (2) the light source is in the form of a streak rather than a spot.

Concave mirror

The modern retinoscope incorporates both a plane mirror and a concave mirror (although the term *concave mirror* is used, the concave mirror effect is usually achieved by displacement of the light source with respect to the mirror). The effect of the concave mirror is to place the effective light source slightly in front of (rather than behind) the plane of the mirror, so when the instrument is tilted, the illumination on the patient's face (and hence also on the retina) will move in the direction opposite to that of the mirror. As a result, when the concave mirror is used, myopia (with respect to the plane of the peephole) will result in "with" motion, and hyperopia will result in "against" motion. The advantage of the concave mirror is that the examiner can confirm the type of motion present by switching the mirror from one position to the other. For example, if the examiner is using the plane mirror and observes "with" motion, the correctness of the observation is confirmed if, by switching to the concave mirror, "against" motion is observed.

Streak retinoscope

The bulb of the streak retinoscope is constructed so that it provides a beam in the form of a streak

Figure 8.24   The Copeland streak retinoscope.

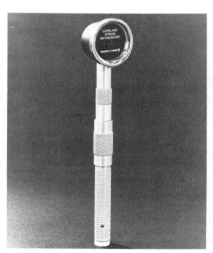

Figure 8.25   Streak retinoscopy: (a) scoping the vertical meridian and (b) scoping the horizontal meridian. In each drawing, the streak is shown as it appears within the patient's pupil (narrow portion) and as it appears on the front of the refractor (wide portion).

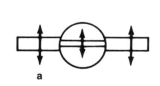

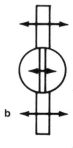

rather than a round spot (see Figure 8.24). The instrument is provided with a mechanism (usually a knurled ring) that makes it possible to rotate the streak into any desired meridian. The orientation of the streak across the patient's face is always at right angles to the meridian of the eye being scoped. Thus, when scoping the vertical meridian (see Figure 8.25a), the examiner moves the instrument vertically, with the streak oriented horizontally. In scoping the horizontal meridian, the instrument is moved horizontally while the streak is oriented vertically (see Figure 8.25b).

In addition to the mechanism for rotating the streak, the streak retinoscope also has a mechanism for varying the width of the streak. This same mechanism also allows the examiner to quickly change from the plane mirror to the concave mirror, and vice versa. When the streak is used at its greatest width, it can be used essentially as if it were a spot retinoscope. As the width is narrowed down, however, the examiner can more easily pin down the two principal meridians.

Procedure

Working distance

Before beginning retinoscopy, the examiner must choose a working distance. The working distance depends somewhat on the length of the examiner's arms. If arm length permits, a 67cm working distance (requiring a working distance lens of

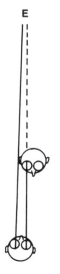

Figure 8.26 The examiner's head is positioned so that it almost blocks the patient's view of the letter _E_ with the eye not being scoped.

+1.50D) is desirable, but otherwise a 50cm working distance (requiring a working distance lens of +2.00D) can be used.

Fixation target

Practitioners vary in the choice of a fixation target for retinoscopy. There is little point in using small letters as a fixation target, as the working distance lenses (when neutrality has been reached) will ensure that the letters are 1.50 or 2.00D out of focus. The author's preference is to use the 20/400 _E_ with the bichrome filter in place (so that one-half of the letter has a red background and one-half has a green background). The advantage of the bichrome filter is that it reduces the illumination on the screen, therefore reducing the illumination of the bothersome reflections formed by the lenses in the refractor. However, such reflections will not be present if the examiner is scoping on the patient's line of sight, as described in the following paragraph.

Patient instructions

The patient is instructed to watch the letter _E_ on the distant chart (usually at 6m). The examiner scopes the patient's right eye with the right eye and the patient's left eye with the left eye. To make sure the scoping is on or close to the patient's line of sight, the examiner's head should be positioned so that it _almost_ blocks the fixation target (see Figure 8.26). The patient is told to be sure to let the examiner know if his or her head blocks the letter _E_. One way to make sure the examiner's head _almost_ blocks the letter _E_ is to instruct the patient (for the right eye) that "it is all right if my head blocks the green side of the letter _E_, but be sure to tell me if my head blocks the red side." In scoping the left eye, the examiner's head can block the red side of the letter _E_ but not the green side.

Starting point

Clinical experience shows that, in using the plane mirror, "with" motion is much easier to observe than "against" motion. If the old prescription or poor distance visual acuity indicates the patient is highly myopic, the practitioner might choose a moderate amount of minus lens power for the starting point. Otherwise, the procedure is begun with no lenses at all—not even a working distance lens—in the refractor. When this is done, "with" motion typically is found in both principal meridians, indicating that the patient is (1) hyperopic, (2) emmetropic, or (3) myopic by less than 2.00D (assuming a working distance of 50cm).

Procedure for spherical ametropia

If it were not for the fact that the majority of people have at least a small amount of astigmatism, retinoscopy would be a relatively simple procedure. Assume that a hypothetical patient has no astigmatism, and the examiner uses a working distance of 50cm. With no lenses in the refractor, "with" motion would be seen in both the vertical and horizontal meridians, using the plane mirror. Plus lens power would then be added in steps of 0.50 or 0.75D, the reflex being observed with each added lens power until a definite "against" motion is observed in all meridians. Plus lens power would then be reduced 0.25D at a time until neutral motion is observed. Due to the aberrations of the eye and other factors, neutral motion of the retinoscope reflex is not as easily found as a "textbook" explanation might lead one to believe. Therefore, when the examiner believes that neutral motion has been observed, a useful procedure is to (1) reduce plus lens power 0.25D, which should result in the observation of "with" motion; and (2) increase plus lens power to 0.25D more than when neutrality was thought to be observed, which should result in the observation of "against" motion.

If neutrality is found to occur with a +2.00D lens in the refractor, the conclusion is that the patient is emmetropic, since the +2.00D sphere corresponds to the working distance lens (for the 50cm distance). If neutrality is found with a +2.75D lens in the refractor, the patient is a +0.75D hyperope; if neutrality is found with a +1.00D lens in the refractor, the patient is a −1.00D myope.

Procedure when astigmatism is present

Because most people do have astigmatism, with each addition of spherical lens power the examiner must scope both the vertical and horizontal meridians. Assume again that the examiner uses a 50cm working distance, and that with no lenses in the refractor, "with" motion is found in both the vertical and horizontal meridians. Plus sphere power is added, 0.50 or 0.75D at a time, until neutrality is found in the least plus meridian. At this point, "with" motion would still be observed in the opposite meridian. If, for example, neutral motion is found in the vertical meridian (bracketing in both directions, as described above), and if "with" motion is still present in the horizontal meridian, the presence of with-the-rule astigmatism would be indicated. This is because the vertical meridian, requiring the least plus lens power for its neutralization, is the meridian of greatest refraction or greatest vergence. The horizontal meridian, requiring the most plus power for its neutralization, will be the meridian of least refraction or least vergence.

The examiner should next make a mental note that neutrality has been found in the vertical meridian and then count the number of "clicks" as additional plus lens power is added to neutralize the motion in the horizontal meridian. If, for example, five clicks of plus lens power are added to neutralize the most plus meridian (each click being 0.25D), the practitioner should make a mental note that this eye has 1.25D of astigmatism. When the most plus (horizontal) meridian has been neutralized, the examiner will find that the vertical meridian now shows "against" motion. Minus cylinder power is then added with the axis horizontal (at 180 degrees) to neutralize the "against" motion in the vertical meridian. In this case, it would be expected that 1.25D (five clicks) of minus cylinder power would be required to neutralize the motion in the vertical meridian. If at the end of the procedure the lenses in the refractor were a +3.00D sphere combined with a −1.25D cylinder, axis 180, after subtraction of +2.00D for the working distance lenses, the finding would be recorded as +1.00 −1.25 × 180.

The examiner is then ready to scope the left eye. Because the patient may have been accommodating while the right eye was scoped, the examiner should briefly recheck the right eye after having finished scoping the left eye.

Locating the principal meridians

The preceding discussion tacitly assumes that the two principal meridians of the patient's eye fall at 180 and 90 degrees. Although this often occurs, the examiner's procedure has to take into account that the principal meridians may *not* be at (or even near) 180 or 90 degrees.

The examiner should carefully observe the orientation of the reflex in the patient's pupil as the beam is moved horizontally and vertically. Referring to Figure 8.27a, assume that the examiner is in the process of neutralizing the motion in the least plus meridian of an eye having what appears to be with-the-rule astigmatism. As neutralization of the horizontal meridian is approached, movement of the retinoscope beam horizontally across the patient's face results in the reflex in the patient's pupil being oriented 20 or 30 degrees from vertical, rather than being oriented vertically. The orientation of the streak is then altered in the direction corresponding to that of the streak in the patient's pupil, and the instrument is moved back and forth in the direction

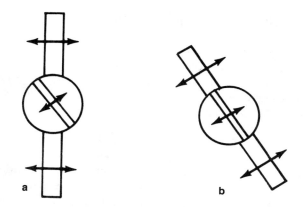

Figure 8.27 Locating the principal meridians (from Brooks, 1975).

perpendicular to that of the streak's orientation. If necessary, additional changes in the orientation of the streak are made to find the orientation that results in the reflex in the patient's pupil appearing to be perpendicular to the direction of movement of the retinoscope.

Referring to Figure 8.27b, assume that it was necessary to orient the streak in the 120-degree meridian for the movement of the reflex in the patient's pupil to be perpendicular to the orientation of the streak. In completing the neutralization of the vertical meridian, the streak should be moved in the 120-degree meridian (while oriented in the 30-degree meridian) until neutralization of the 120-degree meridian has been achieved. The 30-degree meridian is then neutralized, after which "against" motion will be seen in the vertical (120-degree) meridian. The minus cylinder axis should then be set at 30 degrees and minus cylinders added until the 120-degree meridian is again neutralized. At any point in the process, the examiner can decide to make small changes in the orientation of the streak as well as in the axis of the minus cylinder.

Although some examiners take pride in being able to refine the cylinder axis to the nearest degree during retinoscopy, failure to do so creates no serious problem. During the subjective portion of the refraction, the examiner will have ample opportunity to further refine the cylinder axis. Although the procedure may seem complicated to the beginning student, accomplished retinoscopists can complete retinoscopy of both eyes in as little as 2–3 minutes. Many examiners spend only enough time in retinoscopy to determine the cylinder axis to the nearest 10 or 15 degrees, knowing that they can quickly refine the axis during subjective testing.

Control of the patient's accommodation

The patient constantly should be reminded to watch the letter *E* or other fixation target to make sure that accommodation is relaxed throughout the procedure. It should be understood that retinoscopy is a *monocular* procedure. Because the examiner blocks the eye that is being scoped, any accommodation exerted by the eye that fixates the distant target will also be present in the eye being scoped, since both eyes accommodate equally. Some examiners attempt to avoid the possibility of the fixating eye accommodating by beginning the retinoscopy procedure with 2.00D or more of plus power before each eye. Some prefer not to do this, however, unless a concave mirror is used, as it involves working with "against" motion. As already pointed out, the examiner can avoid the problem of accommodation by rescoping the right eye after the left eye has been scoped. In this way, when each eye is scoped, the opposite eye is fogged by the +1.50 or +2.00D working distance lens.

Varying the width of the streak

As noted earlier, the mechanism that controls the width of the streak also allows the examiner to switch from the plane mirror to the concave mirror. With the Copeland streak retinoscope, for example, when this mechanism, located just beneath the head of the instrument, is all the way up, the plane mirror is in position with a wide streak. As the mechanism is gradually lowered, the streak decreases in width, becoming a narrow slit and then widening again. As this widening begins, the instrument is in the concave-mirror mode, and at the lowest adjustment the streak is again at its maximum width (but with the concave-mirror effect). Other retinoscopes, including the American Optical and Welch-Allen instruments, are in the plane-mirror mode when the mechanism is all the way down rather than all the way up.

Brooks (1975) has suggested that lining up the streak so it coincides with the direction of the reflex in the pupil is made easier by slowly changing the mirror setting of the retinoscope, from the plane-mirror position to the concave-mirror position, while watching the width of the reflex band within the pupil. The reflex will narrow somewhat (when the cylinder is larger than 0.75D) until it reaches a minimum width. As the mirror continues to move, the band reflex will begin widening again. The examiner then finds the position where the reflex is at its narrowest, as shown in Figure 8.28.

When working with cylinders under 0.75D,

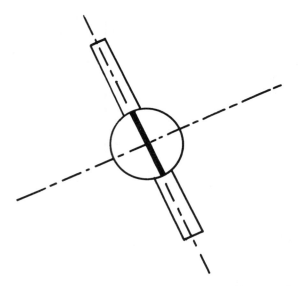

Figure 8.28 The narrowing effect: the position of the mirror is found where the reflex has a minimum width (from Brooks, 1975).

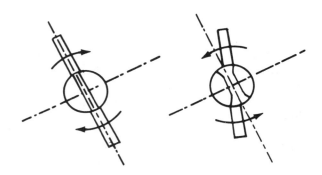

Figure 8.29 Broadening and fluting of the retinoscope reflex (from Brooks, 1975).

where narrowing of the reflex does not occur, Brooks (1975) suggests the examiner note that the reflex band in the pupil increases in brightness and intensity the closer the streak is to the principal meridian. With the pupil reflex band at its narrowest position, the examiner should turn the streak slightly both clockwise and counterclockwise. Using no scanning motion, the reflex band is observed: it will broaden and become slightly fluted at both ends (see Figure 8.29). The narrower the band, the closer the retinoscope streak is to the desired position. The axis position may be confirmed by once again moving the streak back and forth across the pupil while observing the direction of movement in the pupil reflex band, looking for oblique motion.

Brightness and speed of motion of the reflex

The experienced examiner will find that the reflex's brightness and speed of motion serve as important clues in the process of neutralizing the movement of the reflex. As Keller (1977) has pointed out, the peephole of the retinoscope serves as the field stop of the optical system under consideration. The area of the patient's retina observed as filling the pupil of the eye is related to the size of the peephole and the sharpness of focus of the light on the patient's retina. Therefore, when the patient's retina is not conjugate with the peephole of the retinoscope, the illuminated area of the patient's retina is usually larger than the observed area. Thus, in high myopia or hyperopia, the reflex seen in the patient's pupil is not only dull (because it is badly out of focus) but larger than the diameter of the patient's pupil. This being the case, the examiner cannot see a boundary between light and shadow, making it impossible to judge the speed of movement of the reflex (or, for that matter, whether the reflex is moving) as the retinoscope is rotated back and forth. Only by adding enough minus or plus power to reduce the size of the illuminated area of the retina (which will also increase the brightness of the reflex), will the examiner be able to discern that the reflex in the patient's pupil is moving and in what direction.

As the reflex approaches neutrality, the illuminated area of the retina becomes increasingly smaller. This increases the amount of light reflected per unit area of the retina and, therefore, causes the reflex to appear increasingly brighter to the examiner. Keller (1977) calculated that, for a 5mm-diameter peephole and a 40cm working distance, the diameter of the illuminated area of the patient's retina at neutrality would be 0.23mm. It is this highly concentrated area of focused light that fills the patient's pupil at neutrality.

Spot versus streak retinoscopy

Before the invention of the streak retinoscope by Copeland, spot retinoscopy was the only technique available. As the advantages of streak retinoscopy became known, many practitioners switched to the new method and schools of optometry placed heavy emphasis on streak retinoscopy (if they did not abandon spot retinoscopy altogether). Having originally been taught spot retinoscopy, the author used the spot retinoscope in practice for a number of years before entering graduate school. Finding that instruction in spot retinoscopy had been abandoned in favor of instruction in streak retinoscopy, the author converted to the streak retinoscopy method.

From time to time the literature reminds those who care to listen of the presence of the spot retinoscope. For example, in the early days of soft contact lens fitting, Bausch & Lomb Soflens representatives encouraged practitioners to use the spot retinoscope to judge the fit of soft lenses. A poorly fitting lens would cause a shadowy appearing reflex, whereas a well-fitting lens would provide a bright, clear reflex. More recently, Dougal, Hoeft, and Dowaliby (1980) have spoken in favor of spot retinoscopy. They presented the following arguments for its use:

1. In dealing with *pediatric patients*, the practitioner must obtain the greatest possible amount of information in the shortest time. The spot scope provides information concerning the presence or absence of astigmatism in a minimum length of time, simply on the basis of the shape of the reflex. The presence of any significant amount of myopia or hyperopia can be determined in seconds. When children are examined without the use of a phoropter, retinoscopy by means of hand-held lenses can be done much more quickly than would be possible with the manipulation of a streak retinoscope.

2. In *vision-screening programs* involving large numbers of schoolchildren, spot retinoscopy affords more information than streak retinoscopy and in a shorter time.

3. In *progress evaluations* of patients wearing newly prescribed spectacles, spot retinoscopy with a working distance lens enables the practitioner to judge quickly the effectiveness of the new lenses.

4. In the assessment of the fit of *contact lenses*, the spot scope can be used to judge power correction, centration, tear layer, and other factors for hard lenses; and to assess soft lenses for signs of lens buckling, lens transparency, and for signs of steep or flat corneal correspondence.

Accuracy of Retinoscopy

Richards (1977) reviewed a large number of studies comparing retinoscopy with subjective refraction procedures and found no consistent tendency for retinoscopy to result in either higher or lower findings. Bearing in mind that a retinoscopy finding is a monocular finding and should be compared with monocular rather than binocular subjective findings, experience indicates that there are many possible causes of inaccurate retinoscopy findings, including the following.

1. *Incorrect working distance.* An incorrect working distance can cause a significant error in retinoscopy findings. If the examiner works at too close a distance, the findings will be in error in the direction of too much plus or too little minus, whereas working at too great a distance will cause an error in the opposite direction. For example, if an examiner thinks he or she is working at a distance of 50cm (requiring a +2.00D working distance lens) but is actually working at 40cm (requiring a +2.50D working distance lens), the retinoscopy findings will be in error by 0.50D too much plus or too little minus. The examiner should check the working distance from time to time, using a meter stick or the reading rod attached to the refractor.

2. *Scoping off the patient's visual axis.* As long as the examiner works within 2 or 3 degrees of the patient's visual axis, no significant error is likely to result. However, if the examiner is amblyopic in one eye and is thus forced to observe both of the patient's eyes with either right or left eye, he or she will be working somewhat more than 5 degrees off the patient's visual axis (when scoping the patient's right eye with the left eye or the patient's left eye with the right eye). When this occurs, errors of 0.25D or more will be made in spherical or cylindrical power, and small errors will be made in cylinder axis.

3. *Failure of the patient to fixate the distant target.* Occasionally a patient (usually a child) will fixate on and accommodate on the retinoscope source rather than the distant target, causing the refractive finding to be in error by as much as 1.00 or 2.00D in the direction of too much myopia or too little hyperopia. This can be avoided by continually reminding the patient to watch the letter *E* and to let you know if your head gets in the way. Some patients tend to be shy about telling the examiner to move his or her head: it is helpful for the examiner to purposely get his or her head in the way once or twice to test the patient's response.

4. *Failure to obtain a reversal.* Inexperienced examiners occasionally fail to detect moderate or even high with-the-rule astigmatism during retinoscopy. This is usually due to the failure to obtain a reversal in the vertical meridian (not adding enough minus cylinder power to reverse the "against" motion) after having neutralized the horizontal meridian.

5. *Failure to locate the principal meridians.* This can occur if the examiner expects to find the two principal meridians at or near 180 and 90 degrees

and, therefore, fails to twist the beam to look for the meridians at which the reflex most nearly follows the plane in which the instrument is rotated. If keratometry is routinely done prior to retinoscopy, the principal meridians found by means of keratometry can be used as a starting point in retinoscopy.

6. *Failure to recognize scissors motion.* If the pupil is reasonably large, spherical aberration may be present and "scissors motion" will occur. The central band of the reflex will appear to move in one direction while the peripheral portion moves in another direction. When this occurs, the examiner should base the interpretation on the bright central band rather than on the darker peripheral portion of the reflex.

Origin of the Retinoscopic Reflex

The exact location of the reflecting surface within the eye that is responsible for the retinoscopic reflex is a matter of controversy. One possibility is that the interface between the vitreous and the retina is responsible for the reflex. Because this surface is located in front of the receptor layer (and because it is expected that the subjective refraction would be based on the position of the receptor layer), the retinoscopic finding would be expected to be more hyperopic than the subjective finding. Other possibilities are that the reflecting surface is the pigment epithelium of the retina or Bruch's membrane just beneath the retinal pigment epithelium. Either of these possibilities would mean that the retinoscopic finding should be slightly more myopic than the subjective finding. However, the possibility that Bruch's membrane is the reflecting surface seems remote, because much of the light has already been absorbed by the pigment epithelium before reaching Bruch's membrane.

Millodot and O'Leary (1978) compiled data for a total of 1,078 eyes from the practices of three optometrists. They found that the relationship between retinoscopic and subjective data is a function of age: retinoscopic findings were more hyperopic than subjective findings for patients below the age of 55 and less hyperopic than subjective findings for older patients. The increase in hyperopia found in retinoscopy as compared with subjective refraction varied from an average of 0.35D at ages 5–15 to an average of 0.05D at ages 46–55. The authors explained these data by suggesting that the reflecting surface responsible for the retinoscopic reflex is the interface between the retina and the

vitreous. They proposed that with increasing age there is an increase in the index of refraction of the vitreous (conceivably reaching that of the retinal index), so light reflected from Bruch's membrane or from the pigment epithelium would constitute the main reflecting surface, leading to an apparent myopia.

DYNAMIC RETINOSCOPY

In dynamic retinoscopy the patient is instructed to fixate on a letter, group of letters, or other objects in the plane of the retinoscope, or even on the retinoscope itself; no working distance lens power is added to or subtracted from the finding. Those practitioners who perform dynamic retinoscopy usually do so immediately after completing static retinoscopy. Although there are many methods of dynamic retinoscopy, usually the working distance lenses are removed so that at the start of the test, the static retinoscopy finding is in place. The procedure is then to instruct the patient to focus on the letters or other fixation object or objects, and to neutralize the motion of the reflex. If the patient were to fully accommodate for the distance of the retinoscope, the dynamic finding would be the same as the static finding (i.e., no plus or minus lenses would have to be added to the static retinoscopy lenses to obtain neutrality). However, most people fail to accommodate fully for the distance of the retinoscope, exhibiting a lag of accommodation of 0.50 to 1.00D or even more. Therefore, a certain amount of plus lens power must be added to the static retinoscopy finding to obtain neutrality, and the amount of plus lens power that must be added represents the patient's lag of accommodation. For example, if a patient's static retinoscopy finding is +0.50D sphere for each eye, and if the total power required to bring about neutrality in dynamic retinoscopy is +1.25D for each eye, the lag of accommodation is 0.75D.

Early Methods

The pioneer in the field of dynamic retinoscopy (which he called *dynamic skiametry*) was a New York optometrist, Andrew J. Cross. In *Dynamic Skiametry in Theory and Practice* (1911), Cross recommended his procedure as an alternative to cycloplegic refraction in latent hyperopia and also for determining the correction in cases of astigmatism, presbyopia, and subnormal accommodation in young patients. Cross's procedure was to start with the static retinoscopy finding after removal of the working distance lenses (therefore, working with "with" motion) and to add plus lenses to the point just beyond the neutral point until a reversal occurred. In his discussion of latent hyperopia, which he referred to as *ciliary spasm*, he reasoned that, although a patient with ciliary spasm is unlikely to fully relax accommodation when refracted at 20 feet without a cycloplegic, when the same patient is refracted by dynamic retinoscopy the increased muscular effort required will bring about a more normal relationship between accommodation and convergence, bringing out the full amount of the hyperopia. Cross recommended prescribing the full amount of plus found in the dynamic retinoscopy finding.

Charles Sheard (1920), whose research in the areas of clinical refraction and anomalies of binocular vision formed the basis for much of what is taught in optometry schools in the United States, developed his own method of dynamic retinoscopy which differed in some respects from that of Cross. Sheard recommended that plus lens power be added only to the point of neutrality, contending that Cross's method of adding plus lens power to obtain a reversal was actually a measurement of *negative relative accommodation:* the amount of plus power recommended by Cross was so great that patients would not persist in wearing their lenses.

It was Sheard (1920) who introduced the concept of "lag of accommodation." He defined this as a lag of accommodation behind convergence, occurring during dynamic skiametry. He considered this lag of accommodation to be a normal condition, saying that an emmetropic patient possessing a normal amplitude of accommodation and normal amplitudes of fusional reserves will require from 0.50 to 0.75D of plus lens power for neutrality to be obtained in dynamic skiametry. Sheard used a second method to investigate the lag of accommodation behind convergence. He provided a fixation target at a certain distance from the patient and performed retinoscopy behind the plane of the fixation target (without the use of lenses), finding the point at which the retinoscope must be placed for neutrality to be obtained. A sample set of data cited by Sheard, using this procedure, indicated that for fixation distances of 13, 10, and 8.5 inches, the position of the retinoscope for neutrality was found to be 15, 12, and 10 inches, respectively. Lags of accommodation behind convergence were calculated to be 0.40, 0.70, and 0.70D for the three distances.

In performing dynamic retinoscopy, Sheard (1920) selected the patient's usual reading distance as his working distance, adding plus lens power (to the distance retinoscopy lenses) until neutrality occurred. Because he believed that the normal lag of accommodation was 0.50D or slightly more, he routinely subtracted 0.50D from the dynamic finding. For example, if static retinoscopy resulted in a finding of +1.25D, and dynamic retinoscopy resulted in +2.50D, the dynamic finding of +1.25D (dynamic minus static) would be reduced by +0.50D for the "normal" lag, leaving a remainder of +0.75D. Presumably, a part (or all) of the +0.75 would be considered as a correction for near work.

Working at a distance of 33cm, Tait (1953) used what he referred to as Sheard's method of dynamic retinoscopy on 712 patients below the age of 40 years. Tait found an average lag of accommodation (difference between dynamic and static findings) of 1.12D for the whole group, but a lag of only 0.75D for patients between the ages of 20 and 25 years. Using a second technique on 300 of his patients, Tait fogged each patient with a considerable amount of plus lens power and then approached the neutrality point by reducing plus lens power. Using this fogging method, he found an average of approximately 1.50D more than he found with the Sheard system, or a total lag for these patients (using the fogging method) averaging +2.25D. This is of interest in that it is close to the value of +2.50D expected for a *negative relative accommodation test* (the "plus-to-blur" test done at 40cm, in which plus lens power is added 0.25D at a time, beginning with the distance subjective finding, until the patient reports that the letters are blurred).

OEP Method

For many years the Optometric Extension Program (OEP) has advocated the performance of dynamic retinoscopy in its "21-point technique," including dynamic retinoscopy at 50cm (the no. 5 finding) and at 1m (the no. 6 finding). For both of these findings, the OEP has followed Sheard's example by deducting a standard amount of lag of accommodation. As described by Lesser (1969), after static retinoscopy the examiner is positioned at 50cm from the patient and, while the patient fixates letters in the plane of the peephole, adds sufficient plus lens power to bring about "against" motion and then reduces the plus power until neutrality is found. This procedure is a modification of Tait's method since the patient is fogged at the start of the test.

Other Methods of Retinoscopy

Book retinoscopy

An early reference to book retinoscopy is in *Vision: Its Development in Infant and Child*, by Gesell, Ilg, and Bullis (1949). These authors reported on their observations of many aspects of visual behavior in a group of children studied at the Yale Clinic of Child Development, from birth to the age of 10 years. Optometrists Vivian Ilg and Gerald Getman took part in the study.

One form of observation of visual behavior used by Gesell et al. (1949) was retinoscopy. The fixation target used for retinoscopy in most cases was a rectangular aluminum screen on which simple pictures were projected in sequence. Observations were made with the retinoscope at distances of 15 feet, 7 feet, and approximately 20 inches. In addition, for children aged 2 years and older, retinoscopy was performed while the child was shown pictures in a book. The child was brought to the examination room by a guidance teacher, and the child's attention to the pictures on the screen or in the book was guided by questions or suggestions concerning the pictures. The examiner observed (1) the dullness or brightness of the reflex; (2) the color of the reflex; (3) the speed, range, promptness, pickup, and release of motion; and (4) meridional differences. Gesell et al. reported that the reflex increased in brightness the moment a child identified an object, coincidentally registering an "against" motion and indicating an increase in accommodation. They described the color and brightness of the reflex as occurring in the following sequence:

1. *Dull red.* High plus (or minus); low recognition or awareness; "flop" period (neither good quantity nor quality of "effector set").
2. *Bright pink.* Low minus; higher recognition or awareness than when the dull-red reflex occurred; a quantity of set, but only of periodic or episodic quality.
3. *Dull pink.* Low plus; first indication of quality development.
4. *White pink.* Plano; neither plus nor minus, because the effector set is now approximating the point of regard; better quality than before.
5. *White.* Plus (+0.50 or +0.75D); higher grade cortical control; now set with good quality and consistency (Gesell, Ilg, and Bullis, 1949, p. 183).

Gesell et al. (1949) pointed out that this sequence is only a schematic summary that may serve as a frame of reference. Examples given elsewhere in the book indicate that this is a *developmental* sequence: the farther the child's visual development has progressed, the more likely it is that the reflex will be found to be white pink or white. It is of interest that the white reflex, representing the highest stage of development, involves 0.50 or 0.75D of plus: this corresponds exactly to the lag of accommodation found by Sheard (1920) and by Tait (1951) for 20- to 25-year-old subjects.

Book retinoscopy was investigated by Pheiffer (1955) using as subjects ten University of Houston optometry students. Retinoscopy was performed on the students while they read material varying in difficulty from the *Reader's Digest* anthology *Getting the Most out of Life* to textbooks on statistics and optics. On the basis of the study, Pheiffer arrived at the following conclusions:

1. When material is read with interest or there is a search for meaning, the reader accommodates for a distance closer than the plane of regard. Accommodation increases when the material becomes difficult to comprehend and decreases when the material is readily comprehended.
2. When the material is so far beyond the comprehension level of the reader that he or she cannot secure meaning, or when it is readily comprehended but is not interesting to the reader, accommodation is maintained at or beyond the plane of regard (the latter indicating the familiar lag of accommodation behind convergence).
3. When reading material is at 16 inches, the reader cannot accommodate for a distance closer than 10 inches without a blur or a demand to move the material closer to the reader.
4. When reading material is at 16 inches, the reader cannot accommodate for a distance farther than 20 inches.

Referring to conclusion 3, note that when reading material is presented at 16 inches (demanding 2.50D of accommodation) but accommodation is postured at 10 inches (4.00D of accommodation being in play), the subject is overaccommodating 1.50D. However, when accommodation is postured at 20 inches (2.00D of accommodation being in play), the subject is underaccommodating by only 0.50D. This relatively low lag of accommodation beyond convergence, as compared with lags of 1.00D and more found by Tait (1953), is possibly due to the fact that the subjects were actively reading and attempting to secure meaning as opposed to the usual clinical situation in which the patient is fixating on a line of letters.

The changes in the brightness and color of the

retinoscopic reflex during book retinoscopy have engendered some controversy among optometrists. Statements such as "the cortex probably releases an effector impulse which influences the total dioptric apparatus" (Gesell, Ilg, and Bullis, 1949, p. 176), and "a relationship between cognitive processing and changes in the luminance of the fundus reflex" (Kruger, 1977, p. 450) have been interpreted by some as indicating that book retinoscopy is enveloped by an aura of witchcraft. However, the observations made by Gesell, Ilg, and Bullis (1949) regarding the changes in brightness and color of the reflex, and Pheiffer's (1955) conclusions regarding the state of the subject's accommodation while reading materials of varying levels of difficulty, can be interpreted on the basis of well-known principles of optics and visual physiology.

In a critical evaluation of book retinoscopy, Keller (1977) accounted for changes in brightness and color of the retinoscopic reflex on the basis of the size, speed of motion, and extent to which the reflex is out of focus with respect to the peephole of the retinoscope. He pointed out that, due to the eye movements occurring when the patient reads a paragraph of printed material, the circle of light seen by the examiner in the patient's pupil will pass along the surface of the retina as far nasalward as the optic nerve head and the retinal vessels. Therefore, the nerve head and vessels may be responsible for some of the observed changes in brightness and color of the reflex.

Bell retinoscopy

Apell (1975) and others have described a method of dynamic retinoscopy that they call *bell retinoscopy*. Although the procedure was originally done by dangling a small bell in front of the examiner's forehead, a one-half-inch chrome steel ball attached to a thin metal rod was used rather than a bell.

As described by Apell (1975), the examiner is positioned so that the retinoscope is 20 inches (50cm) from the patient's face. The examiner holds the retinoscope with one hand and the ball, suspended on its handle at eye level, with the other hand. No lenses are used. The patient is asked to look at his or her own reflection in the ball; the examiner, while observing the direction of motion of the reflex in the patient's pupil, slowly moves the ball toward the patient's face until neutral motion is observed in each principal meridian. The position of the ball at neutrality is determined by the use of a yardstick, one end held by the patient (by making the "zero" end touch the cheek) and the other end held by the

examiner (by balancing it over the ear or shoulder or by holding it with the hand that also holds the retinoscope). Apell reports that neutrality usually occurs when the ball is located about 15–16 inches from the patient's face (or about 37–40 cm), resulting in a lag of accommodation from 0.50 to 0.75D.

Apell (1975) uses bell retinoscopy as one of his preliminary tests, with the patient wearing his habitual near correction. In his 1975 article, Apell discusses the following responses, along with guides to prescribing: (1) normal response, (2) delayed shift in "against" motion, (3) always "with" motion, (4) always "against" motion, (5) astigmatic motion, (6) anisometropic motions, (7) intermittent esotropia, and (8) intermittent exotropia.

The variability of bell retinoscopy findings was investigated by Streff and Claussen (1971). Each examiner performed bell retinoscopy on a group of children, using the procedure described by Apell (1975), with the exception that testing was done at 67, 50, and 40cm. Data for the two examiners were found to vary by as much as 3.69D for one subject when testing at the 40cm distance. The authors explained this variability by noting that one examiner was measuring the light-shadow edge of the beam with rather larger sweeps of the instrument, whereas the other was watching the center of the beam with small, rapid sweeps of the instrument.

MEM retinoscopy

The monocular estimation method (MEM) of dynamic retinoscopy differs from other methods (such as the OEP method) in that the fixation target is placed at the patient's customary reading distance rather than at an arbitrary distance, such as 50cm.

Bieber (1974) gave the following explanation of the MEM retinoscopy technique. The fixation target is a white card containing a one-half-inch hole, having letters, words, or pictures appropriate to the child's age level printed within one-half inch of the hole (see Figure 8.30). The card is attached to the retinoscope by means of a clip, so the retinoscope beam passes through the hole in the card. The examiner is seated on a stool slightly below the patient's eye level, so the patient's eyes are in a moderate downward gaze when looking at the target, as would occur when reading. No refractor is used: the patient wears his or her own distance correction, a tentative near correction, or possibly no correction at all. The reading distance is determined either by observing the patient while reading or looking at pictures, or by using the "Harmon distance," (equal to the distance from the elbow to the knuckles). According

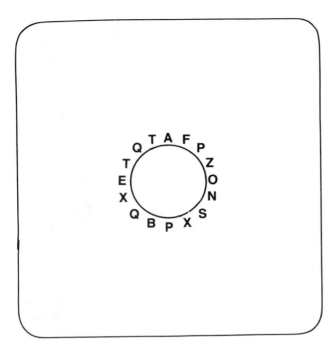

Figure 8.30　Dynamic retinoscopy card.

to Bieber, for the young child this distance is usually from 8–10 inches.

The child is instructed to read the words aloud or describe the pictures, and the examiner quickly moves the vertical streak across the pupil, noting whether "with" or "against" motion is present. If the patient is wearing distance correction, "with" motion will usually be observed due to the expected lag of accommodation beyond the plane of convergence. Using a hand-held trial lens, the examiner again quickly moves the vertical streak across the pupil and also checks the vertical meridian using a horizontal streak. As described by Bieber, the estimation of the direction of movement is always made quickly to keep from disturbing the patient's accommodative response or to avoid interfering with binocular alignment of the eyes.

Interpretation of MEM results. Bieber (1974) notes that there should be no movement of the observed reflex. Due to the thickness of the retinoscope, the fixation target is far enough in front of the retinoscope mirror so there is a "hidden" lag of accommodation as high as 0.50 or 0.75D when neutrality is observed. If we assume that the fixation card is placed at a distance of 10 inches from the patient's spectacle plane (representing a stimulus to

accommodation of 4.00D), placement of the retinoscope peephole at a distance of 11.5 inches (representing a stimulus to accommodation of approximately 3.50D) would cause a "hidden" lag of accommodation of 0.50D. Greenspan (1975) and others have studied MEM retinoscopy, particularly with regard to its utilization in prescribing near-point lenses for children. [The discussions of Bieber (1974) and Greenspan (1975) are recommended reading for those interested in more information on the various possible applications of MEM retinoscopy.]

Near retinoscopy

Mohindra (1977b, 1980a, 1980b) has advocated a form of retinoscopy—which she calls *near retinoscopy*—for use in determining the refractive state of infants and children. Near retinoscopy differs from other forms of dynamic retinoscopy in the following ways: (1) it is performed in complete darkness, the only illumination in the room being that supplied by the retinoscope, with the child fixating the retinoscope light; (2) it is a monocular procedure, the eye not being examined being occluded; and (3) an adjustment factor of −1.25D is algebraically combined with the spherical component of the gross spherocylindrical lens powers. The factor of −1.25D (which is equivalent to subtracting 1.25D due to a lag of accommodation, although Mohindra apparently does not view it as a lag of accommodation) was determined by comparing near retinoscopy findings with static retinoscopy and subjective findings.

Mohindra (1977b, 1980a) suggests that the child be seated on the parent's lap, facing the examiner, and that the intensity of the retinoscope light be kept to a minimum. The examiner encourages the child to fixate the light by ringing bells or by making animal sounds. In studies comparing near retinoscopy results with results of subjective refraction in adults (Mohindra, 1977a), and in studies comparing near retinoscopy results with those of cycloplegic retinoscopy in schoolchildren (Mohindra and Molinari, 1979), extremely high correlation coefficients have been reported. Mohindra (1977b) has concluded that near retinoscopy is a reliable and valid technique for the refraction of adults and infants.

In a study reported by Maino et al. (1984), results of Mohindra's (1977b) method of retinoscopy were not found to agree with the results of cycloplegic retinoscopy. These investigators examined 311 children between the ages of 18 and 48 months, using both Mohindra's near retinoscopy method and standard cycloplegic retinoscopy. Maino et al. found that the predictive value (percent agreement with cycloplegic retinoscopy) of near retinoscopy was very low and concluded that it was not a good predictor of refractive error. In addition, they concluded that the method was not capable, as a screening procedure, of identifying children having hyperopia of 3.00D or more or astigmatism of 1.00D or more. Maino et al. concluded that noncycloplegic retinoscopy as described by Mohindra should not be used in place of cycloplegic retinoscopy.

Chromoretinoscopy

Chromoretinoscopy, as described by Bobier and Sivak (1980), is a procedure whereby retinoscopy is carried out in the usual way except that the light entering the examiner's eye is limited to a specific band of wavelengths. This form of retinoscopy allows the examiner to determine the wavelength in focus in the plane of the retina when a patient fixates a target at a given distance. As described by Bobier and Sivak, the appropriate filter is placed between the retinoscope and the examiner, so the light stimulus to the patient's eye is not affected by the filter. Under these conditions the source must have a higher luminance than is ordinarily used in retinoscopy; a halogen source in conjunction with Kodak Wratten filters no. 55 and no. 25 is recommended.

In a study involving young adults, Bobier and Sivak (1978) found that when fixating a distant object the eye is focused for red light, but when focusing a near object the eye is focused for green light. This was interpreted by the authors as indicating that the eye uses its chromatic aberration to spare accommodation: focusing for red light at distance indicates an incomplete relaxation of accommodation for the distance target, whereas focusing for green light at near indicates a lag of accommodation for the near target.

In another study, Sivak and Bobier (1978) performed retinoscopy at 6m and 33cm on a group of 26 children between the ages of 2 and 6 years. Findings were taken without the use of filters and with filters having wavelengths of 615nm (red) and 530nm (green). For the older group of children (between the ages of 48 and 80 months), results were similar to those found for young adults, the children focusing for the red light at the 6m distance and for the green light at the 33cm distance. For a group of children between the ages of 40 and 61 months (note that there is some overlap in age groups), the red wavelength was found to be in focus both at 6m and at 33cm, indicating that an excessive amount of

accommodation was used at the 33cm distance. For a third group of children (between the ages of 31 and 45 months), accommodative responses were found to be mixed. For example, the youngest child focused on the green wavelength at 6m and on the red wavelength at 33 cm, thus underaccommodating at distance and overaccommodating at near; other children accommodated for an intermediate wavelength at both testing distances. On the basis of these results, Sivak and Bobier concluded that the focusing mechanism is not fully developed until the fourth year of life and that this development appears to occur in three stages: (1) in the first stage there is haphazard focusing within the chromatic aberration interval; (2) in the second stage there is selective focusing for the red end of the interval; and (3) in the third stage there is selective focusing to spare accommodation.

Although chromoretinoscopy has not yet been established as a routine clinical procedure, it appears that the results of Bobier and Sivak (1978) can provide us with a basis for understanding the sometimes confusing results found in performing both static retinoscopy and the various forms of dynamic retinoscopy, including book retinoscopy and near retinoscopy.

Radical Retinoscopy

Because of small pupils, a cataract, or other opacity of the media, the retinoscopic reflex sometimes is so faint and indistinct that it is impossible to perform static retinoscopy at the usual working distance of 67 or 50cm. When this occurs, the practitioner may find that by moving closer to the patient, an observable reflex can be obtained. This may involve a working distance as close as 20cm or even 10cm. At such close working distances, the practitioner must be careful to stay as close as possible to the patient's visual axis; otherwise rather large errors, particularly in cylinder power and axis, can be introduced.

If, for example, the examiner finds that retinoscopy is possible at a 20cm working distance, +5.00D (instead of the usual +1.50D or +2.00D) is subtracted from the lens power in the refractor. If the lens power in the refractor is $+2.00 -1.00 \times 90$, the finding is recorded as $-3.00 -1.00 \times 90$.

Retinoscopy in Screening Programs
String retinoscopy

In school visual screening programs, where speed is important and equipment needs must be kept to a

Table 8.3 Positions of beads for string retinoscopy (with patient wearing +3.00D spheres).

Myopia	3.00D	16.7cm
	2.00D	20.0cm
	1.00D	25.0cm
Emmetropia		33.3cm
Hyperopia	0.50D	40.0cm
	1.00D	50.0cm
	1.50D	66.7cm

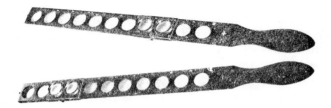

Figure 8.31   Lens bars for retinoscopy.

minimum, string retinoscopy can be used. The child wears +3.00D lenses in a plastic frame and watches a cartoon movie at a distance of 6m or more while retinoscopy is performed. The examiner uses a string attached to the retinoscope, calibrated by means of colored beads. The distance to each bead is measured from the plane of the retinoscope mirror, and the examiner moves to whatever working distance is necessary to neutralize the motion in the principal meridians of each eye. As each meridian is neutralized, the examiner holds the free end of the string up to the child's forehead, determines the finding on the basis of the position of the nearest bead, and calls off the finding to a recorder.

With the +3.00D lenses worn by the child, it is obvious that the child is emmetropic if neutrality is found at a distance of 33.3cm. A large bead is placed at that distance on the string, and smaller beads are placed at positions indicating various amounts of myopia in 1.00D steps and various amounts of

hyperopia in 0.50D steps. The positions for each of the beads are shown in Table 8.3.

Lens-bar retinoscopy

Another method of retinoscopy useful for visual screening programs involves the use of a *lens bar*, a wooden or plastic bar in which a number of lenses are mounted, designed to be moved vertically in front of the child's eye until the lens is found that produces neutrality in a particular meridian (see Figure 8.31). Two lens bars typically are used, one containing plus lenses and one containing minus lenses. For example, if a child wears +2.00D spheres while watching the cartoon, and if the examiner works at a constant distance of 50cm, the occurrence of neutrality with no lens in place (other than the +2.00D lens worn by the child) will indicate emmetropia. The use of two lens bars—one calibrated in 0.50D steps from +0.50 to +3.00D and the other calibrated in 0.50D steps from −0.50 to −3.00D—would take care of the great majority of refractive errors.

Study Questions

1. If the keratometer finding for a patient's right eye is 42.00D at 180 and 43.50D at 90, (a) what are the radii of curvature in each of the two principal meridians, using the index of refraction of 1.3375? (b) Does this eye have with-the-rule or against-the-rule astigmatism?

2. For the keratometer findings given in question 1, what would be the expected refractive astigmatism, using Javal's rule?

3. Using the plane-mirror retinoscope, in what direction does the spot of light on the patient's retina move as compared with the direction of the light on the patient's face (or on the front of the refractor) (a) if the patient is myopic with respect to the position of the retinoscope mirror? (b) if the patient is hyperopic with respect to the position of the retinoscope mirror?

4. What are two possible methods of improving keratometer accuracy?

5. If a patient has a large amount of uncorrected myopia or hyperopia, why is it difficult to see the motion of the reflex in retinoscopy?

6. What keratometric findings would lead the practitioner to suspect that a patient may have keratoconus?

7. In dynamic retinoscopy, the examiner can use either of two methods to determine the patient's lag of accommodation. Describe the two methods.

8. What advantages has the use of a refractor or phoropter as compared with the use of a trial frame and trial lenses?

9. To what extent and why is astigmatism corrected or eliminated (a) by spherical hard contact lenses? (b) by spherical soft contact lenses?

10. Using the plane-mirror retinoscope, in what direction does the reflex in the patient's pupil move, with respect to the spot or streak of light on the patient's face or on the refractor, (a) if the patient is myopic with respect to the position of the retinoscope peephole? (b) if the patient is hyperopic with respect to the position of the retinoscope peephole?

11. For what types of patients may the use of a trial frame and trial lenses be more appropriate than the use of a refractor or phoropter?

12. What would be the effect on the static retinoscopy finding (either too much plus power or too little plus) of (a) scoping at too close a working distance? (b) scoping at too great a working distance? (c) the patient looking at the retinoscope or the examiner's face rather than at the distant target?

13. What are possible sources of error in performing retinoscopy, in addition to those discussed in question 12?

14. When using the Bausch & Lomb keratometer, once the telescope eyepiece has been focused, what mechanism ensures that the telescope is kept in focus on the keratometer mire images? Describe how this mechanism works.

15. How could an examiner who is blind or amblyopic in one eye determine a patient's distance PD?

16. What should be recorded as the static retinoscopy finding if the examiner, working at a distance of 67cm, finds neutral motion in the 180-degree meridian with +2.25DS and in the 90-degree meridian with +3.50DS?

17. When calibrating a keratometer by taking a series of three readings on a ⅝-inch steel ball, what would the examiner conclude if the three readings were (a) 42.50D, 42.12D, and 42.87D? (b) 42.00D, 42.12D, and 42.00D? (c) 42.50D, 42.62D, and 42.50D?

18. List four situations in which spot retinoscopy may be superior to streak retinoscopy.

19. What should the examiner record as the static retinoscopy finding if, at a working distance of 50cm, neutral motion is found in the 90-degree meridian with plano and in the 180-degree meridian with +1.00DS?

20. What is radical retinoscopy? In what situations is it used?

21. Using chromoretinoscopy on adults, (a) what did Bobier and Sivak find? (b) what did they conclude on the basis of their findings?

22. In performing string retinoscopy as a vision screening test, the child watches a cartoon movie at a distance of 6m while wearing +3.00D lenses. What would be the refractive error if neutrality was found when the retinoscope mirror was located at each of the following distances: (a) 33cm; (b) 50cm; (c) 25cm.

23. When Bobier and Sivak used chromoretinoscopy on children, (a) how did their findings differ from those on adults? (b) how did they interpret these findings?

24. What would be the expected subjectively determined astigmatism as determined by (a) Javal's rule and (b) the modification of Javal's rule suggested by Grosvenor, Quintero, and Perrigin, for each of the following keratometer findings: (a) 43.00 at 180/42.00 at 90? (b) 42.50 at 180/42.50 at 90? (c) 42.00 at 180/43.00 at 90? (d) 41.00 at 180/43.50 at 90?

CHAPTER 9

Subjective Refraction

PRINCIPLES OF SUBJECTIVE REFRACTION

The purpose of subjective refraction is to determine, by subjective means, the combination of spherical and cylindrical lenses necessary to artificially place the far-point of each of the patient's eyes at infinity. This is the combination of lenses that provides the best possible visual acuity *with accommodation relaxed*. To make sure accommodation is relaxed, each eye is *fogged* by placing enough plus lens power in front of the eye to ensure that the image formed by the eye's optical system will be located in front of the retina (see Figure 9.1a), making the eye artificially myopic. With the image in this position, any effort to accommodate will result in poorer vision rather than better, in that the increased vergence of the light rays due to accommodation will move the image even farther forward. If the eyes were not fogged before the subjective refraction was begun, it is possible that the image formed by the eye's optical system would be located behind the retina. If this were the case (see Figure 9.1b), any effort to accommodate could focus the image sharply on the retina, and the resulting refractive correction would be of insufficient plus or excessive minus lens power.

Refraction with No Astigmatism

If it were not for the existence of astigmatism, subjective refraction would be a relatively simple procedure. All that would be necessary would be for the examiner to place enough plus lens power in front of each eye to fog vision to 20/40 or 20/50 and then reduce the power until clear vision was obtained.

Assume that for a given eye the fogging lens necessary for 20/50 vision is +1.75D sphere. The blur circle for each object point will be large, as shown in Figure 9.1a. As we reduce the plus lens power 0.25D at a time, the patient will be able to read successively smaller rows of letters until the 20/20 or possibly the 20/15 letters can be read. Assume that this occurs when a +0.75D sphere is in the refractor. Further reduction in plus lens power would stimulate the eye's accommodative mechanism, so vision would continue to be clear.

The end-point criterion used in subjective refraction is the "maximum plus lens power for best visual acuity." Once the patient's best visual acuity has been achieved, the removal of additional plus lens power (or the addition of minus lens power) will stimulate accommodation and can (but will not necessarily) make the letters appear smaller. The examiner should return to the maximum plus (or minimum minus) power that provides the patient's best visual acuity.

Figure 9.1 The fogging principle: (a) with sufficient plus lens power, the eye is made artificially myopic, and any attempt to accommodate will increase the size of the blur circle on the retina; (b) an unfogged eye is free to accommodate, making the retinal blur circle smaller.

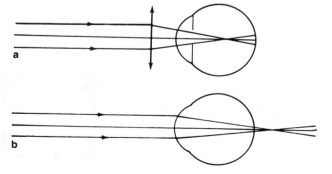

259

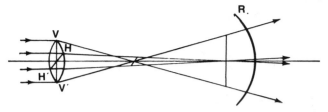

Figure 9.2   Astigmatic imagery. The refraction of the eye is assumed to take place at the aperture VHV'H', and *R* represents the retina.

Astigmatic Imagery

When astigmatism is present, as it is in the great majority of eyes, a point image does not exist for a point object. In Figure 9.2 it is assumed that the refraction of the eye takes place at the aperture VHV'H' and that the refracting power of the eye is at a maximum in the vertical meridian and at a minimum in the horizontal meridian. This is with-the-rule astigmatism.

Inspection of Figure 9.2 will indicate that the rays of light traveling in the vertical meridian will form the horizontal focal line, whereas the rays of light traveling in the horizontal meridian will form the vertical focal line. Because the refracting power is greatest in the vertical meridian (with-the-rule astigmatism), it follows that the horizontal focal line is formed closer to the aperture of the optical system than is the vertical focal line.

For an astigmatic eye, the closest thing to a point image for a point object is the *circle of least confusion*, located at the dioptric midpoint between the horizontal and vertical focal lines. At all image planes other than those occupied by the two focal lines and the circle of least confusion, images are in the form

of *blur ellipses* (note that a blur ellipse for an astigmatic optical system is analogous to a blur circle for a spherical optical system).

Referring again to Figure 9.2, if an eye having with-the-rule astigmatism is fogged sufficiently so both focal lines are located in front of the retina (indicated by *R* in the diagram), the vertical focal line will be closer to the retina than the horizontal focal line. The retinal image for a point object will be in the form of a vertically elongated blur ellipse: if presented with vertical and horizontal line objects, the patient will report that the vertical line is the more distinct of the two.

Astigmatic Chart

The two most commonly used *astigmatic charts* are the *clock dial* and the *rotating T* (see Figure 9.3). Before using either of these charts, sufficient plus lens power is placed in front of the patient's eye to insure that the entire conoid of Sturm will be located in front of the retina. The principles involved in each of these astigmatic charts are the same. Once the examiner has located the two principal meridians of the eye, parallel lines (usually triple lines) are presented in meridians parallel to the eye's principal meridians, and the patient is asked to report which of the two sets of lines appears to be more distinct.

Consider a patient whose principal meridians (right eye) have been found to be 180 and 90 degrees. The patient is asked to observe horizontally and vertically oriented sets of parallel lines, as shown in Figure 9.4. Assume that the patient has with-the-rule astigmatism: the vertical focal line, for a point object, will be closer to the retina than the horizontal focal line (as shown in Figure 9.2). If we consider each line on the chart (Figure 9.4) to be made up of an infinite number of points, it is obvious that each of these

Figure 9.3   Charts for determining cylinder power and axis under fog: *(a)* clock dial chart; *(b)* rotating *T*; *(c)* radial line chart for determining cylinder axis for the rotating *T* test.

Figure 9.4   *(a)* Target consisting of parallel lines oriented at 180 and 90 degrees; *(b)* appearance of target shown in *(a)* for an eye having uncorrected with-the-rule astigmatism.

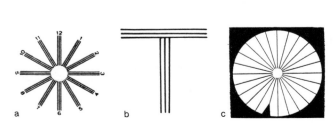

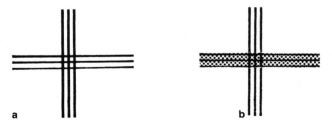

points will form a vertically elongated blur ellipse on the patient's retina. This being the case, each of the three vertical lines will appear to be elongated, while each of the three horizontal lines will appear to be widened (as shown in Figure 9.4b); therefore, the vertical lines will appear to be more distinct than the horizontal lines.

Clock Dial

When the *clock dial* is presented to the patient under sufficient fog, the examiner's first job is to determine the axis of the correcting cylinder. This is done by first asking the patient if he or she can see three lines in any or all of the spokes. If the answer is affirmative, the patient is asked to report in which of the spokes the three lines are the sharpest or most distinct. Most clock dial charts are equipped with numbers similar to those on the face of a clock, and the expected response of the patient is that the spoke from 12 to 6, from 1 to 7, from 2 to 8 o'clock, and so forth, is the most distinct. To determine the axis of the correcting cylinder, the smaller of the two numbers reported by the patient is multiplied by 30. For example, if the patient reports that the 12 to 6 o'clock spoke is the most distinct, the examiner would place the axis of the correcting cylinder at 180 degrees; if the patient reports the 1 to 7 o'clock spoke as the most distinct, the axis of the correcting cylinder would be placed at 30 degrees.

The examiner then begins adding minus cylinder power, 0.25D at a time (with the axis set at the indicated meridian), questioning the patient each time as to the relative sharpness or distinctness of the lines in the spokes representing the two principal meridians of the eye (12 to 6 compared to 3 to 9; 1 to 7 compared with 4 to 10, and so forth). As shown in Figure 9.5, for with-the-rule astigmatism the addition of minus cylinder power, axis 180 degrees, will move the horizontal focal line and the circle of least confusion toward the retina but will not alter the position of the vertical focal line. If sufficient minus cylinder power is added, the horizontal and vertical focal lines will be located in the same plane, so the patient will report that the 12–6 and the 3–9 spokes are equally distinct. This procedure is referred to as "collapsing the conoid of Sturm," and the vertical and horizontal focal lines are replaced by a point image. However, because this point image is not on the retina, the image on the retina will be a blur circle.

When the patient reports that the 12–6 and the 3–9 spokes are equally clear, the examiner adds

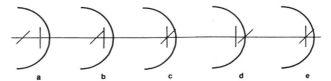

Figure 9.5 *(a)* **Correcting with-the-rule astigmatism under fog. As minus cylinder power, axis 180, is increased *(b)*, the point of equality is reached *(c)*, then a reversal occurs *(d)*, and with a reduction of 0.25D cylinder, equality is again obtained *(e)*.**

additional cylindrical power, 0.25D at a time, until a reversal is obtained (the patient reports that the 3–9 spoke is now more distinct than the 12–6 spoke). A reversal should be expected with the addition of only 0.25D of cylinder power beyond equality in most cases.

The Rotating *T*

When the *rotating T* is used for the determination of the cylinder power and axis under fog, the examiner can determine the axis of the correcting cylinder by either of two methods. The first method involves the use of a radial line chart (see Figure 9.3c) provided with a pointer. As the examiner slowly moves the pointer, the patient is asked to indicate which of the radial lines is the most distinct. For example, if the vertical line is reported to be the most distinct, the examiner leaves the pointer in the vertical position and then orients the rotating *T* in the 90- to 180-degree position (as shown in Figure 9.3b). In the Bausch & Lomb chart projector, the pointer and the rotating *T* are geared together so the orientation of the rotating *T* is similar to that of the pointer.

The second method of determining the axis of the correcting cylinder is by slowly rotating the rotating *T*, and instructing the patient to report when the stem and the crossbar of the *T* are equally distinct. This will occur when the stem and the crossbar are each located 45 degrees from a principal meridian, so when this point is reached, the examiner simply rotates the *T* 45 degrees in either direction to place the two limbs of the *T* parallel to the two principal meridians of the patient's eye.

To determine cylinder power, the same procedure is used as described for the clock dial. Minus cylinder power is added, 0.25D at a time, with the axis in the less distinct of the two meridians until the patient first reports equality and then a reversal. The minus cylinder power is then reduced to the point of equality.

The Jackson Crossed Cylinder

When the cylindrical correction has been determined under fog by means of the astigmatic chart, the fogging lenses are removed and the cylinder power and axis are refined by means of the *Jackson crossed cylinder*. This is a lens having a minus cylinder ground on one side and a plus cylinder ground on the other side, the two axes being located 90 degrees apart. Jackson crossed cylinders are supplied in modern refractors in three powers: ±0.25D, ±0.37D, and ±0.50D.

When the Jackson crossed cylinder, often called the *flip cylinder*, is used to refine cylinder power, it is oriented in front of the refractor lens cell in such a way that the principal meridians of the crossed cylinder are located parallel to the principal meridians of the correcting lens. As shown in Figure 9.6a, if the axis of the correcting cylinder in the refractor is located at 180 degrees, the crossed cylinder is oriented so its two principal meridians are located at 180 and 90 degrees. Therefore, when the ±0.25D crossed cylinder is used to refine cylinder power, in one position 0.25D of minus cylinder is added to the power of the cylinder in the refractor, and in the other position 0.25D of minus cylinder power is subtracted from the cylinder in the refractor. The position is changed simply by flipping the crossed cylinder lens over so the patient looks through the opposite side.

When used as a test for cylinder power, the advantage of the Jackson crossed cylinder is that it can add or subtract cylindrical power relative to the correcting cylinder in the refractor without changing spherical power; that is, the same spherical equivalent power is maintained throughout the test. For example, if the correcting lenses in the refractor have the power

$$+1.00DS \ -0.50DC \ \times \ 180,$$

and a ±0.25D crossed cylinder is used (+0.25DS −0.50DC in one position and −0.25DS +0.50DC in the other position), the power of the combination of the refractor lenses and the crossed cylinder will be

$$+1.25DS \ -1.00DC \ \times \ 180$$

in one position and

$$+0.75DS \ -0.00DC \ \times \ 180$$

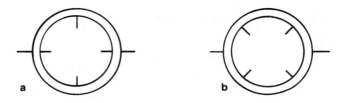

Figure 9.6   **Orientation of Jackson's crossed cylinder when used to refine (a) cylinder power and (b) cylinder axis. In each case the outer circle represents the correcting cylinder (axis 180) and the inner circle represents the crossed cylinder.**

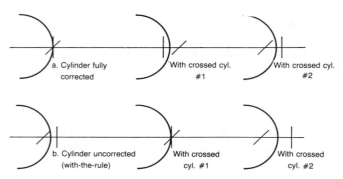

a. Cylinder fully corrected

With crossed cyl. #1

With crossed cyl. #2

b. Cylinder uncorrected (with-the-rule)

With crossed cyl. #1

With crossed cyl. #2

Figure 9.7   **Positions of focal lines when crossed cylinder is used to refine cylinder power. (a) When with-the-rule astigmatism has been fully corrected, views 1 and 2 are equally clear; (b) when with-the-rule astigmatism has not been fully corrected, view 1 (additional cylinder) is reported to be clearer than view 2 (less cylinder).**

in the other position. It is obvious that in each position of the crossed cylinder, the spherical equivalent of the combination is 0.75D.

Figure 9.7 shows what happens to the positions of the horizontal and vertical focal lines, with respect to the retina, when the crossed cylinder is used to refine cylinder power. Because the crossed cylinder test is done without fog, it follows that if the patient's astigmatism were fully corrected in the astigmatic chart test, the horizontal and vertical focal lines would coincide at the retina. As a result, the retinal image of each object point would be a point (although shown as a cross in the first diagram of Figure 9.7). If the crossed cylinder now is placed in front of the refractor lens cell with its minus axis oriented at 180 degrees (the crossed cylinder now having a power of +0.25DS −0.50DC × 180), the vergence of the light rays traveling in the horizontal meridian will increase, while the vergence of the rays in the vertical meridian will decrease. The result will be a vertical focal line located in front of the retina and a horizontal focal line located behind the retina (as shown in the second diagram in Figure 9.7a), thus blurring the image of the letters or other visual acuity target. Flipping the lens over so the minus axis is now located at 90 degrees (the crossed cylinder now having a power of +0.25DS −0.50DC × 90), a horizontal focal line will be formed in front of the retina and a vertical focal line behind the retina, as shown in the third diagram in Figure 9.7a. The retinal image of the chart again is blurred. The patient would be expected to report that the crossed cylinder lens blurred the target equally in positions 1 and 2.

The situation occurring when the patient's astigmatism is not fully corrected, at the start of the test, is shown in Figure 9.7b. In the defogged situation, uncorrected or undercorrected with-the-rule astigmatism would result in the horizontal focal line being located in front of the retina and the vertical focal line behind the retina. Placing the crossed cylinder with the minus axis at 180 (parallel to the axis of the correcting cylinder in the refractor) will cause the vertical focal line to move forward and the horizontal focal line to move backward, as shown in the second diagram in Figure 9.7b. Thus, both focal lines will move toward or onto the retina. When the crossed cylinder is flipped over, each focal line will move farther from the retina, as shown in the third diagram of Figure 9.7b. The result will be that the patient will report that the target is more distinct for position 1 than for position 2.

When the crossed cylinder is used to refine cylinder axis, it is oriented in front of the refractor lens cell so its two principal meridians are located at an angle of 45 degrees from the two principal meridians of the correcting lens. As shown in Figure 9.6b,

if the axis of the correcting cylinder in the refractor is located at 180 degrees, the crossed cylinder is oriented so its two principal meridians are located at 45 and 135 degrees. Therefore, when the ±0.25D crossed cylinder is used to refine cylinder axis, in one position the axis of the combination (the correcting cylinder and the crossed cylinder) is moved in one direction; when it is flipped over to the other side, the position of the axis of the combination of the correcting cylinder and the crossed cylinder is moved an equal amount in the opposite direction.

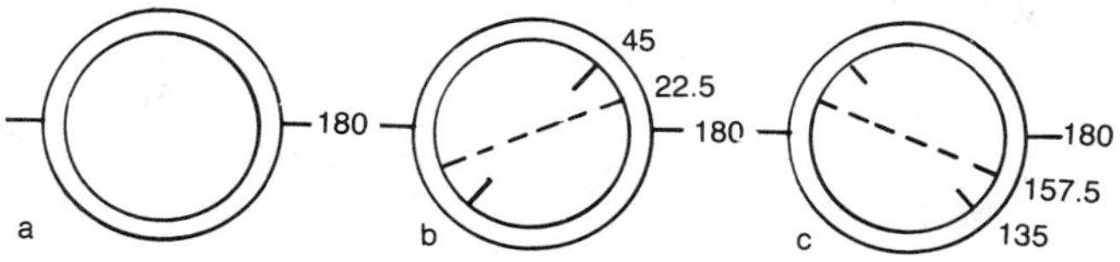

Recall our example using correcting lenses in the refractor having the power +1.00DS −0.50DC × 180 (see Figure 9.8). In one position the combined power of the correcting cylinder and the crossed cylinder would be

$$+1.00DS\ -0.50DC\ \times\ 180$$

combined with

$$+0.25DS\ -0.50DC\ \times\ 45.$$

Using the formulas and graphic construction for resolving obliquely crossed cylinders, this resolves to

$$+0.49DS\ -0.72DC\ \times\ 22.5.$$

In the other position of the crossed cylinder, we have

$$+1.00DS\ -0.50DC\ \times\ 180$$

combined with

$$+0.25DS\ -0.50DC\ \times\ 135,$$

which resolves to

$$+0.49DS\ -0.72DC\ \times\ 157.5.$$

It should be understood that this example is a special case of obliquely crossed cylinders, since the two cylinders are of the same power. In such a case the power of the resultant cylinder is equal to the power of either of the two cylinders multiplied by the square root of 2 (or 1.414), and the resultant axis is halfway between the axes of the two cylinders. If the correcting cylinder and the crossed cylinder are not of the same power, the axis of the combination will be displaced an equal amount in each of the two positions of the crossed cylinder. However, the axis of the combination, as well as the power of the combination, will depend on the individual powers of the correcting cylinder and the crossed cylinder. (The method for resolving obliquely crossed cylinders can be found in most ophthalmic optics textbooks.)

Figure 9.8 *(a)* **Correcting cylinder −0.50 × 180;** *(b)* **combined with +0.25 sphere −0.50 × 45;** *(c)* **combined with +0.25 sphere −0.50 × 135. The resultant cylinder axis in** *(b)* **is 22.5 degrees and in** *(c)* **157.5 degrees.**

MONOCULAR SUBJECTIVE REFRACTION

Monocular subjective refraction consists of the following procedures: (1) determining the cylindrical correction under fog, (2) refining the cylindrical correction without fog, and (3) determining the spherical end-point. Following these procedures, one or more binocular balancing tests are performed.

Determining the Cylinder Under Fog

On completion of static retinoscopy, the patient will be fogged by the plus power of the working distance lenses, either +1.50 or +2.00D. (If dynamic retinoscopy has been performed, suitable fogging lenses will have to be put into place before beginning the monocular subjective refraction.) The left eye is occluded (as a general rule, all optometric tests are done first on the right eye). A block of letters is introduced at the 6m distance, consisting of several lines of letters ranging from 20/50 or 20/40 to 20/20 or 20/15. Plus power in front of the right eye is reduced, 0.25D at a time, until the patient can read all of the 20/40 letters but only a few 20/30 letters. The criterion "all of the 20/40 letters but only a few 20/30 letters" ensures that the eye is fogged by approximately 1.00D, so the entire conoid of Sturm is in front of the retina.

The cylindrical lenses are removed, the astigmatic chart is presented, and the axis of the correcting cylinder is determined. If the clock dial is used, the patient is asked first whether three lines can be seen in any or all of the spokes. If they can be seen, the patient is asked to report in which of the spokes the three lines are the most distinct. The axis of the correcting cylinder in the refractor is set 90 degrees from the position of the sharpest spoke reported by the patient (by multiplying the "o'clock" position by 30). If the rotating T is used, the axis of the correcting cylinder is determined either by instructing the patient to report which of the lines in the radial line target is the most distinct, or by rotating the T until the patient reports that the stem and the crossbar of the T are equally blurred, and then rotating the T to a position 45 degrees away.

Minus cylinder power is then added at the indicated axis 0.25D at a time until equality is obtained. Additional minus cylinder power is then added 0.25D at a time to obtain a reversal, the examiner then returning to the lowest-power cylinder that brings about equality.

The right eye is then occluded, and the procedures are repeated for the left eye. Whereas the experienced practitioner would probably perform the entire monocular subjective sequence on the right eye before proceeding to the left eye, the beginner is advised to perform each of the three parts of the monocular subjective refraction first on the right eye and then on the left eye. If each eye is tested for a prolonged period of time, there is a possibility that the second eye tested (the left eye) will be light adapted at the end of the procedure to the extent that difficulties will be encountered in performing the binocular balancing tests.

Refining the Cylinder Without Fog

On completion of the astigmatic chart test, the left eye is occluded and testing is again begun on the right eye. The right eye is defogged, reducing plus lens power 0.25D at a time, until the best visual acuity line (20/20 or 20/15) is read according to the criterion "maximum plus power for best acuity." When the removal of additional plus power (or the addition of minus power) fails to improve visual acuity, the spherical lens power is returned to the maximum plus or minimum minus power that resulted in the best visual acuity for that eye.

Beginning with the cylinder power and axis found with the astigmatic chart under fog (or in retinoscopy if the astigmatic chart has not been used), the practitioner first refines cylinder axis and then cylinder power. However, if no cylinder was found in retinoscopy or with the astigmatic chart, the practitioner can use the crossed-cylinder test for power before the test for axis to "fish" for cylinder.

Crossed-cylinder test for axis

The crossed cylinder is oriented in front of the lens cell for the right eye so its minus axis is oriented 45 degrees from the minus axis of the correcting cylinder. Because the crossed cylinder will blur the letters somewhat (in either of the two positions), the patient's attention is called to a row of letters somewhat larger than the best acuity line. If the patient's best visual acuity is 20/20 or 20/15, it is convenient to use the 20/30 letters, presenting the patient with a block of letters extending from 20/30 down to 20/15 or 20/10.

The patient is instructed to watch the top (20/30) row of letters and is told that he or she will be shown the letters in each of two positions, that the letters will be blurred somewhat in both positions. He or she is then instructed to report which way the letters are more distinct or easier to read, in position 1 or in position 2. The patient is allowed to observe the letters for a second or two in position 1, after which the lens is "flipped." The patient is then allowed to observe the letters for a second or two in position 2.

If the patient reports that the letters are equally distinct for the two positions of the crossed cylinder, the examiner can conclude that the axis of the cylindrical lens in the refractor is correct, and the test can be discontinued. In this situation, the patient may report that the letters "slant in one direction in position 1 and in the other direction in position 2." This is good evidence that the cylinder axis is correct.

If the patient reports that the letters are not equally distinct for the two positions, the axis of the cylindrical lens in the refractor is rotated 10 or 15 degrees in the direction of the minus cylinder axis for the position in which the letters were more distinct, and the procedure is repeated. For example, if the axis of the correcting cylinder is 180 degrees and the patient reports that the letters are more distinct when the crossed cylinder has its axis at 45 degrees (as opposed to 135 degrees), the axis of the correcting cylinder in the refractor is rotated toward 45 degrees—say to 15 degrees. The crossed cylinder is also moved to the 15-degree position and the test is repeated. (However, with the American Optical Rx-Master phoroptor, the crossed cylinder is geared in such a manner that its axis changes when the axis of the correcting cylinder is changed.)

On repetition of the test, the patient may report that the letters are more distinct either when the minus axis is in the position toward or in the position away from the original cylinder axis. In either case, the axis is moved a smaller amount (usually 5 degrees) in the direction corresponding to that of the minus axis of the crossed cylinder for the more distinct position, and the test is repeated. The end-point of the test occurs when the patient reports that the two positions are equally distinct.

Borish (1972) suggested that instead of being asked to watch only one row of letters during the crossed-cylinder test, the patient should be instructed to begin with the top row of letters and then to look at the letters in the next several rows, reporting on the position of the lens that enables him or her to read *farther down on the chart*. The author has found that this method of patient instruction works well.

Crossed-cylinder test for power

The crossed cylinder is placed in front of the lens well for the right eye so that the axis of the crossed cylinder is either parallel or perpendicular to that of the correcting cylinder. The patient is instructed to watch the 20/30 row of letters and is told that the letters will be shown with the lens in each of two positions. The patient is also told that the letters will be somewhat blurred in each position but that he or she is to report the position in which the letters are more distinct and easier to read. The patient is allowed to observe the letters for a second or two in position 1 before the lens is flipped, and the patient then is allowed to observe the letters for a second or two in position 2.

If the patient reports the letters are more distinct when the axis meridian (indicated by red lines or dots) corresponds to the minus axis of the correcting cylinder, an additional 0.25D cylinder is added to the lenses in the refractor, and the test is repeated. If the patient reports the letters are more distinct when the axis meridian is 90 degrees from the meridian of the minus axis of the correcting cylinder, the cylinder in the refractor is reduced by 0.25D, and the test is repeated. If the patient reports the letters are equally distinct and easy to read in each of the two positions, the cylinder power is considered to be correct, and the test is not repeated. Further, when cylinder power is added during the crossed-cylinder test, +0.25D sphere should be added for each −0.50D cylinder to maintain the same spherical equivalent.

If the astigmatic chart test has been performed correctly, the cylinder power found on the crossed-cylinder test should seldom vary by more than 0.25D from that found with the astigmatic chart. If retinoscopy has been done correctly, the cylinder power found in the crossed-cylinder test should not differ by more than 0.25D from that found in retinoscopy. In some cases the results of the crossed-cylinder test for power depend on whether the patient has previously worn a correction for astigmatism. The patient who has worn a correction for astigmatism for some time will usually accept, in the crossed-cylinder test for power, the full amount of cylinder found in retinoscopy or by means of the astigmatic chart. However, the patient who has never worn a full correction for astigmatism will often reject, in the crossed-cylinder test, some (or all) of the cylindrical power found in retinoscopy or by means of the astigmatic chart.

Patients respond to the crossed-cylinder test for axis and power with varying degrees of difficulty and frustration. Many patients have no trouble "making up their minds," but others have great difficulty and ask the examiner to repeat the test one or more times in each position of the correcting cylinder. It is often helpful to tell the patient who has difficulty responding, that what we are looking for is the position in which there is *no difference* between positions 1 and 2. Many patients are greatly relieved to know this, particularly if all presentations have looked much the same since the beginning of the test.

Additional cylinder check tests

Additional check tests are available for both cylinder power and axis.

Power. As noted earlier, many patients tend to reject cylinder power in the crossed-cylinder test even though it has been evident both in retinoscopy and in the astigmatic chart test. When this occurs, the patient is asked to watch the smallest readable row of letters, with the crossed cylinder removed (usually either 20/20 or 20/15). An additional −0.25D of cylinder is placed in the refractor, and the patient is asked to report which of the two views appears to be more distinct. If the additional −0.25D cylinder does not improve the clarity of the letters (or if it blurs them), the original cylinder power is left in the refractor. However, if the additional cylindrical power causes the letters to be more distinct, the examiner can choose to leave the additional cylindrical power in the refractor. If the difference between the crossed cylinder and the astigmatic chart (or retinoscopy) is more than 0.25D, the examiner may wish to add additional minus cylinder power, 0.25D at a time. However, for each −0.50D of cylindrical power added, +0.25D of spherical power should be added to keep the plane of the image at or near the retina.

Axis. The additional cylinder check test for axis is sometimes referred to as *bracketing*, and it is useful mainly when the power of the correcting cylinder is 1.00D or more. The patient is asked to view a row of 20/20 or 20/15 letters (again, with the crossed-cylinder removed) and to report when the letters blur as the cylindrical lens in the refractor is slowly rotated in one direction. When a blur is reported, the change in the axis is noted mentally, and the test is repeated with the same instructions, the lens being rotated in the opposite direction. The amount of rotation in the two directions is then compared.

For example, if the original correcting cylinder axis is located at 180 degrees and the patient reports a blur at 15 degrees and again at 165 degrees, the examiner can assume that the original axis was correct. However, if a blur is reported at 20 degrees and again at 170 degrees, the original axis is in question, and the test should be repeated after placing the axis of the correcting cylinder at 5 degrees (halfway between the two positions where a blur was reported). Repetition of the test should confirm that the new axis (5 degrees) is correct.

The patient's right eye should now be occluded, and the crossed-cylinder tests for power and axis, as well as additional check tests if indicated, should be performed on the left eye.

Determining the Spherical End-Point

When the tests for refining cylinder axis and power without fog have been completed, each eye is fogged 0.75 or 1.00D and defogged to best acuity, again using the criterion "maximum plus power for best visual acuity." While the fogging and defogging are done, the examiner should continue to present a block of letters extending from 20/40 or 20/30 to 20/15.

The examiner should make a mental note of the patient's acuity for each eye through the +0.75 or +1.00D fogging lens prior to defogging. Even though binocular balancing tests will be done after the monocular subjective finding has been completed, it is important that accommodation be relaxed (and relaxed equally for the two eyes) in arriving at the monocular subjective end-point. For example, +1.00D of fog may blur the right eye to 20/30 (which should be expected), but it may blur the left eye only to 20/20. This is evidence that the left eye is under-plussed (or overminused), and the subjective end-points for both eyes should be determined again.

Patient instructions

In determining the monocular subjective end-point, correct patient instructions are of utmost importance. The examiner should understand that the patient's subjective evaluation of the clarity or distinctness of the letters is not the important consideration. The important, overriding consideration is the ability of the patient to resolve the letters.

As plus power is decreased (or minus power increased) 0.25D at a time, the patient should be asked to read aloud as many letters as possible, proceeding downward from one line to the next. When the point has been reached where an additional decrease in plus power of 0.25D does not make any more letters readable, the previous lens power in the refractor satisfied the criterion "maximum plus for best acuity." On the other hand, if the examiner allows the patient to respond in terms of clarity of the letters or in terms of which lens power is preferred, many young patients will continue to accommodate with each 0.25D of reduction in plus, with the result that the end-point will be completely invalid. In this author's experience, not a semester goes by without a second- or third-year student ending up with a subjective finding of −1.00DS on a patient whose entering acuity (with no lenses) was 20/15!

When minus lens power is added to the point that accommodation is necessary to keep the letters in sharp focus on the retina, many patients will notice that the letters appear to be smaller. This is a purely optical effect, know as *accommodative micropsia*, but patients differ in their ability to detect this decrease in image size. Therefore, the examiner is not advised to count on the patient's report that the letters look smaller to avoid overminusing the patient. It is all right to ask the patient if the letters look smaller as minus power is added in the presence of 20/20 or 20/15 acuity, but the patient's report that the letters are not smaller should *not* be taken as evidence that the patient is not overminused.

Concept of "standard acuity"

In the procedures recommended by the Optometric Extension Program (OEP) as described by Lesser (1969), the criterion for the subjective end-point is 20/20 without a blur. This criterion is based on the notion that 20/20 represents "standard acuity" for everyone, but it overlooks the fact that close to 50 percent of the population is capable of 20/15 acuity, and about 5 percent is capable of 20/10 acuity. The use of this criterion results in overplussing many patients by 0.25D (and occasionally by 0.50D) when compared with the criterion of "maximum plus for best acuity," so few practitioners apply the OEP criterion rigorously.

The examiner is advised to use a projector slide that includes a line of 20/10 letters and to regularly present this line to any patient who reads all of the 20/15 letters with no difficulty. Otherwise, the 1 patient out of 20 who is capable of 20/10 acuity may be overplussed.

BINOCULAR BALANCE

The purpose of binocular balancing tests is not to balance the visual acuity but to balance the *state of accommodation* of the two eyes. If the corrected

visual acuity is the same for the two eyes, the balancing procedure may consist of a comparison of the visual acuity for the two eyes. However, if corrected acuity has not been found to be the same for both eyes, a method not based on visual acuity must be used.

Procedures used for balancing the state of accommodation for the two eyes are often referred to as *equalization tests* or as *binocular balancing tests*. The latter term is used to differentiate these tests from binocular refraction procedures. Binocular refraction typically involves a peripheral fusion lock and a monocularly viewed central area and is discussed in a later section of this chapter and in Chapter 10.

Although some writers have advocated that the accommodative state of the eyes should be balanced while the patient is fogged by 1.00D or more of plus lens power, the recommended procedure is to balance with little or no fog, after which the eyes are fogged binocularly and defogged for best visual acuity.

Balancing with Little or No Fog

On completion of the monocular subjective refraction, the monocular subjective lenses are left in the refractor (the occluders having been removed from both eyes), and the patient's attention is called to a block of letters at 6m. Plus lens power is added in front of both eyes until the 20/20 letters are blurred but the 20/25 letters are easily resolved. This normally requires an increase in plus or a decrease in minus of 0.25 or 0.50D. The patient is then asked to compare the clarity of the 20/25 letters for the two eyes, using either prism dissociation or alternate occlusion.

Prism dissociation

The examiner places 3Δ of base-down prism in front of the right eye and 3Δ of base-up prism in front of the left eye. The patient will see two charts, separated vertically, the upper chart being seen by the right eye. (If the patient has a lateral phoria, the two charts will be separated horizontally as well as vertically.) The patient's attention is called to the 20/25 line of letters (e.g., it can be called "the second line from the top") and is asked to report whether the letters are more distinct or easier to read in the upper chart or the lower chart. If the two 20/25 lines are equally distinct for the two eyes, the accommodative state of the two eyes is considered to be balanced, and the test is over.

If the patient reports a difference in clarity of the

letters for the two eyes, +0.25D is added in front of the eye with the better vision, and the test is repeated. Often the patient fails to report equal clarity for any lens combination. For example, for the first comparison the patient may report that the letters are more distinct for the right eye, but when a +0.25D sphere is added in front of the right eye, the patient reports that the letters are now more distinct with the left eye. This problem can be solved by instructing the patient to report "which of the two lens combinations causes the upper and lower charts to be more nearly equal" or words to that effect while presenting the two arrangements (with and without the additional +0.25D in front of the right eye). Another way of resolving this difficulty is to give the better acuity to the dominant eye. A third approach is to prescribe an additional 0.12D of plus lens power to the eye with the better acuity, which is not a recommended procedure. A number of studies reviewed by Bannon (1977) have indicated that refractive findings have a variability of from 0.25 to 0.50D. It is unlikely that the visual system is able to differentiate between lens powers closer than 0.25D.

Once the patient's acuity is balanced at 20/25, the patient is defogged binocularly to the criterion "maximum plus for best acuity." The comments made in the previous section concerning determination of the spherical end-point in the monocular subjective refraction also apply to the determination of the binocular end-point.

Alternate occlusion

Determining the binocular balance with alternate occlusion differs from the prism dissociation method only in that no prisms are used and the patient is instructed to compare alternate views of the chart while each eye is alternately occluded. Either the cover paddle (used for the cover test) or the occluders in the refractor can be used for occlusion. Otherwise, fogging to 20/25, adding +0.25D to the eye with better vision, and so forth, are done in the same manner described for the prism dissociation test. Carter (1973), who recommends that balancing be done with 20/25 acuity as described here, prefers prism dissociation to alternate occlusion, because it is more difficult for the patient to make a successive comparison judgment than a simultaneous comparison judgment.

Balancing with no fog

Giles (1965) described a balancing test without the use of fog, which makes use of either the prism dissociation or alternate occlusion method. Using either method, the patient is presented a line of 6/6 (20/20) letters for each eye and is asked which of the two lines of letters is clearer. Equalization of acuity is brought about by adding plus lens power in front of the eye with the better acuity. After equalizing the visual acuity for the two eyes, Giles uncovered both eyes. As the patient read the smallest line of letters that could be read monocularly, he added plus lens power 0.25D at a time until the patient reported blurring of the letters. The most plus power that caused no blur of the letters was recorded as the binocular subjective finding.

In the author's experience, balancing with no fog or with a minimum of fog succeeds well as long as the monocular subjective refraction has been completed by "coming out of the fog" with each eye, and the same end-point criterion has been used for each eye. Using this procedure, the eyes are seldom found to be out of balance by more than 0.25D.

Check test for the binocular end-point

Once the examiner is satisfied with the binocular balance, the binocular end-point can be verified by the following procedure.

The patient's attention is called to the 20/20 letters, and he or she is asked if any difference in clarity of the letters is noted as a +0.25D sphere is added in front of both eyes. The same question is again asked as a second +0.25D sphere is added, and again as a third +0.25D sphere is added. Expected responses are that the 20/20 letters will be "slightly blurred" with the first 0.25D of plus, "badly blurred" with the second 0.25D, and "blurred out" with the third 0.25D.

If the 20/20 letters are still easily readable with +0.75D added to the binocular subjective finding, it is obvious that the patient's accommodation was not completely relaxed during the subjective examination. On the other hand, if the 20/20 letters are blurred out with only 0.25D of added plus power, it is possible that the examiner was "pushing plus" in the subjective examination.

Bichrome Test

The prism dissociation and alternate occlusion tests are useful only when the corrected visual acuity is equal or nearly equal for the two eyes. If the maximum acuities found in the monocular subjective refraction differ by as much as several letters (less than a whole line difference), it is imperative that a test not based on visual acuity be used. The most convenient test of this type is the *bichrome test*.

The bichrome test can be used either as a *monocular end-point test*, in which each eye is tested separately, or as a *binocular balancing test*, making use of either prism dissociation or alternate occlusion.

As a monocular end-point test

The bichrome test must be done in an almost completely darkened room. Starting with the results of the monocular subjective finding, +0.50 or +0.75D of spherical power is placed in front of each eye. The red and green filters (red on the left side and green on the right side) are placed in the projector, along with the side-by-side letter charts or the Verhoff circles designed for use with the bichrome test. The rays of light from a green source are refracted to a greater extent than those from a red source: Therefore, if the patient is adequately fogged, the focus of the red rays will be closer to the retina than that of the green rays (as shown in Figure 9.9a), so for each object point the letters on the red side of the chart will form smaller blur circles on the retina than those on the green side.

The patient is asked to report which of the letters (or rings) are "sharper, blacker, or more distinct"—those on the red background or those on the green background. (Because the red and green filters reduce illumination in addition to throwing the optical system of the eye out of focus, the patient's attention is directed to the 20/30 or 20/40 letters. Most patients respond better to the instructions to choose the "blacker, sharper, or more distinct" letters than to choose the "clearer" letters.) As indicated in Figure 9.9a, the patient is expected to report that the letters or rings on the red background are more distinct than those on the green background. As plus lens power is reduced 0.25D at a time, at some point the patient should report that the letters or rings on the red and green backgrounds are equally distinct (see Figure 9.9b). As plus lens power is further reduced, the patient should say those on the green side are more distinct than those on the red side (see Figure 9.9c).

If the original monocular subjective end-point was correct, the patient will typically report that the red letters or rings are more distinct with +0.75, +0.50, and +0.25D of fog. When all fog has been removed, the letters or rings will appear to be equally distinct on both the red and green sides, and when an additional 0.25D of plus power is removed, the letters or rings on the green side will appear to be more distinct. The end-point criterion ordinarily

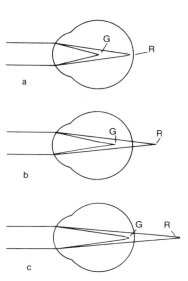

Figure 9.9 The bichrome test: *(a)* patient reports letters or rings on red side of chart are more distinct; *(b)* patient reports those on each side are equally distinct; *(c)* patient reports those on green side are more distinct.

used is the lens power at which the red and green sides of the chart appear to be equally distinct. Occasionally, the patient's response will change from "red" to "green" with only a 0.25D change in power and no report that the two sides appear to be equally sharp. When recording the bichrome test findings, it is a good idea to follow the lens powers recorded with the letters *R*, *S*, or *G*, (for *red*, *same*, or *green*).

As a binocular balancing test

When the bichrome test is used as a binocular balancing test, the prism dissociation method is used. Beginning with +0.50 or +0.75D of fog, the occluders are removed from both eyes, 3△ prism base-down is placed in front of the right eye, and 3△ prism base-up is placed in front of the left eye. The patient's attention is first called to the upper chart (seen by the right eye). The patient is asked to report which of the letters or rings—those on the red side or those on the green side—appear to be blacker, sharper, or more distinct. The expected report is "the red side," and plus lens power is reduced (in front of the right eye only) 0.25D at a time until the patient reports "both the same" and then "the green side." Then +0.25D is added to return to the situation in which the two sides are equally distinct. With each lens change, the patient should be reminded to look at the upper chart. The patient's attention is then called to the lower chart (seen by the left eye), and the process is repeated.

When the end-point has been obtained for both eyes, the lens powers for which the patient's report was "both the same" are left in the refractor. The patient is again instructed to report, first for the upper chart and then for the lower chart, whether the letters or rings are blacker, sharper, or more distinct on the red side or the green side. The expected answer, of course, is "same" for both charts. However, if the report is "same" for one chart and "red" for the other, 0.25D of plus should be placed in front of the eye for which the "same" report was given, with the expectation that "red" will be reported. Likewise, if the report is "green" for one chart and "same" for the other, 0.25D of plus should be placed in front of the eye for which "green" is reported, in the hope that "same" will then be reported. Care must be taken not to add additional minus power at this point, as this may cause the eyes to accommodate, invalidating the test.

Mandell and Allen (1960) have made the following suggestions for improving the accuracy of the bichrome test:

1. The projector screen should be in virtual darkness except for light from the projector, since any stray light will seriously reduce the sensitivity of the test.
2. The projector should be in excellent condition: the optics should be clean, the mirror behind the projector bulb properly adjusted, and the filter clean (and replaced if faded).
3. A highly aluminized projector screen should be used, and it should be angled so maximum reflection from the projector is directed toward the patient.
4. The projector should be matched with the line voltage (e.g., 115 V).
5. The test should always begin with an excess of plus power over the patient's estimated correction.

Comparison of Balancing Techniques

Gentsch and Goodwin (1966) compared a number of balancing tests, using as a basis of comparison an *accommodative response balance* employing an optometer system. With the optometer system, the patient's accommodation is well controlled, so this system is considered an accurate measurement of accommodative response. They computed correlation coefficients for each balancing method as

Table 9.1 Agreement of balancing tests with accommodative response balance procedure (Gentsch and Goodwin, 1966).

Method	Correlation coefficient	Frequency of agreement (%)
Retinoscopy	0.44	18%
Bichrome test	0.54	27
Alternate occlusion	0.61	37
Prism dissociation	0.61	37
Turville	0.69	48

compared with the optometer method, and they also computed the frequency of agreement with the optometer method. The results are shown in Table 9.1.

Surprisingly, Gentsch and Goodwin's (1966) bichrome test results did not compare favorably with the results of the alternate occlusion and prism dissociation tests (frequency of agreement with the optometer method was only 27 percent for the bichrome test as compared with 37 percent for the alternate occlusion and prism dissociation tests). The highest frequency of agreement was found with the Turville infinity balance, a binocular refraction procedure discussed in Chapter 10.

"OVERFOGGING" PROCEDURES

Optometrists have always been aware of the possibility that for some patients, accommodation may not be relaxed completely when refraction is done by routine retinoscopy and subjective refraction without the use of cycloplegic agents. As a result, "overfogging" procedures have been developed, having as their goal the relaxation of a maximum amount of accommodation without the use of a cycloplegic agent.

Delayed Subjective Test

Borish (1945) described what he calls the *delayed subjective test*, an overfogging procedure done after completion of the usual optometric examination routine. This test is performed immediately after completion of the plus-lens-to-blur test conducted at 40cm (negative relative accommodation, or OEP no. 21), with the plus lenses that caused the blur remaining in the refractor.

The near-point card is removed, and the patient's attention is directed to the smallest row of letters on the distance chart that had been readable during the subjective examination. These letters will, of course, be badly blurred. (For a patient who is not a presbyope, the plus-lens-to-blur test usually results in approximately +2.25 or +2.50D more plus power than is found in the subjective refraction.) As plus lens power is reduced binocularly 0.25D at a time, the patient is asked to inform the examiner when the letters clear up; the lens powers remaining in the refractor are recorded as the delayed subjective finding.

Borish (1945) commented that this technique is particularly valuable for a patient who comes in with asthenopic symptoms but whose subjective finding turns out to be little different from the present correction. Further, he found that the plus lens power recorded as the delayed subjective is frequently substantially greater than the amount in the original subjective.

Cyclodamia

An overfogging technique known as *cyclodamia* was reported by Dorland Smith in 1930 and described by Bannon (1947, 1965). Smith developed this technique while examining army recruits. His aim was to provide a means of relaxing accommodation equal to that relaxed by cycloplegic refraction without the use of a cycloplegic. Following retinoscopy, Smith began a subjective examination by leaving the retinoscopy working distance lenses in place, the patient thereby being fogged by approximately +1.50D. Spherical lens power was reduced binocularly until the maximum visual acuity was obtained. The power of the spherical lenses was modified gradually until best vision was obtained, while the patient maintained binocular vision. The cylindrical correction was checked by means of the crossed cylinder under various levels of fog, the eye not tested being uncovered so that, presumably, binocular vision was maintained at all times. Smith referred to this procedure as *maximum accommodation relaxation* and contended that the ametropia revealed compared closely with the refraction determined by cycloplegia.

BINOCULAR REFRACTION

Binocular refraction procedures differ from balancing or equalization procedures in that all or part of the subjective refraction is done with both eyes exposed and without the use of prism dissociation. In the majority of binocular refraction procedures, the peripheral portions of the test chart are seen binocularly and the central portion is seen monocularly. These tests make use of the phenomenon of *fixation disparity*; each eye has its own central area (viewed monocularly), and there is a peripheral fusion lock.

The first binocular refraction procedure was developed by Turville, an English ophthalmic optician who in 1946 published the monograph *Outline of an Infinity Balance* describing the procedure, known as the Turville infinity balance. Turville's system makes use of a chart placed above and behind the patient's head that the patient observes in a mirror. The mirror is provided with a 3cm wide septum, so the left eye can see only the left side and the right eye can see only the right side. The chart has a heavy black border, which serves as a peripheral fusion lock, thus making possible the viewing of separate monocular stimuli for the two eyes while peripheral fusion is stimulated.

In the years following the introduction of Turville's infinity balance system, a large number of additional binocular refraction systems have been developed. (Because binocular refraction procedures include tests for lateral and vertical phorias, fixation disparity, and other binocular vision anomalies, they are described in Chapter 10, "The Binocular Vision Examination.")

ALTERNATIVE METHODS FOR DETERMINING CYLINDER POWER AND AXIS

Many alternative methods have been developed for determining the cylinder power and axis. Those described here include the Robinson Cohen slide, the Paraboline test, variations of the crossed-cylinder test (the Auto-Cross and the Simultantest), and stenopaic slit refraction.

Robinson Cohen Slide

The *Robinson Cohen slide*, available for use with the American Optical Project-o-Chart, is designed for determining cylindrical axis and power under fog and consists of a cross made up of broken black lines on a red background (see Figure 9.10). The red background takes advantage of the chromatic aberration of the eye; accommodation will be relaxed if both principal meridians are in focus in front of the retina. The two principal meridians can be located in either of two ways: (1) the broken-line

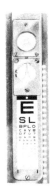

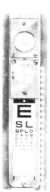

Figure 9.10 The American Optical Robinson Cohen slide.

Figure 9.11 The American Optical Paraboline slide.

cross can be rotated until one of the two lines is in the most distinct position, minus cylinders then being introduced with their axes 90 degrees from the most distinct line, until the two broken lines are equally distinct; or (2) the cross can be rotated until the two lines are equally distinct (or equally blurred) and then rotated 45 degrees, so the two broken lines will be parallel to the principal meridians of the eye.

Paraboline Test

The Paraboline test is a modification of a test designed by Raubitschek in 1929 and described by Eskridge (1958) as being very sensitive for determining cylinder axis but requiring a rather complicated procedure for determining cylinder power. Bannon (1958) added to Raubitschek's test the broken line shown in Figure 9.11 and referred to the new test as the *Paraboline test*. The purpose of the broken line was to determine cylindrical power once the axis meridian was located.

Bannon (1958) suggested that the examiner begin the test by removing all but 0.50D of the working distance lens power from the refractor following retinoscopy, thus providing 0.50D of fog. Using the cylinder axis found in retinoscopy (the cylindrical lenses having been removed), the narrow end of the parabola is set at the meridian 90 degrees from the cylinder axis. The examiner determines which limb of the target appears more distinct by referring to the target as a church steeple or a road becoming narrow at one end. The parabola is then rotated away from the more distinct limb and slowly bracketed back and forth until the patient reports that the two limbs are equally distinct. The examiner then

begins introducing minus cylinder lenses, 0.25D at a time, at the meridian 90 degrees from that of the narrow end of the parabola, until the patient reports that the two broken lines are equally distinct.

Variations of the Crossed-Cylinder Test

Many practitioners routinely forego the use of a test for cylindrical axis and power under fog. They begin the subjective refraction by leaving in the refractor the cylindrical lenses found in retinoscopy, defogging to the criterion of "maximum plus for best acuity," and then verifying the cylindrical axis and power by means of the crossed cylinder. If retinoscopy was reasonably accurate, the axis found by means of the crossed cylinder will usually be within 10 or 15 degrees of that found in retinoscopy for cylinders under 1.00D in power, and within as little as 5 degrees for higher power cylinders. Cylinder power found by the crossed cylinder should not vary by more than 0.25 or 0.50D from that found in retinoscopy.

If no cylinder is found in retinoscopy, and particularly if the patient's pupils are small or the media are cloudy, the practitioner can use the crossed cylinder to "fish" for cylinder. This is done by flipping the cylinder first in the 180- and 90-degree meridians and then in the 45- and 135-degree meridians. If the patient accepts 0.25D or more cylinder in either of these tests, the cylinder is checked for axis. If the resulting axis is very different from the original axis, an additional check test for power should be done. The optical principles involved have been described by Carter (1981). The examiner should use caution, however, when using this procedure, as some patients having a completely spherical refraction (as shown by retinoscopy) will "accept" cylindrical power at an oblique meridian in the "fishing" maneuver.

Auto-Cross and Simultantest

Both the *Auto-Cross* and *Simultantest* were devised for verifying cylindrical axis and power in such a manner that the patient has two simultaneous (rather than successive) views of the test target. Each of these instruments is designed to be attached to the front of the lens well in the refractor (but must be removed when not in use), and each makes use of a prism or mirror system to present simultaneous views of the two positions of the crossed cylinder. Whereas the Auto-Cross is equipped to verify cylindrical axis and power only, the Simultantest also has a +0.25 and −0.25D sphere comparison for use in verifying the spherical endpoint (see Figure 9.12). Borish (1970) criticized the Auto-Cross because its two images are widely separated, requiring the patient to move the eyes back and forth to compare the two targets. The two images formed by the Simultantest are located almost contiguously on the retina, so fixational movements are not necessary. Although based on a valid principle—simultaneous comparison of images—neither the Auto-Cross nor the Simultantest have become popular. One reason for their lack of popularity is the necessity for inserting the device in the refractor.

Stenopaic Slit Refraction

A stenopaic slit is a slit of less than 1mm in width and about 25mm in length, cut into a piece of cardboard, brass, or other material. Most trial lens sets contain stenopaic slits; unfortunately, most refractors do not. It has long been known that the two principal meridians of an astigmatic eye can be located by rotating a stenopaic slit in front of the eye. Referring to Figure 9.9, which shows the vertical focal line closer to the retina than the horizontal focal line in a fogged eye, recall that the horizontal focal line is made up of vertically oriented rays of light. Because most of the vertically oriented rays will be excluded from the eye when the stenopaic slit is oriented along the horizontal meridian, one would expect this patient to report that the letters on a chart at 6m are more distinct when the stenopaic slit is oriented horizontally. Figure 9.2 illustrates the the conoid of Sturm for with-the-rule astigmatism. For

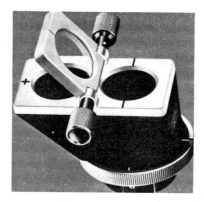

Figure 9.12   The Zeiss Stimultantest.

against-the-rule astigmatism, the patient (with adequate fog) should report that the letters on the chart are more distinct when the stenopaic slit is oriented in the vertical meridian.

Long (1975c) has recommended the following procedure for refraction with a stenopaic slit. First, with the patient fogged and watching the acuity chart, the slit is rotated until acuity is maximized. The slit now lies along the minus cylinder axis. With the slit in this position, the fog is reduced to best acuity. (Best visual acuity through the slit may be a line or two poorer than the patient's best corrected acuity.) The lens in place is the sphere power of the patient's lens formula. Next, the slit is rotated 90 degrees. This will fog the patient again. The fog is again reduced to best acuity. The algebraic difference between the power of the lens in place at the end of this operation and the lens power in place at the end of step one is the minus cylinder power.

Long (1975c) has suggested that the practitioner can easily make a stenopaic slit by placing two pieces of opaque tape on the little-used +0.12D auxiliary cylinder, and mounting it in the phoropter in front of the eye being tested. The small amount of cylindrical power is of little consequence, in that the subjective end-point can quickly be rechecked after the stenopaic slit is removed. Long pointed out that in optometric literature, the use of a stenopaic slit is often recommended for refracting patients with significant optical anomalies, including keratoconus and lenticular distortion.

CYCLOPLEGIC REFRACTION

The history of cycloplegic refraction has been reviewed by Bannon (1947). He noted that Pliny (23–

79 A.D.) discussed the use of various herbs to dilate the pupil for the treatment of corneal ulcers, cataracts, and other ocular conditions. During the 16th century, atropine and other drugs were used to dilate the pupils for cosmetic purposes (as indicated by the name *belladonna*). Atropine's cycloplegic effect, however, was not known until 1811, when Dr. William Wells, a London oculist, found that a patient whose pupils were dilated and had partial ptosis also was found to have a failure of accommodation. It occurred to Wells that this effect might be caused by belladonna, and he convinced a younger physician, Dr. Cutting, to allow him to instill belladonna in his left eye. He found that Dr. Cutting's accommodation was reduced from 7.00D to less than 1.00D in less than 45 minutes, and that the power of accommodation did not return for 8 days. In addition, his refractive state changed from slightly myopic to slightly hyperopic.

As Bannon (1947) noted, it remained for Donders to put cycloplegic refraction on a scientific basis. With his 1864 publication of *On the Anomalies of Accommodation and Refraction of the Eye*, the use of cycloplegics in refraction was universally accepted. Bannon reported that evidence from early ophthalmological journals indicates that the orthodox method of refraction in this country by ophthalmologists entailed the use of cycloplegics. Although as early as 1908 Lucian Howe suggested that refraction was possible without using cycloplegics (pointing out that opticians knew that cycloplegics were unnecessary), ophthalmological training was (and, to a great extent, still is) carried out in hospitals and clinics where patients were often children, illiterate adults, or the aged, whose cooperation level made the use of noncycloplegic refraction methods difficult. Ophthalmologists who learned during their internship or residency to refract only with cycloplegics often did not consider the possibility of refracting without them once they had begun private practice.

With the use of diagnostic pharmaceutical agents now legally permitted in a majority of the 50 states and under consideration in most others, their use is receiving emphasis in optometric training programs both at the undergraduate and continuing education levels.

Cycloplegic Agents

Cycloplegic agents act by antagonizing the muscarinic action of acetylcholine. They do so by blocking its action at structures innervated by postganglionic parasympathetic nerve fibers. These agents paralyze the constrictor pupillae as well as the ciliary muscle, causing mydriasis as well as cycloplegia.

For many years, *atropine* was the only cycloplegic agent available. To bring about full cycloplegia in children, it must be instilled two or three times daily for 3 days before cycloplegic refraction is done. The resulting cycloplegia persists for 7–10 days, and the accompanying mydriasis can last as long as 2 weeks. Atropine is used infrequently—if at all—by optometrists in this country.

Homatropine is a semisynthetic alkaloid. It is not considered to produce sufficient cycloplegia for use in children under the age of 15. Compared with atropine, only a few drops are required, and the cycloplegic effect begins in a matter of 45–60 minutes. Due to the availability of newer preparations (described below), homatropine is used infrequently.

In the following discussion the *italicized* term is the generic name for the drug, whereas the term in parentheses is the trade name. *Cyclopentolate* (Cyclogyl) is a short-duration cycloplegic agent available in 0.5 and 1.0 percent solutions. Cycloplegia occurs within 30–45 minutes and persists for as long as 24 hours. Even though it does not yield as complete a cycloplegia in children as does atropine, Davies (1972) considers it to be a suitable alternative to atropine for children, even under the age of 6, if one or two drops of 1 percent solution are used. For children between the ages of 6 and 16, he recommends one drop of 1 percent solution, and for adults, he recommends one drop of 0.5 percent solution.

A number of reports of central nervous system effects following the use of cyclopentolate, including confusion, ataxia, and personality changes, have appeared in the literature. Hopkins and Lyle (1977) reported that in almost all of these cases, the effects accompanied higher-than-recommended dosage or the combination of cyclopentolate and other antimuscarinic agents.

Tropicamide (Mydriacyl) is also a short-duration cycloplegic available in 0.5 and 1.0 percent solutions. For young adults, three or four drops of the 1 percent solution, separated by a few minutes, will bring about full cycloplegia in about 30 minutes, and recovery occurs within 2–6 hours. Davies (1972) considers tropicamide inadequate for producing cycloplegia in children. Reports of adverse reactions to tropicamide, according to Hopkins and Lyle (1977), are "conspicuous by their rarity." In addition to its use as a cycloplegic, tropicamide is widely used as a mydriatic agent.

Table 9.2 Comparison of cycloplegic action of cyclopentolate and tropicamide.

	Cyclopentolate	Tropicamide
Usual dosage	1 drop of 1% solution	3 drops of 1% solution at 1-minute intervals
Time for onset of maximum cycloplegic effect	30–45 minutes	20–30 minutes
Duration of maximum cycloplegic effect	30–45 minutes	Transient (may be no more than 15 minutes)
Duration of residual cycloplegic effect	6–24 hours	2–6 hours
Possible systemic side effects	Hallucinations, ataxia, disorientation (occurred only with higher-than-the-recommended dosage)	None have been reported

Choice of a cycloplegic agent

There appears to be little doubt that, in children below the age of 6 years, complete cycloplegia can be obtained only with the use of atropine. However, the use of atropine incurs a number of problems and dangers: (1) the parent must cooperate by instilling the ointment in the child's eye twice per day for 3 days; (2) cycloplegia may last as long as 2 weeks; (3) the ointment is poisonous and can cause death if taken by mouth; and (4) for a child with an intermittent convergence strabismus or high esophoria, there is a possibility that complete cycloplegia could cause a constant convergent strabismus (Davies, 1972). Because of these problems, the optometrist should consider the use of a less potent cycloplegic agent, such as cyclopentolate or tropicamide.

If the reason for the cycloplegic refraction is to uncover latent hyperopia that may be responsible for a child's convergent strabismus, the fact that a full cycloplegic effect will not occur is of no great consequence. In any case, when an agent other than atropine is used for cycloplegic refraction, it is not considered necessary to subtract a "tonus allowance," as it is when atropine is used. However, in some cases, the prescription of the full plus found in cycloplegic refracting may result in complaints of blurred distance vision.

On the basis of Davies's (1972) report that 20 patients between the ages of 10 and 14 who were refracted under tropicamide were found to have an average amount of residual accommodation of 3.65D, it is recommended that cyclopentolate (1 percent) be used for children. However, tropicamide will provide an adequate cycloplegic effect for adults. The cycloplegic action of cyclopentolate and tropicamide are compared in Table 9.2.

Indications for Cycloplegic Refraction

Of the three major classes of diagnostic pharmaceutical agents that optometrists are permitted to use, cycloplegic agents are indicated in far fewer cases than is the case with either *mydriatic agents* or *topical anesthetics*. Mydriatics are used frequently by practitioners who use such procedures as binocular indirect ophthalmoscopy and fundus photography; topical anesthetics are used routinely by practitioners who perform applanation tonometry and gonioscopy. Cycloplegic refraction, however, is indicated for only a small percentage of patients.

Older adults

The need for cycloplegic refraction decreases markedly with age. Beyond the age of 40, the amplitude of accommodation decreases rapidly and is essentially nonexistent by the age of 55. Consequently, patients over the age of 40 would not be expected to have latent hyperopia that could not be revealed by routine fogging procedures.

Young adults

For young adults roughly between the ages of 16 and 40, latent hyperopia is sometimes a problem. Its presence should be suspected whenever a patient complains of headaches or other symptoms associated with near work but has little or no uncorrected hyperopia and no other refractive or binocular vision anomaly. The use of overfogging procedures such as Borish's delayed subjective (described earlier in this chapter) can in many cases make the use of cycloplegic refraction unnecessary. If overfogging procedures fail to uncover the expected latent hyperopia, tropicamide (1 percent) is considered to be the best cycloplegic agent because it has virtually no side effects. However, it is necessary to use 3 or 4 drops of 1 percent tropicamide to produce a cycloplegic effect similar to that brought about by 1 drop of 1 percent cyclopentolate.

Children

When a child (often a preschooler) is seen with a convergent strabismus, it is imperative that the practitioner determine whether there is an accommodative element in the strabismus. The only foolproof way to do this is by cycloplegic refraction. If cycloplegic refraction yields little or no uncorrected hyperopia, the condition is not accommodative strabismus, and the prognosis for a nonsurgical cure may be unfavorable. However, if several diopters of uncorrected hyperopia are found, the strabismus is accommodative, and a full correction for the hyperopia (possibly with an addition for near work) will greatly reduce or completely eliminate the esotropia.

The use of a cycloplegic refraction should also be considered for a child whose eyes are normally straight but who has a significant amount of esophoria (a deviation occurring only when fusion has been interrupted), particularly if the esophoria is present at the 40cm distance. Because the combination of hyperopia and esophoria at near is often responsible for asthenopic symptoms and a distaste for reading, any latent hyperopia found in cycloplegic refraction should be corrected. As noted earlier, tropicamide causes insufficient relaxation of accommodation in children, so cyclopentolate (1 percent) should be used.

Comparison of Cycloplegic and Noncycloplegic Refraction

Bannon (1947) reported the results of a study in which both cycloplegic and noncycloplegic refraction were routinely done on 500 patients at the Dartmouth Eye Institute. For all patients the noncycloplegic refraction preceded the cycloplegic refraction, and the same examination procedures were used for both. For children (especially if strabismic), a 1-percent solution of atropine was used, one drop in each eye three times a day for 3 days. For adults, homatropine (5 percent) and *Paredrine* (1 percent)

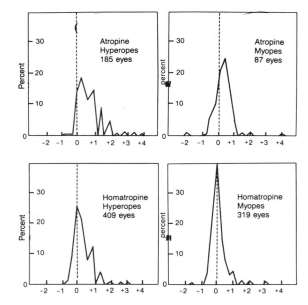

Figure 9.13 Cycloplegic versus noncycloplegic refraction (plotted from data reported by Bannon, 1947).

were used. Completeness of cycloplegia was evaluated, and if more than 2.00D of residual accommodation was found, the subject was not used in the study.

In discussing the results of the study, Bannon (1947) commented that (1) in the younger age groups a definitely greater percentage of cases showed more hyperopia (or less myopia) under cycloplegia; (2) the percentage of cases in which the cycloplegic and noncycloplegic refraction were the same was lowest in the younger group and highest in the older people; and (3) a certain percentage of eyes showed *less* hyperopia (or more myopia) under cycloplegia than without it.

The four graphs in Figure 9.13 are plotted on the basis of data presented in Bannon's report (1947). These graphs show the amount of latent hyperopia or pseudomyopia found in cycloplegic refraction, and they indicate that more latent hyperopia or pseudomyopia was found with atropine than with homatropine. As Bannon commented, this was because atropine was used mainly with the younger patients, and because many of the younger patients had previously worn no correction and, therefore, would be expected to have larger amounts of latent hyperopia. Whereas both graphs for hyperopic patients are skewed toward increased hyperopia in the cycloplegic refraction, both graphs for myopic patients are roughly symmetrical, indicating that there is an about equal chance that a myopic patient will accept more minus as less minus in a cycloplegic refraction.

Later, a study comparing cycloplegic and noncycloplegic refraction was reported by Rengstorff (1966). Manifest and cycloplegic refractions were performed on 122 applicants at Fort Dix, N.J., for a period of 3 years. During the first year, homatropine (5 percent) was used, but during the second and third years, cyclopentolate (1 percent) was used. Almost all subjects were low or medium myopes.

Rengstorff (1966) concluded that the results failed to show that cycloplegics consistently revealed increased hyperopia or less myopia. The mean effect was approximately *no change:* one-third of the subjects had a decrease in myopia averaging 0.37D, one-third showed no significant change, and one-third had an average increase in myopia of 0.36D.

More recently, cycloplegic and noncycloplegic refraction findings were compared on a group of young adults by Grosvenor, Perrigin, Perrigin, Moorehead, and Lamb (1984). The subjects included 60 second-year optometry students having the following spherical equivalent refractions: +0.25 or greater (9 subjects), plano (7 subjects), and −0.25 or greater (44 subjects). A noncycloplegic refraction was first done by the subject's laboratory partner. The amplitude of accommodation was measured, using the push-up method while +3.00D lenses were

Figure 9.14   Typical graphs showing amplitude of accommodation versus time, for tropicamide (upper curve) and for cyclopentolate (Grosvenor, Perrigin, Perrigin, Moorhead, and Lamb, 1984).

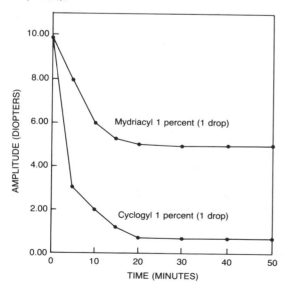

worn in addition to the subjective lenses. After estimating the anterior chamber angle, 1 drop of 1-percent cyclopentolate (*Cyclogyl*) was instilled in each eye. Beginning immediately after instilling the cycloplegic agent, the subject's amplitude of accommodation was measured for each eye, every 5 minutes for a period of 50 minutes, and the subjective refraction end-point was redetermined every 10 minutes for the same period of time.

For the 60 subjects given cyclopentolate, the mean time required to achieve a maximum cycloplegic effect was 20 minutes and the mean residual amplitude of accommodation was 0.75D; for the subjects given tropicamide, the maximum effect was achieved in about the same period of time, but the residual amplitude was between 4 and 6D (Grosvenor et al., 1984). Typical graphs showing amplitude versus time for a cyclopentolate subject and a tropicamide subject are shown in Figure 9.14. A few subjects were given 2, 3, or 4 drops of 1 percent tropicamide, at 1-minute intervals, rather than being given cyclopentolate: it was found that 4 drops of tropicamide were required to provide as great a reduction in amplitude as that caused by cyclopentolate. For 41 of the 60 subjects, the refractive finding under maximum cycloplegia was within ±0.25D of the noncycloplegic finding. Because clinical refraction is known to be accurate to no more than 0.25D, it can be considered that there was no difference between cycloplegic and noncycloplegic refraction for these subjects. However, for 19 subjects, cycloplegic refraction was found to be from 0.50–1.25D more plus than noncycloplegic refraction. When analyzed in terms of noncycloplegic refraction, these subjects were found to be distributed evenly among hyperopia, emmetropia, and myopia. The subject having the greatest cycloplegic effect (1.25D) was a 0.75D hyperope (noncycloplegic refraction) who had long been aware that he was a latent hyperope.

It should be understood that the findings reported by Grosvenor et al. (1984) involved a population group that was not only in the young adult age range but involved a majority of myopes. Although this study and those reported by Bannon (1947) and Rengstorff (1966) indicate that cycloplegic refraction does not necessarily result in more hyperopia or less myopia than noncycloplegic refraction, the fact remains that some young adults will be found to have significantly increased hyperopia under cycloplegia. The practitioner's responsibility, therefore, is to predict the presence of latent hyperopia (or pseudomyopia) so that a cycloplegic refraction can be done.

Study Questions

1. What is meant by *fogging*? What might occur if a patient is not fogged prior to beginning the subjective refraction?

2. Describe Borish's procedure for patient instruction during the crossed-cylinder test for cylinder axis and power.

3. What is the difference between a binocular balancing procedure and a binocular refraction procedure?

4. How do cyclopentolate and tropicamide compare when used for cycloplegic refraction?

5. What is the lens formula for a ±0.50D Jackson crossed cylinder, expressed in (a) crossed-cylinder form? (b) plus-cylinder form? (c) minus-cylinder form?

6. Using the clock dial test for astigmatism under fog, where would you place the cylinder axis if the patient reported that (a) the 12 and 6 o'clock spoke was the most distinct? (b) the 11 to 5 o'clock and 10 to 4 o'clock spokes were equally distinct?

7. Describe a check test for cylinder power other than the Jackson crossed-cylinder test.

8. Starting with the patient fogged by the amount of plus lens power found in retinoscopy including the working distance lenses (the cylindrical lenses having been removed), what is the criterion for ensuring that the patient is adequately fogged prior to beginning the astigmatic chart test?

9. Describe a check test for cylinder axis other than the Jackson cross-cylinder test.

10. (a) What is the criterion for determining the end-point in subjective refraction? (b) What should your instructions to the patient be as you decrease plus lens power or increase minus lens power in arriving at the subjective end-point? (c) Is it a good idea to ask the patient if the letters become smaller as plus power is decreased or minus power increased? Explain.

11. What precautions concerning illumination, the projector, and the screen are important when using the bichrome test?

12. Under what circumstances is it appropriate to use Borish's delayed subjective test? Describe the procedure.

13. In the astigmatic chart test, under fog, describe the positions of the vertical and horizontal focal lines when the patient reports that the 3 to 9 o'clock spoke is more distinct than the 12 to 6 o'clock spoke.

14. What are the disadvantages of atropine for use in cycloplegic refraction for children?

15. If the patient is found to have unequal acuity for the two eyes, what procedure should be used as a balancing test?

16. In using the Jackson crossed cylinder for refining cylinder power for a patient who has with-the-rule astigmatism, where are the vertical and horizontal focal lines (in relation to the retina) when the patient's astigmatism is properly corrected (a) before placing the crossed cylinder in front of the patient's eye? (b) when the minus axis of the crossed cylinder is placed at 180 degrees? (c) when the minus axis of the crossed cylinder is placed at 90 degrees?

17. When a cycloplegic agent is to be used, how can the risk of angle closure be reduced to a minimum?

18. In what situations would you consider the possibility of performing a cycloplegic refraction?

19. Describe a check test that may be used to verify the binocular subjective end-point after the end-point has been determined in the usual manner.

20. On the basis of cycloplegic refraction data reported by Bannon, Rengstorff, and Grosvenor et al., what results could be expected in cycloplegic refraction—as compared to noncycloplegic refraction—(a) with hyperopic patients? (b) with myopic patients?

CHAPTER 10

The Binocular Vision Examination

As noted in Chapter 4, binocular vision anomalies can be considered in terms of two broad categories: (1) anomalies in which binocular vision is maintained, but often at the cost of a considerable amount of stress; and (2) anomalies in which binocular vision is absent. The cover tests, corneal reflex test, and tests of ocular motility that are included in the preliminary examination are designed to detect those anomalies represented in the second category, as well as the more severe anomalies (such as high phorias) in the first category.

The procedures described in this chapter are directed mainly (but not exclusively) toward the first category of anomalies. Phorias, anomalies of accommodation, and anomalies of convergence that were detected in the preliminary examination are further evaluated; more subtle anomalies not detected during the preliminary examination can be discovered and evaluated. Procedures for the evaluation of strabismus and amblyopia are discussed at the end of the chapter.

PHORIA MEASUREMENT

The phoria position of the eyes is the position taken by the two visual axes with respect to one another when all stimuli to fusion have been eliminated. Stimuli to fusion may be eliminated by a number of methods, the simplest of which is to occlude one eye, as is done in the cover test. The method of eliminating stimuli to fusion routinely used for clinical phoria measurement involves the use of a dissociating prism, which is placed in front of one eye so that a measuring prism can be placed in front of the other eye. A vertical dissociating prism is used for the measurement of a lateral phoria, and a horizontal dissociating prism is used for the measurement of a vertical phoria.

If the visual axes are found to be parallel when the patient views a distant object and all stimuli to fusion have been eliminated, the individual is said to have *orthophoria*. If the visual axes converge toward one another (or away from one another) when the eyes are dissociated, the individual has *esophoria* (or *exophoria*); if one visual axis deviates above or below the other, *hyperphoria* is present.

In routine optometric practice, phorias are measured at distances of 6m and 40cm. At 6m the stimuli to both accommodation and convergence are assumed to be zero (although the actual stimulus to accommodation is 0.17D and the stimulus to convergence is approximately 1Δ). At 40cm the stimulus to accommodation is 2.50D and the stimulus to convergence (for an individual with an interpupillary distance of approximately 64mm) is 15Δ.

Distance Phoria

Most people are orthophoric at distance, or very nearly so. This is thought to be due to a "fusion adaptation process" that, as described by Carter (1963, 1965), tends to cause the two visual axes to become (and remain) parallel. According to the fusion adaptation process theory, if an individual is found to have a significant distance phoria, it is because he or she does not possess or has a deficient fusion adaptation process.

Tonic convergence is an important determiner of the distance phoria (Fry, 1943, reprinted 1964). All other things being equal, an excess of tonic impulses to the medial rectus muscles would tend to bring about esophoria at distance, whereas a deficiency in tonic impulses would tend to bring about exophoria.

A number of physical or mechanical factors are also important in determining the distance phoria. These include the positions of the eyes in the orbits, the relative lengths of the ocular muscles, and the positions of the muscle insertions. It is likely that such mechanical considerations are important in the etiology of large distance phorias (particularly when a vertical phoria is also present), just as they are in the etiology of many cases of strabismus.

On the basis of the fusion adaptation theory, we may predict that "orthophorization" (Carter, 1963, 1965) will tend to occur whenever tonic convergence and the physical or mechanical factors are within normal limits. However, when these factors are outside the normal limits or for some other reason the fusion adaptation process fails to develop, a significant heterophoria (esophoria, exophoria, or hyperphoria) may occur. Schor (1980) has described the fusion adaptation process as the *slow component* of the fusional response.

Near Phoria

The near phoria, in contrast to the distance phoria, tends to vary considerably from one individual to another. The norm or expected value of the near phoria is about 3–5Δ of exophoria, but it is not unusual for a patient's near phoria finding to be as high as 10–12Δ of exophoria or 4–5Δ of esophoria. The tendency for asymptomatic individuals to have a moderate amount of exophoria at near is demonstrated by the use of terms such as *physiological exophoria* and *latitude of performance*.

Assuming a given value for the distance phoria, the near phoria is determined by the amount of accommodative convergence the individual possesses. As has been stated, the total amount of convergence required at 40cm is 15Δ. If a patient is orthophoric at 6m and if 15Δ of accommodative convergence are brought into play at 40cm, the convergence demand at 40cm will be completely satisfied by the use of accommodative convergence, and the patient will be found to be orthophoric at 40cm. However, if a patient who is orthophoric at 6m has *less* than 15Δ of accommodative convergence at 40cm, he or she will be found to be exophoric at 40cm; if a patient who is orthophoric at 6m has *more* than 15Δ of accommodative convergence at 40cm, he or she will be esophoric at 40cm.

Vertical Phorias

Vertical phorias seldom occur in isolation. An individual who has a vertical phoria due to the physical or mechanical factors already described will likely have a lateral phoria and will almost certainly have a *cyclophoria* (a condition in which the vertical

meridian of one cornea deviates from the vertical when stimuli to fusion have been interrupted).

Vertical phorias sometimes occur as a result of toxic conditions. A vertical phoria may be found when a patient has a severe cold, sinus infection, or other debilitating condition, but it will disappear when the patient's health returns to normal. In older patients, a vertical phoria may occur—often rather suddenly—as a result of a cerebral vascular accident, or stroke. Due to the intolerable diplopia, the first practitioner to be visited by the patient is apt to be the vision practitioner. Vertical prism can be prescribed to alleviate the diplopia, but in any case the patient should be referred for medical evaluation.

Procedure

The method of phoria measurement described here, in which a dissociating prism is placed in front of one eye and a measuring prism in front of the other eye, is known as the *von Graefe method*. The first decision to be made in phoria measurement by the von Graefe method is how much prism to use to dissociate the eyes. If a weak prism (1 or 2Δ) is placed in front of one eye, with its base in any direction, while the individual fixates a target such as a line of letters, the eyes will make a fusional movement, and single binocular vision will be maintained. However, if a strong prism (about 10Δ or more) is placed in front of one eye, the eyes will be unable to make a sufficiently large fusional movement, and diplopia will result.

The amount of prism necessary to dissociate the eyes varies, depending on the direction of the base of the prism. Most people can fuse only 2 or 3Δ of vertical prism, so as little as 4 or 5Δ of vertical prism would be sufficient to maintain dissociation of the eyes. However, because of the angular size of the line of letters and the projector screen, a prism of 7 or 8Δ is required. As shown in Figure 4.19 (Chapter 4), a base-down prism placed in front of one eye causes the image on the retina to be displaced downward, below the macular area, so the object that formerly was seen straight ahead is now seen as being displaced upward.

When dissociating for the vertical phoria measurement, base-in (rather than base-out) prism is used. This is because the eyes are able to make much larger fusional convergence movements (brought about by base-out prism) than fusional divergence movements (brought about by base-in prism). A prism of 15Δ power is sufficient to bring about dissociation if oriented in the base-in direction, whereas a larger amount may be required to cause dissociation if oriented in the base-out direction.

Lateral phoria at distance

When measuring the lateral phoria at distance, the patient's attention is called to a vertical line of 20/20 letters, and a vertical prism of 7 or 8Δ (the dissociating prism) is placed in front of one eye. A rotary prism is placed in front of the other eye (the measuring prism), and 15Δ of base-in prism is introduced.

It is convenient for the practitioner to establish the habit of always placing the dissociating prism in front of the same eye with the base in the same direction. For example, if the dissociating prism is always placed in front of the left eye, base-up, the practitioner will always know the left eye will see the lower of the two images (unless a large vertical phoria exists). Using a base-up dissociating prism in front of the left eye and a base-in measuring prism in front of the right eye, the patient will see the upper image (seen by the right eye) to the right, as shown in Figure 10.1a. The examiner should ask the patient if the upper image is to the right or to the left of the lower image or directly above it. Unless the patient is highly exophoric, he or she will report that the upper image is to the right of the lower image. At this point, either of the two following procedures can be used.

The "alignment" method. The practitioner instructs the patient to watch the letters in the lower chart, keeping them in sharp focus, and to report when one row of letters is directly above the other. The practitioner then reduces the amount of base-in prism power in the measuring prism until the patient reports alignment. If the two rows of letters are aligned at 0Δ, the patient is orthophoric. However, if the measuring prism indicates base-in prism at alignment the patient is exophoric and if it indicates base-out, the patient is esophoric.

The "flash" method. Using this method, the eye with the measuring prism is occluded (with a paddle) while the power of the measuring prism is changed, and the occluder is removed only long enough to question the patient as to the relative positions of the rows of letters. The practitioner first asks the patient if the upper row of letters is to the right or to the left of the lower row (the expected answer is "to the right"). The practitioner then occludes the right eye

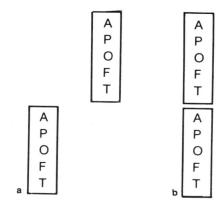

Figure 10.1 Letters seen by the patient during the lateral phoria test. *(a)* **At the beginning of the test, base-up dissociating prism is placed in front of the left eye, and base-in measuring prism in front of the right eye;** *(b)* **at the end of the test, the patient reports that one line of letters is directly above the other.**

while adjusting the measuring prism to, say, 5Δ base-in. The occluder is then removed, and the patient is asked again if the upper row of letters is to the left or right of the lower row. This procedure is repeated until alignment is reported.

A possible disadvantage of the alignment method when compared with the flash method is that continued viewing of both rows of letters may induce attempts at fusional movements, even though the two eyes are dissociated.

During the process of phoria measurement, *no eye movements* occur. As the patient fixates the lower (stationary) row of letters, the upper row simply moves laterally across the visual field until alignment is noted (in the alignment method), or it appears to be in a different position each time the occluder is removed (in the flash method) as the amount of base-in prism is reduced. With this stimulus situation, if the patient has been instructed to watch the upper (moving) row of letters, the right eye would follow the letters as they moved laterally. The lower row would maintain its position as the upper row moved, but the lower row would "move" in the visual field in relation to the position of the (fixated) upper row.

Lateral phoria at near

The patient's attention is called to a vertical row of 20/20 letters on the near-point card at a distance of 40cm, and either the alignment method or the flash method is used. In near phoria testing, the practitioner must emphasize the importance of keeping the letters *in sharp focus*. Otherwise, results will be questionable because of a possible lag of accommodation due to the large amount of depth of focus available at this distance.

The *level of illumination* on the near-point card is important not only for phoria testing but also for the remaining tests done at 40cm. Too high a level of illumination would reduce the pupil size to the extent that the increased depth of focus would adversely affect many of the findings. The recommended light source is a 40-watt incandescent bulb in the refracting unit fixture, located about 18 or 20 inches from the near-point card.

Vertical phorias

Like the lateral phoria, the vertical phoria is also measured at 6m and at 40cm. A base-in prism of 12–15∆ is used to dissociate the eyes, and the measuring prism is oriented so that base-up or base-down prism power can be introduced. If the measuring prism was used in front of the right eye when measuring the lateral phoria, it is convenient to use the prism in front of the right eye for the dissociating prism in measuring the vertical phoria, and to use the prism in front of the left eye as the measuring prism.

The patient's attention is called to a horizontal row of 20/20 letters on the chart at 6m or 40cm as the case may be, and is asked to report when the two rows of letters are on the same level. The test is started with 5 or 6∆ of base-up or base-down prism in the measuring prism, and the amount of prism is gradually reduced until the patient reports alignment. It is not considered necessary to use the flash method for measurement of the vertical phoria, since there is little likelihood of the patient making vertical fusional movements during this test.

When the measuring prism is in front of the left eye, if alignment is reported with base-down in the measuring prism, *left hyperphoria* is present. If alignment is reported with base-up in the measuring prism, *left hypophoria* is present. The presence of a vertical phoria indicates a relationship between the visual axes of the two eyes with respect to one another: a left hyperphoria can also be called a right hypophoria, and a left hypophoria can also be called a right hyperphoria. Conventional usage, however, is to use the term *hyperphoria* rather than *hypophoria*; that is, a patient is said to have either *right hyperphoria* or *left hyperphoria*.

Cyclophoria

As noted, if a patient has a vertical phoria, the presence of a cyclophoria should be expected. One method of detecting and measuring a cyclophoria involves a horizontally oriented Maddox rod on each eye, with a base-in prism in front of one eye. With 12–15∆ base-in (or more, if the patient has a large exophoria), the patient will see a vertically oriented streak with each eye. One streak will be higher than the other, but the streaks formed by the Maddox rods will be long enough so the difference in height will not be a problem. The patient is asked to report whether the two streaks are parallel. If they are not, one of the Maddox rods is rotated slowly until the patient reports that the two streaks are parallel. If the Maddox rod has a protractor scale, the amount of cyclophoria can be read off the scale; if not, it can be estimated.

Cyclophoria is specified as *right encyclophoria*, in which the top of the right cornea tilts toward the nose, as *right excyclophoria*, if the top of the right cornea tilts away from the nose, or as *left encyclophoria* or *left excyclophoria*. For example, if the patient reports that the streak seen by the right eye tilts with respect to that seen by the left eye so the top of the streak tilts toward the right, the patient has right encyclophoria; the amount of rotation of the Maddox rod in front of the right eye that is necessary to cause the two streaks to appear parallel is a measure of the amount of cyclophoria. Unfortunately, there is no treatment for cyclophoria, although the accompanying vertical phoria can be helped by the prescription of prism.

Subjective angle of squint

For a patient having a tropia, the prism dissociation method may be used to measure the lateral or vertical angle of squint in exactly the same manner it is used to measure a lateral or vertical phoria. This is referred to as the *subjective angle of squint*, as opposed to the *objective angle of squint*, which can be measured by the cover test and hand-held prisms. Because many strabismic patients suppress the image seen by the squinting eye, measurement of the subjective angle of squint by the prism dissociation method is often difficult or impossible. If the patient is amblyopic, letters large enough to be seen by the amblyopic eye must be used.

For most strabismic patients a more satisfactory method of determining the subjective angle of squint is measurement with square prisms or a prism bar while performing the alternating cover test, as described in Chapter 5.

Other Methods of Phoria Measurement

Auxiliary methods of phoria measurement include the use of the Maddox rod and the Thorington

I H G F E D C B A ● 1 2 3 4 5 6 7 8 9

Figure 10.2 The Thorington chart for lateral phoria measurement at 6m. With the Maddox rod in front of the right eye, each number represents 1∆ of esophoria and each letter represents 1∆ of exophoria.

method of phoria measurement, which also involves the use of the Maddox rod.

Maddox rod

The original Maddox rod was a single glass rod mounted in a trial lens ring. The Maddox rod now in use consists of a series of glass or plastic rods mounted in a trial lens ring, in a refractor, or in a wooden or plastic handle. Each individual rod acts as a strong convex cylindrical lens; incident light is spread in the form of a streak in a direction 90 degrees to the orientation of the rods. A small, bright source of light (a "muscle light") is used as a fixation object, and the rods are oriented horizontally for lateral phoria measurement and vertically for vertical phoria measurement. A measuring prism is placed in front of the opposite eye.

For example, in measuring the lateral phoria at 6m, the examiner will place the Maddox rod, oriented horizontally, in front of one eye (say, the right eye) and a measuring prism with a large amount of base-in power in front of the left eye. The patient will see a vertical streak with the right eye and a spot of light (the muscle light) with the left eye. The patient will report that the streak is to the right of the spot. As the amount of base-in prism is gradually reduced, the patient is instructed to report when the streak appears to go "right through the spot" (see Figure 4.20 in Chapter 4). The amount of prism present when alignment is reported is a measure of the patient's lateral phoria.

Similarly, in measuring the vertical phoria, the Maddox rod is oriented vertically in front of one eye, and a vertical prism is placed in front of the other. Starting with 8 or 10∆ of base-up or base-down prism, the amount of prism power is gradually reduced until the patient reports that the (horizontal) streak "goes through the spot."

For phoria measurement at 40cm, the examiner can use a bare ophthalmoscope bulb or a penlight as the light source, using the same procedures as described for the test at 6m.

The Maddox rod is of doubtful value in measuring lateral phorias. Because there is no stimulus to accommodation, the patient may localize the streak as being much closer than the 6m testing distance (or either closer or farther than the 40cm testing distance), so the findings tend to be inaccurate. However, a Maddox rod (preferably hand-held) provides a convenient method of screening for vertical phorias.

Thorington method

The Thorington method uses a horizontally oriented distance test chart having a muscle light in the center and numbers or letters extending on either side (see Figure 10.2). The Maddox rod, oriented horizontally, is placed in front of one eye, and the patient is asked to report which number or letter the vertical streak goes through or is closest to. Because each prism diopter of deviation at 6m results in a tangent distance of 6cm, to have 1∆ steps, the numbers or letters must be placed 6cm apart. If numbers are placed to the right, as shown in Figure 10.2, and if the Maddox rod is always placed in front of the right eye, interpretation of the test is simplified. If the patient reports that the streak coincides with a number, the patient is experiencing uncrossed diplopia and has esophoria. If the streak coincides with a letter, the patient is experiencing crossed diplopia and has exophoria. For example, if the response is "5," the patient has 5∆ of esophoria; if the response is "B," the patient has 2∆ of exophoria.

The Thorington test also can be done at 40cm. The near-point card has a hole in its center through which the practitioner projects the light from a penlight, and it has letters and numbers like the distance chart. At 40cm, each prism diopter of power will be represented by a deviation of 0.4cm. Charts can be designed to measure the vertical phoria at both 6m and 40cm by aligning numbers and letters vertically above and below the light source.

Because the Thorington test uses numbers and letters, which exert some control over accommodation, this test does not present the problem of lack of control of accommodation to the extent that the Maddox rod test does. However, it appears to be used infrequently.

FUSIONAL VERGENCE RESERVES

Fusional vergence, also referred to as *reflex vergence* or as *disparity vergence*, is that vergence, stimulated by retinal disparity, that is brought into play to maintain single binocular vision (to keep from seeing double). Fusional vergence movements can be either *positive* (a disjunctive movement of the eyes inward) or *negative* (a disjunctive movement of the eyes outward). *Vertical vergence movements* can also be made, one eye moving upward or downward with respect to the other.

The relationship between fusional vergence and accommodative convergence was investigated by Fry (1937), who varied stimuli to accommodation and convergence by means of a haploscope and measured the state of accommodation by means of a Badal optometer. Fry found that for a given stimulus to accommodation, as the stimulus to convergence was increased, the subject would increase his convergence with little or no increase in accommodation up to a certain point, at which accommodation was found to increase (see Figure 10.3). He found that the point at which accommodation began to increase was related to the subject's report that the target was blurred. Fry concluded that the subject first used positive fusional vergence; when it had reached its limit, he used accommodative convergence to maintain single vision at the expense of clarity.

Fry (1937) also found that as the stimulus to convergence was decreased, the subject would allow the eyes to diverge with no change in accommodation up to a certain point, where accommodation began to decrease. The decrease in accommodation was accompanied by the report of a blur, and this indicated that the patient had reached the limit of negative fusional vergence and had supplemented it with accommodative divergence at the expense of clear vision. However, when the stimulus to accommodation was zero (as would be the case for an infinitely distant object), no blur was reported, as there was no accommodation to be relaxed.

Figure 10.3 Changes in accommodative response, for a given accommodative stimulus, as convergence increases and decreases (redrawn from Fry, 1937).

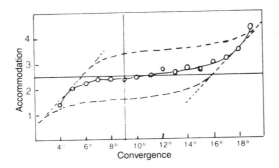

Clinically, either positive or negative fusional vergence can be stimulated by introducing a small amount of horizontal prism before each eye, base-out prism bringing about positive fusional vergence and base-in prism bringing about negative fusional vergence. As shown in Figure 4.24 (Chapter 4), the introduction of a small amount of base-out prism causes the eyes to converge, on the basis of retinal disparity clues, to keep the images of a fixated object on the foveas of the two eyes. Similarly, as shown in Figure 4.25, the introduction of a small amount of base-in prism causes the eyes to diverge to keep the images on the two foveas.

Using rotary prisms, the examiner can gradually increase the amount of base-out prism power before each eye until the patient reports a blur, indicating that the limit of positive fusional vergence has been reached. As the examiner continues to increase the amount of base-out prism power, the patient eventually reports seeing double (a break), indicating that accommodative convergence is no longer being employed, at the expense of clarity, to maintain single binocular vision.

Similarly, as base-in prism power is gradually increased before each eye, the report of a blur will indicate that the limit of negative fusional vergence has been reached and that additional divergence has been brought into play by relaxing accommodation. The eventual occurrence of a break indicates that accommodative divergence is no longer being employed to maintain single vision.

Procedure

Tests of fusional vergence reserves are done both at 6m and at 40cm. Customarily, base-in vergences are tested before base-out vergences. The reason for this is that, because the base-out vergence is a stimulating test, there may be aftereffects that would interfere with the results of the base-in vergence test if the base-out vergence test were done first. A vertical line of 20/20 letters is used to measure the lateral vergences, and a horizontal line of 20/20 letters is used to measure the vertical fusional vergences.

Base-in vergence at distance

For the measurement of negative fusional vergence at distance, the patient's attention is called to a vertical row of 20/20 letters, and as base-in prism is added equally in front of the two eyes, the patient is asked to report if the letters become blurred or break into two rows. The total amount of prism power present when the blur occurs, and then when the break occurs, is mentally noted. After the break occurs, the patient is instructed to report when the two rows of letters have fused into one, as the base-in prism power is gradually reduced.

If the patient reports a blur in the base-in vergence test at distance, this indicates that accommodation is being relaxed to supplement negative fusional vergence with accommodative divergence. However, if the patient's accommodation had been completely relaxed by means of the subjective lenses, no additional accommodation would be available for relaxation. The presence of a base-in blur at distance, therefore, indicates that the subjective finding is in error in the direction of insufficient plus or excessive minus power. The subjective end-point should be rechecked.

In the absence of a blur, the occurrence of a break indicates the limit of negative fusional vergence. However, as pointed out above, when a blur occurs, it also indicates the limit of negative fusional vergence. Therefore, whichever occurs first—a blur or a break—indicates the limit of negative fusional vergence. In the event that a blur occurs, the subsequent occurrence of a break indicates the limit of accommodative divergence. In any case, the occurrence of a break indicates that the eyes are no longer responding to vergence stimuli and have returned to the phoria position. As base-in prism is reduced, when the patient reports that the two rows of letters have come back to one (the *recovery finding*), it indicates that the eyes have made a fusional movement (in this case a negative fusional vergence movement) to reestablish single binocular vision.

Base-out vergence at distance

For the measurement of positive fusional vergence at distance, the patient's attention is again called to the vertical row of 20/20 letters. As base-out prism is gradually added in front of each eye, the patient is asked to report if the letters become blurred and then to report when they break into two rows of letters. A blur on the base-out vergence test indicates that the limit of positive fusional vergence has been reached and that accommodative convergence is being used to supplement fusional vergence; the subsequent occurrence of a break indicates that the limit of accommodative convergence has been reached. In the absence of a blur, the occurrence of a break indicates the limit of positive fusional vergence. After the break is reported, the patient is instructed to report when the two rows of letters have returned to one. Whether or not a blur occurs,

the occurrence of a break indicates that the eyes are no longer responding to vergence stimuli and that the visual axes have returned to the phoria position. When the recovery is reported, it indicates that the eyes have made a positive fusional vergence movement to reestablish single binocular vision.

Base-in and base-out vergences at near

Using a single vertical row of letters on the reduced Snellen chart at 40cm, the base-in and base-out vergences at near are taken in the same manner as the distance vergences. However, interpretation of the base-in vergence finding at near differs from interpretation of this finding at distance. Because 2.50D of accommodation is stimulated when the near findings are taken, the examiner should expect the patient to report a blur, indicating that accommodation is relaxed to supplement negative fusional vergence.

Blur-point criteria

In the graphical method of analysis, all blurs are reported as *first blurs*, the examiner instructing the patient to report when the letters first appear to be blurred (or words to that effect). If further blurring is allowed to occur beyond the first blur, the data will be contaminated by the eyes' depth of focus. In the OEP, or analytical, method of analysis, the patient is not asked to report a blur in the base-in vergence test at distance, but in the base-out test at distance a first blur is requested. However, in both the base-in and base-out findings at 40cm, the OEP system differs from the graphical system in utilizing a *blur-out* rather than a first blur. The patient is instructed to report when the letters are so badly blurred that none can be read. Another difference in the OEP method is that base-out vergence findings are done before base-in vergence findings.

Recording of findings

The blur, break, and recovery findings are recorded in the following manner:

Base-in: *x*/9/5   Base-out: 10/20/8

The *x* recorded for the base-in-to-blur finding indicates that the patient did not report a blur.

Expected Findings

The eyes have only limited ability to diverge beyond parallelism, so divergence findings at distance are typically much lower than convergence findings. At the near testing distance, because the eyes are converging approximately 15Δ at the start of the test, divergence findings are more nearly equal to convergence findings.

Mean values for positive and negative vergence tests have been reported for a clinical population by Morgan (1944a) and for a nonclinical population by Saladin and Sheedy (1978). The following mean values were reported by these investigators:

	Morgan (1944)	Saladin & Sheedy (1978)
Distance		
Base-in	*x*/7/4	*x*/8/5
Base-out	9/19/10	15/28/20
Near		
Base-in	13/21/13	14/19/13
Base-out	17/21/11	22/30/23

Inspection of these mean values indicates that in almost all cases, mean blur and break values were greater for the Saladin and Sheedy nonclinical population than for the Morgan clinical population. One factor that may explain these differences, as pointed out by Saladin and Sheedy, is that their population was younger than Morgan's population. Another factor is that the Saladin and Sheedy subjects were third-year optometry students, who were skilled observers. Therefore, when dealing with the patients seen in the typical optometric practice, the mean values reported by Morgan will serve as a more appropriate guide.

Vertical vergence findings

The procedure for measuring the vertical fusional vergence reserves differs from that for measuring the base-in and base-out reserves in two respects: (1) prism power is introduced in front of only one eye at a time, rather than in front of both eyes; and (2) because vertical prism has no effect on the accommodative mechanism, a blur will not occur. The procedure for measuring vertical vergences is similar for the 6m and 40cm distances. The patient's attention is called to a single horizontal row of small letters. The patient is instructed to report when the letters break into two rows as vertical prism power is introduced in front of one eye, and then to report when the two rows of letters fuse into one as prism power is reduced.

The vertical vergence findings are obtained in the following order: right supravergence (base-down, right eye); right infravergence (base-up, right eye), left supravergence; and left infravergence. The findings are recorded in the following manner:

$$\text{R: } \frac{s\ 3/1}{i\ 4/2} \qquad \text{L: } \frac{s\ 4/2}{i\ 3/1}$$

Because vertical vergence findings indicate the ability of one eye to rotate up or down with respect to the other eye to maintain single binocular vision, the effect of placing a base-down prism in front of one eye is the same as the effect of placing a base-up prism in front of the other eye. Thus, for a given patient, right supravergence and left infravergence should be equal, and right infravergence and left supravergence should be equal (as shown in the preceding recording). It is unnecessary to test vertical vergences unless the patient is found to have a vertical phoria. However, the student clinician is advised to practice the vertical vergence findings on a large number of patients to develop the necessary manual dexterity and to have first-hand knowledge of the *normal* range of findings to be able to recognize an abnormal finding should it occur.

Fusional Vergence Demand Versus Reserve

The procedures discussed here (base-in, base-out, base-up, and base-down findings) are all measurements of *fusional vergence reserves*. The fact that they are referred to as reserves implies that there must be such an entity as a *fusional vergence demand*. The fusional vergence demand is represented by the phoria: exophoria creates a demand for positive fusional vergence, esophoria creates a demand for negative fusional vergence, and a vertical phoria creates a demand for vertical fusional vergence. In all cases the fusional vergence demand is numerically equal to the phoria. An exophoria of 5Δ creates a positive fusional vergence demand of 5Δ, and an esophoria of 3Δ creates a negative fusional vergence demand of 3Δ. The demand can be thought of as the amount of fusional vergence necessary (to be in use at all times) to avoid diplopia. The reserve, on the other hand, can be considered as the amount of fusional vergence not needed to avoid diplopia, as such, but held in reserve.

The relationship between fusional vergence demand and reserve is illustrated in Figure 10.4. Consider a patient whose 6m phoria and fusional vergence findings are as follows: 5 exophoria; base-in *x*/10/5 (blur/break/recovery); and base-out 10/20/8 (blur/break/recovery). These findings are illustrated in Figure 10.4a. In this plot, the zero point indicates the demand on convergence; that is, at 6m the demand on convergence is considered to be zero

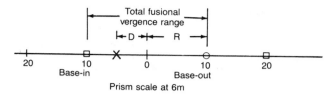

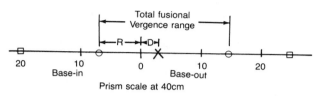

Figure 10.4 Plots of phoria and fusional vergence findings: *(a)* patient who has 5Δ of exophoria at 6m; *(b)* patient who has 3Δ of esophoria at 40cm. Fusional vergence demand is indicated by *D,* and fusional vergence reserve is indicated by *R.*

(even though, for a 6cm interpupillary distance, the convergence demand at 6m would actually be 1Δ). All findings measured by means of base-in prism are plotted to the left of the zero point, and all findings measured by base-out prism are plotted to the right of the zero point. The phoria finding is indicated by an *X,* blur findings are indicated by circles, and break findings are indicated by squares. Recovery findings are not plotted.

The total range of fusional vergence is equal to the distance between the base-in-to-break finding (since there was no blur finding) and the base-out-to-blur finding, whereas the range of accommodative vergence is equal to the distance from the base-out-to-blur to the base-out-to-break finding. In Figure 10.4a, the total range of fusional vergence is 20Δ. However, what interests us in this case, because the patient is exophoric, is the total range of *positive* fusional vergence as well as the relationship between the positive fusional vergence demand (the phoria) and the positive fusional vergence reserve (the base-out-to-blur finding). It is evident that the range of positive fusional vergence is 15Δ, 5Δ of which represents demand and 10Δ of which represents reserve. The fact that this patient has 5Δ of positive fusional vergence demand and 10Δ of positive fusional vergence reserve was evident from looking at the recorded findings and did not require plotting the findings as in Figure 10.4a. However, such a plot is helpful in demonstrating what is occurring.

Consider now a patient whose 40cm phoria and

fusional vergence findings are as follows: 3 esophoria; base-in 7/20/10; and base-out 15/25/12. These findings are illustrated in Figure 10.4b. Although the demand on convergence at 40cm for a patient whose interpupillary distance is approximately 64mm is 15Δ, for simplicity the demand point will be considered zero (to represent the actual convergence demand at 40cm, it would be necessary to add 15Δ to all base-out findings and to subtract 15Δ from all base-in findings). As at 6m, all base-in findings are plotted to the left of zero, and all base-out findings are plotted to the right: an *X,* a circle, and a square are used to represent the phoria, blur findings, and break findings, respectively.

The total range of fusional vergence, extending from the base-in-to-blur to the base-out-to-blur findings, is 22Δ. What interests us in this case, because the patient is esophoric, is the range of *negative* fusional vergence and the relationship between the negative fusional vergence demand (the phoria) and the negative fusional vergence reserve (the base-in-to-blur finding). These ranges are 3 and 7Δ, respectively, as is evident by referring to either Figure 10.4b or the recorded findings. (Further analysis of phoria and fusional vergence findings is presented in Chapter 12.)

Vertical fusional vergence demand and reserve

Compared to lateral phorias, vertical phorias are relatively rare, occurring in less than 5 percent of the general population. The vertical phoria creates a demand on vertical fusional vergence, and the vertical fusional vergence finding in the direction opposite to that of the phoria represents the vertical fusional reserve.

The relationship between vertical fusional demand and reserve is illustrated in Figure 10.5. Consider a patient having the following findings: 2Δ right hyperphoria; right eye vertical vergence findings 5/3 (supravergence), 3/1 (infravergence); and left eye vertical vergence findings 3/1 (supravergence), 5/3 (infravergence). In both diagrams in Figure 10.5, the zero point on the vertical scale indicates that the demand on vertical vergence is zero (this applies to all testing distances). All findings measured by base-down prism are plotted above the zero line, and all findings measured by base-up prism are plotted below zero. The phoria finding is indicated by an *X,* break findings are indicated by squares, and recovery findings are not plotted. It should be noted that, in Figures 10.5a (right eye) and

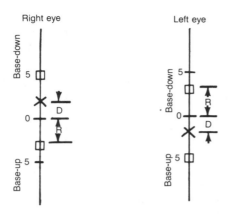

Figure 10.5 Plots of vertical phoria and vertical fusional vergence reserve findings for a patient who has 2Δ of right hyperphoria (left hypophoria). Note that hyperphoria and supravergence are measured with base-down prism, whereas hypophoria and infravergence are measured with base-up prism.

10.5b (left eye), the base-up findings for the right eye and the base-down findings for the left eye (and vice versa) are equal, as expected.

The total range of vertical vergence, for each eye, is 8Δ. However, referring to the plot for the right eye, what interests us is the range of *infravergence* because the patient has a right hyperphoria. The demand for infravergence is 2Δ (the phoria), and the reserve of infravergence is 3Δ (the base-up finding). Similarly, referring to the plot for the left eye, the demand for supravergence is 2Δ (the phoria), and the reserve is 3Δ (the base-down finding).

Effect of prism on the fusional reserves

When a patient has a phoria, one form of treatment (and the *only* form of treatment for a vertical phoria) is the prescription of prism. It is of interest to consider the effect of prescribing prism on a patient's fusional vergence demand and reserve.

When prescribed for a patient with a phoria, prisms are considered to be *relieving prisms*. This is because they reduce the demand on fusional vergence; in doing so, they also increase the fusional vergence reserve an equal amount. Consider the patient who has a distance exophoria of 5Δ and a base-out-to-blur finding of 10Δ (see Figure 10.4a). If the optometrist prescribed 2Δ of base-in prism for this patient, while the prism was worn it would reduce the demand on positive fusional vergence by 2Δ. This can be illustrated, in Figure 10.4a, simply

by moving the zero point (the demand point) 2Δ in the base-in direction. If the phoria and fusional vergence reserves were to be measured while the prism was being worn, the measured phoria would now be only 3Δ of exophoria, and the positive fusional vergence reserve (base-out-to-blur) would be 12Δ. Referring to the 40cm phoria and vergence findings shown in Figure 10.4b, if the practitioner prescribed 3Δ of base-out prism for this patient, while the prism was worn there would be no esophoria at 40cm, and the negative fusional vergence finding (base-in-to-blur) would increase from the former value of 7Δ to 10Δ.

For the patient having 2Δ of right hyperphoria (see Figure 10.5), the practitioner may decide to prescribe 1Δ of vertical prism, base-down, in front of the right eye (or base-up, in front of the left eye). This would have the effect of moving the zero line 1 unit upward (in Figure 10.5); that is, reducing the demand on infravergence 1Δ. The result would be that, while wearing the prism correction, the patient's vertical phoria would be only 1Δ of right hyperphoria, and the base-up-to-break for the right eye would be increased from the former 3Δ to 4Δ. (The prescribing of prism is more fully discussed in Chapter 12.)

TESTS OF ACCOMMODATIVE FUNCTION

Tests of accommodative function that can be included in the binocular vision examination include the monocular and binocular crossed-cylinder findings, the amplitude of accommodation, positive and negative relative accommodation, and the range of accommodation.

Monocular and Binocular Crossed-Cylinder Findings

The monocular and binocular crossed-cylinder findings at 40cm are not ordinarily included in the graphical analysis testing routine, but they are included in the OEP examination routine. These tests provide the practitioner with information about the "posturing" of accommodation at 40cm and can be thought of as a "near subjective." These findings are the subjective analogue of dynamic retinoscopy, discussed in Chapter 8.

The test target for the monocular and binocular crossed-cylinder findings is the *crossed-cylinder grid*, shown in Figure 10.6. For these tests, illumination on the near-point card must be very low. This is easily accomplished by aiming the refracting unit light in such a way that the grid is illuminated from a large angle, so the patient can just make out the lines in the grid. If illumination is too high, the depth of focus will be so great that it will make the results of the test meaningless.

The Jackson crossed cylinders are put into position with the minus axes oriented at 90 degrees, and sufficient fogging lenses are put into place to ensure that both the vertical and horizontal focal lines will be located in front of the retina (see Figure 10.7).

If the patient is not a presbyope, fogging lenses of +1.00D in excess of the binocular subjective finding will usually be sufficient. For a presbyopic patient, however, the fogging lens power must be in excess of the expected total near finding: that is, in excess of the distance subjective finding plus the antici-pated bifocal addition. The author has found that a convenient starting point is +1.00D more than the total plus power for near in the patient's present glasses. For example, if the present glasses have a distance prescription of +1.00D sphere with a +2.00D addition, begin the crossed-cylinder findings with +4.00D of spherical power.

Monocular crossed-cylinder finding

The practitioner can either occlude each eye in turn during the monocular crossed-cylinder finding or use approximately 6Δ of vertical dissociating prism. In the latter situation, the patient's attention can first be called to the image seen by the right eye

Figure 10.6   The crossed-cylinder grid.

Figure 10.7 Positions of vertical and horizontal focal lines at the start of the crossed-cylinder test.

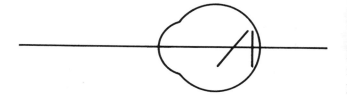

(the upper image if base-down prism is placed in front of the right eye) and then to the image seen by the left eye.

In either case, the patient is asked to report which of the lines are sharper or more distinct, "those going up and down or those going across" (use of the words *vertical* and *horizontal* can result in confusion). At the start of the test the expected reply is that the "up and down" lines are more distinct. Plus lens power is then reduced until the patient reports that the "up and down" and "across" lines are equally distinct. If the reversal occurs directly from "up and down" to "across," with no report of "equally distinct," the finding is recorded as the least plus through which the vertical lines are more distinct than the horizontal lines. Once the finding is completed for the right eye, the patient's attention is directed toward the image seen by the left eye, and the test is repeated.

In the OEP examination routine, a lateral phoria (no. 15a) is taken through the monocular crossed-cylinder finding (no. 14a), using the crossed-grid target and leaving the crossed cylinders in front of the eyes.

Binocular crossed-cylinder finding

The same procedure is used for the binocular crossed-cylinder finding as for the monocular crossed-cylinder finding, with the obvious exception that no occluder or vertical prism is used. If equal distinctness of the vertical and horizontal lines is not obtained, it is recommended that the practitioner stop at the least plus power through which the vertical lines are more distinct. In the OEP proce-dure, the first lens power making the horizontal lines more distinct is recorded.

In the OEP routine, a lateral phoria (no. 15b) is taken through the binocular crossed-cylinder finding (no. 14b). The crossed cylinders are removed prior to taking the phoria, and a vertical line of letters rather than the grid is used as a target.

Interpretation

For a patient who is not a presbyope, the crossed-cylinder findings provide information concerning the lag of accommodation, as does the dynamic retinoscopy finding. In some cases the crossed-cylinder findings identify patients who have latent hyperopia or who could benefit by the prescription of additional plus lens power for near or bifocal lenses. The use of the binocular crossed-cylinder finding with nonpresbyopes sometimes identifies patients who will be found, on the basis of the gradient phoria, to have high AC/A ratios (discussed later in this chapter).

For presbyopic patients, the binocular crossed-cylinder finding provides a rapid and convenient method of determining the tentative addition. If the binocular crossed-cylinder finding is performed as the first near finding, it can be used as a tentative addition for the performance of the subsequent near tests, including lateral and vertical phoria testing, fusional vergence tests, relative accommodation tests, and tests of range of accommodation. (The method of using the binocular crossed-cylinder finding as an aid in determining the bifocal addition to be prescribed for presbyopic patients is described in Chapter 12.)

Amplitude of Accommodation

Accommodation can be stimulated either by moving a test object closer to the eyes or by placing minus lenses in front of the eyes. Either of these procedures can be used to determine the amplitude of accommodation. The first method, called the *push-up*, or *Donders method* (first described by Donders, 1864), is used in the graphical analysis routine. The second method, called the *minus lens method*, is used in either the graphical analysis or the OEP routine.

Push-up method

With the best visual acuity subjective lenses in the refractor, the reduced Snellen chart is placed at a distance of 40cm, and the patient's attention is called to the 20/20 row of letters. The card should be illuminated by a 40-watt incandescent bulb: excessive illumination will greatly increase the depth of focus for some patients and will therefore result in falsely high amplitude findings. The examiner should also make sure, as the card is moved closer to the patient's eyes, that the level of illumination remains relatively constant. In some cases this involves moving the lamp as the card is moved. The test is done first monocularly, for each eye, and then binocularly.

As the examiner slowly moves the card toward the patient's eyes, the patient is requested to report when the 20/20 letters begin to blur and remain blurred. This is the criterion of "first sustained blur." When a sustained blur is reported, the amplitude of accommodation is noted, as indicated on the reading rod, and recorded.

Most patients under the age of 40 will have no difficulty reading the 20/20 letters at 40cm (this, of course, represents 2.50D of accommodation). If a patient is a beginning presbyope and reports that the letters are blurred at 40cm, they will sometimes clear up if the card is moved farther away. The examiner then brings the card toward the patient's eyes until a first sustained blur is recorded.

If moving the card to a distance farther than 40cm does not clear the letters, the card should be moved back to 40cm and plus lenses should be added binocularly until the 20/20 letters are clear. The card is then moved toward the patient's eyes until a first sustained blur is reported. The power of the plus lenses (above the best visual acuity subjective finding) must then be subtracted from the amplitude indicated on the reading rod to determine the patient's actual amplitude of accommodation. For example, if the patient reports a first sustained blur at a distance of 33cm (equivalent to 3.00D) while wearing $+2.00D$ lenses in addition to his or her best visual acuity subjective correction, the amplitude is $3.00D - 2.00D$, or $1.00D$.

Minus lens method

To measure the amplitude of accommodation by the use of minus lenses, the near-point card is placed at a distance of 40cm, and the patient is instructed to watch the 20/20 line of letters first with the right eye and then with the left eye (the opposite eye being occluded), and to report when the letters begin to blur as minus power is gradually added to the patient's subjective correction. To arrive at the amplitude of accommodation, 2.50D (for the 40cm working distance) is added to the minus lens power necessary to blur the letters. For example, if the addition of $-4.00D$ to the subjective correction blurs the letters, the amplitude of accommodation is $4.00D + 2.50D$, or $6.50D$.

If it is necessary to add plus lenses to the subjective lenses to clear up the letters at 40cm, the amount of plus lens power necessary to clear up the letters is subtracted from 2.50D to determine the amplitude of accommodation.

The OEP procedure for determining the amplitude of accommodation by the use of minus lenses differs from this procedure in two ways: (1) the near-point card is placed at 13 inches rather than 40cm (16 inches), although the stimulus to accommodation is considered to be 2.50D rather than 3.00D; and (2) 0.62 *M* type is used rather than reduced Snellen 20/20 letters.

Comparison of the two methods

When the push-up method is used for determining the amplitude of accommodation, the angular size of the retinal image of the 20/20 letters increases in direct proportion to the decrease in distance between the near-point card and the eyes. For example, at 40cm the angular size of a 20/20 reduced Snellen letter is 5 minutes of arc; at 20cm the angular size increases to 10 minutes of arc; at 10cm it increases to 20 minutes of arc. When the minus lens method is used, however, the angular size of the letters remains constant throughout the test (although the retinal image will reduce slightly in size as minus lenses are added, due to accommodative micropsia). When the amplitude of accommodation is determined by the push-up method, it tends to be considerably higher than when determined by the minus lens method. This is particularly true for high amplitudes, in which the push-up test would result in a significant increase in retinal image size. For amplitudes in the presbyopic and near-presbyopic range (i.e., from 1.00 to 5.00D), the difference between the two methods will be small.

According to Donders's table of amplitude of accommodation as related to age—as reported by Borish (1970) and given in Table 2.3 (in Chapter 2)—amplitude of accommodation as determined by the push-up test decreases from 14.00D at age 10 to 2.50D at age 50 and zero at age 75. However, it has been found by Ong, Hamasaki, and Marg (1956) that much of what we think of as amplitude of accommodation in older people is actually due to the depth of focus of the eyes, and that amplitude reaches zero by approximately the age of 54.

Interpretation

The great majority of people in the nonpresbyopic ages (i.e., below the age of 40) will be found to have an amplitude that is within normal limits for their age. However, a few young patients will be found to have lowered amplitudes due to functional or pathological causes, as described in Chapter 4.

As for patients of age 40 or older, a rule of thumb says that to have clear and comfortable vision, an individual should have to use no more than half of his or her accommodation in sustained reading or close work. For a working distance of 40cm, this rule of thumb indicates that a bifocal addition or reading glasses should be considered when a patient's amplitude is found to be below 5.00D. For example, a patient who has an amplitude of 3.50D (the expected amplitude at age 45) should have to use only 1.75D amplitude for sustained near work; if that near work is to be done at a distance of 40cm, an addition of +0.75D would be required. Although other methods are available for determining the bifocal addition,

this simple rule of thumb is useful for beginning presbyopes.

In the OEP system of analysis, the expected finding for the amplitude of accommodation determined by minus lenses is 5.00D. If the amplitude is less than this amount, the patient is considered to be a presbyope.

Relative Accommodation

Positive and negative relative accommodation (minus lens to blur and plus lens to blur) are measured binocularly at 40cm, using as a stimulus the 20/20 letters on the reduced Snellen chart. The starting point for both of these tests, for a patient who is not presbyopic, is the best visual acuity subjective finding. For the presbyope, the starting point should be the tentative addition, as determined by the binocular crossed-cylinder finding or other means. As with the amplitude of accommodation finding, illumination should not be excessive or the findings will be erroneously high due to the increased depth of focus with increased illumination. Because negative relative accommodation (plus to blur) is a relaxing test, whereas positive relative accommodation (minus to blur) is a stimulating test, plus is done first in the graphical routine.

Negative relative accommodation

As plus lens power is added binocularly, 0.25D at a time, the patient is instructed to report when the 20/20 letters begin to blur and remain blurred (a first sustained blur). When this point is reached, the finding is noted and later recorded as the amount of plus lens power added to the best visual acuity subjective lenses, the binocular crossed-cylinder finding, or other starting point. A recommended way to do this is to simply count the clicks as plus power is added: eight clicks equals 2.00D, and so forth.

Positive relative accommodation

This test is done in exactly the same manner as the negative relative accommodation, with the exception that minus lenses instead of plus lenses are used.

OEP method

In using the OEP method, the patient is asked to report when the 20/20 letters are blurred out (i.e., when they are so badly blurred that the patient cannot even read one of the letters). This applies to both the negative relative and positive relative accommodation. In the OEP method, the positive relative accommodation test (finding no. 20) is done before the negative relative accommodation test (finding no. 21).

Interpretation

Because 2.50D of accommodation is stimulated at the 40cm testing distance, the maximum amount of accommodation that would be expected to relax at 40cm would be 2.50D. Therefore, the negative relative accommodation finding (plus lens to blur) should not be expected to be greater than +2.50D. If greater than that amount, the examiner should suspect that accommodation may not have been completely relaxed in the subjective refraction and should repeat the binocular subjective end-point.

As plus lenses are added 0.25D at a time, each 0.25D of lens power reduces the stimulus to accommodation. As accommodation is relaxed, the visual axes would be expected to diverge relative to the point of fixation at 40cm, and this would be expected to bring about diplopia. However, diplopia is avoided by the use of positive fusional vergence. As long as positive fusional vergence is available, the patient can relax accommodation and accommodative convergence, but when the limit of positive fusional vergence is reached, no further accommodation is relaxed, and a blur is reported. The plus-lens-to-blur test, therefore, is considered a test of the limit of *positive fusional vergence*.

Similarly, as minus lenses are added 0.25D at a time, each 0.25D of minus lens power increases the stimulus to accommodation. As accommodation is increased, the visual axes would be expected to converge relative to the point of fixation at 40cm, and this would be expected to cause diplopia. Diplopia is avoided by the use of negative fusional vergence, so the minus-lens-to-blur test is considered a test of the limit of *negative fusional vergence*.

Expected findings

The expected findings for the negative relative accommodation and positive relative accommodation tests depend on a number of factors, including the patient's amplitude of accommodation and the ranges of positive and negative fusional vergence.

As for the negative relative accommodation (plus-to-blur) test, most patients have a sufficient range of positive fusional vergence to enable the relaxation of most—if not all—of the accommodation in play, with the result that the expected value for this finding is about +2.00 to +2.50D. A finding of less than +2.00D would indicate that either (1) the patient's range of positive fusional vergence is severely

limited, in which case the base-out-to-blur finding would also be expected to be below the mean value, or (2) the patient was overplussed in the subjective finding, so less than the normal amount of accommodation (2.50D) was available for relaxation at the 40cm distance.

The limiting factor for the expected value of the positive relative accommodation (minus-to-blur) test is the amplitude of accommodation. If a patient has an amplitude of accommodation of only 1.50D, we would expect the minus-lens-to-blur test to be no greater than −1.50D. For a younger individual having a high amplitude of accommodation, the minus-to-blur finding would tend to be limited by the patient's range of negative fusional vergence. This, in turn, depends to a great extent on the patient's AC/A ratio. In general, the higher the AC/A ratio, the lower the minus-to-blur finding would be expected.

Range of Accommodation

The range of accommodation test is done only if the patient is a presbyope. It is the last test in the binocular vision examination, performed after the plus-to-blur and minus-to-blur tests, and it is done while the patient is wearing the tentative near correction. The patient (using both eyes) is instructed to watch the 20/20 row of letters on the near-point card at a distance of 40cm, and is asked to report when the 20/20 letters blur as the card is moved toward the face along the reading rod. The examiner makes a mental note of where the blur occurred, in centimeters or inches, and then moves the card back to the 40cm position. The patient is then asked to watch the 20/30 letters (the next-to-the-bottom row) and to report when those letters blur as the card is moved away on the reading rod. Again the examiner makes a mental note of the position of the card when the blur was reported and subsequently records the range (e.g., from 25–55cm, or 10–22 inches). Although there may be merit in recording the blur points in centimeters, recording in inches can be advantageous to patient communication. It is then possible to inform the patient that "these lenses will give you clear vision from a distance of 10 inches to 22 inches," as you demonstrate where the 10-inch and 22-inch points are. This gives the patient an opportunity to consider whether or not this range encompasses his or her usual reading or working distances.

For first bifocal or first reading prescription patients, it is advisable to put the reading correction in a trial frame, to seat the patient at a table or desk, and to allow the patient to experiment with the range available with the correction. With previous bifocal wearers, this can be done by placing trial lenses of appropriate power over the present bifocals.

GRADIENT PHORIA AND THE AC/A RATIO

The *AC/A ratio*, when determined clinically, is defined as the ratio of accommodative convergence, expressed in prism diopters, to the stimulus to accommodation, expressed in diopters. The AC/A ratio can be determined by either the *gradient method* or the *calculated method*. The gradient method involves taking more than one lateral phoria at 40cm through differing stimuli to accommodation.

Gradient AC/A Ratio

The *gradient AC/ratio* is determined by taking a near phoria, through the best visual acuity subjective lenses combined with either +1.00 or −1.00D sphere. In each case, the change in phoria brought about by the change in stimulus to accommodation gives us the value of the gradient AC/A ratio. Consider the following phoria findings, taken at 40cm:

> Subjective −1.00DS: 1 exophoria
>
> Subjective: 4 exophoria
>
> Subjective +1.00DS: 8 exophoria

As one would expect, combining minus lens power with the subjective finding brought about a decrease in the exophoria, by stimulating additional accommodation and accommodative convergence; combining plus lens power with the subjective finding brought about an increase in exophoria, by relaxing accommodation and accommodative convergence. In comparing the phoria taken through the subjective with that taken through the subjective −1.00D, the gradient AC/A ratio is 3/1; a comparison of the phoria taken through the subjective with that taken through the subjective +1.00D results in a gradient AC/A ratio of 4/1.

Calculated AC/A Ratio

The *calculated AC/A ratio* is determined on the basis of the relationship between the distance phoria and the near phoria. As noted in Chapter 4, the stimulus to convergence at 40cm, for a person having an interpupillary distance of 64mm, is 15Δ; the stimulus to accommodation at this distance is 2.50D. Again referring to the discussion in Chapter 4, if an individual makes use of 15Δ of accommodative convergence at a distance of 40cm (the total convergence demand therefore being met by accommodative convergence), the AC/A ratio would be

$$\frac{15}{2.5} = \frac{6}{1}.$$

However, when less than 15Δ of accommodative convergence are used at 40cm, the AC/A ratio is less than 6/1, and when more than 15Δ of accommodative convergence are used at 40cm, the AC/A ratio is more than 6/1. For example, if 10Δ of accommodative convergence are used, the AC/A ratio is 10/2.5, or 4/1; and if 20Δ of accommodative convergence are used, the AC/A is 20/2.5, or 8/1.

Convergence is known to have four components: *tonic convergence*, which, as noted earlier, is one of the determiners of the distance phoria; *proximal convergence*, stimulated by the awareness of nearness of the fixated object; *accommodative convergence*; and *fusional convergence*. However, in determining the calculated AC/A ratio, only accommodative and fusional convergence need be taken into consideration.

Consider the individual who has too little accommodative convergence. If only 10Δ of accommodative convergence are available at 40cm, how is the additional 5Δ of convergence demand supplied? It is supplied by fusional vergence. If the individual who has only 10Δ of accommodative convergence at 40cm is orthophoric at 6m, the additional 5Δ of convergence required at 40cm is supplied by positive fusional vergence. As we know on the basis of previous discussions, an individual who must make use of 5Δ of positive fusional vergence to avoid diplopia has 5Δ of exophoria.

On the other hand, for the individual who has an excess of accommodative convergence (20Δ), 5Δ of divergence is supplied by negative fusional vergence, indicating that the patient has 5Δ of esophoria at 40cm.

Formula for calculating the AC/A ratio

The fact that most people are somewhat more exophoric at 40cm than at 6m has led to the concept of *physiological exophoria*. For example, the OEP *table of expecteds* indicates lateral phoria values of 0.5Δ of exophoria at 6m and 6Δ of exophoria at 40cm, resulting in a physiological exophoria of 5.5Δ.

The concept of physiological exophoria can be used in the formula for the calculated AC/A ratio, as follows:

$$\frac{AC}{A} = \frac{15 - \text{physiological exophoria}}{2.5}.$$

For a given patient, the amount of physiological exophoria can be determined by answering the question, how much more exophoria does the patient have at 40cm than at 6m?

For the patient who is orthophoric at distance and has 5Δ of exophoria at near, the physiological exophoria is 5Δ, and the AC/A ratio is

$$\frac{AC}{A} = \frac{15 - 5}{2.5} = \frac{4}{1}.$$

The patient who is orthophoric at distance and has 5Δ of esophoria at near is 5Δ less exophoric at near than at distance, with the result that the physiological exophoria is −5Δ. The *AC/A* ratio is, therefore,

$$\frac{AC}{A} = \frac{15 - (-5)}{2.5} = \frac{8}{1}.$$

It follows that, as long as the distance and near phorias are equal, there is no physiological exophoria and the AC/A ratio is equal to 15/2.5, or 6/1.

Significance of the AC/A ratio

How does it help the practitioner to know the value of a patient's AC/A ratio? Knowing the value of the AC/A ratio is particularly helpful when the practitioner is considering the possibility of altering the spherical component of the patient's spectacle correction to reduce a phoria by stimulating or relaxing accommodation and accommodative convergence. This can be illustrated by the use of two extreme examples.

Example 1. Suppose that our patient is orthophoric at 6m and 10Δ esophoric at 40cm. The calculated AC/A ratio is

$$\frac{AC}{A} = \frac{15 - (-10)}{2.5} = \frac{10}{1}.$$

We would like to prescribe added plus power at near to reduce the esophoria. How much added plus power will be necessary? With an AC/A ratio of 10/1, the addition of 1.00D of plus power would be expected to reduce the near phoria all the way from 10Δ of esophoria to orthophoria.

To find out if the phoria actually will be reduced to orthophoria, we put the +1.00D spheres in the refractor in addition to the subjective lenses, and take the phoria finding. (This, of course, is gradient phoria.)

Example 2. Suppose now that our patient is orthophoric at 6m and has 10Δ of exophoria at 40cm. The calculated AC/A ratio is

$$\frac{AC}{A} = \frac{15 - 10}{2.5} = \frac{2}{1}.$$

In this case, we consider the possibility of prescribing additional minus power at 40cm to reduce the exophoria. How much added minus power would be necessary to make a reasonable decrease in the phoria at 40cm? With an AC/A ratio of only 2/1, the addition of 1.00D of minus power would be expected to reduce the near exophoria only from the present 10 exophoria to 8Δ of exophoria, and it would be at the expense of 1.00D of overaccommodation. A much better way of solving the patient's problem would be to prescribe base-in prism for near work, visual training to build up the amplitude of positive fusional vergence reserve, or a combination of both.

Comparison of Gradient and Calculated AC/A Ratios

Even though the gradient and the calculated AC/A ratios determine the amount of accommodative convergence associated with each diopter of accommodation, there is a fundamental difference between the two. Because the phoria findings used to determine the gradient AC/A ratio are both taken at a distance of 40cm, whatever proximal convergence is operating at 40cm would be expected to affect both phoria findings equally. However, because one of the phoria findings necessary for the calculated AC/A ratio is taken at 6m and the other is taken at 40cm, proximal convergence is operating when one of the phorias is taken, but not when the other is taken. As a result, the calculated AC/A ratio is "contaminated" by proximal convergence; that is, part of what appears to be accommodative convergence in the calculated AC/A ratio is actually proximal convergence, but the gradient AC/A ratio is free of proximal convergence effects.

The lack of proximal convergence effects in the gradient AC/A ratio accounts—at least in part—for the fact that the gradient AC/A ratio is consistently somewhat lower than the calculated AC/A ratio. For example, the patient having orthophoria at 6m and 10 esophoria at 40cm (and therefore a 10/1 AC/A ratio) would probably be found to have a somewhat lower AC/A ratio using the gradient method. The addition of 1.00D of plus lens power to the distance subjective lenses would probably reduce the near phoria not to orthophoria, as indicated by the calculated AC/A ratio, but perhaps to 3 or 4Δ of esophoria. (The use of the AC/A ratio in the diagnosis of and prescribing for binocular vision problems is discussed in Chapter 12.)

BINOCULAR REFRACTION

Binocular refraction systems are not only systems for refraction, but typically include tests for lateral and vertical phorias, fixation disparity, and other binocular vision anomalies as well. Some practitioners consider binocular refraction systems primarily as alternative techniques for balancing the state of accommodation of the two eyes. Except for some patients who have marked anisometropia or amblyopia, a completely satisfactory binocular balance can be obtained by means of the procedures described in Chapter 10.

Binocular refraction procedures, then, can offer the practitioner much more than additional balancing procedures. Those who routinely make use of binocular refraction point out that an important advantage is that both eyes are involved in the procedure, without the use of prisms or other methods of dissociation, so the patient's refraction and binocular vision are evaluated in a more nearly normal, or natural, environment.

The Turville Infinity Balance (TIB)

A. E. Turville (1946) published a monograph describing a binocular refraction procedure known as the *Turville infinity balance (TIB)*. Turville's apparatus was in the form of a reversed illuminated chart with a mirror. The mirror was fitted with a 3cm-wide septum, so the patient saw the right side of the chart with the right eye and the left side of the chart with the left eye. The border of the chart, as well as objects in the visual field surrounding the chart, were seen binocularly. Turville's system can be adapted for use with a projected chart by either of two methods:

1. If the chart is projected onto a mirror, the septum can be a strip of cardboard placed vertically in the center of the mirror, through which the patient views the reflected image of the chart (see Figure 10.8a).

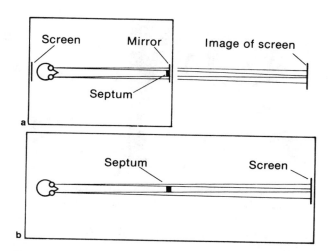

Figure 10.8 The Turville infinity balance arrangement for use with a projector: *(a)* septum placed on a mirror; *(b)* septum placed halfway between patient and the screen.

2. If a mirror is not used, a septum is placed approximately halfway between the patient and the screen. The exact position can easily be determined by trial and error (see Figure 10.8b). The author has used an old-fashioned coatrack for this purpose, but a more professional-looking septum is available from the Bernell Company.

In either case, the projector slide containing side-by-side charts for use with the bichrome test can be used. Turville reported that the TIB technique had been used for 9 years before he wrote his monograph. He said that, in addition to providing a perfect visual balance, the TIB apparatus provides ready means for detecting suppression, suspension, vertical imbalance, lack of stereopsis, cyclophoria, and lateral imbalance (particularly exophoria).

Procedure

The examiner first carries out the conventional refractive procedures of retinoscopy and monocular subjective refraction. The discussion that follows is based on Turville's monograph (1946).

Test 1: Preliminary. Test 1 uses Turville's chart 1a (see Figure 10.9a), which presents the 20/60 letters *L*, seen by the left eye, and *F*, seen by the right eye. The expected response is that the *L* and *F* will be seen as two separate letters, equally clearly and at the same level. A second possible response is that the *L* and *F* will be fused into the letter *E*, and

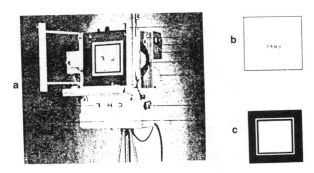

Figure 10.9 The Turville infinity balance test *(a)* **with chart 1a;** *(b)* **chart 1b;** *(c)* **chart 2a. The letters are backward because the chart is designed to be used with a mirror** (Turville, 1946).

a third possible response is that only the *L* or only the *F* will be seen. If the letter *E* is seen, this indicates that the patient's eyes have *diverged* to fuse the *L* and the *F*. The examiner places base-in prism in front of each eye, starting with a total of 2Δ, and increases the amount until the *L* and the *F* remain separate. If only the *L* is seen the patient is suppressing the left eye; if only the *F* is seen the patient is suppressing the right eye.

Test 2: Balancing accommodation. Turville described test 2 for use only if 6/6 (20/20) acuity was obtained with each eye in the original monocular subjective finding. His chart 1b (Figure 10-9b), which presents two small letters for each eye, is used together with a "mask" (chart 2a; see Figure 10.9c), which provides a peripheral fusion lock and prevents the letters from "floating." Although Turville's procedure was to ask the patient to compare the clarity of the letters for the two eyes, Carter (1981) strongly recommends against this, recommending instead that the spherical end-point for each eye be determined independently with the criterion of "maximum plus for best visual acuity."

Test 3a: Lateral imbalance—exophoria. If base-in prisms were required to keep the letters *L* and *F* separate in test 1, after completing test 2 the *L–F* chart should again be used, but with the mask. If base-in prism is still required to keep the letters separate, the patient has exophoria. The amount of prism to be prescribed is the weakest base-in prism that will keep the *L* and the *F* separate.

Test 3b: Lateral imbalance—esophoria. If esophoria is suspected, the examiner should revert

to the target used in test 1 but without the mask. A 2Δ prism, base-out, is placed in front of one eye. If the letters fuse, making an *E*, there is no esophoria of importance. However, if more than 2Δ of base-out prism are required to obtain fusion of the *L* and *F* into an *E*, the amount of base-out prism necessary for fusion is the maximum amount that can be prescribed.

Test 4: Vertical imbalance. If hyperphoria was noted in test 1 (if the *L* and *F* appeared on different levels), test 2 is completed (with the vertical prism removed), and the examiner reverts to the *L–F* target for test 4 without the use of the mask. The weakest prism that will cause vertical alignment of the two letters should be incorporated into the prescription, and, according to Turville, "will be accepted gratefully."

Test 5: Suspension and suppression. If suspension or suppression was noted in test 1, balancing of accommodation is completed as usual. Then the *L–F* chart is reintroduced, the nonsuspending eye being covered to convince the patient that the other letter is really there. As the eye is uncovered, the patient is told to try to keep the letter in view. This may have to be done a number of times. If a satisfactory result is not obtained in test 5, the case is deemed one of *suppression*, and the possibility of orthoptic training should be considered.

Morgan's Adaptation of TIB

Morgan (1949) reported on an investigation in which the side-by-side acuity charts of the American Optical Robinson Cohen slide were used as a basis for the Turville test. Using 215 consecutive patients as subjects, Morgan first performed a regular examination sequence and then examined the patient with the septum in place. Visual acuities were first balanced by asking the patient to compare the clarity of the charts for the two eyes and adding +0.25 and −0.25D spheres to each eye to determine whether or not acuity for the eye improved.

Following this, 20/50 letters were presented, and cylinder power and axis were checked using the flip cylinder method. Next, the patient was presented a 20/30 line of letters for each eye and was asked if the two sides were level. The amount of prism (if any) required to make the two sides appear level was recorded as the hyperphoria (Morgan, 1949).

Morgan next presented the Verhoff circles intended for the bichrome test with the Robinson

Cohen slide and added base-out prism until the two circles fused. He had calculated that 1Δ of base-out prism should make the two circles coincide, but due to peripheral fusion it was found that most patients required 2Δ or more of base-out prism for fusion. Any subject fusing with less than 2Δ was presumed to be exophoric, and base-in prism was prescribed. The subject was then asked if one or the other of the charts disappeared when both eyes were open, indicating suppression.

The results concerning Morgan's 215 patients are shown in Table 10.1. For the first four conditions (involving spherical ametropia and cylindrical correction), the TIB results were compared to those obtained from conventional refraction. Morgan (1949) reported that he prescribed vertical prism for all patients showing a vertical phoria on the TIB (prescribing the amount required to make the two sides of the chart appear level), and that he prescribed base-in prism for all patients requiring less than 2Δ base-out for fusion of the two sides of the chart (the circle target). Of six patients found to be suppressing, two patients had binocular vision restored by means of base-in prism, two by means of vertical prism, one by the addition of +0.75D to the suppressing eye, and one by means of orthoptics.

In a later paper, Morgan (1960) made the following points:

1. When a vertical phoria is found, the patient can be expected to comfortably wear the prism required to level the two halves of the test chart.
2. Prescribing horizontal prism depends to some extent on the particular refracting room setup

because of the variation in stimuli for peripheral fusion. However, as a general rule, (a) if 3Δ base-out are required for fusion of the two targets, no prism is prescribed; (b) if 2Δ base-out are required for fusion, 1Δ base-in is prescribed; and (c) if fusion takes place between 0 and 2Δ base-out, 2Δ base-in are prescribed.

The TIB is enthusiastically used by large numbers of ophthalmic opticians in Great Britain and by many optometrists in the United States. Many who use it consider its major advantage to be in prescribing for vertical phoria; in that the amount of the vertical prism required to cause the two sides of the chart to appear level is the amount of prism to be prescribed. This is a much more direct procedure than the use of a standard prism phoria test with the subsequent need for measuring vertical fusion ranges or prescribing prism by means of a rule of thumb, as is often done (see Chapter 12).

Although it is convenient to speak of the prism found in the TIB as compensating for a vertical or lateral phoria, it should be understood that when the TIB is used, one is dealing with *fixation disparities* rather than phorias. Whereas the measurement of a phoria requires the complete dissociation of the two eyes, any stimulus situation in which a peripheral fusion lock is present involves fixation disparities—not phorias. The prism we are concerned with does not *measure* the fixation disparity: it is the amount of prism necessary to *eliminate* the fixation disparity. (As noted in Chapter 4, fixation disparities are extremely small, measured in minutes of arc; however, the presence of a fixation disparity can permit the visual axes to deviate, under dissociated conditions, by several prism diopters.) It should also be understood that the amount of prism power necessary to eliminate a fixation disparity is usually much less than the measured phoria. A patient found to have 3 or 4Δ of hyperphoria by measurement of the dissociated phoria may require only 1Δ of vertical prism to eliminate the vertical fixation disparity in the TIB, and a patient requiring 8 or 10Δ of base-in prism for alignment in a dissociated phoria measurement may require only 2Δ of base-in prism to eliminate the fixation disparity in the TIB.

To differentiate between phoria and fixation disparity measurements, Ogle, Martins, and Dyer (1967) introduced the term *associated phoria* to designate the measurement of the amount of prism necessary to eliminate fixation disparity, as differentiated from the *dissociated phoria* measured by the von Graefe technique.

Table 10.1   Results of Morgan's TIB study of 215 patients (Morgan, 1949).

Condition	Criterion	Percent
Spherical ametropia	Change of 0.25D	20%
Spherical ametropia	Change of 0.50D	2
Cylindrical correction	Change more than 0.25D	0
Cylindrical correction	Axis change more than 10°	2
Vertical phoria	0.5Δ or more	15
Exophoria	Less than 2 BO for fusion	13
Suppression	One chart disappearing	3

Refraction by Immediate Contrast

Humphriss and Woodruff (1962) described a binocular refracting technique in which the eye not being refracted is fogged by means of a +0.75D sphere. They refer to their method as the *Humphriss Immediate Contrast (HIC)* method, comparing it to the TIB method and characterizing the fogging lens as a "psychological septum."

Refraction is first estimated by retinoscopy or monocular subjective procedures. Humphriss and Woodruff (1962) contend that with the +0.75D fogging lens peripheral fusion takes place, but the macular image of the blurred eye is suppressed in favor of the eye with the clear image. They also note that full binocular vision is present with accommodation relaxed, and any alteration made in vision of the unfogged eye will be appreciated by the patient.

Procedure

The procedure for refraction by immediate contrast, as described by Humphriss and Woodruff (1962), is as follows:

1. Refraction is first determined, leaving the patient in the red, using the bichrome test.
2. The left eye is fogged with +0.75D sphere, and testing is begun on the right eye.
3. The patient is presented with the choice of an additional +0.25 or −0.25D sphere on the right eye and is asked which lens makes an end letter in the 20/30 line clearer. The expected answer is that it is clearer with the −0.25D lens.
4. The −0.25D lens is then placed in front of the unfogged eye and the test is repeated, again presenting +0.25 and −0.25D sphere before the right eye. If the patient was not accommodating before the second +0.25 and −0.25D choice was given, the +0.25D lens would blur the letters, therefore being rejected in favor of the −0.25D lens. On the other hand, if the patient was accommodating before the test was begun, the patient might report that the letters are (a) clearer with the +0.25D lens, (b) equally clear with both lenses, or (c) clearer with the −0.25D lens. The rationale for the HIC procedure is that, if the patient accommodates for −0.50D sphere placed in front of the unfogged eye (in two −0.25D steps), this accommodation will increase the blur in the fogged eye (now fogged by +1.25D sphere) and the blur will be perceived binocularly.
5. Cylinder axis and power are checked with the Jackson crossed cylinder. This can be done at any

point the patient has given any answer other than the immediate rejection of plus (either of the three responses previously given).

6. The +0.75D fogging lens is placed in front of the right eye, and procedures 1–5 are repeated with the left eye.
7. The spherical end-point can now be checked for each eye using the bichrome test. This is done in the usual manner, except that the eye not tested is under +0.75D fog.

Humphriss and Woodruff (1962) made use of two sets of lenses (with three lenses each, mounted on handles) for what they called the *test set* and the *moderating set*. They stressed that the lens should be moved vertically in front of the eye being tested. The test set included a +0.25D sphere, a −0.25D sphere, and a ±0.25D crossed cylinder; the moderating set included a +0.25D sphere, a −0.25D sphere, and a −0.25D cylinder. At the time they published their report, Humphriss and Woodruff stated that the HIC procedure had been used by several experienced optometrists in South Africa on some 5,000 patients, and "all refractionists . . . find the new method superior to any they have used previously" (1962, p. 2173).

Mallett Fixation Disparity Test

The first clinical test designed for the stated purpose of dealing with fixation disparity was described by Mallett (1964, 1966), a British ophthalmic optician. Mallett argued that graphic systems of analysis of heterophorias and fusional vergences are of doubtful value, as they are very time-consuming and lack the necessary accuracy and consistency. Further, he said that the presence or absence of fixation disparity provides a valuable indication of whether the patient is able to cope with heterophoria. The purpose of the Mallett test is not to measure fixation disparity but to detect its presence and then eliminate it by means of prisms or spherical lenses.

Two fixation disparity units ("Mallett boxes") are available: a wall-mounted unit for distance testing and a hand-held unit for near testing. The original distance unit was intended for fixation disparity testing only, but a combined unit for distance testing now includes both a bichrome test and a binocular astigmatic test in addition to the fixation disparity unit.

Both the distance and the near fixation disparity units incorporate a gross foveal fusion lock as well as a peripheral fusion lock; the only monocularly

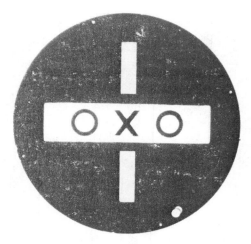

Figure 10.10   Mallett fixation disparity test, distance unit (Mallett, 1966).

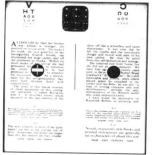 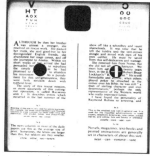

Figure 10.11   Mallett fixation disparity test, near unit (Mallett, 1964).

seen stimuli are in the parafoveal areas. Both units require Polaroid filters in front of the patient's eyes, so the illumination on the testing unit must be strong enough to allow for the filters.

The distance unit

The distance unit is a self-contained, internally illuminated unit (see Figure 10.10). The letters *OXO* are seen by both eyes and constitute a gross foveal fusion lock. The letter *X* subtends an angle of 10 minutes of arc at a distance of 6m, approximately the size of a 20/40 letter. Two red strips are provided—one above and one below the *X*—and are polarized so one strip is seen with each eye. In the position shown in Figure 10.10, the unit is used to measure horizontal fixation disparity; it may be rotated so the strips are oriented horizontally, and the unit may be used to measure vertical fixation disparity. The unit is used in fully illuminated

surroundings to provide paramacular and peripheral fusion stimuli, and a normal visual environment should be provided.

The near unit

As with the distance unit, the near unit presents the letters *OXO* seen by both eyes, providing a gross foveal fusion lock (see Figure 10.11). The letter *X* subtends 18 minutes of arc at a 35cm distance, about the size of a 20/70 letter. The near unit provides separate stimuli for lateral and vertical disparity detection, and green strips are polarized and therefore seen monocularly. Each circle is surrounded by a paragraph of type to provide a stimulus to accommodation and a peripheral fusion lock. Only the *OXO* and the green strips are internally illuminated; the exterior must be illuminated by means of a reading lamp.

Procedure

The patient is told to concentrate on the *X* in the middle of the *OXO* and is asked if he or she can simultaneously see two red (at distance) or two green (at near) strips, one above and one below the *OXO*. The patient is then asked if the top strip is directly above the bottom strip. The patient should be urged to look for a very slight displacement of the two strips. (Remember, no matter how big or how small the heterophoria, the amount of displacement will be no more than about 5–15 minutes of arc.)

If there is no displacement, the patient either has no lateral phoria or has a compensated lateral phoria. If the top strip (seen by the left eye) is to the right of the bottom strip, the patient has exo fixation disparity (see Figure 10.12), and if the top strip is seen to the left, the patient has eso fixation disparity. If both strips are displaced, the fixation disparity is

Figure 10.12   Target appearance during the Mallett fixation disparity test: (a) no fixation disparity; (b) exo fixation disparity; (c) eso fixation disparity. The upper vernier line is seen by the left eye and the lower by the right; the two vernier lines are seen in crossed diplopia in exo fixation disparity (b), and in uncrossed diplopia is eso fixation disparity (c).

 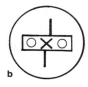 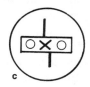

a   b   c

shared between the two eyes; if only one strip is displaced, this is an indication that one eye is strongly dominant (the undisplaced strip belongs to the dominant eye).

Exo disparity. If the patient is found to have exo fixation disparity, the practitioner introduces base-in prism, starting with 1Δ, until the two strips are aligned. The amount of prism to be prescribed is the smallest amount that will bring about alignment. Alternatively, the practitioner can introduce minus spheres until the strips are aligned. A third alternative (in cases of convergence insufficiency) would be to institute base-out training, the criterion being the elimination of fixation disparity. Once the fixation disparity is eliminated, the exophoria can be considered fully compensated.

Eso disparity. If the patient has eso fixation disparity, base-out prism or plus spheres can be introduced until the strips are aligned. The amount of base-out prism or plus spherical power to be prescribed is the smallest amount that will bring about alignment. Occasionally, base-in training may be instituted, the criterion being the elimination of fixation disparity.

Vertical disparity. If vertical disparity is found to exist, the amount of vertical prism to be prescribed will be the smallest amount necessary to eliminate the fixation disparity. This will usually (but by no means always) be much less than the amount of prism measured in the prism dissociation test.

American Optical Vectograph Slide

Grolman (1966) described procedures for binocular refraction using a vectograph projector slide supplied by the American Optical Corporation. Using this slide, Polaroid filters must be placed in front of the patient's eyes, and an aluminized projector screen must be used. The screen must be angled so the normal to its surface bisects the angle between the projector and the patient's eyes. This can be done by placing a small mirror in the plane of the screen and rotating the screen until the patient, seated in the ophthalmic chair, can see the projector reflected in the mirror. If the projector is not aligned at the correct angle, the reflectance of the screen may be reduced to the point that the test will be ineffective. The procedures for use with the vectograph slide, as described by Grolman, are summarized in the following paragraphs.

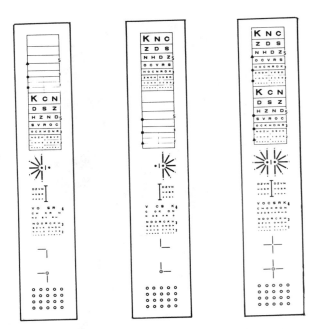

Figure 10.13   The American Optical Vectographic Project-o-Chart slide: *(a)* left eye view; *(b)* right eye view; *(c)* combined view for both eyes.

Acuity testing. Separate acuity charts are provided for each eye (see Figure 10.13), with letters ranging from 20/100–20/15. A parafoveal fusion lock is provided by the line box surrounding each line of letters.

Astigmatism testing. For astigmatism testing a clock dial chart is presented, the right eye seeing the right half of the clock dial and the left eye seeing the left half. A series of symbols is also available for crossed-cylinder testing.

Balancing of accommodation. Balancing of accommodation is done by determining the spherical end-point separately for each eye using the criterion of "maximum plus or minimum minus power for best acuity." Each eye views a chart with 20/40, 20/30, and 20/25 letters; a peripheral fusion lock is provided by the aperture of the chart and the room itself, as well as a central vertical bar.

Fixation disparity. The fixation disparity target consists of a central dot and ring, seen by both eyes, and a cross. The upper and right limbs of the cross are seen by the right eye, and the lower and left limbs are seen by the left eye (see Figure 10.13). If the patient reports that a perfect cross is seen, no fixation disparity is present. Vertical fixation disparity is indicated by a misalignment of the horizontal lines, and horizontal fixation disparity is indicated by misalignment of the vertical lines. If misalignment is reported, the direction and amount of prism necessary to bring about alignment is determined. A second fixation disparity target is provided in the form of a similar cross without the central dot and ring. Grolman (1966) commented that some patients have no difficulty with the target having the dot and ring, but they report misalignment when the target lacking the dot and ring is used.

Fusional vergence and other tests. A target is provided for fusional vergence testing, the left eye seeing the letters *T* and *O* and the right eye seeing the letters *O* and *N*. The central *O* is fused, resulting

in the perception of the word *TON*. Results of this vergence test would not necessarily compare with results of fusional vergence tests done in the customary manner.

Targets for stereo-acuity and testing for suppression are also provided in the vectograph system.

Near-Point Cards

American Optical near-point cards

The American Optical Corporation also has available a series of near-point vectographic cards for binocular refraction and for measurement of the associated phorias and stereopsis. These are illustrated in Figure 10.14.

Borish near-point card

Borish (1978) developed a vectographic near-point card that involves targets seen both binocularly and monocularly (see Figure 10.15). On side 1 of the card a crossed-cylinder grid and a diamond containing 20/40, 20/30, 20/25, and 20/20 letters are seen binocularly. An additional crossed-cylinder grid is seen monocularly (the grid for the right eye on the right side and the grid for the left eye on the left side). On side 2 a reduced Snellen chart with letters ranging from 20/200 to 20/20 and a diamond containing three rows of letters (similar to the diamond on side 1) are seen binocularly. An additional reduced Snellen chart is seen monocularly (again, the chart on the right side seen by the right eye and the chart on the left side seen by the left eye). Side 2 also includes what Borish refers to as a modified Mallett fixation disparity test. A central *X* is seen by both eyes, and there is a cross, the upper and right limbs of which are seen by the right eye and the lower and left limbs seen by the left eye (as with Grolman's American Optical fixation disparity target). Four circles seen by both eyes serve as parafoveal fusion stimuli.

The entire sequence of near-point tests routinely performed by optometrists, plus additional tests, can be done with Borish's card. These tests include the following.

Figure 10.14   American Optical near-point vectographic cards: *(a)* **binocular refraction;** *(b)* **associated phorias;** *(c)* **stereopsis.**

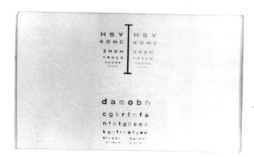

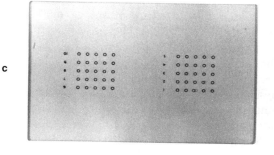

Crossed-cylinder tests. Using the crossed-grid targets on side 1, the monocular and binocular crossed-cylinder tests can be done in the usual manner. This method has the advantage that both eyes are seeing throughout the entire procedure without the use of dissociating prisms.

Acuity determination. Turning now to side 2 of the card, the practitioner determines if acuity is

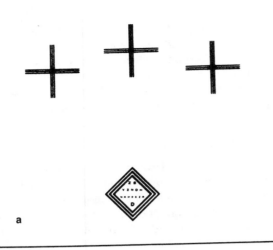

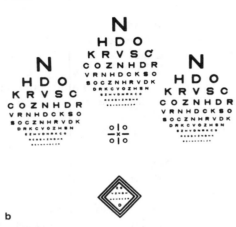

Figure 10.15   The Borish near-point card: *(a)* **side 1 and** *(b)* **side 2** (Borish, 1978).

Phorias and vergences. Using as a target the diamond containing several lines of letters, the von Graefe prism dissociation method can be used to determine lateral and vertical phorias. Using this same chart, base-in and base-out to blur, break, and recovery findings can be obtained.

Amplitude of accommodation and blur findings. Using the visual acuity charts on side 2, amplitude of accommodation can be determined binocularly (central chart) and monocularly (outer charts), using either the push-up or minus lens method. Plus-to-blur and minus-to-blur findings can be obtained in the usual manner, using the central chart (or the outer charts if monocular blur findings are desired).

Suppression. If gross suppression is present, the patient may report that one whole side of the chart is not seen. Less severe suppression may be indicated by the absence of one of the vertical or horizontal lines in the fixation disparity chart.

Because the Borish near-point card can be used for all the near-point tests done by optometrists, it can serve as a convenient, effective, and most welcome substitute for the "old-fashioned" near-point card.

The Disparometer

The first instrument designed for clinical measurement of fixation disparity (as opposed to determination of the prism necessary to eliminate fixation disparity) is the Disparometer, described by Sheedy and Saladin (1977) and by Sheedy (1980a, 1980b). This instrument is designed to fit on the near-point rod of a standard refractor, for use in measuring fixation disparity at 40cm.

As shown in Figure 10.16, the Disparometer includes two stimuli: one for vertical disparity measurement and one for horizontal disparity measurement. Each test stimulus includes a black aperture and two reduced Snellen charts seen with both eyes, and two polarized vernier lines seen in the center of the black aperture (each eye seeing only one of the vernier lines). The outer edge of the black aperture serves as the primary fusion stimulus when the patient views the vernier lines. Rather than presenting a fixed vernier line pattern like that used in tests of associated phoria, the Disparometer is equipped with a series of interchangeable vernier line patterns.

The examiner first presents the patient with the

equal for the two eyes. The expected finding is that acuity will be equal in all three of the charts, or that it will be better in the central (binocularly seen) chart than in the monocularly seen charts. If the acuity in the two monocularly seen charts is not equal, the practitioner may want to do additional testing to determine the cause.

Balancing accommodation. The accommodative balance can be checked by adding plus or minus spherical power to one or the other eye.

Fixation disparity. Using the modified Mallett test on side 2, both vertical and horizontal fixation disparity can be investigated. As with other methods of measuring associated phorias, the amount of prism required to eliminate the disparity is the amount to be prescribed.

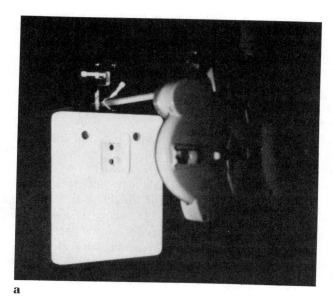

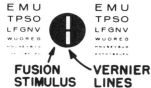

Figure 10.16 *(a)* **The Disparometer;** *(b)* **Test stimuli.**

target in which the vernier lines have no disparity. If the patient reports that the lines are not perfectly aligned, the examiner presents stimuli having varying amounts of disparity until the patient reports alignment. By determining the amount of fixation disparity while forcing vergence with base-in and base-out prisms presented in steps of 3Δ, fixation disparity curves similar to those plotted by Ogle (1950), illustrated in Figure 4.28, Chapter 4, can be plotted. According to Sheedy (1980a, 1980b), the findings necessary to plot a patient's fixation disparity curve can be taken in about 5 minutes.

Once the disparity curve has been plotted, it can be analyzed in terms of four variables, as described by Sheedy (1980a, 1980b):

1. *Type of fixation disparity curve.* About 60 percent of the population is found to have a Type I fixation disparity curve, in which the amount of fixation disparity increases with increasing amounts of prism and levels off at some point as additional prism is introduced. According to Sheedy, patients having Type I curves are generally asymptomatic. Types II, III, and IV curves

(Figure 4.28) tend to be associated with the symptomatic patient.

2. *Slope of the fixation disparity curve.* The slope of the fixation disparity curve indicates how much the fixation disparity changes as prism power is changed. Sheedy (1980a) concluded that because patients whose fixation disparity curves have a high slope tend to have symptoms, a low slope (less than 45 degrees) is desirable.

3. *The y-intercept of the curve.* This is the amount of fixation disparity present with no prism, and it should be less than 10 minutes of arc (although exo fixation disparity is more easily tolerated than eso fixation disparity).

4. *The x-intercept of the curve.* This is the amount of prism required to eliminate the fixation disparity, or the associated phoria, and is the only fixation disparity parameter determined by devices such as the Mallett box, the American Optical vectograph slide, and the Borish near-point card.

Interpretation

Prescribing for a binocular vision problem on the basis of the fixation disparity curve is based on the following principles (Sheedy, 1980a, 1980b): (1) the type of curve can be helpful in deciding whether to train or prescribe prism; (2) the primary sign of poor oculomotor imbalance is a steep slope, and a secondary sign is a large amount of fixation disparity; (3) the primary effect of training usually is to flatten the slope; and (4) prism is prescribed to place the flattest portion of the curve at the zero demand point (by reading the prism value from the x-axis of the graph).

According to Sheedy (1980a), symptomatic patients who have Type I curves with steep slopes respond well to orthoptic training, which has the effect of flattening the slope; patients having Type II curves (who usually have eso deviations) can be helped by the prescription of prisms or plus lenses. (Procedures for prescribing on the basis of Disparometer findings are discussed in Chapter 12.)

STRABISMUS ANALYSIS

Although the primary care optometrist is not necessarily expected to provide therapy for strabismus patients, he or she should be able to fully analyze the strabismus and come to some conclusion concerning the possibility of a functional cure. This analysis should include a pertinent strabismus history (age of onset, any precipitating factors, and any previous surgical or orthoptic treatment) and should enable the practitioner to answer the following questions:

1. How is the patient's strabismus classified in terms of direction, distance, and other factors?
2. Is the strabismus concomitant (functional) or incomitant (paralytic)?
3. Does the patient suppress?
4. Does the patient have amblyopia?
5. Does the patient have eccentric fixation?
6. Does the patient have anomalous retinal correspondence?

The answers to many of these questions in many cases will already have been obtained as a result of tests done in the preliminary examination.

Classification of Strabismus

Whether or not the patient has strabismus will have been determined by the corneal reflex test and the unilateral cover test. In addition, the unilateral cover test will have provided information as to whether the strabismus is unilateral or alternating; constant or intermittent; and occurs for distance fixation, near fixation, or both. The angle of strabismus, at 6m and at 40cm, will have been determined by means of the alternating cover test and the use of square prisms or a prism bar.

Comitancy

Strabismus is said to be *concomitant* if the angle of squint is the same in all directions of gaze and *incomitant* if the angle of squint is not the same in all directions. Cases of concomitant strabismus are *functional* in origin, whereas cases of incomitant strabismus are *paralytic*. Exceptions to this general rule are long-standing cases of paralytic strabismus that have developed comitancy.

Whether an ocular muscle paralysis is present will have been determined in the broad *H* test by a lagging of one eye behind the other in one or more of the six positions of gaze, or in the diplopia field test by the patient's report of diplopia in one or more of the six positions of gaze.

Suppression

The presence of suppression can be detected by means of the Worth Dot test described in Chapter 4.

A strabismus patient who is *not* suppressing would be expected to report that five dots are seen—two red dots being seen with the right eye and three green dots being seen with the left eye. However, if one eye is suppressing, only two red dots or three green dots will be seen.

Another test for suppression involves the use of the Bagolini striated lenses. These lenses are based on the principle of the Maddox rod, but the situations are so fine they do not interfere with visual acuity. The Bagolini lenses are placed in a trial frame with the striations at an angle of 135 degrees for the right eye and 45 degrees for the left eye. A muscle light (at 6m) or a penlight (at 40cm) is used as a stimulus. If there is no suppression, the patient will report seeing two diagonal lines crossing at, above, or below the light source. (If the lines cross above or below the light source, two lights will be seen.) If suppression exists, all or a part of one of the lines will not be seen. If suppression is central, the central portion of one of the lines may be absent but the peripheral portions present.

Amblyopia

The detection of amblyopia should be no problem, as long as the examiner remembers that an amblyope's visual acuity can be deceptively good if single letters or single lines are used (see Chapter 4). If a child is old enough to respond to the Snellen letter chart or the tumbling *E* chart, the whole field of the projector (consisting of four or five lines of letters or tumbling *E*s) should be used.

When refraction is uncertain, the pinhole test can be used to distinguish between amblyopia and poor dioptric correction.

For infants and toddlers below the age of 3, a method of visual acuity testing known as the *preferential looking technique* has been developed (see Figure 10.17). As described by Boltz (1981), this procedure takes advantage of the infant's natural preference to look at the more interesting of two stimuli. The child is shown two pictures, one with black and white stripes and the other a homogeneous gray. The child will look at the stripes, if they can be seen. As the child's fixation pattern is recorded by an observer, the stripes are made progressively narrower until the infant shows no preference, as determined by the observer, to look at the stripes. A commercial version of this apparatus is not available, but it is not difficult to construct.

A second method of testing for amblyopia

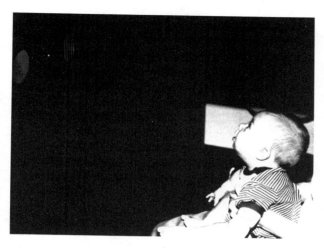

Figure 10.17   Measuring an infant's visual acuity by means of the preferential looking technique (from Boltz, 1981).

described by Boltz involves the use of a vertical prism of approximately 10Δ power placed before one of the eyes. While the child fixates an object such as a toy, the prism is introduced before one eye and the fixation pattern is observed. If the fixation alternates between the two eyes, it is unlikely that amblyopia exists. However, if there is no alternation of fixation, it cannot be concluded that amblyopia is present—the test does not detect amblyopia but can rule it out. Another method of detecting the possible presence of amblyopia described by Boltz is observation of the child's fixation pattern during the cover test. If the child freely alternates the eye used for fixation, it is unlikely that amblyopia is present; if the child presents with a unilateral strabismus, it is likely that the child is amblyopic.

Eccentric Fixation

Both objective and subjective tests are available for the detection of eccentric fixation. The objective procedure, described in Chapter 4, involves the use of a graticule target, with which most ophthalmoscopes are equipped. While the patient fixates a distant object, the examiner projects the center, or bull's-eye, of the target on the patient's fovea and instructs the patient to look at the center of the target. If the position of the foveal reflex changes relative to the target, it indicates an off-foveal fixation point. The position of the foveal reflex indicates the direction and amount of the eccentric fixation.

Subjective tests for eccentric fixation make use of the entoptic phenomena of *Maxwell's spot* and *Haidinger's brushes* (see Figure 10.18). Maxwell's spot can be observed by viewing a diffusely illuminated field through a purple-blue filter. Under these conditions a darkened spot, corresponding to the position of the fovea, is seen. If the diffusely illuminated field is provided with a fixation point, the degree of eccentric fixation can be estimated by asking the subject to describe the position of the gray spot with respect to the fixation point. One problem in using Maxwell's spot clinically is that it fades quickly. This problem can be solved by mounting a rotating disk having alternating sectors of purple-blue and yellow filters in front of the diffusely illuminated field. The yellow filter extinguishes Maxwell's spot, so it is alternately stimulated and extinguished.

Haidinger's brushes can be observed when a diffusely illuminated blue field is viewed through a rotating Polaroid filter. Under these conditions yellow brushlike phenomena are seen radiating from the point of fixation. The brushes are thought to be due to double refraction by the radially oriented fibers of Henle around the fovea. A commercially available test, the Coordinator, makes use of the Haidinger brush phenomena. As the patient observes the phenomena, he or she is instructed to describe the position of the "propeller" with respect to the fixation point.

Figure 10.18   Subjective tests for eccentric fixation: *(a)* **Maxwell's spot;** *(b)* **Haidinger's brushes.**

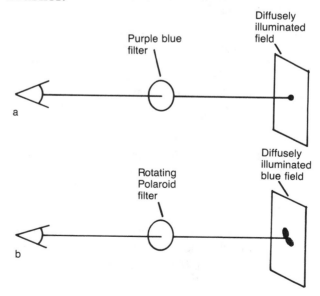

Anomalous Retinal Correspondence (ARC)

Anomalous retinal correspondence (ARC) exists, as an adaptation to strabismus, when an off-foveal point of the deviating eye is associated with the fovea of the fixating eye. Anomalous retinal correspondence is classified as either *harmonius*, *unharmonius*, or *paradoxical*. To classify the ARC in a given case, one must determine the values of three angles: the objective angle of squint, the subjective angle of squint, and the angle of anomaly. The *angle of anomaly* is the angle between the fovea and the anomalously corresponding point of the deviating eye, subtended at the nodal point.

If the objective angle of squint and the angle of anomaly are equal, the ARC is *harmonius*. In this case, the subjective angle of squint is zero, and the ARC can be said to be "successful" in allowing visual direction to be similar for the two eyes with the strabismic eye in its deviating position. If the angle of anomaly is less than the objective angle of strabismus, the ARC is *unharmonius* and can be thought of as partially successful. If the patient has had ocular muscle surgery, a *paradoxical* ARC may be found. This will be the case if the angle of anomaly is greater than the objective angle of squint (paradoxical ARC Type I) or if the subjective angle of squint is greater than the objective angle, and the angle of anomaly is in the direction opposite to the subjective and objective angles of squint (paradoxical ARC Type II).

One of the most straightforward methods of testing for ARC involves the afterimage transfer test, described in Chapter 4 and illustrated in Figure 4.38.

Another method of determining the presence of ARC involves use of the Bagolini lenses already described. Using the Bagolini striated lenses, if the patient reports that the two diagonal lines cross at the light source, it indicates that the subjective angle of strabismus is zero and, therefore, that harmonius ARC exists. According to Parks (1979), interpretation of the Bagolini test requires a level of maturity not often found in a child under the age of 8 years. Both Parks (1979) and Griffin (1976) provide additional information for the interpretation of this test.

Still another method of testing for ARC is to compare the results of the objective and subjective angles measured by means of the alternating cover test and square prisms or a prism bar. In the objective method, the end-point of the test is the amount of prism necessary to eliminate the deviation of the eye (as seen by the examiner). In the subjective method, the end-point is the amount of prism necessary for the patient to report that no movement of the fixation target (a Snellen letter) is seen. For example, if the objective cover test determines that a patient has 20Δ of exotropia, but with no prisms in place the patient reports no target movement, it can be concluded that harmonious ARC is present.

Probability of Obtaining a Functional Cure

Strabismus is often regarded as a cosmetic rather than a functional problem. Unlike heterophoric patients who are able to maintain single binocular vision by the use of excessive amounts of fusional vergence demand, strabismic patients rarely experience symptoms of eyestrain. In most cases the strabismus becomes a problem only when the deviation is great enough so it is cosmetically undesirable. For the strabismic patient, the practitioner may consider the possibility of seeking a cosmetic cure (through ocular muscle surgery) or a functional cure (through a combination of lenses and orthoptics, and possibly with the aid of surgery).

Flom (1963) notes that the view of strabismus as a strictly cosmetic problem is not in the best interest of the patient, and that when a strabismus is corrected so there is normal binocular vision, the cosmetic appearance is almost invariably satisfactory. Flom has discussed the factors involved in the prediction of a functional cure. He defined a functional cure as the maintenance of bifoveal fixation in the ordinary situations of life (loss of bifoveal fixation occurring no more than 1 percent of the time), with vision clear and comfortable, and with the range of bifixation including all fields of gaze and extending from very great viewing distances to only a few centimeters.

In discussing his own percentage of functional cures for nonaccommodative strabismics, Flom (1963) reported higher success rates for exotropes than for esotropes; higher success rates for occasional squints than for constant squints; reduced success rates in the presence of amblyopia; and reduced success rates in the presence of ARC (severely reduced in the case of esotropia). The information shown in Table 10.2 is taken from tables published by Flom (1963).

Analysis of Incomitant Strabismus

If a patient has a vertical deviation that is found to vary with the direction of gaze, the Parks three-step procedure may be more sensitive than the broad *H* test or the diplopia field test for determining the responsible muscle.

Parks three-step test

Parks (1979) described a three-step procedure designed to determine which of the eight cyclovertical muscles (four for each eye) is responsible when a vertical deviation exists. The three steps are as follows:

1. Determine whether right or left hypertropia exists in the primary position. This rules out four of the cyclovertical muscles.
2. Determine whether the vertical deviation increases on gaze to the right or on gaze to the left. This rules out two additional muscles.
3. Use the Bielschowsky head-tilt test to determine whether the faulty muscle is an intorter or an extorter, narrowing the diagnosis down to a single muscle.

The results of the procedure are interpreted on the basis of the following information:

1. Muscles responsible for a right hyper-deviation are the right inferior rectus (RIR), right superior oblique (RSO), left superior rectus (LSR), or left inferior oblique (LIO). Muscles responsible for a left hyper-deviation are the left inferior rectus (LIR), left superior oblique (LSO), right superior rectus (RSR),

Table 10.2 Probability of obtaining a functional cure (Flom, 1963).

Condition	Probability of success (percent)
Constant strabismus	
Exotropia	27%
Esotropia	11
Occasional strabismus	
Exotropia	58
Esotropia	50
Strabismus with amblyopia	
Exotropia	37
Esotropia	10
Normal retinal correspondence	
Exotropia	57
Esotropia	40
Anomalous retinal correspondence	
Exotropia	38
Esotropia	3

or right inferior oblique (RIO). In each case an underacting muscle allows opposing muscles to turn the eye upward or downward. Recall that a right hyper-deviation (phoria or tropia) is also a left hypo-deviation.

2. Muscles responsible for increasing a right hyper-deviation on gaze to the right are the RIR and LIO; those responsible on gaze to the left are the RSO and LSR. Muscles responsible for increasing a left hyper-deviation on gaze to the right are the RSR and LSO; and those responsible on gaze to the left are the LIR and RIO. These statements can be confirmed by considering the effects of the muscle planes of the cyclovertical muscles (See Chapter 6, Figure 6.16) on gaze to the right and left.

3. Muscles responsible for increasing a right hyper-deviation on tilting the head toward the right shoulder are the RSO and LIO; those responsible on tilting the head toward the left shoulder are the LSR and RIR. Muscles responsible for increasing a left hyper-deviation on tilting the head toward the right shoulder are the RSR and LIR; those responsible on tilting the head toward the left shoulder are the LSO and RIO.

In all four cases described in the previous paragraph, the increase in the hyper-deviation is a result of the fact that when the head is tilted, the eyes undergo a *cyclotorsional* movement that tends to keep the vertical meridian of the retina (and thus the visual field) in a vertical position. When the head is tilted toward the right, the right eye makes an encyclotorsional movement (the top of the cornea tilting toward the nose) while the left eye makes an excyclotorsional movement. The upward deviation of the eye occurs because two muscles are involved in any torsional movement of the eyes. Of these two muscles, one is an elevator and the other is a depressor. The faulty muscle involved in this torsional movement allows its fellow intorter (or extorter, as the case may be) to move the eye either upward or downward (in the direction opposite to that in which the faulty muscle would move the eye).

The key to interpreting this final step of the procedure involves remembering that superior muscles (SR and SO) *intort*, and inferior muscles (IR and IO) *extort*. Thus, if it is found that a patient has a right hyper-deviation, ruling out all cyclovertical muscles other than the RIR, RSO, LSR, and LIO (step 1); if the deviation increases on gaze to the left, ruling out all muscles except the RSO and LSR (step 2); and if it is then found that the deviation increases on tilting the head toward the right shoulder (step 3), we conclude that this deviation is due to the action

Table 10.3   Example of results of Parks three-step test (Parks, 1979).

| | Possible responsible muscle(s) | | |
| | Step 1 | Step 2 | Step 3 |
Prior to beginning three-step test	Right hypertropia	Hyperdeviation increases on gaze to left	Hyper-deviation increases on tilting head toward right shoulder
RSR	—	—	—
RIR	RIR	—	—
RSO	RSO	RSO	RSO
RIO	—	—	—
LSR	LSR	LSR	—
LIR	—	—	—
LSO	—	—	—
LIO	LIO	—	—

of the RSR, which is the "fellow intorter" with the RSO, so the faulty muscle is the RSO. This example is illustrated in Table 10.3.

On the other hand, if the vertical deviation is found to increase when the head is tilted toward the left shoulder, the left eye should be considered to deviate downward with respect to the right eye; this is due to either the LIR or the LSO. Because the LSO and the LSR are "fellow intorters" when the head is tilted toward the left, it should be concluded that the downward deviation is due to the LSO and that the LSR is the faulty muscle.

As a final point in the interpretation of the Parks three-step test, note that the two muscles remaining (after the other six have been ruled out) are, in every case, both intorters or both extorters.

Study Questions

1. Why should an elderly person who suddenly develops a vertical phoria be referred for medical evaluation?

2. In measuring a lateral phoria with a base-up dissociating prism in front of the left eye, what eye movements are made if the patient is asked to watch the lower line of letters and to report when one line of letters is directly above the other?

3. If the vertical vergence findings for the right eye are supra 4/1 and infra 2/0, what should you expect the findings to be for the left eye?

4. Why is it necessary to use low illumination when doing the monocular and binocular crossed-cylinder findings at 40cm?

5. A patient has the following phoria findings: phoria through the subjective lenses at 6m, 1 exo; phoria at 40cm through subjective lenses, 5 exo; phoria at 40cm through the subjective lenses combined with +1.00DS, 8 exo. (a) What is the calculated AC/A ratio? (b) What is the gradient AC/A ratio?

6. (a) What is meant by the term *associated phoria*? (b) How does it differ (both in terms of the stimulus situation and in terms of the expected value of the finding) from a dissociated phoria?

7. Which test would you expect to result in a higher finding for the amplitude of accommodations: the push-up test or the minus lens test at 40cm? Why?

8. For a patient who has 10Δ of exophoria and a base-out finding of 12/20/10 at 40cm, what effect would the prescribing of 1.5Δ base-in, each eye, have (a) on the phoria finding? (b) on the positive fusional vergence reserve finding?

9. What disadvantage is there in using the alignment method rather than the flash method in the lateral phoria test?

10. When the vertical vergence findings are being obtained, why is the patient not instructed to report the occurrence of a blur?

11. For a patient who has 4Δ of esophoria at 6m with base-in vergence findings of x/8/4 and base-out vergence findings of 12/22/10, (a) what is the total range of fusional vergence? (b) what is the amount of the negative fusional vergence demand? (c) what is the amount of the negative fusional vergence reserve?

12. What information does the binocular cross-cylinder finding at 40cm provide (a) if the patient is not a presbyope? (b) if the patient is a presbyope?

13. Why is the gradient AC/A ratio usually found to be somewhat lower than the calculated AC/A ratio?

14. As minus lens power is added in front of both eyes at 40cm during the positive relative accommodation test, why is it that the use of accommodative convergence does not result in diplopia?

15. A patient has the following phoria findings: phoria through the subjective lenses at 6m, 2 eso; phoria at 40cm through subjective lenses, 7 eso; phoria at 40cm through subjective lenses combined with +1.00DS, 1 eso. (a) What is the calculated AC/A ratio? (b) What is the gradient AC/A ratio?

16. What is the highest value that you should ever expect to find for (a) the positive relative accommodation finding? (b) the negative relative accommodation finding?

17. A patient is found to have 4Δ of left hyperphoria, and vertical vergence findings R supra 2/0, infra 6/4; and L supra 6/4, infra 2/0. How much prism power (and with the base in what direction) would be necessary to balance the vertical vergence findings?

18. In the lateral phoria test at 40cm, what undesirable result may occur if the patient fails to maintain accommodation on the small letters on the near-point card?

19. Which of the following tests may be used for measurement of both the dissociated phoria at 40cm and the associated phoria at 40cm? (a) Mallett test; (b) American Optical vectograph test; (c) Borish near-point card; (d) Disparometer.

20. What is the significance of each of the following parameters of a fixation disparity curve, as

determined by the use of the Disparometer? (a) the slope of the curve; (b) the y-intercept value; (c) the x-intercept value.

21. When the Worth Dot test is done (red lens on right eye) how would you interpret each of the following reports by the patient? (a) Two dots; (b) three dots; (c) four dots; (d) five dots.

22. When using a 10-prism diopter prism in front of one eye of a child to determine whether the child is amblyopic, how would you interpret the results of the test (a) if fixation alternates between the two eyes while the prism is in place? (b) if there is no alternate fixation between the two eyes?

23. When investigating the possibility of anomalous retinal correspondence by comparing the objective and subjective angles of squint, what would be your diagnosis of each of the following? (a) Objective angle of squint 20 exo, subjective angle zero; (b) objective angle 20 exo, subjective angle 10 exo; (c) objective angle 20 exo, subjective angle 20 exo; (d) objective angle 20 exo, subjective angle 30 exo.

24. What disadvantages does the Maddox rod have when used for a lateral phoria test?

25. What muscle would you consider to be the cause of a vertical deviation if the following results were found in the Parks three-step test? (a) *Step 1:* the patient has a left hyper-deviation in the primary position; (b) *Step 2:* the vertical deviation increases on gazing to the left; (c) *step 3:* during the Bielschowsky head-tilt test, the deviation increases when the head is tilted toward the left shoulder.

CHAPTER 11

Automatic Refraction and Biometry

In recent years, the widespread use of computerization has led not only to the development of objective and subjective automatic refractors but to the introduction of automatic keratometers and A-scan ultrasonic biometers. Computer-assisted refractors represent the most recent stage in the development of the science of ocular refraction, which had its humble beginnings with the invention of spectacles toward the close of the 13th century. As described by Hofstetter (1948), the invention of the movable type printing press in the 15th century resulted in the popularization of reading, and spectacle makers' guilds were formed in England and Germany. Until the invention of the trial lens case by Fronmuller of Germany in 1843, ready-made glasses were sold by spectacle peddlers; as Hofstetter commented, the only refracting was done by the buyer, who selected spectacles from the peddler's tray.

The invention of the trial lens case put the buyer in the position of depending on the peddler for advice. With the incorporation of cylindrical lenses into the trial set (on the suggestion of Donders in 1864) and the development of varieties of frame styles, the practice of what we now call optometry was firmly established.

Marg (1973) relates that the first refractor, invented by De Zang in 1908, evolved into the American Optical 588, 589, and 590 phoropters and into the Rx-Master; in 1931, Hunsicker designed what is now known as the Bausch & Lomb Green's refractor. Prior to the development of computer-assisted refractors, advances in ocular refraction included new charts for the measurement of astigmatism, advances in the design of retinoscopes (particularly with the advent of the streak retinoscope), and procedures for binocular refraction and fixation disparity testing.

Also developed during this period were a large number of optical refractometers, which have been all but ignored by the profession. However, with the development of computer-assisted refraction, these optical refractometers should not be allowed to escape our attention completely.

OPTICAL REFRACTOMETERS

Instruments falling into the category of optical refractometers include the Fincham coincidence optometer, Rodenstock refractometer, Zeiss refractometer, Essel refractometer, and Topcon refractometer. Each of these instruments is based on the principle of the retinoscope, the ophthalmoscope, or the lensometer. They all are objective for the patient and subjective for the examiner, so the examiner sometimes feels that his or her own eyes are being examined. With most of these instruments the measurement of spherical power is relatively straightforward, but small cylinders tend to be difficult to pick up. In addition, the control of accommodation tends to be a problem, so the refractive end-point may be in error in the direction of too little hyperopia or too much myopia.

Topcon Refractometer

The Topcon refractometer is one of the newest optical refractometers. It is about the size and shape of a keratometer and has a range of −20.00 to +20.00D (larger than the range available in many computer-assisted refractors). The cost compares favorably with that of a standard refractor.

When operating the Topcon refractometer, the practitioner and the patient view the same target, except that the patient's target also includes a green ring for fixation. The instrument is operated in much the same way as a lensometer. As the patient fixates the green ring, the operator rotates the optical system of the instrument until the two principal meridians are located, and then clears up the target image in each of the two meridians. The scale readings in each of the two meridians are then converted into the lens formula in the minus cylinder form. Experience with this instrument in the vision screening program at Indiana University indicated that accurate findings (comparable to retinoscopy) can be obtained on older adults, but that accommodation is sometimes a problem when working with children or young adults.

OBJECTIVE COMPUTER-ASSISTED REFRACTORS

A number of objective computer-assisted refractors are now available. These instruments are objective for both the patient and the operator. The operator's only task is to align the patient in the instrument, instruct the patient regarding fixation, and push a button. The patient's refraction is measured using infrared light (which is invisible to the patient), although the patient is presented with a visible fixation object. The first of these instruments to be developed was the Bausch & Lomb Ophthalmetron. This was followed by the Acuity Systems Auto-Refractor, the Coherent Dioptron, and instruments marketed by Canon, Nikon, Humphrey, and others. Although the Ophthalmetron is no longer available, it is described here because it is still in use.

Bausch & Lomb Ophthalmetron

Developed by the ophthalmologist Aaron Safir, the Ophthalmetron was introduced in 1972. The instrument operates on the principle of the retinoscope. A chopper drum rotates about the light source and through the light beam, chopping the beam at 720 slit/scans per second. The light is reflected from the patient's retina and then is brought to a focus by a collimating lens, the focal point representing the eye's far-point. A photodetector assembly detects "with" or "against" motion and moves backward or forward as required while rotating through an angle of 180 degrees, until neutral motion is detected in all meridians. A pen-writer plots a sine-square curve on graph paper previously placed in the instrument by the operator. If the patient maintains steady fixation, the whole procedure takes approximately 3 seconds.

To operate the instrument, the examiner first uses a periscope to align the patient's eye. The patient is then requested to look at a target in the form of a puff of smoke at the end of a rocket. By adjusting the position of a Scheiner disk, the examiner fogs the patient by asking the patient to report when the doubled image of the rocket becomes single. Although the instrument is designed to be examiner objective (in contrast to retinoscopy, in which the examiner must make a series of decisions), the fogging procedure is, in some cases, a crucial step. The author's experience with the instrument has shown that the operator inadvertently may lock in unwanted accommodation before the refracting procedure is begun, thus biasing the refraction in the direction of too little plus or too much minus.

Knoll, Morhman, and Maier (1970) reported on a study in which Ophthalmetron findings were compared with retinoscopy and subjective findings for 100 randomly selected patients. They plotted subjective findings against both retinoscopy and Ophthalmetron findings and concluded that Ophthalmetron data and retinoscopy findings were essentially equivalent. Keech (1979) examined ten optometry students with the Ophthalmetron using both cycloplegic and noncycloplegic refraction, and she found that refraction under cycloplegia resulted in an average of 0.41D more hyperopia than when a cycloplegic was not used. Keech concluded that this was a true difference between cycloplegic and noncycloplegic refraction and was not the result of accommodation.

Acuity Systems Auto-Refractor

The Acuity Systems 6600 Auto-Refractor, which became available in 1973, makes use of the Scheiner disk principle. The instrument has a self-aligning system, and the patient is asked to fixate a diffuse, green blob of light designed for relaxing accommodation. The data are provided in the form of a printout that includes the spherical and cylindrical powers and the cylindrical axis.

Hill (1973) reported on a double-blind study in which Auto-Refractor results were compared with subjective refraction findings on 100 eyes. He found that the results of the two methods were within ±0.50D of each other for 81 percent of the spherical findings and for 92 percent of the cylindrical power findings, and the results were within ±10 degrees of each other for 68 percent of the cylindrical axis findings. Hill concluded that the instrument is highly accurate and provides monocular findings that can be converted quickly into a meaningful binocular correction.

In 1980, Acuity Systems introduced the Rx 1 Auto-Refractor, which was described as an improvement over the 6600 model in that it provides a measurement of spherical power, cylindrical power, axis, and interpupillary distance in 1 second. In addition, a "vertex" button enables the instrument to provide refractive findings referred either to the corneal plane (for contact lens wearers) or the spectacle plane (for spectacle wearers). The Rx 1 was withdrawn from the market by Acuity Systems within months after its announcement but is currently marketed by the Trilogic Corporation.

Dioptron

The original model of the Dioptron, introduced by Coherent in 1973, differed from the Ophthalmetron and the Acuity Systems Auto-Refractor in having a binocularly viewed target (a Snellen chart) and utilizing a fogging technique. The optical system is similar to that of a lensometer. An image-analysis system detects retinal image clarity on the basis of illumination, the measurement being repeated in several meridians within a 20-second period. The readout includes spherical power, cylindrical power, cylindrical axis, and a confidence factor based on the measurement variation during the test period.

Sloan and Polse (1974) reported on a study in which Dioptron findings were compared with retinoscopy and subjective findings on 98 clinic patients. Dioptron findings were taken by an aide using a prototype of the instrument. The authors found correlation coefficients between Dioptron and subjective refraction findings to be 0.978 for spherical power, 0.766 for cylindrical power, 0.594 for cylindrical axis for cylinders of less than 0.50D power, and 0.902 for cylindrical axis for cylinders of −0.50D power or higher.

The Dioptron II, introduced in 1977, was designed to take advantage of more advanced computer technology, allowing the entire refraction procedure to be completed (in six meridians) within a few seconds. The cost of the instrument to the practitioner was considerably less than that of the original Dioptron.

The Dioptron Nova (see Figure 11.1), announced in 1980, has replaced the Dioptron II. It has a monocularly viewed (rather than a binocularly viewed) target but otherwise is similar to the Dioptron II. The original Dioptron has evolved into the Dioptron Ultima. Like the original Dioptron, it has a binocu-

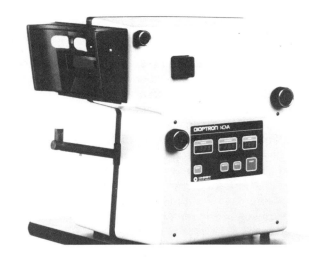

Figure 11.1   The Dioptron Nova.

larly viewed target as well as additional equipment, such as an instrument table, a printer for a permanent "hard copy" of the patient's refraction, and a control for vertex distance for use in overrefraction.

In a three-way comparison of Dioptron Nova results with conventional retinoscopy and subjective findings, Grosvenor, Perrigin, and Perrigin (1985) found that Dioptron Nova and retinoscopy findings compared favorably, mean differences being 0.01D for spherical equivalent power and 0.05D for cylindrical power. However, Dioptron Nova and subjective findings differed by 0.33D for spherical equivalent power and by 0.18D for cylindrical power. It was concluded that the use of this instrument, like retinoscopy, can provide the practitioner with a starting point for subjective refraction but cannot serve as a substitute for subjective refraction.

In 1984, Coherent discontinued both the Dioptron Ultima and Nova. Subsequently, the Nova was redesigned by CooperVision and marketed as the Dioptron V. This instrument, as described by Rassow and Wesemann (1985), has an incandescent light source with a wavelength of 880nm. The infrared pattern is projected onto the patient's retina, and a focus detector determines the sharpness of the retinal image and adjusts the focusing lens for maximum sharpness. The fixation target is a starburst on a white background. The minimum pupil diameter for this instrument is 2.0mm, and the instrument's range is from −10.00 to +15.00DS and ±7.00DC. The readout is in the form of an LED display with a roll-paper printout.

Specifications of Available Auto-Refractors

Rassow and Wesemann (1985) and Wesemann and Rassow (1987) have described and evaluated the then-available automatic infrared refractors. All of the instruments have light sources in the form of one or more LEDs in the 815–900nm wavelength range and provide readings in the form of both an LED display and a roll-paper printout. Although some of the instruments are strictly objective auto-refractors, others have provision for subjective refinement of sphere and cylinder findings. Much of the following information is based on the Wesemann and Rassow (1987) report.

Canon R–10 and Hoya AR–530

The Canon R–10 and Hoya AR–530 auto-refractors are essentially similar, the Hoya instrument being built under license from Canon. The Scheiner double-pinhole principle is used. Each arm of a three-pointed star pattern focused onto the retina is imaged through one of three pairs of Scheiner double-pinholes on one of three linear photodetector arrays. Refraction is measured in each of the three meridians, and astigmatism is determined by fitting a sine-square curve through all data points. The fixation target is a colored picture of a landscape. Minimum pupil diameter is 2.9mm and the range is ±15.00DS and ±7.00DC. Neither instrument has subjective refinement capability.

Humphrey HAR Alpha 500, 505, and 530

The Humphrey HAR Alpha 500, 505, and 530 instruments are equipped with visual-acuity charts.

Figure 11.2　The Humphrey Auto-Refractor.

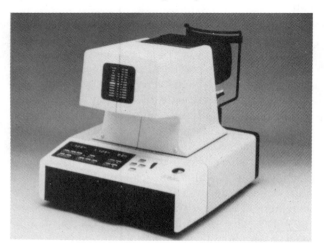

In addition, the 530 provides for subjective refinement of the sphere power, cylinder power, and cylinder axis (see Figure 11.2). The instruments are based on the optical principle that a light spot imaged sharply on the retina will be focused back on itself. A photodetector signals when the retinal image is in focus. All meridians are measured simultaneously, which has the advantage of eliminating errors due to differences in accommodation in different meridians. The fixation target is a blurred light during the initial measurement, and a visual-acuity chart is seen during the automatic fogging step. Minimum pupil diameter is 2.0mm and the range is −12.00 to +20.00DS and ±6.00DC.

Marco and Nidek AR–1600

For the Marco and Nidek AR–1600 instruments, the optical principle is a Scheiner's disc (double-pinhole). There are four fixation targets: a clock dial, a Snellen chart, a cross grid, and a clown face. Minimum pupil diameter is 2.0mm and the range is from −17.00 to +22.00DS and ±7.00DC. The instrument is capable of performing a true computer-assisted subjective refraction. The Nidek AR–1100 is a less expensive instrument, not having the subjective refraction capability.

Nikon NR–7000

The Nikon NR–7000 instrument provides for subjective refinement of the objective findings, with fogging, a clock-dial, and a cross-cylinder test. The optical principle for the instrument is that of the retinoscope: an infrared streak scans the pupil 720 times per second, while a rotating prism allows measurement in all meridians. Five fixation targets are provided: a starburst target, two Landolt ring charts, a bichrome chart, a clock dial, and "minute spots." Minimum pupil diameter is 2.9mm and the instrument's range is ±15.00DS and ±6.00DC. A less expensive instrument, the Nikon NR–5000, does not provide for subjective refraction.

Topcon RM–A 6000 and 6500

The Topcon RM–A 6000 and 6500 instruments are essentially similar with the exception that the RM–A 6500 provides for subjective refinement of the sphere and cylinder findings by means of fogging, a clock dial, and a crossed-cylinder test. The optical system for both instruments is that of the Scheiner double-pinhole. The fixation target for the RM–A 6000 is a starburst pattern, whereas the RM–A 6500 has five fixation targets: a starburst pattern, a letter chart, a bichrome number chart, a clock-dial chart,

Table 11.1   Spherical equivalent power and cylinder power results for seven auto-refractors compared to results of conventional clinical refraction (from Wesemann and Rassow, 1987).

Instrument	Eyes	Spherical equivalent power (mean difference)[a]	Spherical equivalent within 0.50D (percent)	Cylinder power (mean difference)	Cylinder power within 0.50D (percent)
Canon R–10	101	+0.11D	87%	−0.02D	95%
Hoya AR–530	97	+0.11D	87	−0.10D	97
Humphrey 520	105	+0.02D	89	−0.12D	95
Humphrey 530 (Auto + on)	105	0.00D	80	−0.07D	95
Humphrey 530 (Auto + off)	105	−0.16D		−0.12D	
Nidek AR–1600	101	+0.47D	95[b]	−0.11D	97
Nikon NR–7000	109	−0.11D	84	−0.09D	90
Topcon RM–A 6000	109	+0.12D	84	−0.05D	97

[a]Plus sign (+) indicates more plus power for auto-refractor findings.
[b]0.50D has been subtracted from the spherical auto-refractor result.

a cross-grid chart, and a landscape picture. For both instruments, minimum pupil diameter is 2.9mm and the range is ±20.00DS and ±7.00DC.

Evaluation of Auto-Refractors

In their 1987 report, Wesemann and Rassow compared the findings of seven auto-refractors to those of conventional clinical refraction on 55 subjects aged 20–68 years. Their results for spherical equivalent power and cylinder power are summarized in Table 11.1. As shown in the third column of the table, *mean spherical equivalent power* was within 0.12D of that for conventional refraction with two exceptions:

1. The mean difference between the Humphrey 530 (auto + off) and clinical findings was −0.16D. The term *auto +* refers to the automatic fogging sequence built into the instrument's program, which may be turned off as a time-saving measure. Wesemann and Rassow used the instrument both as intended (auto + on) and without the auto +. As a result of these findings, they suggest that the auto + feature should not be bypassed.

2. The mean difference between the Nidek AR–1600 and clinical findings was +0.47D. Wesemann and Rassow noted that the manufacturer of the Nidek instrument purposely calibrated it to "over-plus" 0.50D, with the idea that the finding represents a fogged starting point for a subjective refrac-

tion. For instruments sold in the United States, a readjustment is made to eliminate the 0.50D fog.

As shown in the fourth column of Table 11.1, the spherical equivalent power determined by each of the instruments was within 0.50D of that determined by conventional refraction on 80–95 percent of the eyes tested. The results for cylinder power (noted in the fifth and last columns of Table 11.1) compared even more closely with conventional refraction than was the case for spherical equivalent power. Wesemann and Rassow (1987) reported *cylinder axis* data not in terms of degrees of axis error but in terms of the *power error* induced by an off-axis finding. They found that for 83–90 percent of eyes, the induced power error was less than 0.63D.

Wesemann and Rassow (1987) concluded that, in comparison to their previous studies, there is little difference in accuracy between auto-refractors of different manufacturers; the instruments are so closely matched that it is almost impossible to rate them on the basis of their accuracy with normal ametropic subjects. They further concluded that all of the instruments can be recommended without hesitation for an accurate *preliminary refraction*, but because the instruments occasionally make large errors (of 1D or more) and because none of the instruments is capable of performing a binocular balance, it is *not* possible to *prescribe* directly from an auto-refractor finding. In short, the auto-refractors are capable of serving, as Grosvenor et al. (1985)

note concerning the Dioptron Nova, as substitutes for retinoscopy.

Using an auto-refractor as a substitute for retinoscopy has some advantages but is not without disadvantages. The advantages include:

1. In a busy, high-income practice the cost of the instrument is almost negligible since it can be amortized along with other equipment.
2. Patients tend to be impressed when the practitioner has what appears to be the latest in automated equipment.
3. Because an auto-refractor can be operated as well by an assistant or a technician as by the practitioner, the use of such an instrument saves the practitioner a certain amount of time. The time saved, however, is less than one might imagine, because once the patient is seated in the ophthalmic chair and the refractor is adjusted to his or her face, the time required for the experienced retinoscopist to perform the test is approximately one minute for each eye.

The major disadvantages of the auto-refractor include:

1. It tends to reinforce, in the patient's mind, the idea that the practitioner depends more on "high-tech" instrumentation, operated by an assistant, than on his or her own knowledge and skill.
2. As a result of not performing routine retinoscopy, the practitioner is likely to miss a large number of subtle clues that may be helpful in subsequent testing procedures, including (a) the rapidly changing character of the reflex due to spasm of accommodation in latent hyperopia; (b) the scissors motion of the reflex that occurs when the patient has a large pupil; (c) the "slit"-shaped reflex that occurs when a patient "squints," warning the practitioner that both objective and subjective cylinder findings may be suspect; (d) the presence of early cortical changes in the lens, which may be missed in routine (undilated) ophthalmoscopy and biomicroscopy but observed in retinoscopy because of the greater distance and the larger pupil; and (e) the presence of significant anisocoria that may be missed in the tests of pupillary function.

AUTOTOMATIC KERATOMETERS

Although conventional keratometry requires only a few minutes' time and—in the hands of the experi-

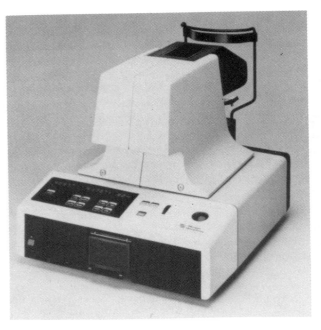

Figure 11.3   The Humphrey Auto-Keratometer.

enced operator—provides valid and reliable findings, the availability of relatively inexpensive microprocessors together with the tendency for eye practitioners to delegate more and more tasks to technicians has encouraged the development of automatic keratometers. These instruments, like automatic refractors, are both patient-objective and examiner-objective.

The Humphrey Auto-Keratometer

In 1981, Humphrey Instruments announced the development of the Auto-Keratometer, an automatic keratometer that detects the eye's optic axis and takes the central reading, specifying both refractive power (in diopters) and radius of curvature (in millimeters) in each of the two principal meridians of the cornea (see Figure 11.3). The instrument also provides the following additional information:

1. The apical keratometer reading, which is usually slightly steeper than the central reading.
2. The corneal "shape factor," which is related to the eccentricity of the cornea: the higher the value of the shape factor, the more the peripheral corneal flattening.
3. The position of the corneal apex in terms of horizontal and vertical displacement.

```
LEFT EYE

CENTRAL K
  DK     mm    AXIS
 43.50  7.76   177
 45.12  7.47    87

ΔK -1.62DK ×177

APICAL K
  DK     mm    AXIS
 43.62  7.73    02
 45.50  7.42    92

ΔK -1.87DK × 02

SHAPE      +.26
APEX        .74OUT
            .21 UP
            .23TOL
HEIGHT    1.54mm
CONF.       88%
```

Figure 11.4 Humphrey Auto-Keratometer printout.

4. A "conformance" factor, which indicates how the cornea being measured conforms to the normal cornea.

This information is provided in the form of a hard copy, as shown in Figure 11.4.

The Canon Auto-Keratometer K-1

The Canon Auto-Keratometer K-1, referred to by the manufacturer as the "Visual Auto-Keratometer," provides an image of the patient's eye in a video monitor by means of which the operator aligns the instrument. A readout, including both radius of curvature (mm) and refracting power (D) in each principal meridian, as well as corneal toricity (mm), corneal astigmatism (D), and axis, is presented at the bottom of the video screen and is also provided as a hard copy.

The Canon RK-1

The Canon RK-1, introduced in 1987, combines auto-refraction and auto-keratometry. The readout provides the auto-refractive finding in terms of sphere, cylinder, and axis, in addition to the auto-keratometric finding expressed as both radius of curvature (mm) and refractive power (D) in each of the principal meridians. The readout also includes

residual (nonkeratometric) astigmatism, which is calculated by subtracting keratometric astigmatism from refractive astigmatism.

The Topcon CK-1000

The Topcon CK-1000 instrument provides for alignment of the patient in the instrument by means of a video screen. The instrument can provide either central keratometric readings (only) or both central and peripheral readings. An audible tone signals that the finding has been taken.

A-SCAN ULTRASONIC BIOMETERS

Until the introduction of A-scan ultrasound instrumentation, no completely satisfactory method was available for measuring the axial distances within the intact human eye. The first method developed for measuring the length of the eye was that devised by Rushton (1938), making use of X-rays. This method was used by Stenstrom (1948) in a study of the refractive components of the eye. However, the X-ray method has two disadvantages: (1) it is a subjective method, requiring the patient to report when a phosphene gradually reduces in size and finally disappears as the X-ray beam is moved farther back toward the posterior pole of the eye; and (2) soon after the method had been developed, it was discovered that X-rays are carcinogenic, with the result that the procedure was no longer considered safe.

Sorsby et al. (1957) developed a method of calculating the length of the eye, which they used in a number of population studies. However, this method has several disadvantages, including the necessity to assume indices of refraction for the ocular media that are assumed not to change with age. With the development of A-scan ultrasonography, however, it is possible to measure not only the total axial length of the eye but also the depth of the anterior chamber, the lens thickness, and the depth of the vitreous chamber.

As described by Millodot (1986), A-scan ultrasonography involves high-frequency ultrasound waves (greater than 18,000Hz) that are emitted by a silicone transducer placed in contact with the eye. The ultrasound waves pass through the media and are reflected backward, in the form of an echo whenever they strike a change in the density of the medium through which they travel. The echos are converted into an electrical potential by a piezoelectric crystal and can be displayed as spikes on an oscilloscope screen. Echos are reflected from the front surface of the cornea, the front and back surfaces of the lens, and the surface of the retina. *A-scan*, or *time-amplitude*, *ultrasonography* measures the time required for the wave to travel to an interface and return; and for each of the ocular media the time of travel is multiplied by a velocity-constant to determine the distance it has traveled. In *B-scan*, or *intensity-modulated*, *ultrasonography*, various scans are taken through the pupillary area, and changes in acoustic impedance are shown as a series of dots on the oscilloscope screen. For measurements of axial distances within the eye, A-scan ultrasonography is used.

A number of manufacturers have marketed A-scan ultrasound instruments for use in laboratory research for some time, but instruments intended specifically for clinical use have been introduced only in recent years. The development of these instruments was motivated by the desirability of measuring the axial length of the eye prior to cataract surgery, in order to calculate the required power of an intraocular lens. Although such an instrument is not considered a necessity in routine optometric practice, there are many occasions when information about the axial distances within the eye is of importance: (1) when a patient is found to have anisometropia, knowledge of the axial lengths of the two eyes enables an estimation of the extent to which an axial-length difference (as opposed to a corneal-power of lens-power difference) is the cause of the anisometropia, thus influencing patient management; and (2) even in routine cases of ametropia, knowledge of the axial lengths of the eyes and their changes with time may be of importance in making future management decisions. For example, the management of a myope may be done differently depending on whether the myopia is thought to be mainly axial or refractive.

Humphrey Ultrasonic Biometer

One of the first A-scan ultrasound instruments to be developed for clinical use is the Humphrey Ultrasonic Biometer (see Figure 11.5). The instrument's transducer is placed in a Goldmann tonometer mount (in place of the tonometer prism) and the instrument is used in connection with a biomicroscope. Because ultrasound waves travel through water, the corneal surface must be kept moist, either with the normal precorneal film or with artificial tears. The eye is first anesthetized with one drop of

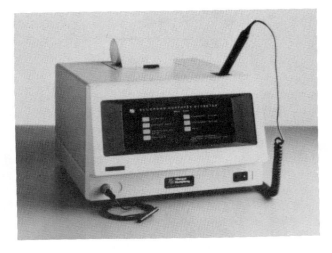

Figure 11.5 The Humphrey Ultrasonic Biometer.

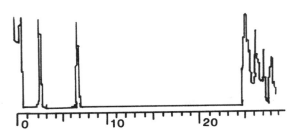

Figure 11.6 A-scan ultrasound recording, showing spikes indicating the position of the corneal surface, the front lens surface, the back lens surface, and the surface of the retina.

0.5 percent proparacaine, and the transducer is disinfected by means of an alcohol preparation. Rather than applanating the cornea, as in Goldmann tonometry, the object of the procedure is to barely touch the cornea. An accurate reading will show the four spikes, indicating the positions of the cornea, front lens surface, back lens surface, and retinal surface (see Figure 11.6). When the correct waveform is seen on the oscilloscope screen, the instrument "beeps" and the reading is "frozen." The instrument is equipped with a printer, which provides a hard copy of the wave-form together with measurements, in millimeters, of anterior chamber depth, lens thickness, and total axial length. If five readings are taken and averaged, the accuracy (assuming no major errors were made in taking the readings) is about 0.1 or 0.2 mm.

SUBJECTIVE COMPUTER-ASSISTED REFRACTORS

Although an increasing number of objective automatic refractors have incorporated provisions for measuring visual acuity and refining the refractive end-point, only a small number of manufacturers have introduced computer-assisted refractors designed only for subjective refraction. Instruments in this category are the Humphrey *Vision Analyzer*, the American Optical *SR–III*, replaced by the *SR–IV*, the Cavitron *Auto-Refractor–7*, and the Bausch & Lomb *IVEX*.

Humphrey Vision Analyzer

The first subjective computer-assisted refractor to be introduced is the Humphrey Vision Analyzer, which, as described at a meeting of the American Academy of Optometry by Humphrey (1974) and Harwood (1974), employs two completely novel concepts.

1. *Variable-focus lenses are used.* Variable-focus spherical lenses were developed by physicist Luis Alvarez in 1962. The lenses consist of two elements shaped in such a way that, when they are moved laterally in the light path in relation to one another, spherical power is introduced. Humphrey later developed cylindrical variable-focus lenses based on the Alvarez system.

2. *There are no lenses in front of the patient's eyes.* While the patient views the image of a projected chart in a concave mirror, lenses for the correction of the patient's refractive error are placed in front of the projector rather than in front of the eyes. The lenses are placed at a distance from the mirror equal to its radius; an aerial image of the lenses is formed in front of the patient's eyes (the patient's spectacle plane also is located at a distance from the mirror equal to its radius), and both the projector and the patient's eyes are located near the optic axis of the mirror.

The development of variable-focus lenses, together with the other steps involved in the development of the Vision Analyzer, are recounted in an interesting and lucid article by Alvarez (1978). Alvarez describes five innovations introduced in the design of the Vision Analyzer: (1) continuously variable spherical lenses; (2) continuously variable cylindrical lenses; (3) measurement of two components of astigmatism instead of astigmatic power and axis; (4) remote refraction, with no lenses in front of the patient's eyes; and (5) separate binocular

channels, without the need for Polaroids or septums.

The method of measuring astigmatism involves the use of two charts, one containing a vertical line and the other containing a line oriented at an angle of 45 degrees. As pointed out by Alvarez (1978), any possible cylindrical lens power can be generated as the optical sum of a spherical lens and two variable power, crossed-cylinder lenses, one with principal meridians at 0 and 90 degrees and the other with principal meridians at 45 and 135 degrees. Alvarez emphasizes the fact that with this system, finding the lens powers to correct the patient's astigmatism involves only two procedures. One uses the vertical line target, and the other uses the 45-degree line target (as opposed to the conventional method in which cylindrical axis is first determined, then power, following which axis and power are both usually rechecked and refined).

Alvarez (1978) compares the new method of measuring astigmatism (making use of only two meridians) to the method used for determining prism to measure a phoria, which is resolved into vertical and horizontal meridians. The conventional method of measuring astigmatism, on the other hand, can be compared to determining the amount of prism with the base-apex meridian at a specific angle rather than resolving the prism into vertical and horizontal meridians (e.g., an individual having 5Δ of lateral phoria and 5Δ of vertical phoria would be found to require 7.07Δ of power with the base-apex meridian at 45 degrees or 135 degrees).

The Humphrey Vision Analyzer (see Figure 11.7)

Figure 11.7 The Humphrey Vision Analyzer.

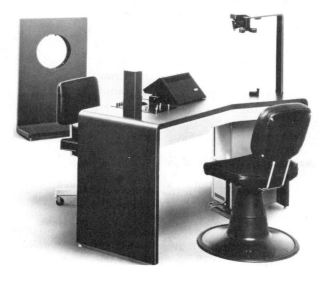

is composed of a desklike, free-standing console, a power-operated patient's chair, an examiner's chair, and a concave mirror mounted on a stand. A forehead rest is located on the patient's side of the chair, and the controls for the lenses and other elements are located on the surface of the console, convenient to the operator. Use of the Vision Analyzer requires no previous refraction by retinoscopy and involves the adjustment of the vertical and oblique lines until the patient reports that each line is in sharp focus. The projecting system is a two-channel system, making it possible to refract the patient binocularly and also to incorporate testing for phorias, fusional vergences, fixation disparity, suppression, and other binocular functions. Refraction can be done with the patient's spectacles in place or while contact lenses are worn. Near-point testing also can be done. A computer converts the refractive data to the standard spherical power, cylindrical power, and cylindrical axis in the form of a digital display.

Kratz and Flom (1977) reported on a double-blind study in which 21 patients were examined both by means of the Vision Analyzer and conventional refraction. Each patient was examined on two separate occasions, once with and once without the use of cylindrical power randomly chosen from a predetermined set of powers and axes. The authors concluded that results with the two different instruments differed by about the same amount as did repeated refraction using the same instrument. In other words, refractive error measurements with either instrument were about as valid as they were reliable.

A comparison of bifocal additions determined by the Vision Analyzer and by conventional refraction was reported by Tiachac and Patella (1979). For an initial group of 25 presbyopes, the authors found an average "minimum subjective add" of +1.72D for conventional refraction compared with +1.79D for the Vision Analyzer. For a later group, the average "minimum subjective add" was found to be +1.77D for conventional refraction and +1.59D for the Vision Analyzer.

American Optical SR–III and SR–IV

Bannon (1977) announced the development of the American Optical Corporation SR–III Subjective Refraction System. The instrument is based on a subjective optometer invented by David L. Guyton and exhibited in 1970 at a meeting of the American Academy of Ophthalmology and Otolaryngology. The original Guyton instrument filled up a large portion of an examining room, but a compact table model (the SR–III) was ultimately developed by American Optical Corporation.

The optical system of the SR–III is that of a spherocylindrical optometer, with spherical power continuously variable from −20.00 to +20.00D and with cylindrical lens powers up to ±8.00D. The instrument is designed to be operated by a trained assistant or technician. However, a control knob is provided for the patient, who manipulates the instrument's optical system on instructions from the operator. Refraction is performed monocularly, at optical infinity.

Test targets include a Snellen chart, two yellow jagged-line targets on black backgrounds for the determination of cylindrical power and axis, and a bichrome test. After the operator aligns the patient's eye in the instrument, the patient is asked to make the letters in the Snellen chart as sharp and clear as possible by turning the control knob, introducing spherical power. The yellow jagged-line targets are then used for the determination of cylindrical power and axis, after which the operator fogs the patient and makes use of the bichrome chart to determine the monocular end-point.

Bannon (1977) reported on a study involving 376 eyes in which SR–III findings were compared with conventional refractive data. The SR–III was operated by a technician who was unaware of the optometrist's refractive findings. Bannon found that for 70 percent of eyes, the sphere measurements agreed within 0.25D for the two methods; for 85 percent of the eyes, agreement was within 0.50D. For cylindrical power, 76 percent of the eyes agreed within 0.25D and 92 percent agreed within 0.50D. Woo and Woodruff (1978) reported on a study in which SR–III findings taken by a trained secretary were compared with conventional refractive data taken on 530 eyes. Their results compared favorably with those of Bannon: spherical measurements agreed within 0.25D for 64 percent of the eyes and within 0.50D for 85 percent, whereas cylindrical power findings agreed within 0.25D for 69 percent of the eyes and within 0.50D for 89 percent. On the basis of their findings and those of Bannon, Woo and Woodruff concluded that SR–III findings are comparable to conventional refractive findings, in that most differences were within tolerances for different examiners and/or different methods.

At the University of Houston, Perrigin, Perrigin, and Grosvenor (1981) compared conventional refractive findings to SR–III findings taken on 119 subjects (238 eyes) by the three authors and by a technician-trainer for American Optical Corporation. Subjects were optometry students, faculty, staff members, and clinical patients. Spherical refractive data were within 0.25D for 72 percent of the subjects and within 0.50D for 91 percent; cylindrical power data were within 0.25D for 75 percent of the subjects and within 0.50D for 91 percent. For cylindrical powers of more than 1.00D, axes were within ±10 degrees for 94 percent of the subjects. In discussing their study, Perrigin, Perrigin, and Grosvenor reported that they enjoyed using the instrument, that the target clarity and contrast were exceedingly good, and that the bichrome test was well designed and easy to use. They questioned the idea, however, that the instrument should be operated by an assistant or technician, suggesting that with certain refinements (some of which were later incorporated in the SR–IV), the optometrist could substitute the SR–III refraction for the usual clinical subjective examination.

The American Optical SR–IV Subjective Refraction System (see Figure 11.8) was introduced in 1980. In this instrument, the yellow jagged-line targets are replaced by a clock-dial chart for determining cylindrical power and axis under fog and by a Simulcross crossed-cylinder system for refining cylindrical power and axis without fog. As with the SR–III, the patient makes the initial spherical power adjustment. The use of the clock-dial chart is not usually necessary if the patient's acuity is 20/30 or better after the original spherical power adjustment.

Using the Simulcross targets (one for power and one for axis), both crossed-cylinder choices are presented to the patient simultaneously. Each target consists of three pairs of Maltese crosses varying in size; the patient's task is to compare Maltese crosses of similar size on the two sides of the chart and to report which of the two is sharper or more distinct. The border of each target is either red or blue, so the patient simply responds by calling out "red" or "blue," as the case may be. The operator pushes a red button (changing the cylindrical axis or power in one direction) when the patient calls out "red," and pushes the blue button when the patient calls out "blue" (changing axis or power in the other direction).

In a study comparing SR–IV refraction to conventional refraction for 131 myopic children, Grosvenor, Perrigin, and Perrigin (1983) found agreement for the two methods within ±0.25D in 79 percent of cases for spherical component refraction, in 67 percent of cases for spherical equivalent refraction,

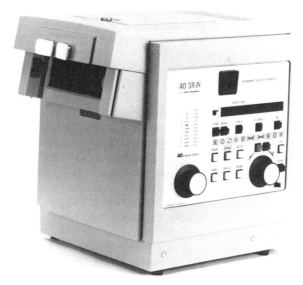

Figure 11.8   The American Optical SR–IV Subjective Refraction System.

in 86 percent of cases for cylindrical power, and within ±10 degrees in 75 percent of cases for cylindrical axis (see the first column in Table 11.2). In a comparison of SR–IV and clinical refractive data on 30 third-year optometry students (1983), the same authors found somewhat better percentages of agreement (see the second column in Table 11.2). In a previous study comparing clinical refractive data taken by the three authors Perrigin, Perrigin, and Grosvenor (1982) on a group of second-year optometry students, comparable percentages of agreement were found (see the third column in Table 11.2). Grosvenor, Perrigin, and Perrigin concluded that the poorer agreement between SR–IV and clinical refraction for the myopic children was to a great extent due to the fact that some of the children overaccommodated during the clinical refraction. For the adult subjects, however, SR–IV refraction was found to be as reliable and as valid as clinical refraction.

Cavitron Auto-Refractor–7

As described by the manufacturer, the Cavitron Auto-Refractor–7 is the first subjective refractor able to assess the patient's accommodative range and lateral phoria, as well as spherical power, cylinder power, cylinder axis, and visual acuity.

Koetting, Akerman, and Koetting (1983) reported on a study in which conventional clinical and Auto-Refractor–7 refractive findings were obtained on 75

Table 11.2   Comparisons of SR–IV and clinical refractive data (Grosvenor, Perrigin, and Perrigin, 1981).

	SR–IV vs. clinical data (children, %)	SR–IV vs. clinical data (adults, %)	Clinical data of three examiners (adults, %)
Spherical component within ±0.25D	79	97	86
Spherical equivalent within ±0.25D	67	90	93
Cylindrical power within ±0.25D	86	100	93
Cylindrical axis within ±10°	75	87	88

soft contact lens wearers, 75 hard contact lens wearers, and 75 spectacle wearers. In the study, the accommodation and lateral phoria features of the instrument were not used. On the basis of spherical equivalent refraction, Koetting et al. reported that about one-half of the subjects accepted about 0.50D more minus spherical power with the Auto-Refractor–7 than with conventional refraction, which they attributed to instrument myopia. In spite of this difference, they reported that 67 percent of the findings were within 0.50D of conventional findings. Koetting et al. concluded that there was no great apparent difference between the three groups tested, and the small discrepancies that existed were scattered among the three groups.

Bausch & Lomb IVEX

The Bausch & Lomb IVEX (Integrated Vision Examination System) is a computerized instrument designed to accommodate the entire refraction and binocular vision testing sequence, including retinoscopy, subjective refraction, phoria and fusional vergence testing, and all near-point testing. The instrument can be operated by the practitioner rather than by an assistant or a technician and, as such, supercedes a refractor or phoropter. Retinoscopy is performed with the practitioner facing the patient (on the opposite side of the instrument) while the patient views a fixation target. The practitioner depresses buttons that position lenses and prisms in front of the eyes for refraction, binocular vision, and accommodation testing.

In a double-blind protocol, Perrigin, Grosvenor, and Perrigin (1985) examined 40 subjects by means of both IVEX and conventional clinical refraction. For most subjects, IVEX cylinder power and axis findings compared well for the two methods, which was reinforced by the examiners' confidence when testing for astigmatism. Spherical equivalent findings varied by no more than 0.25–0.50D from conventional clinical findings for most subjects, but for some subjects IVEX findings yielded as much as 1.00–1.25D more minus or less plus than conventional refractive findings. Two possible reasons for the minus bias suggested by Perrigin et al. are (1) the IVEX optical system is calibrated for infinity rather than for a 6m distance, and (2) the tendency of patients to accommodate while looking through an optical instrument. Because many of the overminused subjects were myopes (from −2 to −8D), a third possibility may be a tendency to refract patients at too great a vertex distance. In another study, Roggenkamp, Richardson, Krebsbach, and Yolton (1985) compared conventional clinical and IVEX findings for 40 subjects. Their results indicated a mean sphere value for the IVEX of 0.32D more minus than for conventional refraction. The authors concluded that the increase in minus power was the result of instrument myopia.

ROLE OF AUTOMATIC REFRACTORS IN OPTOMETRIC PRACTICE

A large number of computerized refractors—both objective and subjective—are currently available. Although the first of these instruments, the Bausch & Lomb Ophthalmetron and the Acuity Systems 6600, were introduced in the early 1970s. There is no evidence that computerized refractors have made a major change in the way optometry is practiced.

Although there is no reason to believe that the quality of patient care would improve with the use of automatic objective refraction, there is also no reason to believe that the quality of patient care would suffer. In either case, the practitioner decides on the lens prescription on the basis of the subjective refractive findings, binocular vision findings, and other considerations.

Even though the use of an automatic objective refractor may be justified in terms of time, money, and quality of patient care, it is difficult to justify the use of a technician-operated automatic *subjective* refractor. Although the manufacturer of one subjective refractor (the American Optical SR–IV) advises the practitioner to have the automatic subjective refraction performed by a technician and to refine the refractive findings using conventional clinical methods, it is possible that many practitioners will find that the SR–IV findings agree sufficiently with their own findings, making their "refinement" of the technician's findings unnecessary. Unfortunately, this paves the way for the abandonment of refraction by eye professionals.

It is possible to make a case for the performance of subjective automatic refraction by the *practitioner* rather than a technician. The author has had sufficient experience with the SR–IV to be convinced that subjective refraction can be done quickly and accurately with this instrument. Without the need for retinoscopy, a subjective refraction can be done "from scratch" in 5–10 minutes (for both eyes); by departing from the programmed refraction sequence, the practitioner has the freedom to do any of the tests—and in any order—that would be done in a conventional monocular subjective refraction. Unfortunately, because the SR–IV is a monocular instrument, it is impossible to perform binocular balance tests, binocular refraction, dissociated or associated phoria tests, or fusional vergence tests. Further, because these tests would have to be done by a phoropter, the patient would have to be moved to the ophthalmic chair after completion of the SR–IV refraction. The most satisfactory solution to this problem would be to redesign the SR–IV to make binocular vision testing possible. A less satisfactory solution would be to mount the SR–IV subjective refractor for use with the ophthalmic chair.

Because the Humphrey Vision Analyzer and the Bausch & Lomb IVEX are binocular instruments with the capacity for performing binocular subjective testing, dissociated and associated phoria testing, and

other procedures, the practitioner who operates one of these instruments is in a position to completely bypass conventional refraction and binocular vision testing. The author's limited experience with the Humphrey Vision Analyzer is insufficient to enable a judgment as to whether it is comparable to conventional refraction and binocular vision testing in terms of the time required for the procedures and the accuracy of results.

COMPUTERIZATION OF CONVENTIONAL REFRACTION

In a series of investigations, Marg and his co-workers (1977, 1978) have analyzed the procedures used by clinicians in performing subjective refraction—including visual acuity measurement and the determination of a reading addition—and have developed and tested a number of computer-actuated refractors. The third instrument developed, called Refractor III, is equipped with spherical lenses ranging from −24.00 to +26.00D and cylindrical lenses from 0.00 to 9.00D (all in 0.12D steps), as well as other devices including crossed cylinders, prisms, Maddox rods, bichrome lenses, and pinholes (Marg et al., 1977). The Refractor III provides a subjective refraction in a manner similar to that performed by a human clinician and is programmed to run on a DEC PDP–8/E digitial computer. The patient responds to recorded instructions, indicating an answer by pressing a button.

In the first study involving Refractor III, 78 patients were refracted both by means of Refractor III and conventional methods using a human refractionist (Marg et al., 1977). Procedures included the determination of visual acuity, monocularly performed subjective refraction, and determination of a reading addition (for presbyopes). Comparing Refractor III results with conventional results, lens prescriptions were categorized as (1) in "good agreement," (2) in "agreement," or (3) "unsatisfactory." Of the 78 prescriptions, 65 (83.4 percent) were found to be in good agreement, 8 (10.3 percent) in agreement, and 13 (16.7 percent) were found to be unsatisfactory. As for the reading additions, 68 percent of the presbyopic patients received a useful addition and 32 percent did not. All but 3 percent of the unsatisfactory reading additions were found to be due to "bugs" in the programming of the flowchart, all of which were correctable.

Although no rigid criteria were used in judging the correctness of the distance prescriptions, it was found (retrospectively) that "good agreement" was considered to be within 0.32D equivalent sphere and 0.28D cylinder, whereas "agreement" was within 0.56D equivalent sphere and 0.50D cylinder. For the reading additions, 0.50D was found to represent "good agreement," and "agreement" was within 0.75 D (Marg et al., "Computer Assisted, VI," 1978).

A second study was conducted comparing Refractor III results with conventional refraction after a number of improvements had been made in the system (Marg et al., "Computer Assisted, VII," 1978). For 80 subjects, 95 percent of the distance prescriptions and 100 percent of the reading additions were found to be satisfactory. Future improvements planned for the system include programming for binocular vision testing; the use of a retroilluminated display chart, making the use of a projector unnecessary; the use of microprocessors to replace hard-wired circuits; the use of a floppy disk storage system rather than digital tapes; a redesign of the stepping motors used to drive lens disks and to set cylinder axes; and a redesign of the Refractor III itself to make it smaller and lighter and to reduce the number of parts by about one-half.

LASER REFRACTION

Laser refraction had its beginnings when Rigden and Gordon (1962) and Oliver (1963) independently described the speckle pattern that results when the coherent light from a gas laser is reflected from a mat surface. If a hyperopic subject moves the head sideways while observing the speckle pattern, the pattern will appear to move in the same direction as the head, whereas for a myopic subject the pattern will appear to move in the opposite direction. For an emmetropic subject, the pattern appears not to move at all.

Knoll (1966) found that the motion of the speckle pattern can be observed more easily if the head is held stationary and the surface on which the speckle pattern is projected is slowly rotated in one direction. This was done by means of a rotating drum 7 inches in diameter and rotated at the rate of one revolution per hour. The drum was mounted on a gimbal so it could be rotated in any meridian (e.g., the two principal meridians of the eye or preselected meridians without regard to the eye's two principal meridians).

Like ordinary subjective refraction, laser refraction is examiner-objective and patient-subjective. Therefore, it can be considered as a substitute for subjective refraction rather than for retinoscopy. The patient's task is to report when the speckle pattern ceases to move as the examiner varies lens power by means of trial lenses or a refractor. Using this procedure, spherical refraction can be done quickly and easily, as can cylindrical refraction if the two principal meridians of the eyes have been predetermined by conventional refractive procedures. However, if the principal meridians have not been predetermined, laser refraction must involve a minimum of three (and usually four or six) *preselected* meridians.

Refraction Using Predetermined Principal Meridians

In a study comparing laser refraction with conventional refraction for seven subjects, Knoll (1966) performed laser refraction in the two principal meridians of each eye predetermined by conventional subjective refraction. He found that the laser measurements tended to show somewhat more hyperopia or less myopia than was found by conventional refraction. Baldwin and Stover (1968) compared laser refraction with conventional refraction, each subject being refracted by each procedure in the horizontal and vertical meridians. Comparing laser refraction with the modified clinical technique (which makes use of retinoscopy) on kindergarten and elementary schoolchildren, they found an inconsistent relationship between the two methods. However, when laser refraction was compared with retinoscopy and subjective refraction using the Turville infinity balance test on 27 adult subjects, the results indicated that laser refraction was a satisfactory technique for determining the subjective refraction of adults.

Dwyer et al. (1972) investigated the reliability of laser refraction by determining the laser refraction for 52 optometry students, making 20 determinations for the dominant eye of each subject. If the subject required a cylindrical correction, the cylinder in the lens prescription was placed in the refractor before the laser refraction was begun. Standard deviations of laser refraction findings varied from 0.198 to 0.336D. However, no comparison with conventional refraction was made. In another study, Dwyer et al. (1973) compared laser refraction with conventional retinoscopy and subjective refraction on 100 clinic patients. Using mean refraction for each of four refractive error groups (low myopes, high myopes, low hyperopes, and high hyperopes), they found correlation coefficients between laser refraction and conventional refraction to range from 0.703 to 0.987. The authors concluded that "both the validity and reliability of the laser refraction are high enough to merit further and serious consideration of its application as a quick and simple method for determining spherical error" (Dwyer et al., 1973, p. 225).

Conventional subjective and laser refractive findings were compared by Phillips, McCarter, and Dwyer (1976) for 75 eyes, using the two principal meridians that had been located by conventional refraction. They concluded that, although laser refraction is highly accurate in a given meridian, even small errors for a given meridian can result in unacceptable variation in the mathematically calculated cylindrical axis and power.

Refraction Using Preselected Meridians

For laser refraction of an astigmatic eye to be done independently of conventional refraction (i.e., without predetermining the principal meridians of the patient's eyes), the examiner can use laser refraction in three or more preselected meridians. Malacara (1974) published a mathematical formulation in which he presented formulas and nomograms for use in laser refraction, using the 0-, 60-, and 120-degree meridians. Phillips, Sterling, and Dwyer (1975) reported on data for 50 eyes, comparing laser refraction in the 0-, 45-, and 90-degree meridians to conventional refraction. They concluded that this procedure was not correlated highly enough with conventional refraction to warrant its use in clinical practice.

Haine, Long, and Reading (1973) reported on a study in which laser refraction was compared with conventional refraction, using three preselected meridians. On the basis of data collected on 12 eyes, these investigators concluded that the axis of the cylindrical correction was not determined within acceptable limits and that a different approach was needed. One approach would be the use of four or more meridians. In a theoretical analysis of meridional refraction, Long (1974) concluded that three meridians are adequate to determine mathematically the resultant spherocylindrical lens, but that the procedure was not experimentally sound due to the variation in clinical findings that occurred when the procedure was used. He found that even a variation as small as 0.12D in clinical data presented a problem, and he suggested that the use of four or more meridians would provide sufficient

redundancy of data to compensate for the effects of experimental error.

Four-meridian and six-meridian laser refraction results were compared for 30 subjects in a later study by Haine, Long, and Reading (1976). Four-meridian laser refraction was done for one eye of each subject, and six-meridian laser refraction was done for the other. Correlation coefficients were then computed between conventional subjective findings and the four- and six-meridian laser data. For spherical power, both four- and six-meridian data resulted in correlation coefficients of 0.99 with subjective findings. For cylindrical power and axis, four-meridian data resulted in correlation coefficients of 0.81 and 0.94, respectively, whereas six-meridian data results in coefficients of 0.89 and 0.97. All coefficients were significant at the 0.00001 confidence level. Haine, Long, and Reading concluded that the four- and six-meridian methods were equally good for spherical power, but that the six-meridian method was better for determining cylindrical power and axis.

Evaluation of Laser Refraction

During the years that have passed since the 1976 report by Haine, Long, and Reading, the literature has included few additional reports on laser refraction. During this period, numerous commercially produced instruments have been introduced for computer-assisted objective and subjective refraction, but none involving laser refraction has been introduced. This lack of popularity of laser refraction undoubtedly reflects the fact that laser refraction, although capable of producing refractive data comparable to conventional refraction, lacks the advantages of saving time for the practitioner or being easily turned over to an assistant or technician.

VISUALLY EVOKED RESPONSE

If trial lenses are introduced before a subject's eye while the subject views an oscillating striped or checkerboard pattern and while the evoked cortical response is recorded, the trial lens that provides the sharpest retinal image also will be the one that causes the greatest cortical response. Thus, the amplitude of the cortical response provides an objective method of determining the refractive status of the eye. This system of refraction is variously known as the *visually evoked response (VER)*, *visually evoked cortical response (VECR), evoked cortical potential (ECP),* or simply *evoked potential (EP).* One disadvantage of the VER is that it requires expensive equipment not normally found in an optometrist's office. The procedure is slow compared with retinoscopy and conventional subjective refraction (even for spherical refraction); spherocylindrical refraction also is a complicated procedure, as is the case with laser refraction.

Spherical Refraction

Millodot and Riggs (1970) determined spherical refraction by recording the VER while making use of an oscillating checkerboard pattern. The checkerboard pattern consisted of oppositely polarized sheets of polarized material and was viewed by the subject through a Polaroid filter, so each of the clear squares of the checkerboard varied from light to dark in a sinusoidal manner. The bright phase of one set of squares coincided with the dark phase of the other, so the total light flux remained nearly constant. The checkerboard field subtended an angle of 9.5 degrees, and the size of an individual square was 14 minutes of arc.

The VER was recorded by means of two electrodes—one placed over the inion and one located 10cm higher. A conventional spherical subjective refraction was performed on each of two subjects, and the lens that provided the best vision of the checkerboard pattern was placed in front of the right eye. The subject was asked to fixate a point in the center of the checkerboard pattern, and lenses varying from +6.00 to −6.00D were placed in the trial frame as the VER was recorded. For both subjects the amplitude of the VER was found to vary with lens power, reaching a maximum at 0.00D power. Millodot and Riggs concluded that their stimulus pattern was effective in eliciting the VER but that the method was more cumbersome and time-consuming than conventional methods of objective refraction. However, they stated that the electrical responses were certain to be valid, in that they depend on the same initial receptive processes as vision itself.

Refraction Using Preselected Meridians

McCormack and Marg (1973) refracted nine subjects using both conventional and VER refraction. They used a target based on that of Millodot and Riggs (1970), with the exception that a bar-grating pattern was used rather than a checkerboard pattern. The reason for the bar-grating pattern was that VER refractions were done meridionally, in each of three preselected meridians, rather than spherically. The investigators found that the sensitivity of the procedure was limited to ±1.00D in any one meridian, and they concluded that there were inconsistencies in the VER method itself, apparently due to a problem in obtaining an adequate signal-to-noise ratio. They found, however, that the VER sensitivity could be increased to ±0.50D if contrast and bar size were optimally controlled.

VER Refraction Using a Stenopaic Slit

By using Fourier analysis of the visually evoked potential, Regan (1973) found that it was possible to perform objective refraction 100 times faster than by the usual signal-averaging procedure. In Regan's procedure, a spherical approximation to the refraction was first done, the subject viewing a checkerboard pattern while the examiner inserted and removed trial lenses until the lens that provided the largest response amplitude was found. The result of changing a trial lens could be seen in 1 or 2 seconds by watching a running-average display of the VER.

A number of methods were employed for the determination of cylindrical axis, the fastest of which proved to be the use of a rotating stenopaic slit. With this method, the two principal meridians could be located in as little as 10 seconds. To determine cylindrical power, the subject fixated the checkerboard pattern through the stenopaic slit while lens power was oscillated between predetermined limits by the use of a lens of continuously variable power. Using this method, lens power in each of the two principal meridians was determined in 18 seconds. Regan stated that the main advantage of the method is that by the use of Fourier analysis, an on-line display of instantaneous VER amplitude is available. The VER amplitude, therefore, can be treated as equivalent to a patient's verbal response in subjective refraction.

Evaluation of VER Refraction

Like laser refraction, VER refraction has been overshadowed in recent years by the rapid development of instrumentation for computer-assisted objective and subjective refraction. However, VER refraction and laser refraction not only complement one another by providing both objective (VER) and subjective (laser) means of refraction; they are similar to the extent that both can be done by refracting four or more meridians. One possible development, therefore, would be an instrument for performing meridional VER and laser refraction, both methods sharing the same hardware and computer facility.

Study Questions

1. What two problems would you expect to find with refractive results obtained by means of an optical refractometer, as compared with conventional clinical refraction?

2. Indicate whether each of the following instruments is patient-subjective or patient-objective: (a) laser refraction; (b) the American Optical SR–IV; (c) the Dioptron; (d) the Humphrey Vision Analyzer; (e) VER refraction.

3. Describe the innovations that were used in the design of the Humphrey Vision Analyzer.

4. In laser refraction, what procedure is used to determine the cylinder axis and power, as described by Haine, Long, and Reading?

5. According to Regan what is the fastest way to determine the cylinder axis when using VER refraction?

6. What optical principle is used in each of the following instruments: (a) the Dioptron? (b) the Ophthalmetron? (c) the SR–IV? (d) the Humphrey auto-refractor? (e) the Topcon auto-refractor?

7. What information does the Humphrey auto-keratometer provide that is not provided by a conventional keratometer?

8. What are the advantages and disadvantages of the subjective refraction capability that is built into a number of objective auto-refractors?

9. Describe the basic principles of A-scan ultrasonography, as used in the measurement of the axial distances within the eye.

10. For what purposes might A-scan ultrasonography be used in the routine practice of optometry?

11. List the advantages and disadvantages of the use of objective computer-assisted refraction in optometric practice.

12. List the advantages and disadvantages of the use of subjective computer-assisted refraction in optometric practice.

PART THREE

Optometric Diagnosis and Treatment

Once the procedures making up the optometric examination (the optometric data base) have been completed, the practitioner lists the patient's problems and, for each problem, formulates an initial treatment plan. It will be recalled that treatment plans, as indicated by Weed (1968 and 1969), include not only plans for therapy but also plans for further diagnostic procedures and patient education. Once optometric treatment has begun, continuing patient care in the form of regularly scheduled progress examinations, with progress notes written in narrative form, completes the closed-loop patient care delivery system.

In the following pages, optometric diagnosis and treatment are discussed in terms of the diagnosis and treatment of anomalies of refraction and binocular vision, prescribing ophthalmic lenses, prescribing contact lenses, and prescribing low vision aids.

CHAPTER 12

Diagnosis and Treatment of Anomalies of Refraction and Binocular Vision

The fact that schools of optometry—as well as optometric textbooks—place a great emphasis on binocular vision anomalies tends to give optometry students the impression that the majority of optometric patients will be found to have binocular vision problems. However, the opposite is true: the majority of patients have refractive anomalies but normal binocular vision. Although the major portion of this chapter deals with prescribing for patients having binocular vision anomalies, it begins with a discussion of the more straightforward procedures involved in prescribing for patients who have refractive anomalies and normal binocular vision.

MANAGEMENT OF REFRACTIVE ANOMALIES

In the absence of binocular vision anomalies, prescribing for anomalies of refraction is a reasonably routine matter. Many patients consulting an optometrist will be found to have relatively small refractive errors; in these cases, the problem may not be that of deciding what lenses to prescribe, but whether to prescribe lenses at all. Once the decision to prescribe lenses has been made, in most cases the practitioner simply prescribes the lens powers determined on the basis of objective and subjective refractive findings. However, there are cases in which, for one reason or another, the full spherical or cylindrical power will not be prescribed. For example, a patient may have an uncorrected (or undercorrected), long-standing refractive error, and the practitioner may feel that the patient would have difficulty adapting to a full correction. For other reasons, a less-than-full correction may sometimes be prescribed for anisometropia or presbyopia.

Another consideration is whether the lenses should be in the form of ophthalmic lenses or contact lenses. In most cases where contact lenses are prescribed, it is because the patient requests them. The majority of patients who request contact lenses are myopic young adults or adolescents who have worn glasses for several years and would like to discontinue them in favor of contact lenses. There are some conditions, however, for which contact lenses provide a superior optical correction compared with glasses. The most important of these conditions are keratoconus and aphakia.

Chapters 13 and 14 discuss the prescribing of ophthalmic lenses and contact lenses, respectively. In this chapter, any reference to the prescribing of lenses is assumed to apply to ophthalmic lenses unless there is a specific reference to contact lenses.

Prescribing for Myopia

Most people who will become myopic do so during the school years. As discussed in Chapter 3, only a small percentage of children are myopic when entering school, but during the school years the prevalence of myopia steadily increases from less than 2 percent in grade 1 to 15 or 20 percent (or even higher) in grade 12. Once a child becomes myopic, the myopia typically increases at the rate of from 0.25 to 0.50D per year, leveling off by about the age of 18. However, a small percentage of people become myopic beyond the age of 18 (e.g., cadets in military academies, students in such fields as accounting, law, medicine, or optometry, and workers involved in occupations involving prolonged work at unusually close working distances). Workers who assemble electronic components and those who work at computer terminals are particularly prone to develop myopia during the adult years.

The common and usually the *only* complaint of

the myope is blurred distance vision. However, myopic children (either those whose myopia has never been corrected or those whose lenses no longer fully correct the myopia) are often not aware of blurred vision and are examined only because of a school vision screening test or a routine optometric or ophthalmological examination. Providing the myope with clear distance vision by providing ophthalmic lenses or contact lenses of appropriate power usually presents no problem.

Procedures for the control of myopia

Some vision practitioners believe that the progression of a child's myopia can be controlled or even eliminated altogether by the use of one or a combination of the following: (1) undercorrection of the myopia, (2) visual training, (3) bifocal lenses, (4) contact lenses, and (5) the use of atropine or other drugs. (These procedures are discussed in Chapter 3.)

Night myopia

Occasionally a patient who is found to have little or no myopia will complain of poor night vision. In such a case, a correction of whatever myopia is found with the addition of 0.50D of minus power (as determined by leaving the patient "two clicks in the green" on the bichrome test) will usually solve the patient's problem. However, the optometrist should be aware that a complaint of poor night vision could possibly occur as a result of retinitis pigmentosa or one of the other receptor degenerations, and a careful ophthalmoscopic examination and peripheral field testing should be done to rule out such a possibility.

Prescribing for Hyperopia

As indicated in Chapter 2, the peak of the refractive error distribution curve is in the neighborhood of 0.50D of hyperopia. Therefore, if we define *hyperopia* as any refractive state greater than plano (0.00D), the majority of people are hyperopic. In the absence of a binocular vision anomaly, whether to prescribe for a hyperopic patient will depend on a number of factors, including age, the amount of hyperopia, and the patient's complaints (if any).

Because low hyperopia (from +0.25 to +1.00D, usually with a small amount of with-the-rule astigmatism), as found by noncycloplegic refraction, is the expected finding for children of school age, lenses are not usually prescribed unless the hyperopia is in excess of +1.00D or the child's history indicates that

the hyperopia is causing a problem. (Remember that we are considering only hyperopia where there is no binocular vision anomaly.) The practitioner should bear in mind that a child may have latent hyperopia that may not be detected in a routine examination, even when the fogging procedure is properly utilized. If the practitioner believes that undetected latent hyperopia may exist, he or she can make use of one of the overfogging procedures described in Chapter 9 (such as the Borish delayed subjective), or can perform a refraction under cycloplegia. If an excess of 1.00D of hyperopia is found by means of the delayed subjective or cycloplegic refraction (using cyclopentolate or tropicamide), and if the child complains of difficulty with reading or schoolwork, the practitioner may consider prescribing lenses to fully correct the hyperopia. In most cases, the lenses will only be required for near work, but often the child will adapt to the lenses more quickly if instructed to wear them constantly for the first 2 or 3 weeks and then to wear them for near work only.

For adults, lenses may be required for smaller amounts of hyperopia. In the absence of a binocular vision problem, a +0.75 or +1.00D hyperope may have no problems until the age of 35 or beyond, when the rapidly receding near-point of accommodation may cause a feeling of eyestrain accompanying close work. In addition, many low hyperopes have a small amount of latent hyperopia that may not become manifest until the late 30s or early 40s. For an adult who engages in a large amount of concentrated near work, as little as 0.50D of hyperopia may require the prescription of lenses for near work.

Sometimes a patient who has as little as 0.50D of hyperopia will have rather pronounced symptoms such as headaches, which could be the result of eyestrain. When this occurs, the patient should be thoroughly questioned concerning these symptoms, to rule out conditions such as migraine, sinus infection, muscular tension headache, or hypertension. As discussed in Chapter 5, in the absence of any other probable cause for the patient's symptoms, the least invasive and often the least expensive diagnostic procedure may be the correction of the patient's refractive error.

Prescribing for Astigmatism

Because astigmatism occurs in conjunction with spherical refractive errors (as simple or compound myopic or hyperopic astigmatism, or as mixed astigmatism), when a patient is found to have astigmatism, the practitioner must determine whether the patient's symptoms (assuming that there are symptoms) are caused by the spherical ametropia, by the astigmatism, or both. In general, children—because of their active accommodation—can easily compensate for 0.50 or 0.75D of uncorrected astigmatism. This is apparently done by focusing back and forth within the conoid of Sturm, near the circle of least confusion. However, as one becomes older, the lowered amplitude of accommodation tends to make it more difficult to compensate for as little as 0.50D of astigmatism, and lenses should therefore be prescribed. Some children and teenagers, particularly those who engage in a large amount of reading or other close work, may require the correction of as little as 0.50D of astigmatism. In the absence of a significant spherical refractive error, lenses are seldom prescribed for astigmatism of less than 0.50D (e.g., plano −0.25D cyl., or +0.25D sphere −0.25D cyl.). However, if a patient requires a correction for myopia or hyperopia and if 0.25D of astigmatism is found to be present, the practitioner may often include the cylinder in the prescription (e.g., −0.75D sphere −0.25D cyl., or +1.00D sphere −0.25 cyl.).

The prescription of cylindrical lenses is usually based mainly on the cylindrical component of the subjective refraction. However, the cylinder found in retinoscopy and keratometry should also be taken into consideration. In general, if the cylinder found in the subjective refraction differs by more than 0.25D from that found in retinoscopy, the retinoscopy finding should be repeated. A general rule is never to prescribe a cylinder that was not seen in retinoscopy. The examiner can create a greater problem for the patient by prescribing for astigmatism that the patient does not have than by not prescribing for a small amount of astigmatism that the patient does have (or can cause a greater problem by overprescribing for astigmatism than by underprescribing). With practice, the student should soon get to the point where the retinoscopy finding usually differs from the subjective finding by no more that 0.25D of cylinder power and by no more than 15 degrees in axis.

Prescribing for Anisometropia

When accommodation is stimulated, the accommodative response is considered to be equal for the two eyes. Therefore, if uncorrected anisometropia exists, it will be impossible for both eyes to have a sharp retinal image at the same time. For this reason, any anisometropia (difference in the refractive state for the two eyes) should normally be fully corrected.

In extreme cases, the practitioner may hesitate to prescribe a full correction for anisometropia. For example, a patient who has been previously uncorrected may be found to have a subjective refraction of right eye, +1.00DS, and left eye, +3.00DS. Because it is impossible for this patient to have a clear retinal image on both retinas at the same time, nothing is to be gained by *not* fully correcting the anisometropia. The possibility of induced aniseikonia comes to mind; however, as shown in the following chapter, if the patient's ametropia in the more hyperopic eye is axial (which is likely to be the case), a full correction for each eye would result in a minimum of induced aniseikonia. An additional consideration is the amount of vertical phoria induced when a patient looks through the lower part of the lenses to read, when the lenses are not of equal power. This, too, is discussed in Chapter 13.

When a large amount of anisometropia is present, often the patient will not subjectively accept the full plus of the retinoscope finding in the more hyperopic eye. For example, the retinoscope finding may be right eye, +0.75DS and left eye, +4.00DS, but the subjective finding may be right eye, +0.75DS, and left eye, +2.50DS. In such a case, it is a good idea to prescribe the lens powers found in the subjective refraction and have the patient return for a progress evaluation in 2 or 3 months to determine whether the full plus of the retinoscope finding can then be accepted in the more hyperopic eye. The foregoing case assumes that corrected visual acuity is normal for the more hyperopic eye. However, if the more hyperopic eye is found to be amblyopic, patching and other forms of training should be considered. [A discussion of training procedures for amblyopia is beyond the scope of this text. Interested readers are referred to Schapero (1971), Griffin (1976), and Parks (1979).]

The examples of anisometropia given thus far have been those in which one eye is more hyperopic than the other. However, it also is possible for one eye to be considerably more myopic than the other. For example, a patient's subjective refraction may be plano for the right eye and −3.00DS for the left eye. Why this occurs is not understood, but it is likely that both eyes were originally emmetropic or slightly hyperopic and, for some reason, one eye became myopic while the other eye remained emmetropic. If this condition is found in a child, a full correction of the anisometropia will restore binocular vision (unless amblyopia or strabismus are present, which is unlikely). However, if the condition is found in an adult approaching presbyopic age (who may have visited the optometrist only for a routine examination or due to failure of a driver's license vision examination), the practitioner may hesitate to prescribe lenses. The patient is skilled at using the two eyes separately (the emmetropic eye for distance and the myopic eye for near) and if uncorrected may never require bifocals or reading glasses. However, if the individual engages in a large amount of close work, correction of the refractive error may be advisable.

Prescribing for Presbyopia

Although the near-point of accommodation gradually recedes from childhood onward, most people are not aware of it until, perhaps in the early 40s, they attempt to read the fine print on a medicine bottle or insurance policy and find to their surprise that it blurs at a distance of 7 or 8 inches. Presbyopia typically begins between the ages of 40 and 45, and the power of the required reading lenses or bifocal addition increases gradually and levels off at about the age of 55 years. During the intervening 10- or 15-year period, the patient may require fairly frequent lens changes.

The fact that latent hyperopia tends to become manifest in the late 30s or early 40s has already been mentioned. It is not unusual for a previously emmetropic patient to require reading lenses even before the age of 40. However, after the lenses have been worn for a year or two, the patient may return with the complaint that the lenses that were originally suitable for near work are now required for distance vision but are of no help for near work. In such cases, what appeared to be early presbyopia was actually latent hyperopia becoming manifest.

Amplitude of accommodation

For a patient who shows symptoms of presbyopia but has not yet worn reading glasses or bifocals, the near-point of accommodation taken through the habitual correction (if any) as a part of the preliminary examination is a valuable test. The patient is handed the reduced Snellen chart at a distance of approximately 40cm and is asked to read the smallest row of letters. Following this, the patient is requested to gradually move the card closer, until the smallest row of letters begins to blur and remains blurred. At this point, the near-point of accommodation is recorded. If the patient cannot read the 20/20 letters at 40cm, the card can be moved farther away in an attempt to clear up the letters and then moved inward again. If the patient's complaint is that "my arms aren't long enough," the patient is very much aware of the appropriateness of this test. If the refraction subsequently indicates the presence of an uncorrected refractive error, the test should be repeated through the subjective lenses and the amplitude of accommodation recorded as the reciprocal of the near-point of accommodation expressed in meters. (The reciprocal of the near-point of accommodation can be specified as the amplitude of accommodation only if the finding is taken through lenses correcting the patient's ametropia.)

The rule of thumb noted in Chapter 10—that a patient should not have to make use of more than one-half of the amplitude of accommodation for a prolonged period of time—is valuable for determining the tentative addition for a beginning presbyope. However, it is of little use for an established presbyope (one who has already worn reading glasses or bifocals). For example, if the near-point of accommodation with the ametropia corrected is 33cm (indicating an amplitude of accommodation of 3.00D), the patient should be required to use only 1.50D of accommodation and, therefore, requires a +1.00D addition for a distance of 40cm.

Determining the tentative addition

There is no value in performing tests at 40cm on a presbyopic patient through the distance subjective lenses, because the near-point card in most cases will be badly blurred. It is essential, therefore, to select a tentative addition for the patient before beginning the near-point tests. One method of determining the tentative addition, as described above, is on the basis of the amplitude of accommodation, leaving one-half of the amplitude in reserve.

Another method is to estimate the patient's amplitude of accommodation on the basis of age, using Donders' table (see Table 2.3, Chapter 2), and then calculate the tentative addition on the basis of leaving one-half of the estimated amplitude in reserve.

A third method is the plus build-up: as the first near test, beginning with the subjective lenses, plus lens power is added 0.25D at a time while the patient looks at the reduced Snellen chart. The letters will gradually become clear and will then begin to blur as additional plus lens power is added; the tentative addition may be considered as the lens that provides the greatest clarity of the 20/20 letters.

A fourth method of determining the tentative addition (and the method that the author uses routinely) involves the use of the binocular crossed-cylinder test.

Binocular crossed-cylinder finding. For the presbyopic patient, the first near test (or the second near test, if the push-up amplitude is done first) should be the binocular crossed-cylinder test. For the beginning presbyope, the crossed-cylinder test will possibly result in a tentative addition that is too high by 0.50 or 1.00D compared with the tentative addition determined on the basis of accommodative amplitude. For the older, "established" presbyope, the push-up amplitude will be so low it will be of little help in determining the tentative addition. However, the binocular crossed-cylinder finding will usually result in a tentative addition that is within about 0.25D of the final addition. The tentative addition as determined by the binocular crossed-cylinder finding is modified on the basis of the plus-and-minus-to-blur findings; the range of accommodation; and other factors, including the patient's occupation and preferred working distance. The procedure involved in performing this test, as well as procedures for the plus-and-minus-to-blur and range of accommodation tests, are described in Chapter 10. The binocular crossed-cylinder finding can be recorded either as the total spherical power in the refractor—"lens in place" (LIP)—or as the added plus over the best visual acuity subjective (ADD).

Plus-and-minus-to-blur findings. The plus-and-minus-to-blur findings (negative and positive relative accommodation) are recorded as the amount of plus above and the amount of minus below the crossed-cylinder finding (or other tentative addition) necessary to cause a first sustained blur. It is necessary only to count the clicks as the lens power is changed (four clicks means a blur finding of 1.00D); there is no need to even look at the refractor dials. For a presbyopic patient, the plus-to-blur finding should be equal to or slightly greater than the minus-to-blur finding for the patient to be able to read with comfort at the distance at which the test is done (40cm). For example, if the blur findings are +1.25 and −1.00D, the amount of plus of the crossed-cylinder finding is about right for the 40cm distance; if the blur findings were +1.00 and −1.25D, it would indicate that the plus of the crossed-cylinder finding was excessive.

Range of accommodation. The range of accommodation through the tentative addition can be determined either through the refractor or with the aid of trial lenses and a trial frame. The latter procedure has the advantage that the test is done in free space, so that the patient is aware of the distance of the test card and can determine whether the range provided by the lenses is adequate. For an early presbyope, a satisfactory range would be from 8–24 inches (8 inches on either side of the 16-inch reading distance), but for an older presbyope, the range may be only from 10 or 11 inches to 21 or 22 inches (5 or 6 inches on either side of the 16-inch distance). The author prefers to specify the range of accommodation in inches, because the patient can then be told the range in inches without having to mentally convert from centimeters.

Patient's working distance. If the patient's usual working distance is 16 inches, the reading lenses or bifocal addition will be the binocular crossed-cylinder finding as amended (if necessary) by the plus-and-minus-to-blur findings and the range of accommodation. If the usual working distance is greater or less than 16 inches, plus power can be subtracted from or added to the lenses in the trial frame and the range of accommodation determined again. If the preferred working distance differs by more than a few inches from 16 inches, the practitioner may find it worthwhile to repeat quickly the crossed-cylinder finding at the new distance.

Reading glasses or bifocals?

Many patients prefer not to wear bifocals and will request reading lenses for their first near correction. If no lenses are needed for distance vision, reading lenses may be satisfactory, as long as the patient understands that the lenses needed for near vision will make distance vision badly blurred. This should be demonstrated to the patient: first, show the patient the letters on the reduced Snellen chart at near with the lenses intended for near vision and then have the patient look at the distance Snellen chart through the same lenses. The point should be made that the reading glasses will have to be removed for vision farther than arm's length. If the patient desires reading glasses, the practitioner can suggest the possibility of half-eye frames.

It is important for the patient to understand that if bifocal lenses are prescribed, it is not necessary to wear them all the time. Bifocals with plano uppers can be prescribed for beginning presbyopes: using an executive or straight-top segment fitted at or slightly above the level of the lower lid margin. Instruct the patient to forget they are bifocals and to wear them only for reading. After a few months the patient may "forget" to take them off when finished with reading or other near work and find that he or she is wearing the glasses most of the time. It is the author's experience that if reading glasses are prescribed for the first presbyopic correction, most patients are happy to change to bifocals when a change in lenses is needed.

When bifocals are prescribed, the practitioner should be particularly careful that the distance prescription is correct. If a patient's hyperopia is undercorrected (or myopia is overcorrected), the patient will almost certainly be unhappy with arm's-length vision; that is, with the vision in the area just beyond the range of the bifocal addition. Even though vision for "a mile away" may be good, the gap at arm's length will often present a problem.

Bifocals or trifocals?

Once patients require a +2.00D addition or more, many will be unhappy with arm's-length vision (even if both the distance and near prescriptions are perfectly correct). This will usually be the case with people who do a large amount of near work, and particularly with those who must have good vision at distances from 2–3 feet. Although the extra dividing line will be a nuisance for the first several weeks, the improvement in intermediate distance vision will usually motivate the patient to persevere with the lenses.

Progressive addition lenses and other multifocals

Lenses available for presbyopic patients, in addition to bifocals and trifocals, include progressive addition lenses, "invisible" bifocals, and occupational bifocals or trifocals. (These lenses are described in Chapter 13.)

Prescribing for Aphakia

Optometrists practicing in communities where there are large numbers of older people will see many patients having cataracts and, therefore, will be fitting many of these patients with postsurgical glasses or contact lenses. Aphakic spectacles present many problems, one of which is that the vertex distance of the finished lenses (the distance from the back surface of the lens to the apex of the cornea) must be the same as for the trial lenses through which the refraction is done. Although changes in vertex distance can be safely ignored for lenses of low power, vertex distance assumes importance for lenses of 5.00 or 6.00D and more, and it assumes critical importance for the high powers used in aphakic lenses.

As shown in Chapter 13, an error in vertex distance of 5mm (i.e., refraction at a 15mm vertex distance and finished lenses fitting at a distance of 10mm) can result in an aphakic lens being 0.75D too weak. After completion of the routine examination by means of the refractor, the practitioner should measure the vertex distance for the frame the patient has selected (while the frame fits correctly on the patient's face), and then should refine the refractive end-point using a trial frame at the correct vertex distance, with the strongest lens in the back cell. An alternative procedure is to refine the refractive end-point by using the patient's frame and Halberg clips, as shown in Figure 15.3 (Chapter 15).

If contact lenses are to be fitted this problem is avoided because trial contact lenses will be used. A close approximation of the correct power for a contact lens to be used as a trial lens can be predicted by a table (see Appendix C) or by calculation either by formula or by use of the step-along method. Using either of these methods, a patient requiring a +13.00D lens at a vertex distance of 15cm will be found to require a +16.00D contact lens. (Aphakic spectacle lenses are discussed in Chapter 13 and contact lenses in Chapter 14.)

Long-Term Patient Care

Many years ago, Barstow (1959) made the point that once a patient visits an optometrist, that optometrist should be prepared to assume responsibility for the patient's vision care for the patient's life-time. He recommended what he called the *perpetual appointment system*, based on a "short hop" progress visit scheduled from 3–4 weeks after the patient's glasses are dispensed and a "long hop" progress visit scheduled 6 months later. Long hop progress visits are then scheduled once each 6 months, indefinitely, and lens changes are made whenever needed.

When in practice, the author used a modified form of Barstow's system and found it to be satisfactory. Most patients appreciate the fact that the practitioner is willing to take the time (even though only a few minutes may be needed) to make sure their correction is serving its intended purpose; they appreciate the practitioner's interest in their long-term visual welfare. From the practitioner's point of view, the short hop progress visit is a valuable form of feedback—if for no other reason than that the practitioner soon learns that when patients are dissatisfied it is usually because of poorly fitting glasses rather than because of an incorrect prescription. Barstow's 6-month hop progress visit cycle is probably based on the successful public relations programs of dentistry (carried on mainly by toothpaste companies). However, the 6-month period proved to be too short a time for vision care patients, many of whom may not require a change of lenses for a number of years.

Enough is known about expected changes in refraction and about the incidence of eye disease for patients of various age groups to enable the practitioner to make specific recommendations to patients concerning the future need for vision care services. These recommendations are made mainly on the basis of the patient's age, but they may be influenced by the patient's refractive state and other factors.

Children and teenagers

Relatively few preschool children require vision care services. Of those who do, many are high hyperopes, possibly with esotropia, and the practitioner will want to decide on the frequency of visits on an individual basis. In most cases, the practitioner will want to see the patient at least once each year.

The majority of patients of school age are myopes. Because myopia is known to progress at the rate of from 0.25 to 0.50D per year, yearly examinations should be recommended throughout the elementary and high school years. Of those children who are not myopes, many will have borderline hyperopia, astigmatism, or binocular vision anomalies and may not require a correction on the first visit; however, they should be monitored on a yearly basis.

Many concerned parents arrange to have their children's visual status evaluated prior to entering school or during the first year of school, in the absence of any apparent complaints or problems. If the child is found to be perfectly normal visually, the practitioner may recommend reexamination in two years, or sooner if symptoms develop.

Young adults

It is a well-known fact that changes in refraction occur more slowly for young adults, as a group, than for people of any other age group. (A possible exception to this rule is the adult aphakic. Because changes in refraction during the adult years are to a great extent due to lens changes—both to increasing thickness of the lens and to the fact that latent hyperopia may become manifest—there is little that can change in the aphakic eye.) In a survey involving refractive changes of 111 optometrists between the ages of 20 and 40 years (Grosvenor, 1977c), it was found that (1) emmetropes at age 20 were usually still

emmetropic at age 40; (2) myopes at age 20 had about the same amount of myopia, or slightly more, at the age of 40; (3) hyperopes at age 20 had about the same amount of hyperopia, or slightly more, at age 40; and (4) astigmatism changed little and in no predictable manner between the ages of 20 and 40. Experienced practitioners are aware that were it not for contact lenses and fashion frames, young adults would seldom require their services. Reexamination for patients in this age group should be recommended about every other year.

Ages 40–55

Changes in refraction of people aged 40–55 have already been discussed but will be summarized here. Many previously uncorrected hyperopes will need lenses in their early 40s, either because of latent hyperopia becoming manifest or because the amplitude of accommodation has decreased to the point where near visual tasks cannot be maintained for long periods of time with comfort. Most people require their first correction for presbyopia between the ages of 40 and 45 and will require periodic increases in reading lens or bifocal addition power (and possibly increases in plus power for distance) for a period of about 10 years before leveling off at a +2.25 or +2.50D addition. Because of the increasing possibility of ocular disease during this period, Hirsch (1969) suggested that the patient be scheduled for a complete optometric examination every other year and for an ocular health examination in the intervening years.

Age 55 and over

On the basis of refractive data reported by Hirsch (1958), the practitioner can expect to find many patients to change little in refraction beyond the age of 55, a smaller number to become more hyperopic, and a still smaller number to become more myopic. Hirsch's data on 820 patients over the age of 45 indicate that the prevalence of emmetropia (between −1.12 and +1.12D) decreased from 59 to 37 percent from ages 55–75 and over, the prevalence of hyperopia increased from 35 to 48 percent, and the prevalence of myopia increased from 5 to 15 percent during the same period. Hirsch warned against the practice of telling a patient who requires a +2.50D bifocal addition that no further lens changes will be needed, as the available evidence indicates that this is frequently not true.

Finally, it is of interest to compare Barstow's (1959) perpetual appointment system to Weed's (1968) concept of health-care delivery as a closed-loop system. Barstow's short hop progress visit usually requires only brief progress notes; however, the long hop progress visit may require only progress notes or it may in some cases require repetition of a large portion of the optometric data base.

MANAGEMENT OF BINOCULAR VISION ANOMALIES

The majority of patients who have binocular vision anomalies have been able to maintain binocular vision but at the cost of varying amounts of stress. These are patients who have heterophoria, fusional vergence anomalies, fixation disparities, unusually high or low AC/A ratios, and other anomalies involving the accommodation or convergence systems as well as the relationships between the two systems. Most of these anomalies can be managed by a system of analysis that has become known as *graphical analysis*, because binocular vision findings can be plotted on a graph. The remainder of this chapter is concerned with the diagnosis and management of binocular vision problems by means of graphical analysis and fixation disparity analysis.

A small minority of patients having binocular vision problems do not possess binocularity, having strabismus, and usually have developed one or more adaptive mechanisms, including suppression, amblyopia, eccentric fixation, and anomalous retinal correspondence. The primary care optometrist should be able to diagnose these conditions and make a reasonably accurate prognosis in terms of their management with lenses, prisms, orthoptics, surgery, or a combination of these. However, the supervision of orthoptic training programs is not included in the scope of most primary care practices and as such is not presented here. [Procedures for the diagnosis of strabismus are discussed in Chapters 6 and 10. For information about orthoptic training of strabismus and amblyopia, see Griffin (1976) and Schapero (1971).]

GRAPHICAL ANALYSIS OF BINOCULAR VISION FINDINGS

Although the graphical method of analysis was originated by Donders and further developed by Sheard, the system of analysis now in use stems largely from the work of Fry (1937), Hofstetter (1945), and Morgan (1948, reprinted 1964). Fry (1937) used a haploscope to vary the stimulus to both accommodation and convergence and was also able to measure the accommodative response by means of a Badal optometer. He found that, for a given stimulus to accommodation, as the stimulus to convergence was increased, the subject would increase convergence without increasing accommodation up to a certain point, where accommodation was found to increase. Fry found that the point where accommodation began to increase was related to the subject's report that the target was blurred. He interpreted this as meaning that the subject first employed positive fusional vergence, but when this reached its limit, the subject used accommodative convergence to maintain single vision (but at the expense of clarity).

Similarly, as the stimulus to convergence was decreased, the subject would allow the eyes to diverge with no change in accommodation up to a certain point, where accommodation began to increase. The decrease in accommodation was accompanied by a report that the target was blurred. This was interpreted as meaning that the subject first used negative fusional vergence; when its limit was reached, accommodative divergence was used at the expense of clear imagery. Fry's (1937) results are shown in Figure 10.3 in Chapter 10.

In Fry's graph, convergence is plotted along the x-axis, and accommodation is plotted along the y-axis. The graph resembles the graph used for clinical data, except that when dealing with clinical data we must plot accommodative stimulus rather than accommodative response. This is because we have no method of measuring accommodative response in clinical work while taking binocular vision findings. Inspection of Figure 10.3 shows the following characteristics: it is shaped like a parallelogram (rounded off at the lower right and upper left corners); the width of the graph at any level of accommodation represents the total amplitude of convergence; and the slope of the graph represents the AC/A ratio (the ratio of accommodative convergence to accommodation).

Plotting Clinical Data

The graph used for plotting clinical data is shown in Figure 12.1. Similar to the graph of haploscopic data, convergence (in prism diopters) is plotted along the x-axis. Note that convergence at 6m is indicated along the bottom of the graph, and convergence at 40cm is indicated along the top of the graph. The stimulus to accommodation is indicated along the y-axis.

A horizontal dotted line is supplied at the 2.50D stimulus to accommodation level, as this represents the stimulus to accommodation at 40cm. A vertical dotted line is supplied at the 15Δ base-out level, representing the convergence required at 40cm (for an individual with an interpupillary distance of approximately 64mm). The slightly curved, diagonal line is known as the demand line. Points along this line represent the demand on both accommodation and convergence at all levels of stimulus to accommodation. Another way to describe the demand line is to say that if the patient were orthophoric at all distances, all of the patient's phoria findings would be plotted along the demand line.

As shown in Figure 12.1, phorias are plotted by means of an *x*, blurs are plotted by means of a circle, and breaks are plotted by means of a square. Although a triangle can be used to plot recoveries, these are seldom plotted. The amplitude of accommodation is plotted as a horizontal line, forming the upper limit of the graph; the amplitude of convergence is plotted as a vertical line, forming the right-hand limit of the graph.

A typical set of findings is shown plotted in Figure 12.2. The findings are as follows:

Distance	Phoria: ortho
	Base-in: *x*/10/5
	Base-out: 10/15/7
Near	Phoria: 5 exo
	Base-in: 15/20/10
	Base-out: 6/13/7
	Plus-to-blur: +2.25D
	Minus-to-blur: −3.00D
	NP Accom.: 11cm
	NP Conv.: 7cm

The first step in plotting the graph is to place a line across the graph at the level of the amplitude of accommodation, which constitutes the upper limit of the graph. The second step is to place a vertical line to indicate the amplitude of convergence, which constitutes the right-hand limit of the graph. The amplitude of convergence is determined by converting the near-point of convergence (measured from an imaginary line joining the centers of rotation of the two eyes) to *meter angles* (MA) of convergence by taking its reciprocal, in meters, and multiplying this by the interpupillary distance expressed in centimeters. Assuming an interpupillary distance of 6cm, the amplitude of convergence will be

Amplitude of convergence

= (MA of convergence) (PD)

= (14.3) (6) = 86Δ.

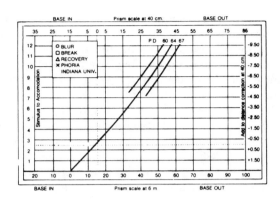

Figure 12.1. The graphical analysis form (Grosvenor, 1975b).

A vertical line, therefore, is plotted as 86Δ base-out.

The distance and near phorias are plotted next and are connected by a straight line, forming the phoria line. Note that the phoria line (like all other lines) is extended to the line representing the amplitude of accommodation. Next, the base-out-to-blur findings are plotted and connected with a straight line and the base-out-to-break findings are plotted and connected. Similarly, the base-in-to-blur and base-in-to-break findings are plotted and connected. In the event that a blur does not occur for a given test (as is the expected situation for the base-in finding at distance), the line that would otherwise go through the blur finding is plotted through the break finding (as shown in Figure 12.2 for the base-in-to-break finding at distance).

The plus-lens-to-blur finding, because it represents the limit of positive fusional vergence as plus

Figure 12.2 A typical set of clinical findings. The shaded area represents the zone of clear, single binocular vision (Grosvenor, 1975c).

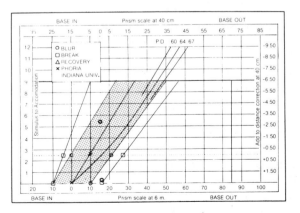

lenses are added, should line up with the base-out-to-blur findings. (See the discussion of plus-and-minus-to-blur findings in Chapter 10.) Similarly, the minus-lens-to-blur finding, because it represents the limit of negative fusional vergence, should line up with the base-in-to-blur findings. However, in the majority of cases, the minus-lens-to-blur finding is much too low to be plotted on the base-in line. This is obviously the case with the present data. When this occurs, it is due to the fact that, as minus lens power is increased, the minus lenses cause the letters to appear smaller and thus farther away.

Interpretation of the Graph

The graph is interpreted in terms of the five fundamental variables in the relationship between accommodation and convergence.

Five fundamental variables

The five fundamental variables were described by Fry (1943, reprinted 1964). Each of the variables has an easily recognized counterpart on the graph:

Variable	Graph
1. Distance phoria.	1. Origin of the graph.
2. AC/A ratio.	2. Slope of the graph.
3. Amplitude of accommodation.	3. Upper limit of the graph.
4. Positive fusional vergence.	4. Right-hand limit of the graph.
5. Negative fusional vergence.	5. Left-hand limit of the graph.

Zone of clear, single binocular vision

As shown in Figure 12.2, the *zone of clear, single binocular vision* is bounded by the base-in and base-out-to-blur lines, the zero stimulus to accommodation line, and the line representing the amplitude of accommodation. Whereas the height of the zone of clear, single binocular vision depends only on the amplitude of accommodation, its width at any level of stimulus to accommodation depends on the amplitude of fusional vergence (both positive and negative) at that level.

AC/A ratio

The *AC/A ratio* is indicated by the slope of the phoria line. The greater the slope, the lower the AC/A ratio; and the lower the slope, the greater the AC/A ratio. For the data plotted in Figure 12.2, the AC/A ratio can be calculated as follows:

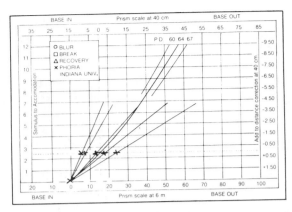

Figure 12.3   AC/A ratios of 2/1, 4/1, 6/1, 8/1, and 10/1. Note that the greater the slope of the phoria line, the lower the AC/A ratio (Grosvenor, 1975c).

$$\frac{AC}{A} = \frac{15 - \text{physiological exophoria}}{2.5}$$
$$= \frac{15 - 5}{2.5} = \frac{4}{1}.$$

The effect of the AC/A ratio on the phoria line is shown in Figure 12.3. In this diagram, the distance phoria is zero in all cases. Going from the greatest to the least slope, near phorias are 10 exo, 5 exo, ortho, 5 eso, and 10 eso. The corresponding AC/A ratios are 2/1, 4/1, 6/1, 8/1, and 10/1.

Use of the Graph in Prescribing

Once the patient's data have been plotted on the graph form, a casual inspection of the graph will indicate the width of the zone of clear, single binocular vision and the approximate values of the AC/A ratio. In addition, inspection of the graph gives an indication of the validity and reliability of the findings. The extent to which the graph indicates validity and reliability is limited, however, because the phoria line and the base-in and base-out lines are each plotted by means of only two points. Additional points can be supplied by plotting a third set of findings taken at a third distance (say, 25cm), but this has the effect of prolonging the examination and unnecessarily fatiguing the patient. Validity and reliability are indicated if the graph has the shape of a parallelogram—fanning out slightly at the top—and if the phoria line and the blur and break lines are roughly parallel.

If a patient is found to have a phoria of significant amount, the practitioner should first determine whether the phoria presents a problem, such as diplopia, headaches, fatigue when reading, or other subjective symptoms. (Occasionally a patient will claim to have no symptoms whatsoever, but on further questioning it will become apparent that the patient does little or no reading or other close work. Such a patient obviously needs help.) If such symptoms are present and are not likely to be relieved by the correction of the refractive error, the practitioner can conclude that the problem is one of excessive fusional vergence demand. The demand on fusional vergence can be relieved by the use of one (or a combination of three) procedures.

1. Prescribing prism. The prescribing of prism increases the fusional vergence reserve while decreasing the fusional vergence demand (the phoria) by an amount equal to the power of the prism. Assume that a patient has 8Δ of exophoria and a base-out-to-blur (positive fusional vergence reserve) of 12Δ. If we prescribe 2Δ of base-in prism, the positive fusional vergence reserve will be increased to 14Δ, and the phoria will be decreased to 6Δ (while the prism is worn).

2. Prescribing visual training. Visual training can be prescribed with the intention of building up the positive fusional vergence reserve (in exophoria) or the negative fusional vergence reserve (in esophoria). The problem of the patient described in the previous example could be handled by prescribing base-out training, with the idea of building up the base-out (positive fusional vergence) reserve until it is sufficient to meet the demand created by the phoria.

3. Alteration of the spherical portion of the correction. If the AC/A ratio is sufficiently large, the provision of additional plus lens power at near can greatly reduce a patient's esophoria and, therefore, decrease the demand on negative fusional vergence. It is also possible that additional minus power at near can be used to reduce a patient's exophoria and thus reduce the demand on positive fusional vergence. However, this is seldom a viable alternative, as most people who have exophoria at near have low AC/A ratios.

Sheard's criterion

Sheard (1925, reprinted 1957) proposed that for comfortable binocular vision, the fusional convergence reserve should be at least twice the demand.

For example, if a patient has 10Δ of exophoria, the positive fusional vergence reserve should be at least 20Δ. Sheard's criterion can be used to determine (1) the amount of prism to be prescribed or (2) the increase in fusional vergence reserve that should be achieved by visual training.

When Sheard's criterion is used to determine the amount of prism to be prescribed, the prism power can be computed by the following formula:

$$\text{Prism} = \frac{2(\text{phoria}) - \text{compensating vergence finding}}{3}.$$

Using this formula, if a patient has 8Δ of exophoria and a base-out-to-blur finding of 10Δ, the amount of prism required would be 2Δ base-in.

Most practitioners find it easier to determine the amount of prism by trial and error than by using the formula. Using the previous example, the prescribing of 1Δ base-in would reduce the phoria from 8 to 7Δ of exophoria and would increase the fusional vergence reserve from 10 to 11Δ. Because 11 is not twice 7, 1Δ would obviously not be sufficient, but 2Δ base-in would reduce the phoria to 6Δ and increase the fusional vergence reserve to 12Δ, thereby satisfying Sheard's criterion. Sheard's criterion should not be regarded as an exact, scientifically determined formula, but rather as a guide that can help the practitioner in solving a patient's problem.

Percival's criterion

Percival's (1928) criterion is known as the "middle third" criterion. It states that the point of zero demand should be in the middle third of the total fusion range, without regard to the phoria (Sheard, 1930, reprinted 1957). For example, if the base-out-to-blur finding for a given patient is 30Δ, and the base-in-to-blur finding is 10Δ, the total range of fusional vergence is 40Δ, and the point of zero demand is not in the middle third of the total fusional range (see Figure 12.4). Using a trial and error

Figure 12.4   Application of Percival's criterion. To move the convergence demand (the zero point) to the middle third, 4Δ of base-in prism would be required.

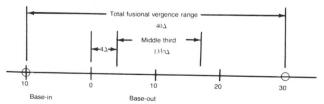

method, the provision of 4Δ of base-out prism would increase the base-in finding to 14Δ and decrease the base-out finding to 26Δ, satisfying the middle third criterion (each third of the total fusion range being 13 1/3Δ in this case). The amount of prism to satisfy Percival's criterion can also be determined by the use of the following formula:

$$\text{Prism} = \frac{1}{3}G - \frac{2}{3}L,$$

where

G = the greater of the two fusional vergence findings

L = the lesser of the two fusional vergence findings.

Percival's criterion appears to be used infrequently. It is not only cumbersome to apply, but the logic of prescribing prism without regard to the phoria is questionable.

Evaluation of Sheard's and Percival's criteria

Sheard's (1925) criterion was used in optometric practice for many years before it was evaluated in a controlled clinical study. Worrell, Hirsch, and Morgan (1971) reported on a study in which 43 patients with muscular imbalance and asthenopic complaints were each fitted with two pairs of glasses—one with no prism and the other with the amount of prism required to satisfy Sheard's criterion. Each patient wore one pair of glasses for one week and the other pair for the following week. Neither the experimenters nor the patients knew which pair of glasses had the prism. At the end of the second week, each patient was asked to choose the pair of glasses that helped the most.

The patients were considered in terms of four categories for the purpose of analyzing the results:

	N	Preferred prism	Preferred no prism
Exo at 6m	2	0	2
Eso at 6m	13	11	2
Exo at 40cm	24	11	13
Eso at 40cm	8	3	5

Only in the second category (eso at 6m) was there a statistically significant preference for the glasses with prism. The preference for prism of patients with exophoria at 40cm (the third category) appeared to be related to age: of the 19 patients under the age of 45, only 6 preferred the glasses with the prism, whereas of the 5 patients over the age of 45, 4 preferred the prism (Worrell et al., 1971).

The investigators concluded that their findings were contrary to the "conventional wisdom," for it is usually assumed that base-out prism for esophoria at 6m must be used with caution, whereas base-in prism at near is usually assumed to be clearly warranted (Worrell et al., 1971).

Sheedy and Saladin (1977) compared binocular vision findings of 28 asymptomatic optometry students and 32 orthoptics patients with symptoms associated with binocular oculomotor difficulties. Using discrimination analysis to determine which tests discriminated best between the two groups of subjects, they found that Sheard's criterion was the best discriminator for exophoric subjects, whereas the amount of phoria was the best discriminator for esophoric subjects; fixation disparity was the second-best discriminator for both exophoric and esophoric subjects. However, the authors pointed out that the "second-best" rating of fixation disparity may have been a result of the way the subjects were selected. Fixation disparity findings were not available on patients at the time they were referred for orthoptics treatment, and, therefore, referrals were made on the basis of phorias and fusional vergence findings.

In another study, Sheedy and Saladin (1978) compared binocular vision findings of 44 asymptomatic optometry students with those of 33 symptomatic optometry students. Again using discrimination analysis, they found that Sheard's criterion was the best discriminator for all subjects as a group (including both exophores and esophores). However, when exophoric and esophroic subjects were considered separately, the best discriminator for the exophores was the y-intercept of the fixation disparity curve as determined by the Disparometer (i.e., the actual amount of fixation disparity at the near testing distance); the best discriminator for the esophores was Percival's middle third criterion (using break points rather than blur points). The fact that Sheard's criterion was a much better discriminator for exo deviations than for eso deviations was interpreted as indicating that positive vergences are a more active process than negative vergences. This agrees with the clinical impression that positive vergences are more easily trained than negative vergences.

Prescribing on the basis of the AC/A ratio

Gradient and calculated AC/A ratios are discussed in Chapter 10, and the representation of the AC/A ratio on the graph is described earlier in this chapter. Inspection of the formula for the calculated AC/A ratio,

$$\frac{AC}{A} = \frac{15 - \text{physiological exophoria}}{2.5},$$

in which the term *physiological exophoria* indicates how much more exophoric the patient is at near than at distance, indicates the following:

1. If the distance and near phorias are equal, the AC/A ratio is equal to 6/1 (i.e., there is no physiological exophoria).
2. If the patient is more exophoric at near than at distance (the usual situation), the AC/A ratio will have a value of less than 6/1.
3. If the patient is more esophoric at near than at distance, the AC/A ratio will have a value greater than 6/1.

An AC/A ratio of 6/1 has been considered by some to be a "normal" AC/A ratio. However, a much more desirable situation occurs when the patient is orthophoric or near-orthophoric at distance and has a small amount of exophoria at near, resulting in an AC/A ratio of about 4/1.

The majority of patients are orthophoric or near-orthophoric at distance, but many people are found to be either esophoric or exophoric at near. When this occurs, the practitioner may consider the possibility of altering the spherical component of the patient's near correction to reduce the near phoria and, therefore, reduce the demand on fusional vergence. The following examples illustrate the importance of the AC/A ratio in predicting whether altering the spherical lens powers will be effective in reducing the near phoria.

Example 1. Suppose that a patient's phoria findings are orthophoria at distance and 10Δ of esophoria at near. The AC/A ratio is, therefore, equal to

$$\frac{15 - (-10)}{2.5} = \frac{10}{1}.$$

We would like to prescribe added plus power at near to reduce the esophoria. How much added plus will be necessary? With an AC/A ratio of 10/1, the addition of 1.00D of added plus power at near would be expected to relax accommodation and, therefore, accommodative convergence sufficiently to reduce the near phoria all the way from 10Δ of esophoria to orthophoria.

To determine if the phoria actually will be reduced to orthophoria, we put the +1.00D spheres in the refractor, and take the phoria finding. This is equivalent to determining the gradient AC/A ratio,

and we would predict that the phoria would change somewhat less than 10Δ, because proximal convergence is a constant factor when two phorias are both taken at the same distance.

Example 2. Suppose that a patient's phoria findings are orthophoria at distance and 10Δ of exophoria at near. The AC/A ratio is equal to

$$\frac{15 - 10}{2.5} = \frac{2}{1}.$$

We are considering the possibility of prescribing added minus power at near to stimulate accommodation and accommodative convergence and thereby reduce the exophoria at near. However, with an AC/A ratio of only 2/1, a whole diopter of minus power would be expected to reduce the exophoria at near only from the original 10Δ of exophoria to 8Δ of exophoria. A much easier way to solve this patient's problem would be to prescribe base-out training to increase the amplitude of positive fusional vergence, or to prescribe base-in prism for near work.

The only situation in which a practitioner may seriously consider prescribing added minus power at near for an exophoric patient is when the patient is exophoric at both distance and near, thereby having a sufficiently high AC/A ratio so the added minus power will materially reduce the exophoric at near. Even then, the added accommodation necessary may fatigue the patient in spite of the reduction in fusional vergence demand.

BINOCULAR VISION SYNDROMES

As noted by Borish (1970), Duane and White described a number of binocular vision syndromes of particular interest to optometrists; they easily lend themselves to graphical representation and can be explained in terms of anomalies of accommodation and convergence. Borish (1970) pointed out that these syndromes were originally applied to strabismic conditions rather than phorias, but they have been modified to some extent by Tait (1951), who described them in terms of accommodation and convergence.

Convergence Insufficiency

In convergence insufficiency, the patient is usually orthophoric or near-orthophoric at distance and has a high exophoria at near, indicating a low AC/A ratio.

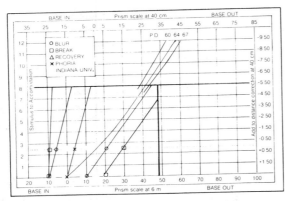

Figure 12.5 Convergence insufficiency (Grosvenor, 1975d).

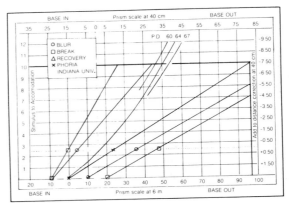

Figure 12.6 Convergence excess (Grosvenor, 1975d).

There is usually a poor near-point of convergence, and there is likely to be a low positive fusional vergence reserve. The patient may complain of visual fatigue, drowsiness, and even transitory diplopia accompanying prolonged close work.

A typical case of convergence insufficiency is plotted in Figure 12.5. The graph has a high slope, which indicates a low AC/A ratio. In addition, the base-out zone is somewhat narrower than the base-in zone, and the graph is of limited extent to the right because of the poor near-point of convergence. With orthophoria at distance and 10Δ of exophoria at near, the AC/A ratio is found to be 2/1.

Base-out training is usually an effective method of treating convergence insufficiency. It requires no expensive instrumentation and often requires only a small number of training sessions to increase the base-out zone sufficiently to solve the patient's problem. It can be done easily as a home training procedure using the Keystone Base-Out series, the Bausch & Lomb Ortho-Fuser, or other inexpensive instrumentation that can be loaned to the patient. "Pencil push-ups" are often all that is required. Sheard's criterion can be used to determine the amount of increase that is needed in the base-out zone.

If the patient's symptoms are not alleviated by the base-out training (an infrequent occurrence), it may be necessary to prescribe a small amount of base-in prism for close work only.

Convergence Excess

Convergence excess is the typical high AC/A ratio case. The patient will have orthophoria or near-orthophoria at distance and a high esophoria at near. An example of convergence excess is plotted in

Figure 12.6. With orthophoria at distance and 10Δ esophoria at near, the calculated AC/A ratio will be found to be 10/1. As described earlier, one would expect that a $+1.00D$ addition would bring the phoria all the way down to orthophoria. The way to find out is simply to add $+1.00D$ spheres in the refractor and measure the near phoria again (in effect measuring a gradient phoria).

If the patient requires no correction for distance, only reading glasses will have to be prescribed. If the distance correction is for hyperopia, bifocals (or two pairs of glasses) must be prescribed. If the patient has a small amount of myopia, often the problem can be solved easily by having the patient remove the glasses for prolonged close work. For example, when a myopic patient removes a pair of $-1.00D$ spheres for close work, this is the equivalent of wearing a $+1.00D$ addition.

Experience has shown that the provision of added plus power at near is an effective method of managing convergence excess. An alternative approach, if needed, is to prescribe base-out prism power for close work. A third possibility is base-in training to increase the amplitude of negative fusional vergence; however, experience indicates that this form of training often is not effective.

Divergence Insufficiency

As described by Tait (1951), divergence insufficiency can occur in either of two forms: (1) the patient may have a high esophoria at distance with a lesser esophoria at near, indicating excessive tonic convergence but normal accommodative convergence; or (2) the patient may have a higher esophoria at near than at distance, indicating that both tonic and accommodative convergence are excessive. The two

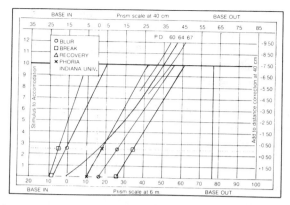

Figure 12.7 Divergence insufficiency with excessive tonic convergence but normal accommodative convergence (Grosvenor, 1975d).

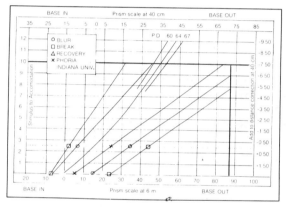

Figure 12.8 Divergence insufficiency with excessive tonic and accommodative convergence (Grosvenor, 1975d).

forms of divergence insufficiency are shown in Figures 12.7 and 12.8. If a patient has the first form of divergence insufficiency and complains of headaches or other forms of asthenopia, the practitioner should consider prescribing base-out prism. In the second form of divergence insufficiency, the use of base-out prism with added plus at near should be considered.

Divergence Excess

A patient with divergence excess has a high exophoria at distance and a lower exophoria or orthophoria at near, and may complain of occasional diplopia at distance. However, as Giles (1949) pointed out, the patient may have learned to suppress, so will have no complaint of diplopia but will be told by friends that one eye sometimes turns out. As

shown in Figure 12.9, divergence excess is a condition in which there is a high AC/A ratio: the slope of the phoria line is similar in that in Figure 12.6, but the whole graph is shifted to the left.

Several approaches can be taken in the management of divergence excess. Because the AC/A ratio is high, an overcorrection of minus power (or undercorrection of plus power) will reduce the exophoria at distance; however, it can create an esophoria at near unless a bifocal addition is prescribed. Base-in prism may be prescribed for distance, but this would also create an esophoria at near. In mild cases of divergence excess—in which the amount of exophoria at distance is not greatly less than the exophoria at near—base-in prism for full-time wear (both distance and near) may be effective. Clearly, each case of divergence excess must be handled on its own merits.

"False" convergence insufficiency

"False" convergence insufficiency is not included in the syndromes described by Duane and White but it is a syndrome that is observed with great regularity in optometric practice. The patient has orthophoria or near-orthophoria at distance and a high exophoria at near, usually accompanied by a low near-point of convergence—all of which would be expected in convergence insufficiency. However, false convergence insufficiency differs from classical convergence insufficiency in that the zone of clear, single binocular vision has a normal slope, while the phoria line has the high slope indicative of a low AC/A ratio (shown in Figure 12.10).

As pointed out by Heath (1959), the most likely explanation for this condition is that the patient fails to accommodate sufficiently during the near-phoria test. Even though the patient is admonished to "keep

Figure 12.9 Divergence excess (Grosvenor, 1975d).

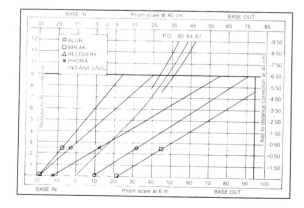

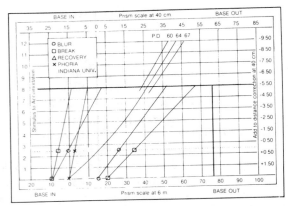

Figure 12.10   "False" convergence insufficiency (Grosvenor, 1975d).

the letters clear," he or she apparently makes use of the eyes' depth of focus and accommodates as little as possible, resulting in a falsely high exophoria finding. Heath suggests that this is really a problem of accommodation rather than of convergence, and that training procedures should be aimed at improving the facility of the accommodative response. After training, the phoria line swings into line with the other findings, indicating a normal AC/A ratio.

Effects of Depth of Focus and Proximal Convergence on the Zone of Clear, Single Binocular Vision

Both depth of focus and proximal convergence can affect the shape of the zone of clear, single binocular vision.

Depth of focus

Due to the depth of focus of the eyes, an object (even as small as a 20/20 letter) can be considerably out of focus but still be seen clearly. Even though an effort is made to minimize depth of focus effects by using first blurs rather than blur-outs, depth of focus effects are sufficient to alter the shape of the graph.

If we were to measure the amount of accommodation in play (by means of an optometer or dynamic retinoscopy) as the amount of base-in and base-out prism is increased at various levels of accommodative stimuli, the results could be plotted as in Figure 12.11. As shown in the figure, when base-in prism is added, as much as 1.00D or more of accommodation is relaxed (dashed lines) before a blur is reported (solid circle); when base-out prism is added, as much as 1.00D or more of accommodation is in play before a blur is reported. Therefore, the base-in-to-blur

findings indicate points on the graph for which the eyes are underaccommodated for the stimulus, and base-out to blur findings indicate points on the graph for which the eyes are overaccommodated for the stimulus. Figure 12.11 shows that the greater the stimulus to accommodation, the more the accommodative mechanism goes out of focus before a blur is reported.

The solid lines in Figure 12.11 show the base-in and base-out lines as they would occur if the patient reported a blur as soon as the accommodative mechanism were out of focus (i.e., if there were no depth of focus); the circles show the base-in and base-out limits of the zone as they would be plotted for a routine clinic patient. A comparison of these two zones—the one plotted by the solid lines and the one indicated by the blur points—demonstrates the effect of the depth of focus on the shape of the zone of clear, single binocular vision. The effect is a *fanning out* of the base-in and base-out limits of the zone, indicating that the widening of the graph due to depth of focus is greater when accommodation and pupillary constriction are in play than when they are relaxed.

Proximal convergence

One method of studying the effects of proximal convergence on the shape of the graph, as suggested by Abel and Hofstetter (undated), is to plot a given patient's phorias, base-in limits, and base-out limits by two methods. In the first method, all tests are done at 6m, first through the subjective finding and then through −1.00, −2.00, and −3.00DS combined with the subjective finding. In the second method, all tests are done at 33cm, first through the subjective finding and then through +1.00, +2.00, and

Figure 12.11   The effect of depth of focus on the zone of clear, single binocular vision (Grosvenor, 1976e).

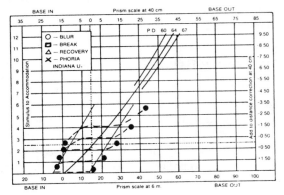

+3.00DS combined with the subjective finding. The result is findings at four different levels of stimulus to accommodation, and at each level we have one set of findings taken at 6m and one set of findings taken at 33cm.

The findings are plotted on a graph, as shown in Figure 12.12, with 6m findings plotted by solid lines and 33cm findings plotted by dashed lines. As shown in the figure, the base-in findings are essentially the same for the 6m findings and the 33cm findings; however, the phoria line is displaced about 3Δ to the right for the 33cm findings, and the base-out line is displaced about 6Δ to the right for 33cm findings. If the six findings taken through the subjective refraction are replotted (omitting the other findings), it is evident that the zone "fans out" as it goes upward.

We can conclude that both depth-of-focus effects and proximal convergence effects result in a fanning out of the zone of clear, single binocular vision.

Can the AC/A Ratio Change?

Whether the AC/A ratio is inborn and remains the same throughout life or it is a learned relationship subject to change has been a matter of controversy in optometry for several decades. Those who believe the AC/A ratio remains constant throughout life—and cannot be changed as a result of training—are mainly researchers who deal with the *response AC/A ratio*. They use a haploscope and an optometer system, which enables them to measure the accommodative response. Those who believe the AC/A ratio is subject to wide fluctuations—particularly as a result of training—are mainly practitioners who deal with the *stimulus AC/A ratio*. They use clinical methods and have no way to measure accommodative response while measuring clinical phoria findings.

Because of the large depth of focus of which the eyes are capable, a patient's near-phoria findings can vary considerably, depending on whether the patient is correctly accommodated, underaccommodated, or overaccommodated for the plane of the test card. As discussed in connection with false convergence insufficiency, some patients will accommodate at a considerable distance beyond the plane of regard, and thus, show an artificially high exophoria at near (as indicated by the fact that the base-in and base-out limits of the zone have a lower slope than the phoria line). If visual training is given, the resulting decrease in the exophoria at near can then be interpreted as meaning that the AC/A ratio increased as a result of training. An alternate conclusion is that

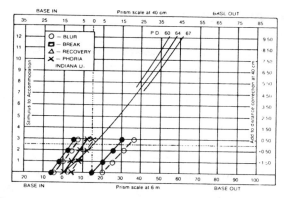

Figure 12.12   Effects of proximal convergence on the zone of clear, single binocular vision (Abel and Hofstetter, undated).

in the original examination the AC/A ratio was falsely low, and therefore it did not really change as a result of training.

As an example of false convergence insufficiency, suppose a patient who is orthophoric at distance is found to have 10Δ of exophoria at near, resulting in the following AC/A ratio:

$$\frac{15-10}{2.5} = \frac{2}{1}.$$

If the patient had actually used only 1.25D of accommodation, the response AC/A ratio would have been

$$\frac{15-10}{1.25} = \frac{4}{1}.$$

If, after accommodative facility training, the patient actually makes use of 2.50D of accommodation, he or she will be found to have only 5Δ of exophoria at near, and the AC/A ratio will appear to have increased to 4/1:

$$\frac{15-5}{1.25} = \frac{4}{1}.$$

It is of interest that Flom (1960) found that even the response AC/A ratio can undergo a significant change as a result of training. He monitored both haploscopic and clinical AC/A ratios for a group of eight subjects during a series of orthoptics sessions lasting 8 weeks. Flom found that the haploscopic AC/A ratio increased by an average of 0.66/1 during the training period, whereas the clinical AC/A ratio increased by an average of only 0.32/1. He concluded that the increase in the AC/A ratio with orthoptics was probably genuine and could not be attributed to practice effects or to an increase in accommodative response or proximal convergence.

Prism Adaptation

Prism adaptation is the phenomenon in which a patient's phoria increases as a result of wearing prisms. The increase in the phoria is usually equal to the amount of prism prescribed. For example, an optometrist may prescribe 2Δ of base-in prism for constant wear by an exophoric patient. The patient returns in 1 year for a routine examination; the optometrist finds that the phoria has increased 2Δ and prescribes an additional 2Δ of base-in prism. A year later, the same thing happens, so at the end of 2 years the patient is wearing 6Δ of base-in prism. If the optometrist went back through the patient's original history, he or she would almost certainly find that the patient had had no symptoms to indicate that the prism was needed in the first place, and that in the two succeeding examinations he or she prescribed additional prism in the absence of any complaints on the part of the patient.

Fusion adaptation phenomenon

In graphical analysis theory we talk of *tonic convergence* as being one of the determiners of the distance phoria. Too much tonic convergence can cause esophoria and too little can cause exophoria. For a given distance phoria, the near phoria is determined by the amount of accommodative convergence in play for a given fixation distance. Too much accommodative convergence can cause esophoria, and too little can cause exophoria. However, there are many factors other than tonic convergence that help determine the distance phoria. These include the positions of the eyes in the orbits, the lengths of the extraocular muscles, the positions of the check ligaments, the position of the muscle insertions, and other factors. In view of all these factors, it is surprising that the range of distance phoria findings in the population is so small. Morgan (1944) found that for a large group of patients, the distance phoria fell between 1Δ of esophoria and 3Δ of exophoria for 76 percent of the patients. Carter (1963) concluded that some factor must be acting to maintain approximate orthophoria for distance fixation. He pointed out that Sato coined the term *orthophorization* to describe the phenomenon, which he believed to be an adaptive process causing a large percentage of persons to be orthophoric or near-orthophoric at distance.

Referring to this process as the *fusion adaptation phenomenon,* Carter (1963) suggested that there is also an adaptive process that tends to keep the *near* phoria somewhere near orthophoria at the downgaze position. He also suggested that this adaptive process probably operates on the basis of proximal convergence. More recently, Carter (1981) suggested that the usual situation for near work is 3Δ of exophoria through the phoroptor or orthophoria in the normal downgaze reading position. Carter further proposed that when a patient is found to have a high distance phoria, it is because of the absence of the fusion adaptation phenomenon (in addition to the presence of a combination of anatomical and physiological factors that would be expected to produce a phoria). This is the patient who is most likely to benefit from the prescription of prism and obviously is unlikely to adapt to the prism by building up additional amounts of phoria.

Carter (1965) studied prism adaptation by making both fixation disparity measurements and phoria measurements immediately after fitting subjects with varying amounts of prism, and at intervals from 15–30 minutes after fitting. He used 13 subjects in the experiment, and amounts of prism varying from 10Δ base-in to 32Δ base-out. Carter found that the subjects exhibited marked changes in fixation disparity after wearing prisms for only 5 minutes, and he concluded that these changes in fixation disparity indicated that the subjects had a change in the tonicity of the motor centers as a result of the prolonged demand on motor fusion. Carter proposed that the change in tonicity resulted in a reduction of the demand on fusional vergence, and, therefore, probably prevented the occurrence of discomfort from the effort of prolonged vergence.

Carter's (1965) research confirmed the clinical impression that prism adaptation will occur only for patients whose symptoms did not warrant the prescription of prism in the first place. For the patient whose symptoms indicate that the prism is necessary, the prism is likely to alleviate the symptoms, and adaptation to the prism is not likely to occur. As Carter suggested, for those practitioners who are concerned about prism adaptation there is little gamble involved in prescribing prism for a patient who may not need it. If future testing indicates adaptation, the prismatic component of the prescription can be left as it is or removed. The problem is not in prescribing the original prismatic correction but in subsequently increasing the amount of prism prescribed for a patient who did not really need it.

Phoria and AC/A Ratio Changes in Myopia

It is often found that an uncorrected (or undercorrected) myope exhibits a change in the near phoria in the direction of increased esophoria when lenses are prescribed for the correction of the full amount of myopia. There may also be a change in the distance phoria in the same direction; however, this is usually relatively small, so there is an increase in the clinically determined AC/A ratio. This has caused some writers to question the stability of the AC/A ratio.

Flom and Takahashi (1962) investigated this phenomenon by measuring distance and near phorias of 28 previously uncorrected or undercorrected myopes. Phoria findings were taken when the full correction for the myopia was first worn and after the correction had been worn for a week or longer. For 14 of the subjects who were esophoric at near on the initial phoria measurements, the average change after wearing the correction for a week or longer was 3.01Δ in the direction of decreased esophoria at near. There was also a change in the distance phoria, averaging 0.64Δ of decreased esophoria and resulting in an average decrease in the AC/A ratio of 0.96/1.

Flom and Takahashi (1962) reasoned that the abnormally high AC/A ratio of the previously incompletely corrected myope occurs as a result of the fact that before correction, the stimulus to accommodation at the reading distance is reduced by the amount of the undercorrection. This reduction in accommodative demand at the reading distance results in a relative exophoria; bifixation is possible only with the use of positive relative vergence (convergence not associated with accommodation), which becomes conditioned through use over a long period of time. When the myopia is fully corrected, the conditioned convergence remains in play. However, with continued wearing of the correction, this conditioned convergence will be extinguished, and the AC/A ratio (along with the near phoria) will return to its previous level.

This means that the practitioner need not be overly concerned about the newly corrected myope who is found to be esophoric at near. The esophoria is only temporary and can be expected to reduce by about 3Δ with the continued wearing of the lenses.

Prescribing Vertical Prism

The management of vertical phorias differs from that of lateral phorias in that the prescription of prism is the only available form of therapy. Visual training and the alteration of spherical lens power are of no value in the management of vertical phorias.

A patient found to have a vertical phoria should be questioned concerning any possible symptoms. One obvious indication that prism is needed is a complaint of occasional vertical diplopia. Other indications are an aversion to prolonged, concentrated visual tasks; extreme sensitivity to bright light (often accompanied by a tendency to partially close one eye); car sickness; and a habitual head tilt. Fannin (1962) observed that the patient may complain of a "pain in the neck" and may even trace the problem to an occurrence like stepping on a stone or twisting the neck.

When the prescription of prism is based on a von Graefe phoria measurement and vertical fusional reserves, the usual procedure is to prescribe the amount of prism that equalizes the vertical reserves, as indicated by the following relationship:

$$\text{Prism} = \frac{\text{base-down-to-break} - \text{base-up-to-break}}{2}.$$

Base-down prism is prescribed if the answer is positive and base-up prism is prescribed if the answer is negative. The recommended procedure is to take the vertical phoria and the vertical fusional reserves for each eye. If they are not equal (i.e., equal vertical phoria but in opposite directions, and base-up vertical fusional reserve for one eye equal to base-down fusional reserve for the other eye), a likely cause is inaccurate prism calibration.

The use of this formula is demonstrated by the following example. Consider a patient found to have 2Δ of right hyperphoria (measured by 2Δ base-down, right eye, or 2Δ base-up, left eye) and the following vertical fusional reserve findings (s = supravergence, and i = infravergence):

$$R \frac{s\ 4/3}{i\ 2/1} \qquad L \frac{s\ 2/1}{i\ 4/3}.$$

Using the formula, for each eye the correcting prism would be

$$R \frac{4-2}{2} = 1\Delta, \text{ base-down, or}$$

$$L \frac{2-4}{2} = 1\Delta, \text{ base-up.}$$

The amount of prism required to equalize the vertical fusional reserves can also be determined without the formula by inspecting the vertical fusional reserve findings. Inspection of the findings for the right eye immediately indicates that 1Δ, base-down, would equalize the findings. Inspection of the findings for the left eye indicates that the findings would be equalized by 1Δ, base-up. The practitioner could prescribe either 1Δ, base-down for the right eye or 1Δ, base-up, for the left eye; also, the prism could be split equally between the two eyes.

Associated phoria measurement (described in Chapter 10 and further discussed in this chapter) is an increasingly popular method of determining the amount of vertical prism to be prescribed.

PRESCRIBING ON THE BASIS OF FIXATION DISPARITY TESTS

Fixation disparity tests available for use in optometric practice include the Mallet fixation disparity tests (distance- and near-testing units), the American Optical Vectographic system (a vectographic projector slide for distance testing and a set of vectographic cards for near testing), the Borish near-point card, and the Sheedy and Saladin Disparometer. As described in Chapter 10, all of these tests, with the exception of the Disparometer, are for measuring the associated phoria (i.e., for determining the direction and amount of prism necessary to eliminate the patient's fixation disparity). Only the Disparometer is designed to measure the patient's fixation disparity. The Disparaometer also enables the practitioner to determine the changes in fixation disparity that occur with forced vergence and to plot a fixation disparity curve, which can be used as a basis for diagnosing and prescribing for the patient's binocular vision problem.

Recall that the discussion of the procedure for using the Mallett distance and near units in Chapter 10 describes not only prescribing lateral or vertical prism but also determining the need for orthoptic training and the amount of added plus that may be needed for a patient who is esophoric at near. These uses also apply to the American Optical vectographic system, the Borish near-point card, and the Disparometer. It is obvious that with any one of these tests making use of fixation disparity, it is possible to prescribe all of the treatment modalities for which graphical analysis is designed. Although some practitioners are willing to discard the graphical analysis system in favor of the tests involving fixation disparity, many practitioners (and probably all schools of optometry) are incorporating the fixation disparity procedures while retaining the graphical analysis method.

One practitioner in favor of discarding the graphical analysis system is Mallett (1964 and 1966), the British ophthalmic optician who developed the first clinically useful test involving fixation disparity.

Mallett argued that the amount of heterophoria measured in a dissociated phoria test provides no indication of the patient's ability to cope with the phoria; that the measurement of fusional vergence reserves is an unreliable procedure; that the use of graphical systems of analysis is time-consuming; and that the need to correlate so many variables (few of which can be measured with the accuracy and consistency demanded for such an analysis) makes their usefulness doubtful.

Mallett (1964) contended that the important matter is not how much phoria the patient has, but whether the phoria is compensated; he said that the presence of a fixation disparity is an indication that the phoria is uncompensated. He further contended that when a dissociated phoria is measured, the visual apparatus is presented with an unnatural set of circumstances. Fixation disparity must be detected under the conditions the patient will have to contend with when reading or pursuing a similar task requiring fine adjustment of accommodation and convergence. In addition, Mallett said that the amount of fixation disparity is small—limited to the size of Panum's fusional area at the fovea (about 5 minutes of arc)—and that the amount of disparity is much the same whether it is caused by a phoria of 1 or 20Δ.

Comparison of Associated Phoria Test Results

In comparing the relationship of the dissociated phoria with the associated phoria using the Mallett and American Optical tests, the author has found that the Mallett system (both distance and near units) results in associated phoria findings that are usually much smaller than the dissociated phoria findings for the same patient, whereas the American Optical system (particularly the target not having the central dot and ring) results in associated phoria findings that are in some cases almost as large as the dissociated phoria findings. As stated in Chapter 10, the practitioner using the Mallett system prescribes the amount of prism necessary to eliminate the fixation disparity. If this is done with the American Optical system, much larger amounts of prism would be prescribed than with the Mallett system.

The difference in associated phoria findings can be accounted for on the basis of the much stronger peripheral fusion lock and a weaker central fusion lock that the Mallett units provide. The Mallett distance unit is designed to be used in a fully lighted room, and objects in the room provide stimuli for peripheral fusion. In addition, the frame of the chart itself provides further clues for peripheral fusion. The Mallett near unit is also used in a fully lighted room and is provided with a background of reading material, which acts as a strong stimulus to peripheral fusion. As contrasted to the Mallett units, the American Optical Vectographic system (both the distance slide and the near-point cards) provides weak peripheral fusion clues. In some cases, the patient may completely dissociate, the result being a dissociated phoria finding rather than an associated phoria finding.

The Borish near-point card differs from the American Optical near-point cards in a number of ways. The American Optical card, designed to measure the associated phoria, has only a cross in the center of an otherwise unstructured card (the upper and right limbs seen by the right eye and the lower and left limbs seen by the left eye). The Borish card (side 2) presents the patient with an almost confusing array of detail, including three reduced Snellen charts (one seen by both eyes, and one each seen by the right and left eyes) and a heavily bordered diamond at the bottom of the chart containing letters for use in measuring phorias. The associated phoria test, in the center of the chart, is similar to the American Optical associated phoria test, but with the addition of four small circles forming a structured background for the cross. This amount of detail provides a much stronger peripheral fusion stimulus than is provided by the American Optical card.

Evaluation of the Mallett Technique

The Mallett technique was evaluated by Payne, Grisham, and Thomas (1974), who used the Mallett test to prescribe prism for ten clinic patients, all of whom showed fixation disparity at near and reported symptoms. Two pairs of glasses were prescribed for each patient, one containing the prism required to eliminate fixation disparity and the other containing no prism. Using a double-blind technique so neither the clinician nor the patient knew which pair of glasses contained the prism, each patient was asked to wear one pair of glasses for the first week and the other pair for the second week, and each was then asked to report which pair of glasses was preferred.

Nine of the patients had exo fixation disparity, and one had eso fixation disparity. All ten of the patients reported that they definitely preferred the pair of glasses containing the prism. Payne et al. (1974) reported that dissociated phoria and fusional vergence findings showed little correlation with the prism actually prescribed. There was also little similarity to the prism that would have been prescribed on the basis of Sheard's criterion.

Prescribing on the Basis of Disparometer Findings

As described in Chapter 10, the Disparometer is an instrument designed to fit on the near-point rod of a standard refractor (see Figure 10.16, Chapter 10), and it can be used not only for measuring fixation disparity but also for determining the changes in fixation disparity as a result of forced vergence. On the basis of this information, a *fixation disparity curve* can be plotted.

The majority of patients will be found to have a Type I fixation disparity curve (see Figure 4.28, Chapter 4). While most of these patients will be asymptomatic, Sheedy (1980a, 1980b) reported that patients having a Type I curve with a steep slope (roughly, 45 degrees or greater) have oculomotor imbalance and respond well to orthoptic training. The effect of the training is to reduce the slope of the curve.

Sheedy (1980a, 1980b) usually found patients having Type II fixation disparity curves to have esophoria. He recommends prisms or plus lenses for these patients rather than orthoptic training. The prism power or plus lens power should be such that the patient will be able to "operate" on a flat portion of the fixation disparity curve. To find this amount of prism, the practitioner reads the prism value from the x-axis of the graph corresponding to the flat portion of the curve and prescribes that amount of prism. This is usually less than the amount of prism required to eliminate fixation disparity (as determined in an associated phoria measurement).

Sheedy (1980a, 1980b) does not say how he determines the amount of plus lens power to be prescribed in the case of an esophoric patient having a Type II curve. An appropriate way to do this would be to repeat the fixation disparity curves with plus lens additions (based, for example, on the patient's AC/A ratio), selecting the amount of plus power that places the flattest portion of the curve nearest the point of demand (i.e., the y-axis).

Sheedy (1980a, 1980b) reports that patients having Type III curves can be trained, but not as easily as those having Type I curves. The results of training patients having Type IV curves (representing only about 5 percent of the population) have not been reported.

BINOCULAR VISION ANOMALIES IN PRESBYOPIA

Presbyopes seldom complain of asthenopia. Although a presbyopic person may still have the same distance phoria, fixation disparity, or fusional vergence anomaly that the patient had before becoming presbyopic (with or without symptoms), it has been widely recognized that the occurrence of presbyopia is seldom a source of asthenopia. It is even possible that preexisting near-point problems (particularly in the exophoric direction) cease to be problems once presbyopia is established.

Presbyopes tend to be highly exophoric at near while wearing their bifocals or reading glasses. This exophoria has been explained on the basis that the presbyope makes no effort to accommodate while wearing near correction and, therefore, brings no accommodative convergence into play. The fact that the presbyope maintains single binocular vision at near, apparently without the use of accommodative convergence, has been variously accounted for on the basis of the use of proximal convergence or the use of positive fusional vergence. However, until recently there has been no convincing explanation of the almost complete lack of asthenopia in spite of the high exophoria.

Sheedy and Saladin (1975) compared near phorias, fusional vergences, and fixation disparity curves on 13 nonpresbyopes and 10 presbyopes. As expected, they found that the presbyopes were more exophoric than the nonpresbyopes (having average near phorias of 8.7Δ as compared with 2.8Δ of exophoria) and had much smaller fusional vergence ranges than the nonpresbyopes. However, the presbyopes were found to have no greater fixation disparity at near than the nonpresbyopes; in addition, their fixation disparity curves were found to have lower slopes than those of the nonpresbyopes. As Sheedy and Saladin commented, the lower slope of the fixation disparity curve is associated with efficient and comfortable vision. In questioning the subjects, they found that none of the presbyopes complained of eyestrain associated with close work and that the presbyopes worked at a closer distance and for longer periods of time than the nonpresbyopes.

On the basis of these results, Sheedy and Saladin (1975) concluded that fixation disparity curves provide a truer picture of the presbyope's binocular vision system at near than do phoria and fusional vergence findings, in addition to correlating better with the lack of symptoms than do phoria and fusional vergence findings. They further concluded (quoting Drs. Glenn A. Fry and Ronald Jones) that the presbyope maintains single binocular vision by the use of accommodative convergence and, in fact, has *nearly unrestricted use of accommodative convergence.* Presbyopes are in an ideal situation, because they can use accommodative convergence without getting the normal dosage of accommodation as dictated by the AC/A ratio. Even though presbyopes are unable to accommodate due to the hardening of the lens and the aging of the ciliary muscle, the innervation for accommodation remains. This enables presbyopes to use as much accommodative convergence as necessary to maintain bifixation without the reflex occurrence of accommodation.

Study Questions

1. What are two possible causes of a patient's complaint of poor night vision?

2. How is each of the following tests used in determining the (tentative or final) bifocal addition? (a) the push-up amplitude of accommodation; (b) the binocular crossed-cylinder test; (c) the plus- and minus-to-blur tests; (d) range of accommodation.

3. (a) What are the five fundamental variables in the relationship between accommodation and convergence? (b) What is the counterpart of each of these variables on the graphical analysis form?

4. A patient is found to have 10Δ of exophoria at 40cm, base-in findings of 18/28/12, and base-out findings of 10/16/8. (a) How much prism (and in what direction) would have to be prescribed to satisfy Sheard's criterion? (b) How much prism (and in what direction) would have to be prescribed to satisfy Percival's criterion?

5. What effect does depth of focus have on the shape of the graph?

6. What is the calculated AC/A ratio for each of the following? (a) orthophoria at 6m and orthophoria at 40cm; (b) 2 exophoria at 6m and 8 exophoria at 40cm; (c) 2 esophoria at 6m and 8 esophoria at 40cm.

7. In convergence insufficiency, (a) what symptoms would you expect the patient to report? (b) what binocular vision findings would indicate the presence of this condition? (c) what form(s) of treatment would you consider?

8. Can either the stimulus AC/A ratio or the response AC/A ratio be changed as a result of visual training? Briefly discuss.

9. What is the best way to convince a newly presbyopic patient that lenses required to correct near vision will blur distance vision?

10. What effect does proximal convergence have on the shape of the graph?

11. (a) What is the fusion adaptation phenomenon?

(b) What does the fusion adaptation phenomenon have to do with adaptation to prism?

12. A patient is found to have 5Δ of esophoria at 6m, base-in findings of 5/16/10, and base-out findings of 13/24/10. (a) How much prism would have to be prescribed (and in what direction) to satisfy Sheard's criterion? (b) How much prism would have to be prescribed (and in what direction) to satisfy Percival's criterion?

13. In convergence excess, (a) what symptoms would you expect the patient to report? (b) what binocular vision findings would indicate the presence of this condition? (c) what form(s) of treatment would you consider?

14. (a) On the basis of the explanation of Flom and Takahashi, how can the esophoria at near, found when a previously uncorrected or undercorrected myope is corrected, be accounted for? (b) Is this esophoria a matter of concern? Why or why not?

15. According to Mallett, what tells the practitioner if a patient is able to cope with phoria?

16. Why does a presbyope seldom complain of asthenopia accompanying near work in spite of the presence of a high exophoria at near?

17. In divergence insufficiency, (a) what symptoms would you expect the patient to report? (b) what binocular vision findings would indicate the presence of this condition? (c) what form(s) of treatment would you consider?

18. When prism is prescribed for a phoria, how can the practitioner predict whether prism adaptation will take place?

19. What form of treatment is recommended if a patient's fixation disparity curve, as determined by the Disparometer, (a) is a Type I curve, and the patient has symptoms? (b) is a Type II curve?

20. In divergence excess, (a) what symptoms would you expect the patient to report? (b) what binocular vision findings would indicate the presence of this condition? (c) what form(s) of treatment would you consider?

CHAPTER 13

Prescribing Ophthalmic Lenses

In the past, optometrists took pride in being able to provide complete vision care for their patients—not only examining and prescribing for them but also personally supervising frame selection, ordering and verifying the materials, dispensing the finished eyewear, and performing any subsequent adjustments and repairs. The great majority of optometrists now turn over the responsibility for ophthalmic dispensing to trained assistants or technicians, and some have even given up ophthalmic dispensing altogether.

All optometry schools provide courses in ophthalmic optics and dispensing, and the purpose of this chapter is not to fully cover these subjects. The topics addressed are those of importance to the practitioner when ophthalmic lenses are to be prescribed, whether the actual dispensing is to be done by the practitioner, a trained assistant or technician, or an outside dispenser.

SPECIFICATION OF POWER

The power of an ophthalmic lens can be specified in terms of approximate power, back vertex power, or front vertex power. The *approximate power* of a lens is determined simply by adding the refracting powers of the front and back surfaces of the lens, neglecting the effect of lens thickness on the power. For example, a lens having a front surface power (F_1) of +6.00D and a back surface power (F_2) of −5.00D obviously has an approximate power of +1.00D. When a lens measure (often called a *lens clock*) is used to determine the power of a lens (see Figure 13.1), the power is specified in terms of approximate power. For lenses of low power, the use of approximate power involves a negligible error; for higher powered lenses, however (particularly plus lenses), the error is too large to be neglected.

It should be understood that lens measures are calibrated for the index of refraction of ophthalmic crown glass, and therefore they can be used with plastic lenses or lenses made of high-index glass only if a conversion factor is used.

The *back vertex power* is the power of an ophthalmic lens specified as if the refraction occurred at the back surface of the lens, with light incident on the front surface. When the power of a lens is measured by means of a lensometer or vertometer (see Figure 13.2), back vertex power is measured. The formula for back vertex power is

Figure 13.1   The lens measure.

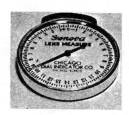

Figure 13.2   American Optical Lensometer.

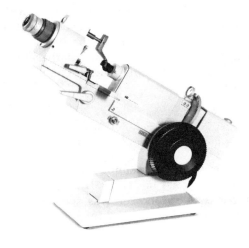

$$F_v' = \frac{F_1}{1 - \dfrac{t}{n}F_1} + F_2.$$

In this formula, t indicates the center thickness of the lens (expressed in meters), and n indicates the index of refraction. The formula shows that back vertex power depends not only on the surface powers and thickness of the lens but also on the *form* of the lens, the front surface power making a large contribution to the back vertex power. The use of the formula is illustrated by the following examples.

Example 1. Given $F_1 = +6.00D$, $F_2 = -1.00D$, $t = 0.005m$, and $n = 1.523$, the approximate power of this lens would be $+5.00D$. The back vertex power is

$$F_v' = \frac{6}{1 - \dfrac{0.005}{1.523}(6)} - 1 = +5.120D.$$

Example 2. Given $F_1 = +1.00D$, $F_2 = -6.00D$, $t = 0.002m$, and $n = 1.523$, the approximate power would be $-5.00D$. The back vertex power is

$$F_v' = \frac{1}{1 - \dfrac{0.002}{1.523}(1)} - 6 = -4.999D.$$

These examples show that the convex lens, because of its stronger front surface power and greater center thickness, has a back vertex power about 0.12D stronger than its approximate power. The concave lens, having a relatively weak front surface and being much thinner than the convex lens, has a back vertex power that is essentially the same as the approximate power.

The *front vertex power* is the power of an ophthalmic lens specified as if the refraction occurred at the front surface of the lens, with the light incident upon the front surface. When hand neutralization is used to determine the power of a lens, front vertex power is measured; therefore, it is also known as *neutralizing power*. The formula for front vertex power is

$$F_v = F_1 + \frac{F_2}{1 - \dfrac{t}{n}F_2}.$$

For the lenses used in examples 1 and 2, the front vertex power would be $+5.003D$ and $-4.95D$. For the first lens, if the power was specified in back vertex power and measured by the use of front

vertex power (e.g., by putting the lens in the lensometer backwards), an error of 0.12D would result. For an aphakic lens having a front surface power of $+12.00D$, a back surface power of zero, and a thickness of 0.009m, the error would be 0.85D (back vertex power being $+12.85D$ and front vertex power being $+12.00D$).

Effective Power

The effective power of a correcting lens varies with the distance of the lens from the cornea and is given by the formula

$$F_e = \frac{F}{1 - dF},$$

where

$d =$ the distance, in meters, through which the lens is moved (see Figure 13.3).

This is positive if the lens is moved to the right and negative if it is moved to the left (with light traveling from left to right).

Example 1. Assume that a patient is refracted at a vertex distance of 15mm and is found to require a $-6.00D$ lens, but that the correcting lenses will be fitted in a frame that will result in a vertex distance of 10mm. What will be the required lens power at the new vertex distance?

$$F_e = \frac{-6}{1 - (0.005)(-6)} = -5.83D.$$

This formula indicates that at the 10mm distance, only a $-5.83D$ lens is required; if the $-6.00D$ lens is mistakenly prescribed, the lens will be 0.17D too strong. Fortunately for the myope, most frames

Figure 13.3   A change (d) in vertex distance changes the effective power of a lens.

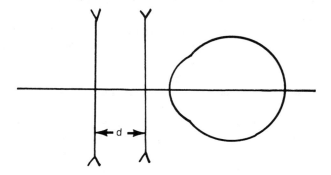

result in a vertex distance smaller (if anything) than the vertex distance at which the refraction is done. Therefore, if the change in vertex distance is ignored (as in example 1), the lenses will be too strong rather than too weak. Long (1976) has shown that changes in effective power are proportional to the distance the lens is moved and proportional to the square of the lens power. The result of doubling the lens power is shown in example 2.

Example 2. If refraction at 15mm requires a −12.00D lens, what power lens would be required at 10mm?

$$F_e = \frac{-12}{1 - (0.005)(-12)} = -11.32D.$$

The change in effective power (0.68D) is just four times that of the change in effective power (0.17D) for the −6.00D lens.

Example 3. An aphakic patient, refracted at 15mm, is found to require a +12.00D lens. What power lens will be required at a vertex distance of 10mm?

$$F_e = \frac{+12}{1 - (0.005)(+12)} = +12.77D.$$

Therefore, the patient will be undercorrected by more than 0.75D if the change in vertex distance is ignored.

Effective power at near

Because ophthalmic lenses are worn several millimeters in front of the eyes, it is necessary for the spectacle-wearing hyperope to make use of more accommodation than is required by the emmetrope or the myope for a given reading distance. Long (1976b) has shown that for a 33cm reading distance, an 8.00D hyperope must accommodate about 0.75D more than an emmetrope, and that an emmetrope must accommodate about 0.75D more than an 8.00D myope. This means that a high hyperope should require reading lenses or a bifocal addition at an earlier age than a high myope. However, Long has found that, because myopes are usually in the habit of reading at a relatively close distance, they often require reading lenses or bifocals at an age equal to or even earlier than a hyperope of the same degree.

Effective power differences reach their greatest extreme when a patient switches from glasses to contact lenses (or vice versa). This applies for both distance and near vision. (This topic is discussed in Chapter 14.)

PRISM IN OPHTHALMIC LENSES

Prism can be obtained in an ophthalmic lens either by *grinding* or by *decentration*. For relatively large amounts of prism, grinding is usually necessary, but small amounts of prism power (or even moderate amounts in lenses of high refracting power) can be obtained by decentration. When the patient's prescription calls for spherical lenses, the problem of decentration to obtain prism power is a simple one, but for spherocylindrical lenses the problem can be more complex.

Spherical Lenses

A common problem occurs when a myope requires base-in prism at distance or near (or both) because of exophoria or exo fixation disparity. If prism is needed at near only, a small amount of base-in prism can be provided at near simply by centering the lenses for the patient's distance PD. The amount of prism that can be provided by this method can be easily determined by the use of Prentice's rule:

$$P = dF,$$

where

P = prism power

d = decentration (in centimeters)

F = refracting power of the lens.

For a 6.00D myope having a distance PD of 64mm and a near PD of 60mm, the resulting prism (for each eye) at near, when the lenses are centered for distance, will be

$$P = 0.2(-6) = -1.2\Delta.$$

The minus sign indicates that the base of the prism is in the direction opposite to that of the decentration, which in this case is outward in relation to the near PD. The total prismatic effect at near, therefore, is 2.4Δ base-in (see Figure 13.4).

If a myope requires base-in prism at distance as well as at near, base-in prism at distance can be provided by decentering the lenses outward relative to the patient's distance PD. For example, if a 5.00D myope requires 2Δ base-in for each eye, the required amount of decentration for each lens will be

$$d = \frac{P}{F} = \frac{2}{-5} = -0.4cm = -4mm.$$

Again, the minus sign indicates that the base of the

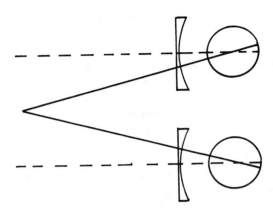

Figure 13.4 For a myope, if lenses are centered for the distance PD, base-in prism power is induced for near viewing.

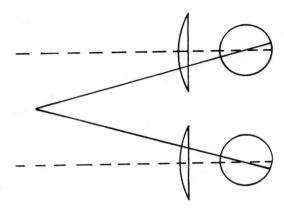

Figure 13.5 For a hyperope, if lenses are centered for the distance PD, base-out prism is induced for near viewing.

prism is in the direction opposite to that of the decentration. Therefore, a total prismatic effect of 4Δ base-in (2Δ for each eye) will be obtained by decentering each lens outward 4mm. Remember that an additional amount of base-in prism will be present for near vision. If the near PD is 4mm less than the distance PD, the additional base-in prism at near will be

$$P = 0.2(-5) = -1.00\Delta,$$

resulting in a total added prism (for both eyes) of 2Δ base-in.

Fortunately for the exophoric myope, today's large lens sizes allow for large amounts of outward decentration. A patient having a 64mm distance PD who will be fitted with a frame having a lens width of 52mm and a distance between lenses of 18mm (therefore having a "frame PD" of 70mm) will require 3mm of decentration inward to have the lenses properly centered for distance. Failure to decenter the lenses inward will result in unwanted base-in prism for the myope and, as will be discussed, base-out prism for the hyperope. Depending on the patient's PD and the size of the lens blank, as much as 5 or 6mm of outward decentration (relative to the patient's PD) can often be achieved for each lens. However, large lens sizes are of no help in allowing inward decentration unless a patient has an unusually large PD, so only small amounts of inward decentration are usually possible. Therefore, the myope who requires base-out prism or the hyperope who requires base-in prism (both of whom require inward decentration) can be provided with relatively little prism by decentration; if prism is required, it may have to be ground into the lens.

As an example of a hyperope who requires base-

out prism because of esophoria or eso fixation disparity at distance, consider a 6.00D hyperope requiring a total of 3Δ of base-out prism, or 1.5Δ for each eye. The amount of decentration required for each lens will be

$$d = \frac{P}{F} = \frac{1.5}{6} = +0.25\text{cm} = +2.5\text{mm}.$$

The plus sign indicates that the direction of decentration is the same as that of the base of the prism (see Figure 13.5). Again, remember that an additional amount of prism will be present for near vision. If the near PD is 4mm less than the distance PD, the additional amount of base-out prism at near for each lens will be

$$P = 0.2(6) = +1.2\Delta,$$

resulting in a total added prism for both eyes of 2.4Δ base-out.

Spherocylindrical Lenses

For spherocylindrical lenses in which the two principal meridians are at 180 and 90 degrees, calculation of the decentration necessary to provide a given amount of prism is complicated only slightly. Using as an example the myope who requires base-in prism at distance because of exophoria or exo fixation disparity, consider a myope requiring the lens power −5.00 −1.00 × 180 for each eye and requiring 2Δ of base-in prism for each eye. Because the −1.00D cylinder has its refracting power entirely in the vertical meridian, it will have no effect in the horizontal meridian, and the amount of decentration required for each lens will be

$$d = \frac{P}{F} = \frac{2}{-5} = -0.40\text{cm} = -4\text{mm}.$$

However, if the myope's distance prescription is $-5.00 -1.00 \times 90$, the -1.00D cylinder will have its full refractive power in the horizontal meridian. The amount of decentration required for each lens to provide 2Δ of base-in prism will be

$$d = \frac{P}{F} = \frac{2}{-6} = -0.33\text{cm} = -3.3\text{mm}.$$

Spherocylindrical Lenses with Oblique Axes

For spherocylindrical lenses whose principal meridians are oblique, it is tempting to use the familiar sine-square formula to determine the power of the cylinder in the horizontal meridian, and then to substitute this power in Prentice's rule. However, Long (1975b) pointed out that this is an incorrect procedure which will yield the wrong answers: Prentice's rule applies only to circular cross sections and, therefore, can be used only with principal meridians.

For a spherocylindrical lens having oblique meridians, the formulas given by Long (1975a) or the graphical solution given by Jalie (1974, pp. 95–103) can be used to determine the amount of decentration required to provide a given amount of base-in or base-out prism power. However, such decentration will also result in a certain amount of unwanted vertical prism power. For this reason, the preferred method of providing horizontal prism when an oblique cylinder is involved is to have the prism ground into the lens.

Vertical Prism

When a small amount of vertical prism is required to compensate for a vertical phoria or a vertical fixation disparity, it can often be obtained by decentering the lens upward or downward, using Prentice's rule. For example, if a 5.00D myope requires 1Δ of base-down prism for the right eye, the required amount of decentration will be

$$d = \frac{P}{F} = \frac{1}{-5} = -0.20\text{cm} = -2\text{mm}.$$

The minus sign indicates that the lens will have to be decentered upward relative to the other eye to induce base-down prism.

For spherocylindrical lenses having their principal meridians at 180 and 90 degrees, the amount of vertical decentration required to bring about a specific amount of vertical prism power can again be easily calculated. However, if the principal meridians are oblique, providing prism by decentration would result in an unwanted horizontal prism component, so the recommended method is to have the prism ground into the lens.

Vertical Prismatic Effect at the Reading Level

One of the problems experienced by the anisometropic patient is the induced vertical prismatic effect that occurs when the individual looks through the lower portions of the lenses during reading or other close work. Consider a patient whose distance correction is right eye: -4.00DS, and left eye: -6.00DS, and whose reading level is 10mm below the distance center, or major reference point, of each lens. The amount of vertical prismatic effect for each eye is

$$\text{Right eye: } P = dF = 1(-4) = -4\Delta;$$
$$\text{Left eye: } P = dF = 1(-6) = -6\Delta.$$

The minus sign indicates that the base of the induced prism is in the direction opposite to that of the decentration, and because the major reference point is located upward in relation to the reading level of each lens, the induced prism is in the base-down direction (see Figure 13.6). The left eye, therefore, is subject to 2Δ more base-down prism than is the right eye.

The ability of the eyes to make vertical fusional movements is not great, most patients dissociating with as little as $2–3\Delta$ of vertical prism (e.g., during the vertical fusional vergence reserve tests). Therefore, a patient having as little as 1 or 2Δ of induced vertical prism at the reading level would be expected to have discomfort or even diplopia accompanying reading or other near visual tasks.

Figure 13.6 When looking through the lower portion of a lens for reading, a minus lens induces base-down prism. In this example, the left lens, having more minus power, induces more base-down prism.

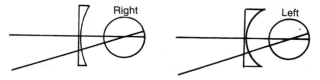

This problem may not be as evident for wearers of single vision lenses as for wearers of bifocal lenses. A single vision lens wearer habitually turns the head downward when reading, probably looking through the lenses at a level not greatly different than the level used for distance vision, whereas the bifocal wearer is forced to read through the lower portions of the lenses. One way to manage the problem for the single vision lens wearer is to have the major reference points (i.e., distance optical centers) of the lenses located somewhat lower than usual, at what can be considered as the "most-used portion of the lens." The correct level can be determined by having the patient wear the habitual correction and using a grease pencil or felt pen to mark the portion of each lens used for distance vision and for reading. This procedure, however, induces some vertical prism at both distance and near.

Another way of handling the problem for a single vision lens wearer is to prescribe two pairs of glasses: a pair for general use, having the major reference points in their usual locations, and a second pair for close work, having the major reference points located at the level used by the patient when reading. This method can also be used for a presbyope who is willing to wear separate pairs of single vision lenses for distance and near rather than wear bifocals.

An additional method of compensating for differential vertical prismatic effects at near for a single vision lens wearer involves the use of a *slab-off lens*. As described later in the chapter in the section on bifocal lenses, a slab-off lens is one in which vertical prism has been induced in the lower portion of the lens by means of *bicentric grinding*. Because bicentric grinding induces base-up prism, the more minus or less plus lens is the one that is slabbed off. Further, because bicentric grinding results in a noticeable dividing line in one lens but not in the other, it should be used (in single vision lenses) only when other methods (placing major reference points lower in the lenses or prescribing separate pairs of glasses) prove to be unsatisfactory.

ABERRATIONS AND LENS DESIGN

Any lens or optical system is subject to the following aberrations: chromatic aberration, spherical aberration, coma, oblique astigmatism, curvature of image, and distortion. Chromatic aberration is present whenever light of more than one wavelength is involved, and it is a property of the material of which the lens is made. The remaining aberrations are often referred to as the *monochromatic aberrations* and are due not to the lens material but to the form of the lens.

Chromatic Aberration

For any optical medium, the index of refraction varies with the wavelength of the incident light. *Axial chromatic aberration* of an ophthalmic lens is so small that it is of little consequence. *Transverse chromatic aberration* is of greater significance, as it can cause the wearer of a relatively high-powered ophthalmic lens to see color fringes when looking through the edge of the lens. However, there is no lens material available that can eliminate transverse chromatic aberration. Cameras and other instruments use compound lenses for this purpose, but such lenses are impractical as ophthalmic lenses.

Spherical Aberration

Spherical aberration is a problem only for large-aperture optical systems and constitutes little problem for ophthalmic lenses, as the pupil of the eye allows entrance of only a relatively small bundle of rays. Bechtold (1958) has shown that for a $-20.00D$ plano concave lens, the spherical aberration (i.e., the difference in focus between the marginal and the peripheral rays) for a 5mm pupil amounts to only 0.21D.

Coma

Coma, like spherical aberration, requires a large aperture, so it is of little importance in ophthalmic lenses. Rays from an off-axial point are focused by different zones of the lens in such a way that the resulting image is shaped like a comet. For a single lens, this aberration is at a minimum when spherical aberration is at a minimum. When coma is present, placing a small aperture behind the lens will eliminate the coma; however, oblique astigmatism (astigmatism due to obliquity of incidence) may be present.

Oblique Astigmatism

The aberrations of most concern in the design of ophthalmic lenses are *oblique astigmatism* and *curvature of image*, also referred to as *curvature of field*.

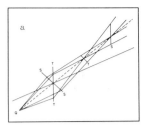 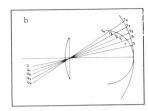

Figure 13.7 *(a)* Oblique astigmatism; *(b)* image shell diagram (Grosvenor, 1976b).

When a bundle of rays of light from an off-axial object point is incident on an ophthalmic lens, oblique astigmatism (see Figure 13.7a) can result. Referring to Figure 13.7b, rays of light traveling in the plane of the paper (the tangential plane) form tangential line foci at points T, T_1, and so forth, whereas rays of light traveling in the plane perpendicular to that of the paper (the sagittal plane) form sagittal line foci at points S, S_1, and so forth. If the off-axis point Q is successively moved to points Q_1, Q_2, and so forth, the tangential and sagittal foci will move to points T_1, T_2, and so forth, and S_1, S_2, and so forth. The surface traced by T and S, as Q is moved outward from the axis of the lens, is known as the *image shell diagram* and is also referred to as the *teacup and saucer diagram* (see Figure 13.7b). The tangential focal lines run in a circumferential direction, forming the rim of the teacup; the sagittal focal lines run in a radial direction, forming the saucer.

The lens form necessary for a minimum of astigmatism was determined by Jalie (1974) for a thin lens of power +5.00D having an index of refraction of

Figure 13.8 Power errors as a function of back surface power for tangential and sagittal foci, for a +5.00D lens (data from Jalie, 1976b).

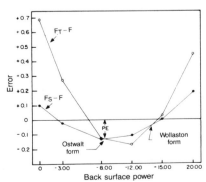

1.5, for a distant object, assuming that a stop (the center of rotation of the eye) is located 25mm behind the lens. In the resulting graph (see Figure 13.8), which shows power error as a function of back surface power for the tangential ($F_T - F$) and sagittal ($F_S - F$) foci, the two curves cross at approximately −8.00D and at approximately −15.00D. This indicates that a lens with either of these back surface powers (the *Ostwalt* and the *Wollaston forms*) would have no astigmatism for a point 22 degrees off the axis. A lens that has been corrected for astigmatism is known as an *anastigmatic lens*, or *point-focal lens*. Because the Wollaston form of point-focal lens is always much more steeply curved than the Ostwalt form, the Wollaston form is not used in the design of ophthalmic lenses. Where the S and T curves cross, it will be noted that the resulting power is weaker (by about 0.12D for the Ostwalt form) than the axial power. Bechtold (1958) pointed out that in the point-focal form, the oblique power of a lens is always weaker than the axial power. As a result, when viewing obliquely through the lens, a hyperope can obtain clear vision by accommodating; however, for a myope, accommodation only makes vision more blurred.

Curvature of Image

For paraxial rays, a flat object surface is assumed to result in a flat image surface. However, for an object of large extent (neglecting the other aberrations) we should expect the image surface to be *curved*, in that every pair of object points and image points should be equidistant. The fact that the expected image surface is curved was first pointed out by Petzval, and the image surface is therefore known as *Petzval's surface*. For a single lens in air, the radius of curvature, r_p, of Petzval's surface is given by the relationship

$$r_p = -nf,$$

where

  n = index of refraction of the glass

  f = back focal length of the lens.

When oblique astigmatism exists, the distance from the sagittal focus to Petzval's surface is equal to one-half the distance from the sagittal focus to the tangential focus (see Figure 13.9). When oblique astigmatism has been fully corrected, the tangential and sagittal image shells coincide with the Petzval surface. The Petzval surface is a property of the *refracting power* of the lens, each lens power having

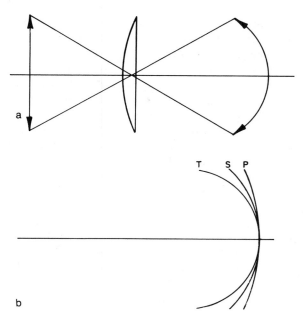

Figure 13.9 *(a)* **Curvature of image;** *(b)* **relationship between tangential** *(T)* **and sagittal** *(S)* **image shells and Petzval's surface** *(P)* (Grosvenor, 1976c).

its own secondary focal length and its own Petzval surface. Bending the lens (changing the base curve) does not alter the curvature of the Petzval surface.

Distortion

If a stop such as the pupil of the eye is placed at some distance behind a lens, the only rays from an off-axis object point that can be included in the image are those entering the periphery of the lens. As shown in Figure 13.10, those rays coming from point Q that would otherwise enter the central portion of the lens are blocked by the stop, so the image point Q' is formed entirely by rays coming through the periphery of the lens. Because rays entering the periphery of the lens are subject to prismatic effects that increase as the distance from the pole of the lens increases, magnification either increases (for a convex lens) or decreases (for a concave lens) toward the periphery of a lens. Therefore, a convex lens causes the peripheral portions of a square object to extend outward, resulting in *pincushion distortion*. A concave lens causes the peripheral portions of a square object to extend inward, resulting in *barrel-shaped distortion*.

Distortion is a problem only for ophthalmic lenses of very high power, such as aphakic lenses. It can be

minimized but not eliminated by lens bending. Unfortunately, the base curves required to minimize distortion are much steeper than those required to minimize oblique astigmatism. Because patients adapt rapidly to small amounts of distortion, this aberration can be safely neglected in the design of most ophthalmic lenses.

Lens Design

Recall that the far-point of a hyperopic eye is located behind the eye and is conjugate with the retina. Rays of light converging toward the far-point, after refraction by the optical system of the eye, will come to a focus on the retina. As the eye rotates to fixate a peripheral object, the far-point also rotates (as shown in Figure 13.11), tracing out the *far-point sphere*. Because the far-point sphere has its center of curvature at the center of rotation of the eye, its radius of curvature is given by the relationship

$$r_{FPS} = s - f,$$

where

s = the distance from the lens to the center of rotation of the eye

f = the secondary focal length of the lens.

It is important to note that the far-point sphere is a property of the eye—not of the lens—and that no amount of lens bending can alter the far-point sphere's curvature. It is also important to recall that

Figure 13.10 Distortion. *Upper diagram: the only rays making up the image point Q' for the object point Q are those entering the periphery of the lens. Lower diagram: (a) no distortion; (b) pincushion distortion caused by a strong convex lens; (c) barrel-shaped distortion caused by a strong concave lens* (Grosvenor, 1976c).

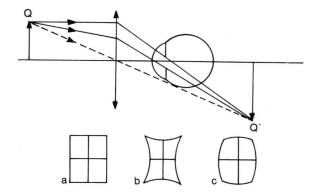

the Petzval surface is a property of the lens and not of the eye, and that because it depends on the secondary focal length of the lens, its curvature cannot be changed by bending of the lens. However, the curvature of the tangential and sagittal image shells *can* be altered by bending the lens.

The function of an ophthalmic lens is to provide, for any angle of rotation of the eye, a sharply focused image on the far-point sphere. This image then acts as an object that is sharply focused on the retina by the eye's optical system. For this to occur, the ophthalmic lens should provide a Petzval surface that will coincide with the far-point sphere. Because the radius of Petzval's surface is equal to $-nf$, and the radius of the far-point sphere is equal to $s - f$, it follows that the two surfaces will coincide only when

$$- nf = s - f,$$

or when

$$f = \frac{s}{1 - n}.$$

If we substitute values of 25mm for s and 1.5 for n,

$$f = \frac{-0.25}{0.5}, \quad \text{and} \quad F = -20.00D.$$

Therefore, it is possible to have the far-point sphere coincide with the Petzval surface *only* when a patient requires a $-20.00D$ lens. For all minus lenses weaker than $-20.00D$ and for all plus lenses, the curvature of the far-point sphere is greater than that of the Petzval surface.

Figure 13.11 Far-point sphere: *(a)* hyperopic eye; *(b)* myopic eye (Grosvenor, 1976d).

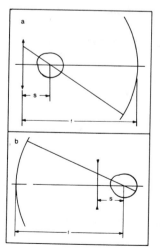

Because it is ordinarily impossible to make the Petzval surface correspond to the far-point sphere, the lens designer can do any of the following:

1. Design the lens in such a way that the tangential and sagittal image surfaces coincide with the Petzval surface—the *point-focal*, or *no-astigmatism*, lens.

2. Design the lens in such a way that oblique astigmatism remains uncorrected but the midpoint of the astigmatic interval falls on the far-point sphere—the *no-curvature error*, or *no-power error, lens.*

3. Choose to compromise between the no-astigmatism and no-curvature error lens forms.

As noted earlier, when oblique astigmatism is fully corrected, the hyperope can have clear vision for oblique rays by accommodating slightly (only about 0.12D for a 5.00D hyperope). However, the myope can do nothing to clear up oblique rays unless he or she is slightly overcorrected for axial rays and, therefore, can accommodate for peripheral rays. However, when curvature error is corrected at the expense of astigmatism, no amount of accommodating will reduce the astigmatism for oblique rays. For these reasons, lens designers have historically emphasized the correction of oblique astigmatism rather than curvature error.

The first "corrected curve" lenses, designed by von Rohr in 1911 and sold by Zeiss as the Punctal series, were completely corrected for astigmatism using the Ostwalt curves. Each lens in the series had its own base curve. In 1928, Bausch & Lomb introduced the Orthogon series of lenses, also designed to correct astigmatism but making use of only 15 base curves at the expense of allowing a certain amount of astigmatic error. The series of lenses designed by Tillyer of American Optical Corporation, and bearing his name, allows some oblique astigmatism to remain uncorrected while providing a partial correction for curvature error.

With the exception of high plus lenses for aphakia and low vision (discussed later in this chapter), relatively little research has been devoted to comparing the merits of the various forms of corrected curve lenses. There appear to be two reasons for this neglect: (1) for the great majority of ophthalmic lens wearers (certainly more than 90 percent), the axial lens power is so small that the oblique aberrations are insignificant; and (2) although in everyday life one's eyes are constantly moving, when an eye movement of 20 degrees or more is made (a movement large enough to introduce astigmatism and curvature errors), the movement is usually followed by a head movement during which the fovea continues to fixate the object of interest. The result of this head movement is that any critical inspection of the object is done more or less through the central portion of the ophthalmic lens.

As a final comment concerning lens design, lens designers must choose between correcting the oblique aberrations for distance vision or near vision. Because large eye movements are often made during distance vision, while reading and other near vision activities involve rather small eye movements, lens designers have chosen to correct the oblique aberrations for distance vision. An additional consideration is that during reading, the oblique aberrations can be minimized by changes in accommodation.

LENS MATERIALS AND THICKNESS CONSIDERATIONS

Ophthalmic lenses are available in various materials, including *crown glass*, having an index of refraction of 1.523; high-index glass such as *Hi-lite* glass, having an index of refraction of 1.70; and *CR–39 plastic*, having an index of refraction of 1.498. Prior to the last decade or so, the great majority of lenses were made of crown glass. Plastic, although resistant to breakage, was easily scratched and was not often used. With the development of more scratch-resistant plastic materials and larger frame sizes, plastic lenses have become increasingly popular. From the point of view of the laboratory, an important advantage of plastic lenses is that heat tempering or chemical tempering is not required. An additional impetus to the increasing popularity of plastic lenses has been the availability of easily applied "fashion tints." Compared with crown glass and plastic, high-index glass is used very little.

The use of crown glass, plastic, and high-index glass also can be compared from the point of view of lens weight and lens thickness. Plastic lenses are obviously much lighter than crown glass lenses and thus are particularly desirable when large lens sizes are used. On the other hand, because of the low index of refraction compared with crown glass, plastic materials require a greater difference between front and back surface curvatures (a greater *sag*) than is required by crown glass to achieve a given amount of power. This means that minus lenses, for a given center thickness, will have greater edge thickness if made of plastic; plus lenses,

for a given edge thickness, will have a greater center thickness if made of plastic. The increased center thickness for a plus lens is of no real consequence, since it is not apparent to an observer. In fact, most wearers of plus lenses would agree that the decreased weight is a far more important factor than the increased center thickness (if they indeed were aware of the increased thickness when changing from glass to plastic lenses). However, the increased edge thickness for a minus lens can create a serious cosmetic problem for lenses of 5.00 or 6.00D or more. This problem is most evident when rimless lenses are prescribed and is least evident when a plastic frame is used, when the bevel is placed entirely at the back of the edge, or when the "hide-a-bevel" technique is used.

The most important use for high-index glass is for a myope of 9.00 or 10.00D or more; here even crown glass lenses will have edges that are so thick they are cosmetically unacceptable. Even though high-index glass lenses are noticeably heavier than crown glass lenses, many high myopes will not object to the increased weight of the lenses because the cosmetic appearance is more acceptable. Both the lens weight and the lens thickness can be minimized by choosing a moderately sized lens that is more or less round or oval in shape and lacks any relatively sharp corners. If the myope happens to have exophoria at distance, decentering the lenses outward to provide base-in prism will not only relieve the strain on fusional vergence but will usually place the major reference point of the lens closer to the geometrical center of the lens (unless the patient has a large PD), thereby decreasing the thickness of the temporal edge of the lens. Hi-lite and other high-index lenses, however, do have disadvantages other than their added weight. They tend to scratch easily, and the color dispersion is higher than for crown glass.

Predicting Edge Thickness

The difference between the center thickness and edge thickness of a lens—called the *sagitta*, or sag, of the lens—can be determined by the following formula:

$$s = \frac{y^2 F}{2{,}000\,(n - 1)},$$

where

y = the semidiameter of the lens (expressed in milli-meters)

F = the power of a lens surface

n = the index of refraction of the lens material.

Jalie (1974) simplified this relationship by introducing the constant k, which is defined as the rate of change of lens thickness per diopter of power, resulting in the formula

$$k = \frac{s}{F} = \frac{y^2}{2,000\,(n-1)},$$

where

F = the power of the lens rather than the power of a surface.

To determine the edge thickness of a lens of a given power and a given center thickness, we need only know the value of k for the material of which the lens is made. Values of k for lenses of various semidiameters made of ophthalmic crown glass, high-index glass, and plastic are shown in Table 13.1. Determination of edge thickness can best be demonstrated by two examples.

Example 1. A 5.00D myope is to be fitted with 48mm round lenses, on center. If center thickness is to be 2.2mm, what will be the edge thickness for (1) ophthalmic crown glass, (2) high-index glass, and (3) plastic?

(1) $k(F) + 2.2 = 0.55(5) + 2.2 = 4.95$mm.

(2) $k(F) + 2.2 = 0.41(5) + 2.2 = 4.25$mm.

(3) $k(F) + 2.2 = 0.90(8) + 2.2 = 9.40$mm.

Note that in examples 1 and 2, the symbol F represents the power of the lens without regard to sign.

Example 2. A patient requiring the prescription $-7.00 -1.00 \times 90$ is to be fitted with a frame with a horizontal width of 52mm. Each lens will be decentered in 4mm. What will be the thickness at the temporal edge of the lens for (1) ophthalmic crown glass, (2) high-index glass, and (3) plastic? Assume the center thickness to be 2.2mm. (Note that $y = (52/2) + 4 = 30$mm.)

(1) $k(F) + 2.2 = 0.86(8) + 2.2 = 9.08$mm.

(2) $k(F) + 2.2 = 0.64(8) + 2.2 = 7.32$mm.

(3) $k(F) + 2.2 = 0.90(8) + 2.2 = 9.40$mm.

Note that in examples 1 and 2, an identical center thickness is specified for lenses of all materials. Although the minimum center thickness of a glass lens is usually considered to be 2.2mm, the use of a smaller center thickness for a plastic lens can minimize the differences in edge thickness between crown glass and plastic.

Gentax Corporation has introduced a series of

Table 13.1 Values of k based on lens diameter and material.

Semidiameter	Crown glass (1.523)	High-index glass (1.70)	Plastic (1.498)
20mm	0.38	0.28	0.40
22mm	0.46	0.35	0.48
24mm	0.55	0.41	0.58
26mm	0.65	0.48	0.67
28mm	0.75	0.56	0.78
30mm	0.86	0.64	0.90

plastic lenses made of coated *polycarbonate* material. This material has an index of refraction of 1.586, with the result that for high minus lenses of equal center thickness, edge thickness will be less (rather than greater) than that of a crown glass lens of equal power. The specific gravity of this material is 1.20 (which may be compared with 1.31 for CR–39 and 2.53 for crown glass). A disadvantage is a low nu value, which may result in wearers of high powered lenses seeing color fringes.

Long (1976c) published four computer-drawn graphs (shown in Figure 13.12) for use in predicting edge thickness. Each graph is intended for a different value of PD – distance between lenses (DBL), and the ten curves on each graph represent maximum edge thicknesses for spherical lenses of 1.00 to 10.00D in 2.00D steps. Each of the three abscissa scales on each graph corresponds to a different *shape factor*: the upper scale is for a shape factor of 1.14, typical of an aviator frame; the middle scale is for a shape factor of 1.12, typical of a common rectangular frame; and the lower scale is for a shape factor of 1.00, that of a round frame.

The use of the graphs can be demonstrated by an example taken from Long's (1976c) discussion. An 8.00D myope with a 60mm PD selects an aviator frame having a 52mm eyesize and a DBL of 18mm. Because PD – DBL = 42mm, the graph in Figure 13.12b is used. This shows that the difference between maximum edge thickness and center thickness of the lens blank is 10mm. Adding to this the center thickness of 2.2mm, the maximum edge thickness (i.e., the thickness at the thickest part of the edge) will be 12.2mm.

The object of using the graphs, as discussed by Long (1976c), is to get the most pessimistic estimate of edge thickness. For spherocylindrical prescriptions, he suggests that the thickness corresponding

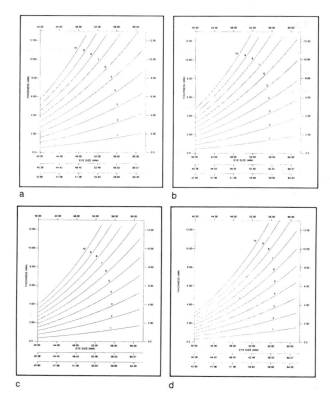

Figure 13.12 Graphs for predicting edge thickness; *(a)* **PD − DBL = 38;** *(b)* **PD − DBL = 42;** *(c)* **PD − DBL = 46;** *(d)* **PD − DBL = 50** (Long, 1976c).

to a sphere with a power equal to that in the most powerful meridian in the prescription be used.

MAGNIFICATION CHARACTERISTICS OF OPHTHALMIC LENSES

The practitioner is usually not concerned with the magnification characteristics of ophthalmic lenses unless a patient has anisometropia or high astigmatism, the correction of which (in either case) can result in *induced aniseikonia. Aniseikonia* is defined as a difference in the sizes or shapes of the retinal images for the two eyes. In the majority of cases it is possible to predict not only whether or not aniseikonia will be induced for a given patient but also *how much* aniseikonia will be produced. Measures to minimize the aniseikonia include altering the lens base curves, thicknesses, and vertex distances; and, in some cases, recommending contact lenses rather than glasses. Before discussing aniseikonia, the

magnification characteristics of ophthalmic lenses are discussed in terms of spectacle magnification and relative spectacle magnification.

Spectacle Magnification

When a patient's ametropia is corrected by a spectacle lens, the lens brings about a change in retinal image size. The ratio of the retinal image size with the correcting lens to that without the correcting lens is known as *spectacle magnification (SM)*. For any given lens, the spectacle magnification depends on both the form, or shape, of the lens and the power of the lens. This is shown by the spectacle magnification formula, in which the first term is known as the *shape factor* and the second term is known as the *power factor:*

$$\text{SM} = \left(\frac{1}{1 - \frac{t}{n} F_1} \right) \left(\frac{1}{1 - dF'_v} \right)$$

where

F_1 = power of the front surface

F'_v = back vertex power of the lens

t = thickness of the lens

n = index of refraction of the lens material

d = distance from the back vertex of the lens to the entrance pupil of the eye.

It is usually assumed that the distance from the front surface of the cornea to the entrance pupil is equal to 3mm. This formula makes use of the ray, for each object point, passing through the center (*E*) of the entrance pupil (the chief ray, as shown in Figure 13.13). Retinal image size, therefore, is measured from the center of each blur circle, with the result that the formula applies even though the uncorrected retinal image may be badly blurred.

Figure 13.13 The chief ray method of determining the size of the retinal image of an uncorrected ametropic eye. The size of the retinal image is measured from the centers of the two blur circles.

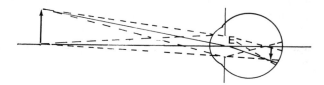

Shape factor

Inspection of the shape factor shows that spectacle magnification increases with an increase in front surface power or with an increase in lens thickness, and it decreases with an increase in the index of refraction of the lens material.

Power factor

Inspection of the power factor shows that spectacle magnification varies directly with back vertex power of the lens, the retinal image size increasing with increasing plus lens power and decreasing with increasing minus lens power. It is evident that any spectacle lens, by virtue of its power, will bring about a change in retinal image size. As a plus lens is moved closer to the eye, decreasing the value of d, there is a decrease in retinal image size. The opposite occurs when a minus lens is moved toward the eye.

Example 1. A patient is found to require $-6.00D$ spheres for both eyes. What will be the change in retinal image size with the lenses compared with that without the lenses (i.e., the spectacle magnification) if the front surface power is $+4.00D$, center thickness is 2.2mm, index of refraction is 1.523, and vertex distance is 12mm?

$$SM = \left(\frac{1}{1 - \frac{2.2(4)}{1523}}\right)\left(\frac{1}{1 - \frac{15(-6)}{1000}}\right)$$

$$= (1.0058)(0.91743)$$

$$= 0.923.$$

$$\% \ SM = -7.7\%.$$

Example 2. What would be the contact lens magnification if the same patient were to be fitted with contact lenses having a power of $-5.62D$ (allowing for the change in effective power due to the change in vertex distance), front surface power of $+58.00D$, center thickness of 0.1mm, index of refraction of 1.490, and vertex distance of zero (and, therefore, a d value of 3mm)?

$$SM = \left(\frac{1}{1 - \frac{0.1(58)}{1490}}\right)\left(\frac{1}{1 - \frac{3(-5.62)}{1000}}\right)$$

$$= (1.0039)(0.9834)$$

$$= 0.9873.$$

$$\% \ SM = -1.3\%.$$

The results of examples 1 and 2 show that while spectacle lenses reduce the retinal image size by 7.7 percent compared with the retinal image size with no lenses, contact lenses for the same patient reduce the retinal image size by only 1.3 percent. This illustrates why high myopes notice that "everything looks bigger" when they change from glasses to contact lenses.

Comparable examples for a hyperopic patient would show that the retinal image size increases considerably with glasses but relatively little with contact lenses. The spectacle magnification formula makes no assumptions concerning the nature of the patient's ametropia (whether axial or refractive) and provides the practitioner with no information that can be used to predict aniseikonia. It provides only an "after-correction" image size related to a "before-correction" image size for the eye in question.

Relative Spectacle Magnification

Relative spectacle magnification (RSM) is the ratio of the retinal image size of the corrected eye to that of the schematic emmetropic eye. It can be expressed as follows:

$$RSM = \frac{F_S}{F_A},$$

where

F_S = the equivalent power of the schematic emmetropic eye

F_A = the equivalent power of the system made up of the correcting spectacle lens and the power of the ametropic eye.

The denominator of this formula can be expanded, resulting in the following expression:

$$RSM = \frac{F_S}{F + F_E - xFF_E},$$

where

F = the equivalent power of the spectacle lens

F_E = the equivalent power of the eye

x = the distance between the second principal plane of the spectacle lens and the first principal plane of the eye (Jalie, 1974)

Axial ametropia

If the eye's ametropia is purely axial (due to an abnormally short or long axial length), the relative spectacle magnification formula can be written as follows:

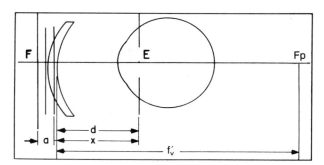

Figure 13.14　Diagram of the eye showing measurement parameters for axial and refractive ametropia (Grosvenor, 1976f).

$$RSM = \frac{1}{1 + aF},$$

where

a = distance between the primary focal plane (F) of the eye and the secondary principal plane of the correcting lens (see Figure 13.14).

In Figure 13.14, d is the distance from the entrance pupil (E) of the eye to the back surface of the lens, x is the distance from the entrance pupil of the eye to the secondary principal plane of the correcting lens, and f'_v is the distance between the far-point (F_p) of the eye and the back surface of the correcting lens.

If it is assumed that the refracting power of the schematic emmetropic eye is +60.00D and that the distance from the cornea to the first principal plane (or, with negligible error, the entrance pupil) of the eye is 3mm, the anterior focal plane of the axially ametropic eye can be considered to be 14mm from the cornea. (It should be remembered that for the purely axially ametropic eye, the optical system of the eye is of normal focal length, so the primary focal length is the same for the axially ametropic eye as for the schematic emmetropic eye.)

Fortunately, the secondary principal plane of the correcting lens is often very close to the eye's primary focal plane. When this occurs, the value of a can be considered equal to zero, and the previous formula reduces to

$$RSM = 1.$$

This indicates that for a purely axially ametropic eye, if the secondary focal plane of the correcting lens is placed at the primary focal plane of the eye, the retinal image size is that of the schematic emmetropic eye. This expression is known as *Knapp's law*.

Refractive ametropia

If an eye has a "normal" axial length but is ametropic by virtue of an optical system having an abnormally long or short focal length, the relative spectacle magnification is given by the following formula:

$$RSM = \frac{1}{1 - xF} = \left(\frac{1}{1 - \dfrac{t}{n}F_1}\right)\left(\frac{1}{1 - dF'_v}\right),$$

where

x = the distance from the secondary principal plane of the spectacle lens to the entrance pupil of the eye (see Figure 13.14).

This is the same expression as that for the magnification caused by the lens (the spectacle magnification) and indicates that the correcting lens is likely to bring about a marked change in image size, in contrast to the situation in axial ametropia, in which a "normal" retinal image size often results.

Consideration of this formula shows that magnification increases with increasing values of x. The value of x will be at a minimum when a contact lens is worn; thus, in purely refractive ametropia, the relative spectacle magnification can be minimized by the use of a contact lens.

Predicting Image Size Differences in Anisometropia and Astigmatism

To summarize the preceding discussions on axial and refractive ametropia: (1) if a patient's anisometropia is due to differences in axial length for the two eyes, correction with spectacle lenses is expected to result in a minimum of retinal image size difference for the two eyes; (2) if a patient's anisometropia is due to differences in the media of the two eyes (i.e., refractive anisometropia), correction with contact lenses is expected to result in a minimum of retinal image size difference for the two eyes. If spectacle lenses are to be used in refractive anisometropia, retinal image size differences can be minimized by careful selection of front surface curves and vertex distances.

How can we predict which patients will have axial ametropia and which will have refractive ametropia? Sorsby et al. (1957) have shown that eyes having ametropia of less than ±4.00D are ametropic not because of any abnormal constituents (such as abnormal axial lengths) but because of faulty correlation of axial length, corneal refracting power, lens refracting power, and anterior chamber depth. In eyes having ametropia in excess of ±4.00D, axial lengths are usually abnormal (being abnormally short in hyperopia and abnormally long in myopia).

On the basis of this information, if a patient is emmetropic or has a small amount of ametropia in one eye and more than ±4.00D of ametropia in the other eye, there is a good chance that the ametropia in the second eye is *axial* and that correction with spectacle lenses would result in a minimum of aniseikonia. However, if the second eye has less than ±4.00D of ametropia, it is more likely that its ametropia is *refractive* and that if spectacle lenses are to be prescribed, front surface powers and axial lengths will have to be carefully selected to minimize image size differences for the two eyes.

This is not to be interpreted as indicating that ±4.00D is a cutoff point and that all ametropia below this point is refractive and all ametropia above it is axial. What we must do in these cases is to think in terms of probabilities. For example, if a patient has a refractive error of +0.75D in one eye and +3.00D in the other eye, it is unlikely that the difference in ametropia for the two eyes is entirely axial; therefore, adjustments in front surface powers and vertex distances should be considered if spectacle lenses are to be prescribed. If a patient has a refractive error of +0.75D in one eye and +5.00D in the other eye, it is much more likely that the difference in ametropia for the two eyes is entirely axial and that correction with spectacle lenses should result in a minimum of aniseikonia with no adjustments in lens curves or vertex distances.

In addition to basing predictions on the amount of anisometropia, another possible method of predicting whether the difference in refraction between the two eyes is axial or refractive is to consider the keratometer findings for the two eyes. If the findings are about the same for the two eyes, it reinforces the suspicion that the ametropia is axial. If they differ by 1.00D or more and if the difference is in the direction of higher corneal refracting power for the more myopic or less hyperopic eye, refractive ametropia is probably present. However, the author's experience has been that, in cases of anisometropia not involving high astigmatism, the keratometer findings for the two eyes usually agree rather closely. However, even when keratometer findings agree closely, the patient's anisometropia could be due mainly to differences in refracting power of the crystalline lenses (which, unfortunately, cannot be easily measured by clinical means).

Fortunately, there are some situations in which the practitioner can accurately predict whether a patient's ametropia is axial or refractive. If an older patient has one normal eye but has a nuclear cataract in the other eye (that eye being more myopic than the other eye), there is no doubt that the cataractous eye has refractive ametropia (see Figure 13.15a.) In such a case the practitioner should be concerned not only with the problem of induced aniseikonia but also with the problem of the induced vertical prismatic effect at the reading level (discussed earlier in this chapter). However, in many of these cases the visual acuity of the eye with the cataract is lowered to 20/30 or 20/40, so neither the image size difference nor the prismatic effect at the reading level seems to cause a problem for the patient.

The second situation in which one can accurately conclude whether the patient's anisometropia is due to axial or refractive differences between the two eyes is the case of the unilateral aphakic patient. There is no doubt that the difference in refractive error for the two eyes (which is usually about 10.00 to 12.00D) is due to the fact that one eye has a crystalline lens and the other eye does not (see Figure 13.15b.) As shown in Chapter 14, the retinal image size difference for the two eyes will be about 25–30 percent if spectacles are worn, and no amount of adjusting lens surface powers or vertex distance will help the situation significantly. For this reason, the only successful method of optometric management for this patient would be to prescribe a contact lens for the aphakic eye. (*Ophthalmological* management may include implanting an intraocular lens.)

The third situation in which the source of ametropia can be accurately predicted is when a patient has high astigmatism in both eyes, resulting in induced aniseikonia due to the fact that the retinal images have different shapes for the two eyes. Because the source of high astigmatism is almost

Figure 13.15 Refractive ametropia: *(a)* Nuclear cataract; *(b)* Aphakia.

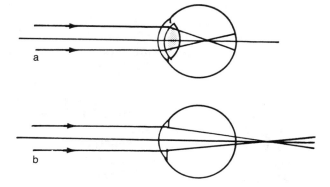

always the cornea, spectacle lenses would result in a maximum of aniseikonia, and contact lenses would result in a minimum. It should be understood that the axes of the correcting lenses for the two eyes are of great importance in predicting aniseikonia. For example, if a patient requires a spectacle correction of +1.00DS −2.50DC axis 180 for each eye, there will be no induced aniseikonia. However, if the axes were 30 degrees for one eye and 150 degrees for the other, correction of the astigmatism with spectacle lenses would cause a difference in the shapes of the retinal images for the two eyes. It should be understood that correction with contact lenses, although optically superior to spectacles in cases like the example just given, often is not a viable alternative. Although an excellent optical result can often be obtained with hard contact lenses the presence of high corneal astigmatism tends to cause "rocking" or other problems with hard lenses, making them uncomfortable. Toric soft lenses however, provide good vision with greatly increased comfort. Fortunately, many patients who have high corneal astigmatism adapt to the induced aniseikonia and complain of subjective symptoms only if a significant change is made in the cylinder power or axis.

Minimizing Image Size Differences

There are three possible methods of predicting the aniseikonia that will be induced by a spectacle correction: (1) *measurement* of the aniseikonia, using an eikonometer, while the patient wears the new correction in a trial frame; (2) *calculation* of the magnification differences for the two eyes, as described earlier in this chapter, and then estimation of the presence (and amount) of or absence of induced aniseikonia based on whether the ametropia is thought to be axial or refractive; and (3) the use of a *rule of thumb* for estimating the induced aniseikonia, followed by the use of magnification tables.

The only commercially produced eikonometer in the United States was the American Optical Space Eikonometer, which has not been available for many years, so the use of an eikonometer is not a viable alternative for most practitioners. Calculation of magnification differences is a time-consuming task, but with the availability of programmable calculators and microcomputers, this procedure can be greatly simplified. Jalie (1974, pp. 427–439) described the procedure for calculation and the necessary equations. Linksz and Bannon (1965) published tables showing approximate magnification changes associated with changes in front surface power and vertex

distance for lenses of various powers (see Tables 13.2 and 13.3).

To make use of the Linksz and Bannon tables, there are a number of rules of thumb to estimate the magnification per diopter of change of lens power. Ryan (1975) estimated that the retinal image size changes at about the rate of 1.4 percent per diopter of lens power for refractive ametropia, and 0.25 percent per diopter of lens power for axial ametropia. Although Knapp's law predicts that there would be no aniseikonia in axial ametropia, the law does not hold perfectly in the clinical situation for a number of reasons. For example, (1) most spectacle lenses have their back vertex located at least 2 or 3mm inside the primary focal plane of the eye, and (2) the less ametropic eye cannot be expected to have the optical characteristics of the schematic emmetropic eye. In regard to the use of his rule of thumb, Ryan has made the point that axial-refractive combinations are more the rule than the exception, and if the correcting lens is worn closer to the eye than the primary focal plane of the eye, the magnification effects of the axial and refractive components are in the opposite directions and, therefore, tend to compensate for one another.

The use of Table 13.2 is demonstrated by the following example. Suppose a practitioner determines (by measurement or by estimation) that a patient's right lens, having a back vertex power of +2.00D and a center thickness of 2.7mm, requires an increase in magnification of 1 percent. Table 13.2 shows that for this lens, an increase in magnification of 1.1 percent will result if the front surface power is increased by 4.00D. The table takes into consideration the change in vertex distance that results when the front surface power is changed. For example, the table shows that for a −3.00D lens, an increase in front surface power of 2.00D actually causes a minification of 0.2 percent due to the increase in vertex distance that accompanies the steepening of the front surface.

Magnification changes associated with changes in vertex distance are shown in Table 13.3. Linksz and Bannon (1965) pointed out that the decrease in magnification brought about by increased vertex distance of a minus lens begins to cancel out the magnification due to increased curvature as the power of the lens approaches −2.00D. They suggest that, because strong minus lenses have thick edges, it is possible to change the position of the bevel and thus bring the lens closer to the eye, preserving the magnification achieved by the increase in curvature. The practitioner may decide not to alter the front

Table 13.2 Approximate magnification changes associated with changes in front base curves for various lens powers—percentage (Linksz and Bannon, 1965).

Vertex power of lens (diopters)	Average center thickness (mm)	Change in front base curve (D)					
		−4.00D	−2.00D	+2.00D	+4.00D	+6.00D	+8.00D
+8.00	7.0	−3.5	−1.7	+1.7	+3.5	+5.2	+6.9
+7.00	6.2	−3.0	−1.5	+1.5	+3.0	+4.5	+6.0
+6.00	5.4	−2.6	−1.3	+1.3	+2.6	+3.9	+5.2
+5.00	4.6	−2.2	−1.1	+1.1	+2.2	+3.3	+4.4
+4.00	3.9	−1.8	−0.9	+0.9	+1.8	+2.8	+3.7
+3.00	3.2	−1.5	−0.7	+0.7	+1.5	+2.2	+2.9
+2.00	2.7	−1.1	−0.6	+0.6	+1.1	+1.7	+2.2
+1.00	2.2	−0.8	−0.4	+0.4	+0.8	+1.2	+1.6
0.00	1.8	−0.5	−0.2	+0.2	+0.5	+0.7	+1.0
−1.00	1.4	−0.2	−0.1	+0.1	+0.2	+0.3	+0.3
−2.00	1.0	+0.1	+0.1	−0.1	−0.1	−0.2	−0.3
−3.00	0.9	+0.4	+0.2	−0.2	−0.4	−0.5	−0.7
−4.00	0.9	+0.6	+0.3	−0.3	−0.6	−0.8	−1.1
−5.00	0.9	+0.8	+0.4	−0.4	−0.8	−1.1	−1.5
−6.00	0.9	+1.0	+0.5	−0.5	−1.0	−1.4	−1.9
−7.00	0.9	+1.2	+0.6	−0.6	−1.2	−1.7	−2.3
−8.00	0.9	+1.4	+0.7	−0.7	−1.4	−2.0	−2.7

surface power at all for a minus lens, but to bring about the desired magnification change by changing only the vertex distance. For example, Table 13.3 shows that to bring about a 1.2 percent increase in the magnification of a −6.00D lens, the lens is moved toward the eye (by moving the bevel forward) 2mm.

In any case, when a practitioner orders spectacle lenses for a patient who has anisometropia, the laboratory should be instructed to use *the same front curve* and *the same center thickness* for each lens: this will assure that the shape factor of the spectacle magnification formula is similar for the lenses.

ABSORPTIVE LENSES

The total *electromagnetic spectrum* extends from the extremely short gamma rays having a wavelength of 10^{-12}cm to the extremely long radio waves having a wavelength of 10^6cm. The *visible spectrum* constitutes a small portion of the electromagnetic spectrum in the region between 10^{-4} and 10^{-5}cm (from approximately 390 to 760nm). (A nanometer (nm) equals 10^{-7}cm.) Within the visible spectrum, radiation of all wavelengths is not equally visible. As shown in the photopic luminosity curve in Figure 13.16, the light-adapted eye has its greatest sensitivity to radiation having a wavelength of 555nm (yellow-green); the sensitivity drops off in either

Table 13.3 Approximate magnification changes associated with changes in eyewire distance for various lens powers—percentage (Linksz and Bannon, 1965).

Vertex power of lens (diopters)	Change in eyewire distance			
	Lens moved *toward* the eye			
	−1mm	−2mm	−3mm	−4mm
+ 10D	−1.0	−2.0	−3.0	−4.0
+ 8D	−0.8	−1.6	−2.4	−3.2
+ 6D	−0.6	−1.2	−1.8	−2.4
+ 4D	−0.4	−0.8	−1.2	−1.6
+ 2D	−0.2	−0.4	−0.6	−0.8
− 2D	+0.2	+0.4	+0.6	+0.8
− 4D	+0.4	+0.8	+1.2	+1.6
− 6D	+0.6	+1.2	+1.8	+2.4
− 8D	+0.8	+1.6	+2.4	+3.2
− 10D	+1.0	+2.0	+3.0	+4.0
	Lens moved *away* from eye			
	+1mm	+2mm	+3mm	+4mm
+ 10D	+1.0	+2.0	+3.0	+4.0
+ 8D	+0.8	+1.6	+2.4	+3.2
+ 6D	+0.6	+1.2	+1.8	+2.4
+ 4D	+0.4	+0.8	+1.2	+1.6
+ 2D	+0.2	+0.4	+0.6	+0.8
− 2D	−0.2	−0.4	−0.6	−0.8
− 4D	−0.4	−0.8	−1.2	−1.6
− 6D	−0.6	−1.2	−1.8	−2.4
− 8D	−0.8	−1.6	−2.4	−3.2
− 10D	−1.0	−2.0	−3.0	−4.0

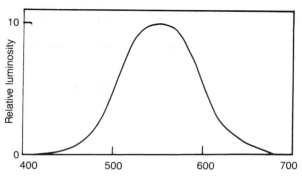

Figure 13.16 The photopic luminosity curve.

direction, being the least at the two extremities of about 390nm (violet) and 760nm (red).

Ultraviolet radiation extends from about 10–390nm, whereas *infrared radiation* extends from about 760–500,000nm. The radiation reaching the earth's surface from the sun, after passing through the atmosphere, extends only from about 290–20,000nm. However, there are artificial sources of both ultraviolet radiation (sun lamps and electric arcs used for welding) and infrared radiation (furnaces used in steelmaking and in glassblowing).

In considering the harmful effects of radiation on the eye, it should be understood that radiation has no effect on an ocular structure unless it is absorbed by the structure. Radiation transmitted by the media of the eye does no harm to the structures involved.

Ultraviolet Radiation

Ultraviolet radiation can be absorbed by the anterior structures of the eye (conjunctiva, cornea, aqueous, lens, and iris) and, therefore, can adversely affect these structures. Subjective effects of short wavelength ultraviolet exposure include photophobia and itching of the eyes as a result of keratoconjunctivitis. Exposure is more likely to occur if ultraviolet light is reflected into the eye by surfaces below eye level, such as snow, the sea, sand, or concrete. Ultraviolet radiation, therefore, is a problem for skiers (both snow and water), fishermen, hikers, and others who spend much time outdoors.

The condition referred to as *snow blindness* is actually two conditions: (1) the keratoconjunctivitis already described and (2) a perceptual problem due to an almost complete lack of borders in the visual environment. In everyday life, we "see" objects because of the presence of both brightness-contrast

and color-contrast borders. Stefansson, an arctic explorer, described in some detail the problems encountered in attempting to see objects in the colorless and borderless environment of the arctic. The inability to see changes in terrain—even abrupt ones—constitutes a form of blindness that is further complicated by the presence of photophobia and itching of the eyes due to keratoconjunctivitis.

In a study of the harmful effects of ultraviolet radiation on the eye, Pitts (1978) found that in the rabbit, primate, and human eye, the cornea absorbed ultraviolet radiation between 210 and 325nm, with the absorption greatest at 290nm. He also found that the crystalline lens of the rabbit absorbed radiation in a narrow band between 295 and 320nm. Damage to the rabbit cornea consisted of epithelial deposits, stippling, and haze due to the lower ultraviolet wavelengths, as well as stromal haze and opacities for wavelengths above 320nm at high-exposure levels. Damage to the rabbit lens involved small, dotlike, anterior subcapsular opacities and, with high-exposure levels, permanent anterior subcapsular cataracts. Signs of anterior uveitis were also noted, including ciliary injection, aqueous flare, and keratic precipitates.

Infrared Radiation

The eye is susceptible to damage, as a result of heat, by radiation in the 800–1,300nm range. Depending on the nature of the source of the radiation, damage can occur either to the retina or the crystalline lens.

As shown in Figure 13.17a, infrared radiation from a *point source* such as the sun will be concentrated on the retina and can cause a retinal burn. This is the familiar *eclipse burn* of the retina, or *photoretinitis*. If the radiation is in the form of an *extended source* (see Figure 13.17b) such as a blast furnace the radiation will be concentrated at the

Figure 13.17 Infrared radiation (a) from a point source and (b) from an extended source.

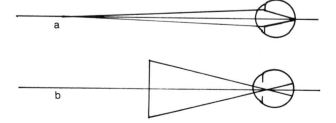

nodal point of the eye and can coagulate the protein of the lens, causing a *glassblower's cataract*. In this situation the iris also absorbs a large amount of heat and transmits it to the lens.

Light Transmission of an Ophthalmic Lens

When light is incident on an ophthalmic lens, some of the light is reflected, some is absorbed, and the remainder is transmitted. The percentage of light that is lost by reflection from each surface (the *reflection factor*) can be determined by Fresnel's law, assuming normally incident light:

$$\left(\frac{n-1}{n+1}\right)^2.$$

For crown glass having an index of refraction of 1.523, the reflection factor would be

$$\left(\frac{1.523-1}{1.523+1}\right)^2 = 0.043, \text{ or } 4.3\%.$$

The amount of light lost by reflection from the front and back surfaces, therefore, would be 2(4.3) = 8.6 percent. The amount of light lost by absorption, for crown glass, is less than 1 percent per centimeter of lens thickness. Therefore, for a lens 0.2cm thick, loss by absorption would be approximately 0.2 percent. The transmission for this lens would be

$$100\% - 8.6\% - 0.2\% = 91.2\%.$$

Crown glass has a relatively sharp cutoff point at about 300nm, so it provides protection against the ultraviolet rays causing much of the damage reported by Pitts (1977). The transmission curve for crown glass is the upper curve in Figure 13.18.

Neutral Density Indoor Tints

A neutral density tint is one that has approximately the same absorptive characteristics for all wavelengths in the visible spectrum. Several lens manufacturers make neutral density absorptive lenses intended for indoor as well as outdoor wear. Transmission curves for two of these lenses—American Optical *Cruxite A* and Bausch & Lomb *Soft Lite A*—are shown in Figure 13.18. These lenses absorb all ultraviolet radiation below about 350nm. Although their transmission of visible light is only about 5 percent less than that of ordinary ophthalmic glass, many patients find that these lenses provide increased visual comfort in indoor situations involving glare or when working under fluorescent lighting.

Outdoor Tints

Absorptive lenses designed for outdoor wear should have high absorption (low transmission) in the ultraviolet and infrared regions of the spectrum as well as in the visible spectrum. Figure 13.19 shows transmission curves for American Optical *Cosmetan* (brown) and *Calobar D* (green), and for Bausch & Lomb *Ray Ban 3* (green) and *G–15* (gray). The Calobar D, Ray Ban 3, and G–15 meet the criterion of low transmission in both the ultraviolet and infrared

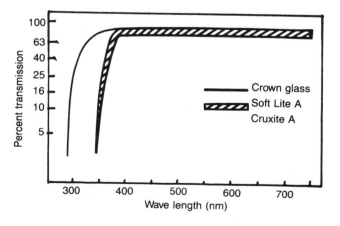

Figure 13.18 Transmission curves for ophthalmic crown glass, Soft Lite A and Cruxite A (redrawn from Kors and Peters, 1972).

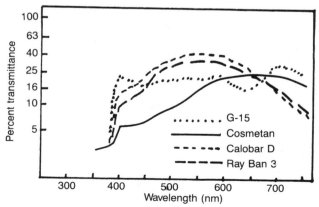

Figure 13.19 Transmission curves for G–15, Cosmetan, Calobar D, and Ray Ban 3 (redrawn from Kors and Peters, 1972).

regions, but the Cosmetan transmission is greater in the infrared region than in the visible region of the spectrum. Transmission curves for plastic lenses and for coated glass lenses show even higher transmission in the infrared region than for the Cosmetan lens.

Clark (1968) made the point that sunglass lenses having higher transmission in the infrared region than in the visible spectrum can be hazardous, because the reduced transmission of visible light can cause pupillary dilation to the extent that the eyes will be subjected to more infrared radiation than they would be without the lenses. In another report, Clark (1969) concluded that *color* in absorptive lenses has no advantages but has disadvantages for both color-normal and color-defective observers. He recommended that absorptive lenses be neutral gray rather than colored.

Photochromic Lenses

Photochromic lenses, developed by Corning in 1965, are made of glass containing silver halide crystals, which decompose into silver and halogen when exposed to long ultraviolet radiation and recombine into silver halide in the absence of long ultraviolet radiation. The crystals are held within the glass, so they can decompose and recombine repeatedly. This process is analogous to that taking place in a photographic emulsion, which also makes use of silver halide. However, in a photographic emulsion the halide diffuses away and the silver remains, whereas in photochromic glass both the silver and the halide remain.

Transmission curves for the *Photogray* lens, in both the completely faded (overnight) stage and the completely darkened stage, are shown in the upper diagram of Figure 13.20. As shown in these curves, the transmittance in the completely faded state is uniform over the visible spectrum and about the same as that of untinted ophthalmic crown glass; the transmittance in the completely darkened stage appears to average about 50 percent but varies greatly with wavelength, ranging from a low of about 40 percent in the 600nm (orange) region of the spectrum to about 60 percent in the 700nm (red) region and to almost 90 percent in the infrared region.

Time characteristics of darkening and fading of the Photogray lens are shown in the lower diagram of Figure 13.20. When exposed to light at 77°F, the lenses darken to a transmittance of about 55 percent within just a few minutes, reaching 50 percent

transmittance by the end of 60 minutes and recovering to a transmittance of about 80 percent or slightly higher within 90 minutes after the stimulating light is removed. It should be understood, however, that recovery to the 90 percent transmittance level occurs only after overnight fading.

Since the introduction of the Photogray lens in the 1960s, Corning has developed additional photochromic lenses. *Photobrown* lenses have transmittances similar to those of Photogray lenses both in the darkened and lightened states, differing mainly in terms of color. The *Photogray Extra* lens differs from the original Photogray in darkening much more quickly when exposed to sunlight (in 60 seconds,

Figure 13.20 *Upper diagram:* spectral transmittance of 2.0mm thick Photogray lens at 77°F *(a)* unexposed; *(b)* after 60 minutes darkening. *Lower diagram:* transmittance of 2.0mm thick Photogray lens with 60 minutes sunlight exposure and 90 minutes recovery *(a)* at 77°F; *(b)* at 32°F. (redrawn from Shaver, 1968).

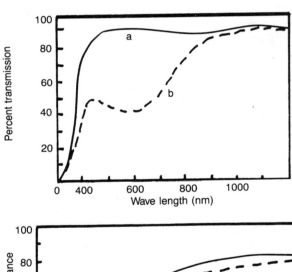

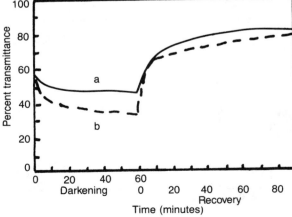

according to the manufacturer) and completing 75 percent of the fading cycle within 10 minutes. *Photosun* lenses are intended as sunglass lenses and are significantly darker than Photogray lenses in both the darkened and faded states, having transmittances of about 23 percent in the darkened state and only 65 percent in the faded state. Fusible photochromic glass, used in making fused bifocals, is available in Photogray, Photobrown, and Photosun. Data published by the manufacturer indicate that fusible photochromic glass has a transmittance of about 7 percent less than the original photochromic glass in the darkened state.

Many people regard a single pair of photochromic lenses as a substitute for two pairs of glasses—sunglasses for daytime outdoor wear and clear lenses for indoor and evening wear. If the lenses are to be worn for night driving, this arrangement is completely unacceptable with Photosun lenses because they have a transmittance of only 65 percent in the completely faded state. Night driving is questionable even with Photogray lenses, since these lenses recover to 90 percent transmittance only after overnight fading.

The high infrared transmittance of photochromic lenses, shown in the upper diagram of Figure 13.20 for the Photogray lens, also makes questionable the use of this lens as a sunglass lens. Chase (1975) measured the transmission characteristics of four types of photochromic lenses and found that transmission for the infrared wavelength of 1,400nm was approximately 90 percent for the Photobrown lens, 87 percent for the Photogray lens, 82 percent for the Photosun lens, and 75 percent for fusible photochromic glass. Stating that infrared is most heavily absorbed by the eye in the vicinity of 1,400nm, he warned that patients should be told that photochromic lenses fail to effectively absorb infrared radiation and, therefore, can be harmful to the eyes. He made the point that photochromic lenses should not be used to take the place of sunglass lenses.

Brooks (1978) called attention to the fact that a photochromic lens turns to its lighter state by exposure to red or infrared light or heat. This is consistent with the fact that the lenses become darker at lower temperatures than at higher temperatures and remain somewhat darker in the faded state. Brooks also made the point that heat tempering results in a reduction of transmittance of photochromic lenses both in the darkened and lightened states, whereas chemical tempering increases the transmittance slightly in both states. Because many people wear Photogray lenses for night driving

or for general evening and indoor wear, chemical tempering is the preferred method for hardening these lenses.

BIFOCAL AND TRIFOCAL LENSES

One of Benjamin Franklin's many inventions was the bifocal lens. As cited by Morgan and Peters (1948), Franklin wrote a letter to a friend in May 1785, stating:

> I imagine it will be pretty generally true that the same convexity of glass through which a man sees clearest and best at the same distance for reading is not the best for greater distances. I, therefore, had formerly two pairs of spectacles which I shifted occasionally, as in travelling I sometimes read and often wanted to regard the prospect. Finding this change troublesome and not always sufficiently ready, I had the glasses cut, and half of each kind associated in the same circle, thus . . . by this means, as I wear my spectacles constantly, I have only to move my eyes up and down as I want to see distinctly far or near, the proper glasses always being ready. (pp. 51).

Franklin's bifocal lens compared well to present-day bifocals, having a large reading field and an absence of "jump." (*Jump* is an abrupt vertical movement of the environment experienced by a bifocal wearer when the line of sight crosses the dividing line.) Following Franklin's invention, the bifocal lens evolved through a number of stages before the development of modern fused and one-piece bifocal lenses early in the 20th century. Early bifocal lenses included the following: the solid upcurve bifocal (1836), an ordinary convex lens with a less convex curve ground on the upper part of the back surface, forming a "distance window"; the Perfection bifocal (1885), similar to the original Franklin bifocal but with a rounded, beveled dividing line; and the cement bifocal (1888), an ordinary convex or concave lens with a glass wafer cemented to the back surface using a cement called *Canada balsam*. Cement bifocals are still used occasionally for special uses such as a temporary bifocal or a double bifocal. Transparent epoxy resin, called *araldite*, is now used for cement. The precursor to the modern fused bifocal was the *cement Kryptok* (the word *kryptok* means "hidden") invented by Borsch in 1899. This was the first bifocal lens using two kinds of glass. A flint ($n = 1.67$) segment was cemented onto a ground-out portion on the back surface (called a *countersink curve*) of an ophthalmic crown glass lens ($n = 1.523$) and was held in place by a cover glass.

Fused Bifocals

The first fused bifocal was the *fused Kryptok* invented by Borsch in 1908. A countersink curve is ground into the front surface of the major lens, a high-index button (flint or other high-index glass) is ground with the same curvature, and the two are fused together in an oven at a temperature of about 650°C. Because the segment is on the front surface, if cylinder is required it must be ground on the back surface. Kryptok bifocals are still available and have the advantage that due to the feather-edge dividing line, the segment is less visible than it is in flat-top fused bifocals or in one-piece bifocals. Modern Kryptoks usually have a 22mm round segment. The Kryptok and other bifocal lenses are shown in Figure 13.21.

The first straight-top bifocal was the *Univis D*, developed in the 1930s. This lens uses a button made of two pieces of glass fused together, the lower part being flint and the upper part being crown. The round button is then fused into a countersink on the front surface of the major lens. The upper dividing line disappears in the fusing process, resulting in a *D*-shaped segment. All ophthalmic lens manufac-

turers now make flat-top bifocals, which are available in segment widths of 22, 28, and 35mm. Univis also makes the *Univis B*, a ribbon segment that has the advantage that some distance vision is available *under* the bifocal segment; and the *Univis R*, a wider ribbon segment. The *Compensated R*, designed for compensating vertical prismatic effects at the reading level, is discussed later in this chapter.

The *Panoptik* bifocal, developed by Bausch & Lomb in 1927, is similar in appearance to the Univis D except that the corners are rounded. Baryta crown ($n = 1.664$) is used instead of flint for the segment. This material has the same dispersive power as ophthalmic crown (nu value = 55) and, therefore, eliminates the chromatic aberration that occurs with flint segments. The American Optical *Fulvue* and the Shuron *Widesite* are similar to the Univis D but have a curved rather than a straight dividing line.

One-Piece Bifocals

The earliest one-piece bifocal that is still in use is the *Ultex* bifocal developed by Continental Optical Company in 1905. This lens uses a single piece of crown glass, and the added power at near is provided by the use of a steeper curvature in the lower part of the back surface. Two or more lenses are produced at a time, using a saucer-shaped blank and a ring tool for surfacing. Several shapes are available, including the *Ultex K*, which is shaped like a Univis D segment. Because the bifocal is on the back surface of the lens, if cylinder is needed it must be ground on the front surface.

The *Executive* bifocal, introduced in the 1950s by the American Optical Corporation, has a horizontal dividing line on the front surface of the lens and a steeper curvature in the lower portion. This lens looks and performs much like the original Franklin bifocal. The dividing line is obvious and causes reflections that most wearers eventually learn to ignore. Like many lenses, the Executive bifocal is now made by many manufacturers under a variety of trade names. Because the bifocal is on the front surface, any required cylinder must be ground on the back surface.

Bifocal Specifications

When bifocals are to be prescribed, in addition to the specifications required for single vision lenses (lens size, distance between lenses, and amount and direction of decentration), the laboratory order must include the following: bifocal style (usually speci-

Figure 13.21   Bifocal types: *(a)* Kryptok; *(b)* Univis; *(c)* Ultex A; *(d)* Executive. The Kryptok and Univis are fused bifocals, whereas the Ultex A and Executive are one-piece bifocals. In each case the dot indicates the optical center, or pole, of the segment.

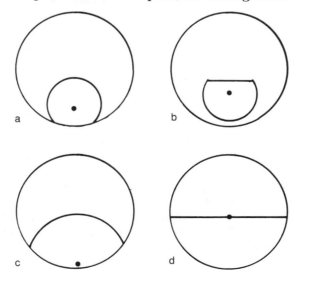

fying company trade name), segment height, segment width, and segment inset.

Segment height

Segment height is determined while the patient wears a sample frame of the style, size, and shape that will be used for the finished lenses. While the patient looks straight ahead at the examiner's eye, the examiner measures the distance from the top of the patient's lower lid to the lower eyewire (where the bevel of the lens will fit into the groove). If the patient has an unusually low lower eyelid, with sclera showing underneath the limbus, the measurement should be from the lower limbus rather than the top of the lower lid. The position of the segment top is usually specified as no more than 1 or 2mm below the top edge of the lower lid. For example, if the distance from the top edge of the lower lid to the lower eyewire is 20mm, the segment height will be specified as 18 or 19mm. Segment height depends on a large number of factors, including head position and the tasks for which the lenses will be used. A person who habitually holds the head high ("looks down the nose") will need a lower segment height than a person who slouches a bit and habitually tips the head downward. Assuming a normal head position, an individual who works at a desk all day long will prefer an unusually high segment (at or even above the top edge of the lower lid) and will learn to tip the head downward, if necessary, for certain distance vision tasks. The novice should be aware that he or she is much more likely to make a mistake in the direction of having the segment height *too low* rather than too high. The well-intentioned act on the part of some practitioners and optical dispensers of trying to keep the segment "out of the patient's way" has resulted in many a patient getting a stiff neck as a result of tilting the head backward to try to see through the bifocals.

Segment width

Segment widths are usually available (for straight-top segments) in 22, 25, 28, and 35mm widths. Whereas the wider segments were formerly thought of as "occupational" bifocals, many patients given a choice prefer the widest segment possible. Because the Executive bifocal encompasses the full width of the lens, it is obviously not necessary to specify segment width when this lens is prescribed.

Segment inset

Segment inset is specified as the difference between the patient's distance and near PD. In the normal range of PDs, the near PD for a reading distance of 40cm is 4mm less than the distance PD. Segment inset, therefore, is usually specified as 2mm for each lens.

There are two reasons for insetting bifocal segments: (1) to ensure that the patient's line of sight will go through the segment at its optical center and (2) to ensure that the reading fields for the two segments will coincide with one another. As discussed later in the chapter, the lines of sight will go through the resultant optical centers of the near portions of the lenses only when the distance lenses have no power in the horizontal meridian.

Optical Characteristics of Bifocal Lenses

Optical characteristics vary widely from one bifocal style to another, so they should be taken into consideration when selecting a bifocal segment style for a given patient.

Image jump

The abrupt upward movement of the environment experienced by a bifocal wearer when the line of sight crosses the dividing line is caused by the base-down prismatic effect induced by the segment, and it is accompanied by the presence of a scotomatous, or "blind," area. The only way the wearer can see objects in the scotomatous area is by moving the head upward or downward. The magnitude of the jump (as well as the angular size of the scotomatous area) can be found by multiplying the power of the bifocal addition by the distance from the segment top to the segment pole. (The word *pole* is used here to indicate the optical center, or major reference point, of the major lens—usually referred to as the distance lens—or of the bifocal segment.) Referring to Figure 13.22, in which the bifocal segment is shown as if it were a separate lens,

$$\text{jump} = d(F_A),$$

where

d = the distance from the segment top to the segment pole expressed in centimeters

F_A = the power of the bifocal addition.

The amount of jump can be minimized by placing the pole of the segment as close to the dividing line as possible. Franklin's bifocal and its modern counterpart, the Executive bifocal, have no jump, because the pole of the segment is at the dividing line. It follows that the amount of jump will be at

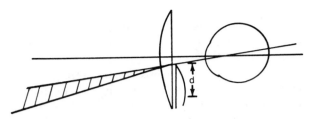

Figure 13.22 Image jump. In this diagram, the distance lens and the segment are considered as two separate lenses. The shaded area is the scotomatous area. Jump, expressed in prism diopters, is equal to the distance from the segment top to the segment pole (in centimeters) times the power of the addition.

maximum when the pole of the segment is at or near (or even beyond) the lower edge of the lens. For the lenses shown in Figure 13.21, the distances from the segment top to the segment pole are 11mm for the Kryptok bifocal, 5mm for the Univis D or straight-top bifocal, 19mm for the Ultex A bifocal, and 0mm for the Executive bifocal. For a +2.00D addition, the respective amounts of jump for these four lenses would be 2.2, 1.0, 3.8, and 0Δ base-down.

For a given bifocal addition, the amount of jump varies *only* with the distance from the segment top to the segment pole and is not affected by the power of the distance prescription.

Segment-induced prismatic effect

When a wearer of single vision lenses turns the eyes downward to read, prismatic effect is encountered. For example, if a 3.00D hyperope reads at a level of 10mm below the pole of the lens, a prismatic effect of 3Δ base-up is encountered when reading (see Figure 13.23a). When bifocal lenses are worn, the prismatic effect will change. If the 3.00D hyperope is given a +2.00D addition in the form of an Executive bifocal, and if the reading level is 5mm below the segment top, how would the segment alter the prismatic effect? Remembering that the pole of an Executive segment is at the dividing line, the prismatic effect induced by the segment at the reading level would be

$$0.5(2) = 1.0\Delta \text{ base-up.}$$

Of course, this would be added to the prismatic effect induced by the distance lens (see Figure 13.23b).

As demonstrated in this example, the prismatic effect induced at the reading level by the segment is

equal to the power of the bifocal addition times the distance from the segment pole to the reading level. It follows that if the segment pole is at the reading level, no prismatic effect will be induced by the segment. This condition is met with a straight-top bifocal if the dividing line is 5mm below the distance pole, the segment pole is 5mm below the dividing line, and the reading level is 10mm below the distance pole.

A relevant question to ask at this point is, which is the greater problem—jump or segment-induced prismatic effect at the reading level? We have just seen that a bifocal free of jump (the Executive) will induce a certain amount of prismatic effect at the reading level, while one that induces no prismatic effect at the reading level (the straight-top) is subject to a certain amount of jump. For the long-term spectacle wearer who is accustomed to a certain amount of vertical prismatic effect at the reading level, the amount (and possibly the direction) of prismatic effect will change when bifocal lenses are first worn. Adaptation to this new prismatic effect should not be difficult, as the wearer would be expected to easily "forget" the learned prismatic displacement. However, jump manifests itself each

Figure 13.23 The effect of the bifocal segment on prismatic effect at the reading level: *(a)* prismatic effect with a +3.00D single vision lens; *(b)* prismatic effect with a +3.00D distance lens combined with a +2.00D addition in the form of an Executive bifocal whose segment pole is at the dividing line.

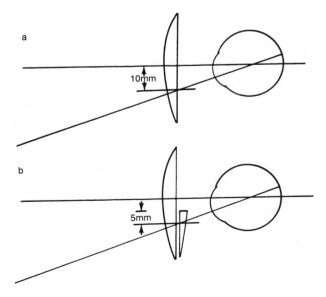

time the wearer directs the line of vision downward across the dividing line. Even though the patient will learn to ignore the displacement of the environment, it will never cease to occur. Consequently, we should expect jump to be a greater problem for the wearer than segment-induced prismatic effect.

Total prismatic effect at the reading level

The total vertical prismatic effect at the reading level is found by adding the prismatic effect induced by the distance lens to that induced by the segment. For a patient who wears a +3.00D sphere at distance with a +2.00D addition in the form of an Executive bifocal and reads at a level 5mm below the dividing line, the prismatic effect due to the distance lens would be

$$0.5(3) = 1.5\Delta \text{ base-up,}$$

and the prismatic effect due to the bifocal addition would be

$$0.5(2) = 1\Delta \text{ base-up,}$$

for a total of 2.5Δ base-up.

For minus lenses the Executive bifocal provides a minimum of prismatic effect, whereas for plus lenses the Ultex 38 provides a minimum of prismatic effect. For the straight-top bifocal (which has a segment pole coinciding with the reading level), the vertical prismatic effect at the reading level is that due to the distance power only; therefore, it does not change when the wearer switches from single vision lenses to bifocals.

The total vertical prismatic effect at the reading level is of practical importance, because it determines the amount of transverse chromatic aberration to which the wearer will be subject.

Chromatic aberration

Axial chromatic aberration is expressed as the dioptric difference between the red and blue foci for white light along the optic axis of the lens. It presents little problem for lenses made of ophthalmic crown glass (whether single vision or bifocal lenses) because it adds to or subtracts from the axial chromatic aberration of the eye. Even when flint glass is used, axial chromatic aberration can be safely ignored.

Transverse chromatic aberration is a potential problem for wearers of single vision lenses as well as bifocal lenses, since it can cause the wearer to see *color fringes* when looking through a point in the lens some distance from the lens pole. Transverse chromatic aberration varies directly with the power of the lens and the distance from the pole of the lens

to the point in question, and it varies inversely with the nu value (V) of the lens, as shown by the formula

$$\text{Transverse chromatic aberration} = \frac{P}{V} = \frac{dF}{V}.$$

For bifocal lenses, transverse chromatic aberration may be considered in either the vertical or the horizontal meridian. Confining our discussion to the vertical meridian, transverse chromatic aberration for a one-piece bifocal lens can be determined by considering the distance lens and the segment as two separate lenses, adding the prismatic effect (for any point on the lens) of the distance lens and that of the segment, and dividing by the nu value of the lens material:

$$\text{Transverse chromatic aberration} = \frac{d_D F_D + d_s F_s}{V},$$

where

F_D and F_s = the powers of the distance lens and the segment

d_D = the distance from the point in question to the distance pole

d_s = the distance from the point in question to the segment pole.

To determine the transverse chromatic aberration of a fused bifocal, Jalie (1974) suggested that the lens be considered as having three components, the transverse chromatic aberration being the total of that due to each of the three components:

Transverse chromatic aberration

$$= \frac{d_D F_D}{V_D} - \frac{d_s F_s K}{V_D} - \frac{d_s F_s (K + 1)}{V_s},$$

where

d_D, d_s, F_D, and F_s have the same meanings as before

V_D = the nu value of the distance lens

V_s = the nu value of the bifocal segment.

K is a constant whose value is given by the expression

$$K = \frac{n_D - 1}{n_s - n_D}.$$

The use of these formulas is demonstrated by examples 1–5.

Example 1. An Executive bifocal has a distance power of +2.00D sphere and an addition of +2.00D. The dividing line is 5mm below the geometrical center of the lens, and the reading level is 10mm below the geometrical center (or 5mm below the dividing line). Recalling that the distance pole and the segment pole of an Executive bifocal are both located at the level of the dividing line, the transverse chromatic aberration at the reading level for this lens is

$$\frac{0.5(2) + 0.5(2)}{60} = 0.033\Delta.$$

However, for a point 10mm below the reading level, the transverse chromatic aberration for this lens would be

$$\frac{1.5(2) + 1.5(2)}{60} = 0.10\Delta.$$

If we consider chromatic aberration of 0.10Δ or more to be sufficient to cause the wearer (under certain conditions) to see color fringes, the chromatic aberration at the reading level would be no problem for the wearer but that resulting for a point near the lower edge of the lens conceivably could cause a problem.

Example 2. An Executive bifocal has a distance power of -2.00D sphere and a $+2.00$D addition. The chromatic aberration at the reading level for this lens is

$$\frac{0.5(-2) + 0.5(2)}{60} = 0.$$

For a point 10mm below the reading level, it would be

$$\frac{1.5(-2) + 1.5(2)}{60} = 0.$$

It is obvious that for a distance power of more than -2.00D, some chromatic aberration would result. We can conclude that for the Executive bifocal, a hyperope is likely to encounter a significant amount of transverse chromatic aberration when looking through the lower part of the lens, while the chromatic aberration experienced by a myope is not likely to be significant.

Example 3. A straight-top fused bifocal has a distance power of $+2.00$D sphere and an addition of $+2.00$D. The segment pole is at the reading level (5mm below the segment top and 10mm below the distance pole). The nu value of the segment glass is 36, and the value of K is 4. The transverse chromatic aberration at the reading level for this lens will be

$$\frac{1(2)}{60} - \frac{0(2)(4)}{60} + \frac{0(2)(5)}{36} = 0.033\Delta,$$

or the chromatic aberration due to the distance portion of the lens only.

For a point 10mm below the reading level, the chromatic aberration would be

$$\frac{2(2)}{60} - \frac{1(2)(4)}{60} + \frac{1(2)(5)}{36} = 0.210\Delta,$$

or more than twice that found for the same point on an Executive bifocal lens of the same power.

Example 4. For a similar straight-top bifocal with a distance power of -2.00D sphere and a $+2.00$D addition, chromatic aberration at the reading level would be

$$\frac{1(-2)}{60} - \frac{0(2)(4)}{60} + \frac{0(2)(5)}{36} = -0.033\Delta,$$

or, as with the $+2.00$D lens, that of the distance portion of the lens only (but opposite in direction to that for the plus lens). For a point 10mm below the reading level, the transverse chromatic aberration would be

$$\frac{2(-2)}{60} - \frac{1(2)(6)}{60} + \frac{1(2)(5)}{36} = 0.078\Delta.$$

As with the Executive bifocal, the myope experiences less chromatic aberration than the hyperope when looking through the lower part of the lens.

Example 5. Chromatic aberration for a fused bifocal can be decreased by the use of a "no-chrome" bifocal having a segment made of a material with a higher nu value. For the lens considered in example 3 (straight-top fused bifocal with a distance power of $+2.00$D sphere and an addition of $+2.00$D), the use of a segment having a nu value of 50 and a constant (K) having a value of 6 would result in the following transverse chromatic aberration at a point 10mm below the reading level:

$$\frac{2(2)}{60} - \frac{1(2)(6)}{60} + \frac{1(2)(7)}{50} = 0.147\Delta,$$

thus reducing the chromatic aberration by about one-third.

Fortunately, even with Kryptok or straight-top fused bifocals with flint segments and with a moderately high-distance correction—what might be considered the "worst case" for chromatic aberration when looking through the lower part of the segment—few patients complain of seeing color fringes.

Vertical prismatic effect at the reading level

If bifocal lenses are to be prescribed for a patient whose distance lenses have different powers in the vertical meridian, any of three methods can be used to compensate for the induced differential prismatic effect at the reading level.

1. The Univis R-compensated bifocal.
Recall that the Univis R bifocal is a fused bifocal having a ribbon segment, 14mm high. With the *R-compensated segment*, the center of the segment can be placed at any level from 4–10mm below the top of the segment. The amount of vertical prism that can be compensated by this method depends on the power of the bifocal addition and can be determined by means of Prentice's rule. For a +2.50D addition and a reading level 10mm below the distance major reference point, the maximum amount of prism that can be compensated is

$$P = dF = 0.6(2.50) = 1.5\Delta.$$

The lens for the less myopic or more hyperopic eye (requiring base-down prism) would have the segment center located 10mm below the segment top, whereas the lens for the other eye would have the segment center located 4mm below the segment top (explaining the 0.6 in the equation). In this case, the bifocal segment for the least myopic eye would look like an upside down *D* segment, whereas the one for the more myopic eye would look like an ordinary *D* segment.

2. Prism segment bifocals.
A relatively small number of bifocal styles (including the Univis, the Panoptik, and the Executive) are available with vertical prism segments. The amount of prism that can be incorporated in these segments is limited to about 3Δ.

3. Bicentric grinding.
By the use of bicentric grinding, a *slab-off lens* can be made. The lower part of the more minus or less plus lens is "slabbed off," resulting in a lens having a horizontal dividing line across the middle, above which there is no prism but below which there is base-up prism. If a one-piece (Executive) bifocal is used, the dividing line will coincide with the dividing line between the distance and near portions of the lens, so the slabbed-off lens will have the same general appearance as the patient's other lens. If a fused flat-top bifocal is used, the dividing line on the slabbed-off lens will be more noticeable; however, the use of as wide a segment as possible (35mm) will make the dividing line less conspicuous than would a narrower segment. As much as 5 or 6Δ of vertical prismatic effect at the reading level can be provided by the use of bicentric grinding.

In determining the amount of prismatic effect to be compensated when any of the three methods (R-compensated, prism segment, or bicentric grinding) is to be used, the power of the bifocal addition need not be taken into consideration as long as it is the same for both lenses. It is necessary only to determine the amount of power difference for the two eyes in the vertical meridian and the patient's customary reading level, and then to use Prentice's rule to determine how much prism should be compensated. When bicentric grinding is used, base-up prism is prescribed for the less plus or more minus lens.

If the patient has not previously worn a correction with compensation for the vertical prismatic effect at near, it may be wise to slightly undercorrect the compensating prism. A patient is usually better able to adapt to an undercorrection than to an overcorrection.

Provision of horizontal prism power

When a patient has esophoria (or eso fixation disparity) or exophoria (or exo fixation disparity) at near but not at distance, the practitioner may consider the possibility of providing base-out or base-in prism at near by prescribing "prism segments." Many manufacturers make available prism segment fused straight-top bifocals allowing for a maximum amount of prism of 2 or 3Δ (or a total of 4 to 6Δ base-in or base-out for both lenses).

Prism segments are not often prescribed, and for good reason. Although presbyopic patients tend to be highly exophoric at near, they seldom complain of asthenopia. Sheedy and Saladin (1975) found that presbyopic patients, although exophoric at near, have no greater fixation disparity at near than nonpresbyopes who have less exophoria. In addition, they found the fixation disparity curves of presbyopes to have a lower slope than nonpresbyopes' fixation disparity curves. A low slope is associated with comfortable binocular vision. Sheedy and Saladin hypothesized that, because the crystalline lens does not respond to innervation for accommodation, the presbyopic individual has almost unrestricted use of accommodative convergence; it is this accommodative convergence that allows the presbyope to easily compensate for large amounts of exophoria at near.

Horizontal prism at near induced by the distance prescription

Except in rare cases, when the distance portion of a bifocal lens has no power at all in the horizontal meridian, the near portion of any bifocal lens—whether fused or one-piece—contains horizontal prism power induced by the distance portion of the lens. Although this induced prism can be minimized or eliminated by decentration of the segments or by the use of prism segments, most practitioners do nothing to compensate for it (and many are probably not even aware of its existence). The extent of the induced prism is demonstrated in examples 1 and 2.

Example 1. A patient's distance prescription is +2.50D sphere, each eye, with a +2.50D addition. The distance PD is 66mm, and the near PD is 62mm. Assuming that the lenses have been decentered correctly for distance and that the segment inset is correct, what horizontal prismatic effect would the wearer experience when reading through the near portion of the lens?

The answer to this question has two parts. First, how much horizontal prismatic effect would be due to the addition? If the segments were properly inset for a 62mm PD, the +2.50D addition would result in no induced horizontal prismatic effect. Second, how much prismatic effect would be induced by the distance lens power? With respect to the near PD, the distance portion of each lens is decentered outward, so (because the distance power is plus) base-out prism will be induced at near. The amount of induced prism can be determined by applying Prentice's rule:

$$P = dF = 0.2(2.50) = 0.5\Delta \text{ base-out.}$$

This is the induced prism for each eye, so the total would be 1.0Δ base-out. Because most presbyopes are exophoric at near, this induced prism would simply add 1.0Δ to the exophoria that would exist if the patient looked through perfectly centered distance and near lenses.

In example 1, the base-out prism induced at near by the distance lenses could be eliminated by providing an additional amount of segment inset, thus inducing base-in prism. If the segment inset were increased to 4mm for each lens, when the patient used the reading portion of the lenses he or

she would be subject to—in addition to the 0.5Δ base-out for each eye due to the distance lens—the following amount due to the segment itself:

$$P = dF = 0.2(2.5) = 0.5\Delta \text{ base-in.}$$

For each eye, the amount of base-in prism induced by the segment just equals the amount of base-out prism induced by the distance portion of the lens. Equal values for the distance portion and the addition were chosen to demonstrate that in this special case, one needs only to double the amount of segment inset to eliminate the prismatic effect at near induced by the distance lenses.

Unless distance lens powers are very large, increased segment inset is not usually considered necessary. For example, for a distance prescription of +10.00D (and distance and near PDs of 66 and 62mm), the base-out prism at near induced by the distance lens power would be 0.2(10) = 2.0Δ for each eye, or 4Δ for both eyes. To eliminate this prismatic effect by additional segment inset, each segment would have to be inset an additional 8mm for a +2.50D addition because 0.8(2.5) = 2Δ for each eye. This amount at decentration, if a fused bifocal were used, would have the disadvantage that the reading fields for the eyes would not overlap.

Example 2. A patient's distance prescription is −2.50D sphere, each eye, with a +2.50D addition. The distance PD is 66mm, and the near PD is 62mm. Assuming that the lenses have been decentered correctly for distance and that the near inset is correct, what is the horizontal prismatic effect through the near portion of the lens?

As in example 1, if the segments are correctly inset for a 62mm PD, no prismatic effect will occur due to the +2.50D addition. Because the distance lenses will be decentered outward with respect to the near PD, the minus powers of these lenses will induce base-in prism at the near PD. The amount of induced prism will be

$$P = dF = 0.2(-2.50) = 0.5\Delta \text{ base-in,}$$

for a total of 1.0Δ base-in, for both eyes. Because the patient probably will be exophoric at near, the 1.0Δ of base-in prism will reduce the exophoria by that amount, thus relieving the strain on fusional vergence.

On the basis of these examples, it is clear that plus power in the patient's distance prescription induces base-out prism at the near PD (which will aggravate an exophoria at near), and that minus power in the distance prescription induces base-in prism at the near PD (which will reduce an exophoria at near).

However, because presbyopic patients seldom complain of asthenopia due to exophoria at near (apparently due, as already indicated, to the almost unrestricted use of accommodative convergence) the induced base-out prism seldom presents a problem.

Verifying segment inset for a bifocal correction

When verifying the distance correction in a pair of glasses received from the laboratory, the lenses are centered in the lensometer, "spotted" by means of the inked marking device mounted in the instrument, and the distance between the centers is measured with a millimeter ruler. This is the correct procedure to use for verifying the distance centers, or the "distance PD of the glasses," but it is not appropriate for verifying the segment inset (except in the rare case when the distance lens has no power in the horizontal meridian). As described earlier, the distance lens will induce horizontal prism in the segment: the induced prismatic effect will cause the lensometer mire image to be decentered inward or outward from the pole of the segment.

We must think in terms of the distance lens existing *behind* the bifocal segment. It actually does exist behind the bifocal segment in a fused bifocal,

whereas in an Executive bifocal, the distance portion of the lens and the segment are a single piece of glass. However, the same principle applies.

There are two correct ways of verifying segment inset. One, which can be done with any fused bifocal, is simply to measure the distance from the temporal edge of one segment to the nasal edge of the other (in the finished glasses) with a millimeter ruler (see Figure 13.24a). This should result in the near PD (the distance PD minus the total segment inset for the two segments). This system does not work with an Executive bifocal because the segment continues to the edges of the lens. With this lens, the method of verifying segment inset is to look at a vertical line through the lens and to find the position of the lens relative to the vertical line where the line does not deviate in passing through the lens (as shown in Figure 13.24b). At this point, a dot is placed at the upper edge of the segment where the line intersects it, and the distance between the dots on the two lenses is measured to determine the near PD (see Figure 13.24c). This method of verifying segment inset can be used not only with the Executive bifocal but with any type of bifocal.

Field of view of a bifocal segment

For a given bifocal add, vertex distance, and pupil size, the field of view of a bifocal segment depends only on the segment size. Years ago, many manufacturers attempted to make bifocal segments as small as possible. Kryptok bifocals came in 19 and 22mm widths, and many practitioners routinely used the 19mm segments. Very small (12mm-wide) "button" Kryptok segments were popular with some practitioners; the Univis B segment (9mm high and 22mm wide) was a further manifestation of the desire for the bifocal segment not to intrude more than absolutely necessary into the distance portion of the lens.

By a simple geometric construction (see Figure 13.25), it can be shown that if a lens is at a vertex distance of 13mm and if the center of rotation of the eye is located 14mm behind the corneal apex, a 20mm round bifocal segment would provide a macular field of view measuring approximately 35 degrees in all directions. However, many people engage in occupations requiring a wide field of view at near (working at a desk is one example), and many find it annoying to make a quick eye movement to one side and find that vision is blurred by the segment edge. As a result, bifocal segments have increased from 19 or 20mm to 22, 25, 28, and, finally,

Figure 13.24   Determining the segment PD: (a) for fused bifocals; (b) and (c) for the Executive bifocal (from American Optical Corporation, 1975).

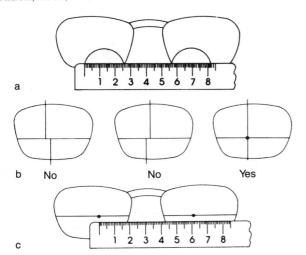

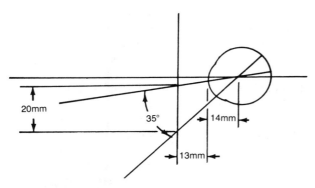

Figure 13.25 Macular field of view (constructed to scale) for a 20mm round bifocal segment assuming plano power at near. The field of view would be somewhat smaller for plus power at near and somewhat larger for minus power at near.

35mm. For the Executive bifocal, the width of the segment is the width of the lens. Wide bifocal segments appear to be here to stay.

Meridional magnification of bifocal lenses

The spectacle magnification formula (given earlier in this chapter) shows that the power of the front surface of a lens is an important factor in determining the magnification brought about by the lens. Therefore, when a toric surface (for the correction of astigmatism) is ground on the front surface of the lens, magnification differences between the two principal meridians will be greater than if the toric surface were ground on the back surface of the lens. In recent years, most single vision lenses have been in back toric form, therefore minimizing these magnification differences. However, bifocal lenses having the bifocal segment on the back surface of the lens necessitate the use of front surface toric curves. Fortunately, all bifocals (with the exception of the Ultex bifocal) have front surface segments, allowing back surface toric curves.

Plastic Bifocal Lenses

With the large lens sizes currently in use, plastic lenses have become increasingly popular because of their considerably lighter weight. One-piece plastic bifocal lenses are available in the Executive style and also in straight-top and round (similar in appearance to Kryptok) styles. The straight-top and round styles, as well as the Executive, are front surface bifocals. In the case of the straight-top and round bifocals, the

bifocal segment creates a ridge at the segment edge.

Most calculations relative to bifocal lenses are independent of the material of which the lens is made, and therefore they apply to plastic lenses as well as glass lenses. These include calculations of image jump, segment-induced prismatic effects, total prismatic effect at the reading level, differential vertical prismatic effects at the reading level, and horizontal prism at near induced by the distance correction. Plastic lens materials have a nu value close to that of ophthalmic crown glass, so chromatic aberration compares closely with that of one-piece bifocals made of ophthalmic crown.

Blended Bifocals

Blended bifocals are one-piece bifocal lenses having round segments, in which the line of demarcation between the distance portion of the lens and the bifocal segment has been obliterated by a polishing process. This results in an "invisible" bifocal segment. There is a blurred area surrounding the segment, 1 or 2mm in width, in which neither distance nor near vision is clear. These lenses are marketed under various trade names, including the Beach Blended bifocal and the Younger Seamless bifocal.

Blended bifocals are designed for no purpose other than to render the bifocal segment invisible; they cater strictly to the wearer's vanity. Some bifocal wearers are willing to put up with the blurred area between the distance and near portions of the lens, as well as the rather small reading field, to avoid the stigma of wearing bifocals.

Trifocal Lenses

A patient requiring only a +1.00 or +1.50D bifocal addition still has sufficient accommodation to have acceptably clear vision—with appropriate corrective lenses for distance and near—for distances ranging from infinity to 8 or 10 inches. However, when an addition of about +2.00D or more is required (usually indicating an amplitude of accommodation of 1.00D or less), appropriate distance and near correction by means of bifocal lenses results in unacceptable arm's-length vision at distances from about 24–36 inches. Clear vision at this intermediate range can be obtained by the provision of a reading lens or addition about one-half that required for the usual 40cm (16-inch) reading distance.

The first trifocal lens was introduced by the Univis Lens Company. As shown in Figure 13.26, the intermediate segment "sits on top of the bifocal," encroaching on what would otherwise be the distance portion of the lens. Univis originally offered a choice of 6 and 8mm-high intermediate segments, but after several years it settled on a 7mm-high segment. Most bifocal manufacturers now offer trifocal lenses (including fused lenses, such as the Panoptic and other straight-top lenses, and one-piece lenses, such as the Executive). Trifocals are also available in plastic in both the Executive and the one-piece straight-top style. In almost all cases, intermediate segments are 7mm high, and the intermediate addition is one-half the power of the near addition.

Prescribing and fitting

Trifocal lenses should be considered for any patient requiring a +2.00D addition or more, particularly if the individual's life-style includes the frequent use of intermediate vision. Although a short period of adaptation to the intermediate segment is necessary, most patients conclude that the adaptation period was well worth the trouble. If on reexamination a year or two later a trifocal wearer requests to switch back to bifocals, the request is due to the fact that (1) the patient has little need for intermediate vision in everyday life or (2) the lenses were incorrectly prescribed or fitted.

Prescribing. Many practitioners are accustomed to undercorrecting hyperopic presbyopes for distance vision and compensating for the undercorrection at distance by prescribing a higher addition than would otherwise be necessary. This may be satisfactory for a beginning presbyope who is still able to make use of some accommodation. As a matter of fact, it sometimes is necessary to avoid complaints of poor vision at night due to night myopia. (However, one problem with undercorrecting at distance—even for the beginning presbyope—is that the distance lenses provide insufficient help for arm's-length distances.) For the older

presbyope who no longer attempts to accommodate, night myopia is less of a problem, and there is no reason not to fully correct the hyperopia. If trifocals are fitted with less than a full plus correction at distance, the intermediate portion of the lens just will not perform the way it was intended to.

Consider a hyperopic presbyope who is given a 0.50D undercorrection at distance with a +1.00D intermediate addition and a +2.00D near addition. Due to the 0.50D undercorrection at distance, the +1.00D intermediate addition is really only a +0.50D addition, providing clear vision (without the help of accommodation) at a distance of 2m. Although the near addition may provide clear vision for the usual range of about 12–24 inches, the intermediate addition will be useless for the 24-to-36-inch distance for which it was intended. Similarly, a myopic presbyope should not be overcorrected at distance.

Fitting. If a patient needs an intermediate lens, it is needed "on top of" the bifocal lens rather than in place of it. The biggest mistake made in fitting trifocals is to fit the intermediate segment (and, therefore, the near segment also) too low. If a bifocal segment height of 18mm in a specific frame is required, the patient will need an 18mm-high bifocal in the same frame (with a 25mm-high intermediate segment height) if trifocals are fitted. There are exceptions to this rule, but in the majority of cases it is a mistake to fit the near segment any lower when trifocals are fitted than when bifocals are fitted. The 7mm intermediate segment means that the top of the intermediate segment may split the pupil, and the patient will soon learn to tilt the head down slightly when clear distance vision is needed.

Occupational Bifocals and Trifocals

The most commonly used occupational lens is the double D or similar lens having a bifocal addition for the usual reading distance and an intermediate addition (or near addition) located at the top of the lens, with a 12-to-14mm-high distance portion between the two segments. This lens is indicated for electricians, painters, and other workers who must routinely work above eye level. The double D and the double-segment Executive are shown in Figure 13.27. For an individual whose work requires clear near vision above eye level but distance vision at and below eye level, an ordinary bifocal lens can be placed upside down so the segment is at the top of the lens. A presbyopic painter, who must look at a

Figure 13.26   Trifocal lenses: (a) Univis; (b) Executive. For each lens, the intermediate segment is 7mm high.

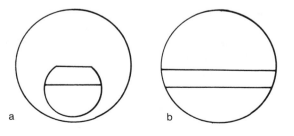

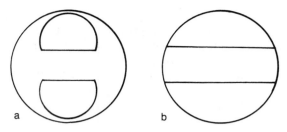

Figure 13.27 Occupational bifocals: *(a)* **double D;** *(b)* **double-segment Executive. The distance portion (between the upper and lower segments) usually is from 12–14mm high.**

model or distant object on one side of the visual field and at the canvas on the other side, may be pleased with a sideways bifocal segment of the appropriate power.

PROGRESSIVE ADDITION LENSES

Progressive addition lenses not only have invisible segments but, as the name implies, the power of the addition gradually increases as the line of vision sweeps downward through the lens. Although the stated reason for recommending these lenses is the availability of clear vision for all distances, practitioners as well as patients often are attracted to these lenses because their segments are invisible. However, many wearers of progressive addition lenses, including the writer, wear them not for cosmetic reasons but because they provide clear vision for all desired distances *without the annoyance of the dividing lines* that are present in trifocal lenses.

The first progressive addition lens available in the United States was the *Omnifocal*, developed by Volk in 1962. The *Varilux* lens was developed by Maitenaz of France in the 1950s, but was not available in the United States until 1965. The original Varilux lens has now been replaced by the *Varilux 2*. In 1973, the American Optical Corporation introduced the *Ultravue* lens, a CR–39 plastic lens having a near "segment" width of 25mm. In recent years, a large number of progressive addition lenses have been introduced.

Optical Properties

Progressive addition lenses have aspheric front surfaces that provide a gradual increase in plus

power as the line of vision sweeps downward through a *progressive corridor* (see Figure 13.28), at the expense of blurred vision on either side due to the presence of astigmatism. As described by Davis (1978), the Varilux 2 and Ultravue handle the problem of astigmatism in different ways (see Figure 13.29). Varilux 2 spreads the power change in the vertical meridian over the entire lens, from top to bottom, minimizing the amount of astigmatism but resulting in a relatively narrow area of maximum addition (at the bottom of the lens) free of astigmatism. The Ultravue, on the other hand, has a well-defined distance portion free of astigmatism; the rate of progression of added plus power increases in the lower portion of the lens, resulting in a relatively wide astigmatism-free area of maximum addition at the bottom of the lens, but at the expense of larger amounts of astigmatism on either side of the "addition."

The choices made by the designers of the Varilux 2 and the Ultravue lens can be summarized by noting that the use of an aspheric surface (which is necessary to provide an increase in plus power from the upper to the lower part of the lens) results in unwanted astigmatism. The designer can either spread this astigmatism throughout the lens (Varilux 2) or concentrate it in areas where it will seem to create the least amount of harm (Ultravue). The differences in vertical plus-power change, "segment" size and shape, and areas of astigmatism are shown by the two grid patterns in Figure 13.29.

Available Progressive Addition Lenses

A large variety of progressive addition lenses are available. The original Ultravue lens was followed in 1978 by the *Ultravue 28*, having a 28mm-wide segment area, and in 1982 by the American Optical Corporation's *TrueVision* lens, having a 15mm-deep progressive corridor (as compared to the 10–12mm corridor of the Ultravue lens), an unaberrated distance area, and a fairly wide segment area but lower in the lens because of the longer progressive corridor. The Younger *10/28* lens was introduced in 1978, having a 10mm-deep progressive corridor and a 30mm-wide segment area. In 1982, Younger introduced the *CPS* (cosmetic parabolic sphere) lens, having an unaberrated distance area, a 12.5mm-deep progressive corridor, and a relatively small segment area. Silor Optical, which originally marketed the Varilux lens, introduced the *Super NoLine* lens in 1980, having a 12mm-deep progressive corridor and a 25mm-wide segment area. Univis Lens company

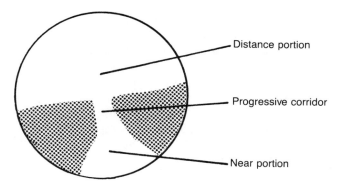

Figure 13.28 **Schematic representation of a progressive addition lens. The shaded areas indicate the presence of varying amounts of astigmatism.**

introduced the *Unison* lens in 1980 (now manufactured by Vision-Ease), which has a spherical distance portion, a 12mm-deep progressive corridor, and a fairly wide segment area. These and other lenses are described in more detail by Fannin and Grosvenor (1987).

Patient Acceptance

To determine the patient acceptance of progressive addition lenses, Borish, Hitzman, and Brookman (1980) fitted both Varilux 2 and Ultravue lenses on each of 54 presbyopic patients. Using a double-masked procedure in which neither the practitioner nor the technician knew which lenses were being worn, each subject wore the Varilux 2 and Ultravue lenses, in identical frames, for one month each. It was found that 93 percent of the subjects preferred progressive addition lenses to ordinary bifocals or reading glasses. Although most subjects had no strong preference for one lens or the other, younger subjects (requiring low- or medium-power additions) preferred the Varilux 2 by a ratio of approximately 2:1. This was interpreted by Borish et al. as due to the fact that the reading portion of the Varilux 2, although physically narrower than that of the Ultravue, has the advantage of only gradually increasing astigmatism on either side. This allows the younger presbyopes to increase the effective reading field by accommodating for the astigmatic image. The older presbyopes, on the other hand, tended to be evenly divided between the two lenses. This was probably because some older presbyopes were unable to clear up the gradually increasing astigmatism lateral to the reading portion of the Varilux

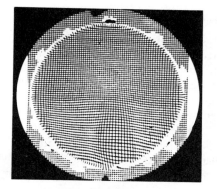

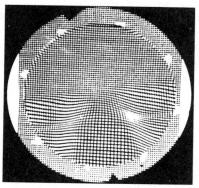

Figure 13.29 **Grid patterns for (a) Varilux 2 and (b) Ultravue** (Davis, 1978).

2 lens and, therefore, were more satisfied with the wider reading portion of the Ultravue (although it has much greater amounts of astigmatism lateral to the reading portion).

The acceptance of progressive addition lenses as compared to conventional bifocal lenses was investigated by Hitzman and Myers (1985), who fitted each of 40 clinical patients with both Younger CPS lenses and with bifocals having straight-top fused, 25mm-wide segments in identical frames. One-half of the subjects wore one correction (progressive or conventional) and one-half wore the other for the first month, wearing the alternate correction for the second month and then wearing the first correction for an additional week. Of the 40 patients, 28 (70 percent) preferred the Younger CPS lenses and 12 (30 precent) preferred the bifocals. The authors concluded that the greater preference for the CPS lenses was because they provide acceptable vision at all distances, with a smooth transition from one distance to another, and that this advantage outweighed the disadvantage of having a relatively narrow segment area.

Fitting and Dispensing

When taking the measurements for progressive addition lenses, it is necessary to (1) measure the interpupillary distance *monocularly*, using one of the "pupillometers" available, since each pupil must be aligned correctly with the progressive corridor; and (2) determine the position of the *center of the pupil* while the patient is wearing the frame (in the correct size) in which the lenses will be mounted. The center of the distance portion of the lens is normally located 2mm below the center of the pupil. If the sample frame contains lenses, the simplest procedure is for the patient to hold the head erect, looking straight ahead, and for the dispenser (at the patient's eye level) to use a felt-tipped pen to mark the point on each lens corresponding to the center of the pupil. If the sample frame is not glazed, a strip of transparent tape can be stretched across the eyewire, and the dispenser can place the mark on the tape.

In selecting the frame, it should provide for a vertical distance of at least 22mm below the level of the center of the pupil: this will allow for a 12mm-deep progressive corridor (which begins 2mm below the pupil center) and an 8mm-deep segment area. For a progressive corridor deeper than 12mm, a vertical distance greater than 22mm will be desirable. A frame fitted with adjustable pads should be used because slight vertical adjustments may be required when the lenses are dispensed. As is the case with bifocal or trifocal lens fitting, dispensers are more likely to fit progressive lenses *too low* than too high: the majority of failures in fitting these lenses are due to placing the lens centers too low or to incorrect monocular interpupillary distances.

Comparison of Optical Characteristics

The Commission of Ophthalmic Standards of the American Optometric Association has recommended a format for displaying the optical characteristics of progressive addition lenses consisting of two diagrams, one showing *isospherical equivalent* lines and the other showing *isocylindrical* lines. Sheedy, Buri, Bailey, Azus, and Borish (1987) used a Humphrey Lens Analyzer to make power measurements every 3 degrees (about 1.5mm on the lens surface), both vertically and horizontally, on ten progressive addition lenses from various manufacturers. This required about 700 measurements per lens. Each of the lenses had a plano distance power and a +2.00D add, was made on the base curve normally used by the manufacturer, and was edged 62mm round. On the basis of these measurements,

two graphs were plotted for each lens, one showing isospherical equivalent lines and the other showing isocylindrical lines together with axis orientation. Graphs for two representative lenses—the Varilux 2 and the TrueVision (both in plastic)—are shown in Figure 13.30.

Sheedy et al. (1987) tabulated the depression of the visual axes (in degrees) necessary to obtain addition powers of +0.25, +0.50, +1.00, +1.50, and +2.00D. In each case, the depression of the visual axes was that required for the most superior location of the stated addition power. Table 13.4 is based on the authors' tabulation for +1.00 and +2.00D additions, and presents depression of the visual axes in millimeters rather than in degrees (using the close approximation that for a 27mm stop distance, 1 degree = 2mm). The figures for +1.00D of add are included in Table 13.4 because they represent the power of the intermediate segment for a +2.00D add trifocal lens. As noted by Sheedy et al., the center of a 7mm intermediate segment for a trifocal lens, fitted at the lower pupil margin, is 5–6mm below the pupil: this can be compared to the values ranging from 4mm (for the Younger CPS lens) to 10mm (for the Varilus plastic lens). It is of interest that for four of the ten lenses, the +2.00D add power was not reached: the authors commented that some fitting guidelines recommend that the near addition be increased by 0.50D to make the lenses more useful for the patient.

Sheedy et al. (1987) listed the advantages of progressive addition lenses as including a much better transition of power from distance to near and the obvious cosmetic advantage, and their shortcomings as unwanted cylinder errors, limited useful field width, and larger required depression of the visual axes to view through the near portions of the lenses. They concluded that the advantages outweigh the shortcomings for many multifocal lens wearers. They suggested that, in order for the prescriber of progressive addition lenses to be able to make informed prescribing decisions, the optical characteristics of the lenses should be available in a format (such as that recommended by the American Optometric Association) that allows comparison of relevant parameters.

OPHTHALMIC LENSES FOR APHAKIA

When ophthalmic lenses are to be prescribed for an aphakic patient, one of the main problems confronting the practitioner is correctly specifying

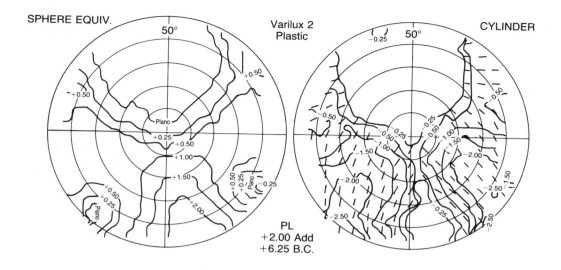

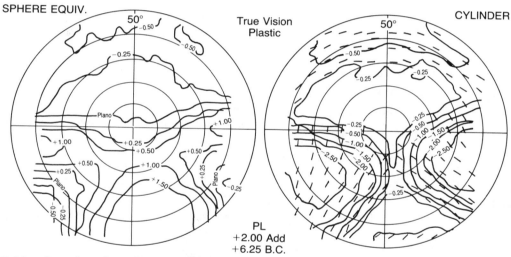

Figure 13.30 Graphs showing isospherical equivalent lines (left) and isocylindrical lines (right) for Varilux 2 (top) and TrueVision (bottom) lenses (Sheedy et al., 1987).

Table 13.4 Depression of the visual axes required to obtain specified addition power (Sheedy et al., 1987).

	Addition power (D)	
	+1.00	+2.00
Progressive R	7mm	14mm
Sola VIP	6mm	13.5mm
Super NoLine	5mm	15.5mm
TrueVision	8.5mm	—
Unison	6.5mm	—
Varilux 2 (glass)	7mm	16mm
Varilux 2 (plastic)	10mm	14.5mm
Varilux 2 (high-index)	9mm	—
Younger CPS	4mm	—
Younger 10/30	5.5mm	10.5mm

the power of the lenses. As shown earlier in this chapter, an error of 5mm in vertex distance for a +12.00D lens will result in an effective power error of 0.75D. Such an error can be avoided by verifying the refraction with trial lenses and a trial frame, and making sure that the strongest lens is in the back cell of the trial frame and that the distance from the back surface of that lens to the corneal apex is equal to the vertex distance that will be used in the patient's new correction.

The main disadvantages of the strong plus lenses that aphakic patients must wear are (1) lens weight,

(2) lens thickness (from the point of view of appearance), (3) magnified appearance of the wearer's eyes, (4) lens aberrations, (5) decreased field of view, and (6) increased retinal image size. All of these problems can be avoided if contact lenses rather than ophthalmic lenses are fitted. The magnified appearance of the wearer's eyes can be eliminated *only* by the use of contact lenses, because image magnification for high plus lenses (no matter which side of the lenses one looks through) is greatly influenced by the distance of the correcting lens from the principal plane of the eye. All the other problems can be minimized by careful selection of ophthalmic lens parameters.

Lens weight can be greatly reduced by the use of plastic rather than glass lenses. The center thickness of an aphakic lens can be reduced by using a *lenticular lens* consisting of a powered central portion about 40mm in diameter and a plano carrier. Lens aberrations can be minimized by the use of an aspheric front surface, along with careful selection of base curves.

Aberrations of Aphakic Lenses

As noted earlier, modern ophthalmic lenses are designed to minimize the effects of oblique astigmatism and curvature of image. Ordinarily, no attempt is made to minimize the effects of distortion, since this aberration presents little problem for low- and medium-powered lenses and its correction would require much steeper lenses than would be needed otherwise.

Recall that distortion occurs when a stop—such as the pupil of the eye—is placed at some distance behind a lens, so the only rays for an off-axis object point that can be included in the image are those entering the periphery of the lens. These rays are subject to prismatic effects, which increase as the distance from the lens pole increases. The amount of distortion, therefore, increases with lens power and also with lens diameter. For a positive lens, the distortion causes a square object to suffer pincushion distortion.

Jalie (1974) showed diagramatically the back surface curves required to minimize distortion for lenses of various back vertex powers. The graph shows that for a +10.00D lens, a back surface power of about −18.00D minimizes distortion; for a +15.00D lens, a back surface power of about −12.00D minimizes distortion. These back surface powers would require front surface powers of about +25.00D, which would be impractical; however,

Jalie's graph shows that the *more steeply curved* an aphakic lens is, the less distortion there will be.

The Visual World of the Aphakic

The spectacle-wearing aphakic is not only subject to distortion, but also must contend with a greatly decreased field of view and a greatly magnified retinal image. As shown in Figure 13.31, the decreased field of view is due to the fact that the high plus lens induces base-toward-the-center prism power, which not only reduces the size of the field of view through the lens but results in a ring scotoma between the outer extent of the field through the lens and the field beyond the edge of the lens. As described by Welsh (1961), when an object presents itself in the peripheral field beyond the lens (and beyond the ring scotoma), the patient turns the head and eyes toward the object, causing the object to disappear momentarily into the blind area and then to reappear in the seeing area. Welsh describes the scotoma as the *roving ring scotoma* and uses the term *jack-in-the-box phenomenon* to describe the confusion experienced by the patient when objects jump into and out of the ring scotoma.

An additional problem is that of *retinal image magnification*. The retinal image magnification for an aphakic wearing spectacles is between 25 and 30 percent, compared with about 7 or 8 percent when contact lenses are worn. This extreme magnification not only causes familiar objects to appear to be much larger than they were formerly, but it also has the effect of causing objects to seem to be much closer than they actually are. As a consequence, the individual has difficulty performing everyday tasks, such as eating, until he or she learns to respond correctly to a whole new set of space perception clues.

The problems that aphakic patients have in adjusting to their spectacles have been cleverly described by an aphakic physician (Anonymous, 1952). The following quotations are typical of this anonymous author's experiences:

> It usually takes several weeks for the neophyte in aphakic vision to accustom himself to the magnified aspect of the outside world, forget his previous and now erroneous concepts of the size of objects, and so to overcome false orientation....The newly aphakic regards a door through which for years he has been accustomed to pass without misadventure and, to his amazement, he finds the jambs in each side curve in toward the middle and leave an aperature only a few inches wide at the center, through which all reason

tells him it will be impossible to wedge his portly person. When mature thought finally persuades him that this is an optical illusion, and he timidly advances to make the test, he finds to his delight that as he approaches the opening the curves recede gracefully and invitingly to his approach and he finds easy and unimpeded passage....Gradually he learns the secret of persuading the outside world to remain in a properly upright position and to abandon its sinuous behavior. The secret consists in holding his eyes motionless, his gaze fixed through the optical center of the correcting lens, and to move his head slowly to look at any desired object not in his direct view. (pp. 119–120)

Aphakic Lenses

The simplest form of aphakic lens is a full-diameter glass lens having a fused bifocal segment. Due to the excessive weight of glass and the presence of aberrations, these lenses are now used little except as temporary lenses to be worn after surgery until the eye stabilizes. The earliest attempt to improve on the full-diameter glass lens was the development of the glass lenticular cataract lens, having a 34mm-wide powered portion with a plano or low-powered carrier lens.

The development of plastic aspheric lenticular lenses was begun about 25 years ago, and at the present time each lens manufacturer has available a lens of this style. Typically, the powered portion of the lens has a diameter of 40mm, the back surface has a power of about −3.00 or −4.00D (and includes the cylinder, which is almost always required in an aphakic lens), and the aspheric curve is on the front surface. Compared with a full-diameter lens, the 40mm diameter of the powered portion allows a significant decrease in both center thickness and lens weight (although lens weight is obviously much less a problem when plastic is used). Although the field of view is limited compared with that of a full-diameter lens, this is not a serious handicap: the oblique aberrations of astigmatism, curvature of image, and distortion are at their greatest when the eye rotates sufficiently to look through the peripheral portion of a full-diameter aphakic lens. If lenticular lenses are fitted as close to the eyes as possible, not only does the angular field of view increase, but image magnification is held to a minimum.

In recent years, two manufacturers have developed full-diameter aspheric lenses having an exaggerated amount of asphericity, or *drop*, in the periphery. The Welsh 4-drop lens is made by Cataract Lens Laboratories, and the HyperAspheric

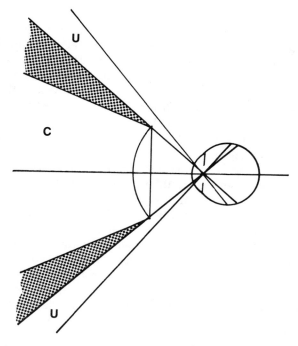

Figure 13.31 The field of view of an aphakic wearing spectacles. _C_ indicates the corrected field of view, seen through the lens, and _U_ indicates the uncorrected field of view, seen outside the lens. The shaded area indicates the roving ring scotoma. If the wearer turns the eyes toward an object in the uncorrected area, the object will disappear momentarily into the blind area and reappear in the seeing area (jack-in-the-box phenomenon). This can be minimized by fitting the lenses as close to the eyes as possible.

lens is made by Signet Optical Company. In describing these lenses, Davis (1978) pointed out that when plano back surface curves are used (which is the case with these lenses), the wearer encounters more spherical error, astigmatism, and distortion than would be the case if −3.00D or −5.00D back curves were used. In addition, flat lenses suffer more from reflections than meniscus lenses do. Davis makes the point that the increased asphericity, or power drop, is sufficient only to overcome the handicap of having a flat back surface.

Fitting procedures

In a discussion of optical considerations in aphakic fitting, Welsh (1971) describes what he calls the *minimal effective diameter system* of fitting full-diameter aspheric lenses. He suggests that the frame size be chosen such that the distance centers will not have to be decentered inward from the mechanical center. For a patient with a 66mm distance PD, he recommends a 48/18 combination frame, with the distance optical center placed 1.0–2.5mm above the mechanical center. Welsh also recommends the use of a pad bridge frame with jumbo pads, so the frames can be adjusted as close to the eyes as possible and can be adjusted downward somewhat (which is usually necessary, because the distance centers are purposely set higher than the mechanical centers). Only a small amount of pantoscopic tilt can be used; otherwise the lenses, because they fit closely, will touch the patient's face. For patients who desire stylish frames, Welsh recommends lenticular lenses rather than full-diameter lenses. For elderly aphakics who may have difficulty getting around if a bifocal is worn, he recommends the use of single vision aspheric lenses, fitted closely: the patient is instructed to push the lenses down on the nose for reading.

Prismatic effects at near

The discussion of bifocal lenses pointed out that even though the segment poles are correctly centered for the patient's near PD, the wearer will be subject to prismatic effects at near due to the power of the distance lenses. Although the induced prismatic effect is negligible for low-powered lenses, for an aphakic correction it will reach significant amounts.

For example, assume that an aphakic requiring a distance prescription of +13.00D sphere −1.00D cylinder, axis 90, each eye, is fitted with bifocal lenses; each has an addition of +2.50D and a segment inset of 2mm. Because the −1.00D cylinder manifests its power in the 180 meridian, the power in that meridian is +12.00D, and the amount of induced prism for each eye is

$$P = dF = 0.2(+12) = 2.4\Delta.$$

Because the distance lenses are decentered outward with respect to the near PD, the prism is in the base-out direction and is a total of 4.8Δ base-out for the two eyes. If the wearer were esophoric at near, the 4.8Δ base-out would be an advantage; however, most aphakics, like presbyopes, are exophoric at near, so the induced base-out prism may place undue strain on fusional vergence. The provision of additional segment inset in this case would be of little help in reducing the induced prism and would serve mainly to keep the fields of view for the two bifocals from coinciding. Aphakics apparently share the advantage of presbyopes (discussed in Chapter 12) of having almost unrestricted use of accommodative convergence. In any case, the presence of a high exophoria at near seldom appears to elicit complaints of discomfort.

Fitting the unilateral aphakic

If cataract surgery has been performed on only one eye, binocular vision with ophthalmic lenses will be impossible because of the large difference in retinal image size for the operated and unoperated eyes. The only way the patient will be able to make use of the operated eye will be for the unoperated eye to be fogged with a high plus lens. Welsh (1971) suggests that rather than order a "balance" lens for the unoperated eye, the practitioner order a lens that will be useful in the future when the cataract is removed from the eye. The lens should have the power that the practitioner predicts will be needed after surgery, and it should be properly centered for the eye. It can then be used as a temporary lens while the eye is healing.

Study Questions

1. A patient has exophoria at 6m, and the practitioner wishes to prescribe 1Δ, base-in, for each eye. If the patient's prescription is R −4.00DS, L −4.00DS, how much decentration (and in what direction) will be required to supply the prism?

2. What is the vertical prismatic effect at the reading level for a patient who wears the correction R +2.00DS, L +2.00DS − 1.00DC × 180 with a +2.50D addition for both eyes, if the patient reads at a level 10mm below the distance centers?

3. Is chromatic aberration likely to cause a problem for the single vision lens wearer? If so, in what way? What can be done to correct or eliminate it?

4. (a) What is a point-focal lens? (b) How does the oblique power of a point-focal lens compare with the axial power? (c) What implications does this have for a fully corrected myope as compared with a fully corrected hyperope?

5. How can lens weight be kept to a minimum for a patient requiring a +10.00 lens?

6. On the basis of the relative spectacle magnification formula for axial ametropia, show that a minimum of aniseikonia will occur in anisometropia due to axial ametropia when spectacle lenses rather than contact lenses are worn.

7. What ocular damage may occur (in humans) as a result of (a) ultraviolet and (b) infrared components of solar radiation?

8. (a) How is segment-induced prismatic effect calculated? (b) With a straight-top bifocal lens, calculate the amount of segment-induced prismatic effect for a +2.00D addition for a distance correction of +4.00D, and for a distance correction of −4.00D (assuming the segment top is 5mm below the distance pole, the segment pole is 5mm below the segment top, and the reading level is 10mm below the distance pole).

9. How do the Varilux 2 and Ultravue progressive addition lenses compare in regard to the progression of power in the vertical meridian of the lens and the areas of unwanted astigmatism?

10. How is segment inset verified, in a pair of finished bifocal lenses, (a) for fused bifocals? (b) for Executive bifocals?

11. A patient requires the correction R −2.00 −1.00 × 180, L −4.00 −2.00 × 180 with a +2.00D addition (each eye). If the differential vertical prismatic effect at the reading level (10mm below the distance centers) is to be fully corrected by using bicentric grinding, how much prism power (and with the base in what direction) must be supplied?

12. List the situations in which one can be sure that a patient's ametropia is axial (rather than refractive), or refractive (rather than axial).

13. Why is it undesirable to use photochromic lenses (a) as "sunglass" lenses? (b) as night driving lenses?

14. On the basis of the relative spectacle magnification formula for refractive ametropia, show that a minimum of aniseikonia (for anisometropia due to refractive ametropia) will occur when contact lenses rather than spectacle lenses are worn.

15. In ophthalmic lens design, do designers correct oblique aberrations for distance vision or for near vision? Why?

16. How can the cosmetic appearance of a lens edge be maximized for a patient requiring a −10.00D lens?

17. Under what condition or conditions is it possible for Petzval's surface to coincide with the far-point sphere?

18. To what extent is distortion a problem for wearers of ophthamic lenses?

19. A patient who will wear a distance correction R +2.00D, L +2.00D requires 1Δ of base-out prism, each eye, because of an esophoria. How much decentration (and in what direction) will be required to supply this prism?

20. Is spherical aberration likely to cause a problem for an ophthalmic lens wearer?

21. How does the use of a correcting lens change retinal image size (as compared with image size without a correcting lens) for a 6.00D hyperope

(a) wearing a spectacle lens having a front surface power of +8.00D, a center thickness of 4.3mm, an index of refraction of 1.523, and a vertex distance of 12mm? (b) wearing a contact lens having a front surface power of 71.50D, a center thickness of 0.28mm, an index of refraction of 1.490, and a vertex distance of zero?

22. By means of the spectacle magnification formula, show that when contact lenses are worn rather than glasses, the size of the retinal image is always greater in myopia and smaller in hyperopia.

23. A patient having a distance correction of R $-3.00 -1.00 \times 180$ and L $-3.00 -0.50 \times 180$ wears lenses centered for distance PD. How much prism power (and with its base in what direction) does the patient experience for near work if the near PD is 4mm less than the distance PD?

24. Is the aberration of coma apt to cause a problem for an ophthalmic lens wearer? Why or why not?

25. (a) What is Petzval's surface? (b) When oblique astigmatism is corrected, how do the sagittal and tangential image shells relate to Petzval's surface? (c) How can the curvature of Petzval's surface be changed?

26. What is Ryan's rule of thumb regarding the estimated percentage change in retinal image size per diopter of refractive ametropia and per diopter of axial ametropia? Why is the estimated percentage not *zero* for axial ametropia?

27. When trifocal lenses are prescribed, where should the intermediate segment of the lens be placed (in relation to the position of the segment top if bifocals rather than trifocals were prescribed)?

28. Define image jump for a wearer of a bifocal lens. How is the amount of image jump determined? Name a bifocal segment that provides a minimum of image jump and one that provides a large amount.

29. (a) What is the far-point sphere? (b) How can the curvature of the far-point sphere be changed?

30. In ophthalmic lens design, do designers concentrate mainly on the correction of oblique astigmatism or on the correction of curvature error? Why?

31. To fit a full diameter aspheric aphakic lens as thin as possible and to reduce aberrations to a practical minimum, (a) what lens shape ideally should be used? (b) how should the distance between the geometrical centers of the correcting lenses (the frame PD) compare with the patient's PD? (c) approximately what should be the back surface power? (d) how close should the lenses be fitted to the patient's eyes?

CHAPTER 14

Prescribing Contact Lenses

CONTACT LENS DEVELOPMENT

Although the suggestion that ametropia could be corrected with a water-filled lens placed directly on the eye was made by Leonardo da Vinci in about 1508 (Hofstetter and Graham, 1953), the development of clinically useful contact lenses has taken place during the working lives of many optometrists now in practice. The development of what we now call *hard* contact lenses has been traced in some detail by Graham (1959), and the descriptions in the following paragraphs are based on his treatise.

The first powered contact lens to have actually been worn was designed by A. Eugen Fick in 1887. It was what we would now call a *scleral* contact lens, having separately ground corneal and scleral portions. *Fluid-containing* scleral contact lenses were developed during the years between World Wars I and II, the first glass lens fitting set being made by Zeiss in 1920 and greatly expanded some 10 years later. Important turning points in the development of scleral lenses were the introduction of the plastic material *polymethyl methacrylate (PMMA)* by Theodore Obrig in 1940 and the development of the minimum-clearance *fluidless* scleral lens by Norman Bier in the year 1943. A plastic fluidless scleral lens known as the Mueller-Welt lens became available in America in 1950: this and other scleral lenses enjoyed a brief period of popularity until they were overshadowed by the rapid development of the *corneal* contact lens.

Working in Obrig's laboratory, Kevin M. Tuohy saw the advantages of the use of PMMA in the manufacture of scleral lenses and conceived the idea of making plastic lenses covering only the cornea. In 1948, he began the manufacture of corneal contact lenses. The lens designed by Tuohy was approxi-

mately 11.5mm in diameter and 0.40mm thick, and it was fitted considerably flatter than the corneal apex. This lens was immediately popular, but it had the disadvantage of riding on the sensitive corneal apex, and due to the thick edges and a large amount of edge standoff, it was responsible for a good bit of "lid bumping." In 1951, William Sohnges, Frank Dickinson, and John Neill improved the original Tuohy lens by developing what they called the *microlens*. This lens was smaller and thinner than the Tuohy lens, being 9.5mm in diameter and 0.20mm thick; like the Tuohy lens, it was fitted several diopters flatter than the corneal apex. The lighter weight of the microlens made it more acceptable than the Tuohy lens for many patients, but it still had the disadvantage of excessive movement and the consequent irritation of the sensory nerve endings in the corneal epithelium and lid margins.

In 1955, Norman Bier introduced a lens, called the *Contour lens*, about the same diameter as the microlens but having a central optical portion 6.5mm in width, fitted parallel to the corneal apex, with one or more flatter curves in the periphery of the lens. Wesley and Jessen, in 1956, developed what they called the *Sphercon lens*. This lens had a diameter (approximately 8.5mm) small enough so it fitted mainly on the optical portion of the cornea, therefore requiring only a narrow bevel at the edge rather than a series of peripheral curves. During the following decade, many variations of the original Contour lens were developed, with the general tendency being toward smaller and thinner lenses.

The first reference to the development of *soft (hydrogel) contact lenses* was contained in a brief review published in *Nature* by Wichterle and Lim (1960). In this article they described their research with plastic materials for use in various prosthetic devices, in particular copolymers of glycomonomethacrylate with several tenths percent of glycol dimethacrylate. In the last sentence of their report, Wichterle and Lim mentioned that promising results had been attained with these materials in the manufacture of contact lenses. The lens developed by Wichterle was a *spin-cast lens* made in a revolving mold; according to reports by Morrison (1966) and by Fisher (1968), it was fitted in large numbers at the Second Eye Hospital in Prague under the supervision of Dr. Dreifus.

The soft contact lens was introduced in the United States by Bausch & Lomb in 1971. Called the *Soflens*, the Bausch & Lomb lens is made by a spin-casting process similar to that used by Wichterle and consists of a three-dimensional network of *hydroxyethylmethacrylate (HEMA)* chains cross-linked with *ethylene glycol dimethacrylate* molecules (about 1 in every 200 monomer units). The first *lathe-cut soft contact lens* available in North America was the Griffin *Naturalens*, introduced in Canada in 1971. The pace of soft contact lens development was much slower in the United States than in most other countries, due to the stringent requirements of the Food and Drug Administration (FDA). Although the Bausch & Lomb Soflens received FDA approval in 1971, it was the only soft lens available in this country until 1974, when the Soft Lenses, Inc., *Hydrocurve* lens was given approval. In recent years, a large number of soft lenses have been approved by the FDA, so the contact lens practitioner now has an ample (and sometimes confusing) array of lenses from which to choose.

Along with the development of soft contact lenses, a number of manufacturers were developing *gas-permeable hard contact lens* materials. The first of these to receive FDA approval were the Danker and

Wohlk *Meso* lens, a *cellulose acetate butyrate (CAB)* lens approved in 1978, and the Syntex *Polycon* lens, a methyl methacrylate and silicone lens approved in 1979. Since that time a large number of additional gas-permeable hard lenses have been approved.

The most recent development in the contact lens field has been *extended-wear lenses*. These are lenses designed for 24-hour-per-day wear for an extended period of time, and they were originally intended primarily for use by elderly aphakic patients who are unable to handle their lenses on a daily basis. However, they are now available also for the correction of myopia and hyperopia. The first extended-wear lenses to receive FDA approval were the Cooper *Permalens* and the Soft Lenses *Hydrocurve*, in 1979.

OPTICAL PRINCIPLES OF CONTACT LENSES

Power Considerations

In terms of power, hard and soft contact lenses differ in that hard lenses are considered to be rigid enough so the lens tends to retain its shape while on the cornea, whereas soft lenses are considered to be flexible enough so they completely conform to the corneal surface. However, there are exceptions in both cases. Hard lenses are often sufficiently flexible so they fail to retain their shape while on the cornea, and soft lenses (particularly in the high plus powers required in aphakia) can be sufficiently rigid to fail to completely conform to the corneal surface. The main consequence of this difference (to be discussed below) relates to the need for the provision of toric surfaces for the correction of astigmatism. If a hard contact lens is rigid enough so it does retain its shape while on the cornea, the use of a spherical lens eliminates, for all practical purposes, corneal astigmatism. On the other hand, if a soft lens is flexible enough so it conforms to the corneal contour, the lens fails to eliminate corneal astigmatism, and therefore a toric refracting surface may be necessary.

Power considerations that apply equally to hard and soft contact lenses are effective power, back vertex power, and lens surface power.

Effective power

As described in Chapter 13, when a correcting lens is moved from the spectacle plane toward or away from the eye, the required power of the lens changes. As shown in Figure 14.1, when a lens is

Figure 14.1 *(a)* **For a myopic eye, a contact lens has a longer secondary focal length (and thus a lower power) than a spectacle lens for the same eye.** *(b)* **For a hyperopic eye, a contact lens has a shorter secondary focal length (and thus a higher power) than a spectacle lens for the same eye** (Grosvenor, 1963).

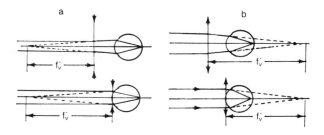

moved from the spectacle plane to the plane of the cornea, the power of a minus lens must be decreased and the power of a plus lens must be increased for parallel rays of light to be refracted in such a way that the refracted rays diverge from the far-point (myopia) or converge toward the far-point (hyperopia).

If the power of the required spectacle lens is known, the power of a contact lens required to correct the same eye can be determined by means of the *effective power formula,*

$$F_{CL} = \frac{F_s}{1 - dF_s},$$

where

F_s = the power of the spectacle lens

F_{CL} = the power of the contact lens

d = the vertex distance expressed in meters.

As shown in the following examples, contact lens power begins to differ by as much as 0.25D from spectacle lens power when spectacle lens power is about ±4.50D. If we assume that a prospective contact lens wearer's refraction, done at a 12mm distance, results in a need for a −4.50D lens, the required contact lens power would be

$$F_{CL} = \frac{-4.5}{1 - 0.012(-4.5)} = -4.27D.$$

If we assume that the refraction, again at a 12mm distance, results in a need for a +4.50D lens, the required contact lens power would be

$$F_{CL} = \frac{4.5}{1 - 0.012(4.5)} = +4.76D.$$

Back vertex power

A lens can be considered a "thin lens" if its radii of curvature are large compared with its thickness. In such a case, the *approximate power formula* can be used:

$$F_a = F_1 + F_2.$$

However, the surfaces of a contact lens are so highly curved that in spite of the small thickness value, the use of the approximate power formula results in a significant error. Contact lens power, therefore, must be specified in terms of the *back vertex power formula:*

$$F'_v = \frac{F_1}{1 - \dfrac{t}{n}F_1} + F_2.$$

The necessity for using this formula can be demonstrated by considering a lens with front and back surfaces of equal but opposite power. If for a given PMMA lens, $F_1 = +62.50D$, $F_2 = -62.50D$, $t = 0.10mm$, and $n = 1.490$, the approximate power of the lens would obviously be plano, but the back vertex power would be

$$F'_v = \frac{62.5}{1 - \dfrac{0.0001}{1.490}} - 62.5$$

$$= +0.26D,$$

or +0.26D more than the approximate power.

Minus lenses (both hard and soft) often are fitted in thicknesses of 0.10mm or less, so the difference between approximate power and back vertex power is in most cases equal to or less than that shown here for a plano lens. However, plus lenses (particularly lenses for the correction of aphakia) tend to be much thicker than 0.10mm, so the difference between approximate power and back vertex power is much greater than that for a plano lens.

Surface power

The refracting power of a contact lens surface in air can be determined by the use of the familiar formula

$$F = \frac{n - 1}{r}.$$

For a PMMA lens whose back surface radius of curvature (determined by an instrument like a Radiuscope) is 7.5mm, the refracting power would be

$$F = \frac{1.490 - 1}{-0.0075} = -65.33D.$$

Many practitioners think of contact lens curvature in terms of *keratometer value* rather than radius of curvature. When keratometer value is used, it must be multiplied by a conversion factor to obtain refracting power, because the keratometer has been calibrated for an index of refraction other than that of the contact lens. The conversion factor is the ratio of the refraction between air and plastic to that between air and the cornea, using the index of refraction for which the keratometer is calibrated. For a hard lens having an index of refraction of 1.490, the conversion factor is

$$\frac{1.490 - 1}{1.3375 - 1} = 1.452.$$

The lens used in the previous example, having a back

surface radius of curvature of 7.5mm, if checked in the keratometer, would be found to have a keratometer value of −45.00D. Using the conversion factor, the back surface power would be

$$F_2 = (1.452)(-45.00) = -65.34D,$$

differing from the previous value by only 0.01D.

Hard Contact Lens Optics

Refraction by the tear layer

The refraction we ordinarily think of as taking place at the cornea (as measured by the keratometer) actually takes place at the interface between air and the tear layer. When a contact lens is placed on the cornea, the lens will often alter the curvature of the *air-tear interface* (described later in the chapter) but is not expected to alter the refraction taking place at the *tear-cornea interface*.

Consider the refraction taking place between air and the tear layer for a typical cornea, assuming a tear layer radius of curvature of 8.0mm and an index of refraction of 1.336:

$$F = \frac{0.336}{0.008} = 42.00D.$$

Because the keratometer is calibrated for an index of refraction of 1.3375 (rather than the cornea's true index of 1.376), the resulting keratometer finding would be

$$\frac{0.3375}{0.008} = 42.19D,$$

or 0.19D more than the tear layer's true refracting power. This is an error of only 0.45 percent.

What about the refraction taking place at the tear-cornea interface? If we assume that the tear layer is infinitely thin, the refraction at the tear-cornea interface would be

$$\frac{1.376 - 1.336}{0.008} = 5.00D.$$

The total refraction (air-tears-cornea) is consequently 42.00D plus 5.00D, or 47.00D, rather than the 42.19D shown by the keratometer. Let us now consider the effect of a contact lens on the curvature of the tear layer, first for a spherical tear layer and then for a toroidal tear layer.

Spherical tear layer. If the tear layer is spherical (as shown by the keratometer), and if a contact lens is firm enough so it will retain its curvature while on the eye, the curvature of the tear layer will

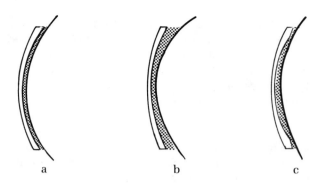

Figure 14.2 Effects of contact lens back surface (base curve) on the tear layer (a) for a back surface parallel to the tear layer; (b) for a back surface flatter than the tear layer; (c) for a back surface steeper than the tear layer.

(1) not change if the radius of curvature of the back surface of the lens is the same as that of the tear layer (see Figure 14.2a); (2) steepen if the radius of curvature of the back surface of the lens is steeper than that of the tear layer (see Figure 14.2b); and (3) flatten if the radius of curvature of the back surface of the lens is flatter than that of the tear layer (see Figure 14.2c).

What effect does steepening or flattening the tear layer have on the power of a contact lens required to correct the eye's refractive error? Referring to Figures 14.2b and 14.2c, it is obvious that when the curvature of the tear layer is steepened, the eye is made more myopic, and that when the curvature is flattened, the eye is made more hyperopic. How much more myopic or more hyperopic is demonstrated in the following example.

Consider a spherical tear layer having a radius of curvature of 7.90mm that is fitted first with a contact lens having a 7.90mm (42.75DK) base curve radius (the radius of the central portion of the back surface of the lens) and then with one having a 7.80mm (43.25DK) base curve radius. The designation *DK* indicates the power of the contact lens surface as indicated by the keratometer (which is in error because the keratometer is calibrated for an index of refraction other than that of the contact lens). Assuming that in each case the lens maintains its curvature while on the cornea, what will be the required lens powers if the refractive error at the corneal plane is 4.00D of myopia?

This problem can be best solved by considering that a thin layer of air is interposed between the contact lens and the tear layer, as shown in Figure

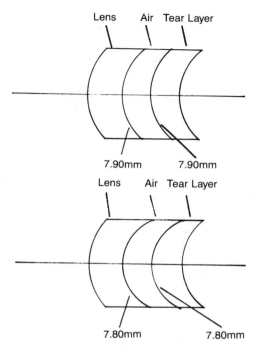

Figure 14.3 The effect of a change of tear layer curvature on refraction. When the back surface of the lens is steeper than the tear layer, the tear layer curvature is steepened, making the eye more myopic and requiring a contact lens of greater power.

14.3. While wearing the 7.90mm lens, the refraction between the (hypothetical) thin layer of air and tears would be

$$\frac{0.336}{0.0079} = 42.53D,$$

and the refraction while wearing the 7.80mm lens would be

$$\frac{0.336}{0.0078} = 43.08D.$$

The steeper lens results in an increase of 0.55D in the eye's myopia (that is, 43.08 − 42.53), which means that the power of the correcting lens must be increased from −4.00 to −4.50D.

This example illustrates the following rule of thumb. If a contact lens base curve is specified as steeper or flatter than the corneal curvature (i.e., the tear layer curvature), the power of the lens must be specified 0.50D more minus for each 0.10mm (0.50DK) of lens steepening, or 0.50D more plus for each 0.10mm of lens flattening.

Toroidal tear layer. What happens if a contact lens having a spherical base curve is placed on a toric cornea? Consider a tear layer having a refracting power, as measured by the keratometer, of 43.00D in the horizontal meridian and 45.00D in the vertical meridian (the tear layer radii being 7.85 and 7.50mm). If a hard lens having a 43.50DK spherical back surface is fitted, what will be the effect on the corneal astigmatism?

Again, considering a thin layer of air to be present between the contact lens and the tear layer, we find that the front surface of the tear layer now has a refracting power of 43.50D in all meridians (as a result of the spherical back surface of the contact lens) and that the patient's corneal astigmatism has been eliminated. This last statement should be amended to note that all the corneal astigmatism measured by the keratometer has been eliminated, because the astigmatism at the tears-to-cornea interface would be

$$\frac{0.040}{0.0075} - \frac{0.040}{0.00785} = 5.33 - 5.10 = 0.23D.$$

The presence of this small amount of uncorrected astigmatism need not concern us, particularly because it is possible that it is compensated by the astigmatism at the cornea-to-aqueous refraction.

In summary, as long as the hard contact lens maintains its spherical curvature while on the cornea, the tear layer surface will no longer be toroidal but will have the same radius of curvature as the back surface of the contact lens; therefore, corneal astigmatism as measured by the keratometer will be eliminated.

Internal astigmatism

Because a hard contact lens having a spherical back surface eliminates corneal astigmatism, only internal astigmatism remains. Internal astigmatism has been found to average −0.50D × 90, so we should expect to find approximately this amount of uncorrected astigmatism present when a patient wears a spherical base curve contact lens. The amount of uncorrected astigmatism can be determined easily by performing retinoscopy or subjective refraction while the lens is worn. If 0.75D or more of uncorrected astigmatism is found to be present, consideration should be given to prescribing a toric front surface lens.

It has been assumed that a hard contact lens maintains its curvature while on the cornea. This is true of plus lenses and of minus lenses thicker than about 0.13mm (center thickness), but minus lenses in the thicknesses now usually fitted are flexible enough so when fitted on a toric cornea, the lenses tend to conform to the shape of the corneal surface. This can easily be determined by taking a keratometer finding while the patient wears the lens. The mire images seen will be those reflected from the front surface of the contact lens, and while a relatively thick lens will maintain its spherical curvature while on the cornea, a thin lens may have a toric front surface while on the cornea.

Harris and Chu (1972) have shown that when a lens having a center thickness of less than 0.13mm is fitted on a with-the-rule astigmatic cornea, the flexure of the lens reduces the amount of uncorrected astigmatism. In many cases this flexing is sufficient to eliminate or substantially reduce the cylindrical power that would otherwise be found as a result of internal astigmatism.

Specifying power of spherical hard lenses

Because hard contact lenses tend to eliminate corneal astigmatism, the great majority of hard contact lenses are fitted with spherical front and back surfaces. When spherical hard lenses are fitted, specification of lens power is a relatively simple matter and is made even simpler if the base curve radius is fitted parallel to the flattest meridian of the cornea, a method referred to as *on K fitting*. For example, if a patient having the keratometer finding 42.00 at 180; 43.00 at 90 is to be fitted with a spherical hard contact lens, the base curve of the lens (the curvature of the central, or optical, portion of the back surface) will be specified as 42.00DK, or 8.04mm, radius. (The radius is determined by using the index of refraction for which the keratometer is calibrated, 1.3375.)

It should be obvious that the presence of the contact lens on the cornea does not change the refracting power of the tear layer in the horizontal meridian, but it does change the refracting power of the tear layer in the vertical meridian from the original 43.00D to 42.00D, thereby rendering the tear layer spherical in curvature.

Because the patient will have a spherical tear layer surface while wearing the lens equal in refracting power to that of the horizontal meridian for the tear layer without the lens, the power to be specified is that of the patient's spectacle correction in the horizontal meridian (corrected, if necessary, for the change in vertex distance).

If the patient in our example is found to require a spectacle correction of −3.00DS −0.50DC × 180, the lens power to be specified would be −3.00DS. The −0.50DC × 180 is ignored. However, we would expect in this case to find about −0.50D × 90 of uncorrected astigmatism due to the internal astigmatism of the eye.

In our example, the power of the spectacle correction is not sufficient to make necessary a correction for vertex distance. However, for the spectacle correction −4.50DS −0.50DC × 180, the use of the vertex distance formula would show (assuming that the refraction had been done at a distance of 12mm) that the required contact lens power would be only −4.25DS.

Fitting steeper or flatter than K. For one of a number of reasons, a practitioner may decide to fit a contact lens with a base curve steeper or flatter than the flattest meridian of the cornea. As described earlier and shown in Figure 14.3, when this is done the curvature of the tear layer is changed, a steeper lens making the eye more myopic and a flatter lens making the eye more hyperopic. Let us return to our original example of the eye to be fitted with a lens having a 42.00DK, or 8.04mm, base curve radius and requiring a power of −3.00D. If for some reason the base curve were changed to 43.00D (1.00D steeper), the power of the lens would have to be increased to −4.00D. On the other hand, if the base curve were changed to 41.00DK (1.00D flatter), the power of the lens would have to be decreased to −2.00D.

The foregoing discussion is based on what may be called the "mail order" method of contact lens fitting. It is possible to order contact lenses for a patient without the use of trial lenses by specifying the keratometer finding in the flattest meridian (assuming an *on K* fit is desired) and the spherical power of the spectacle correction (corrected for the change in vertex distance, if necessary). This method of fitting was advocated by contact lens manufacturers in the early days of PMMA lens fitting and is still used by some practitioners. However, the majority of practitioners make use of trial contact lenses, using the keratometer finding and the patient's spectacle correction to determine the starting lens and making whatever changes necessary to meet the fitting criteria for the lens in question.

Specifying power of toric hard lenses

Hard contact lenses having toric surfaces can be prescribed for two entirely different purposes: (1) for the strictly optical purpose of correcting for internal astigmatism, in which case a toric front surface is used; and (2) for the purpose of providing an adequate physical fit on a highly toric cornea, in which case a toric back surface is used. In many cases, the provision of a toric back surface will serve as an additional source of uncorrected astigmatism, in which case a toric front surface can be provided to eliminate this astigmatism (resulting in a *bitoric lens*).

Toric front surface lenses. The distribution curve for internal astigmatism has a mean of about 0.50D, against the rule, and is highly leptokurtic (peaked). Therefore, few people have with-the-rule internal astigmatism, and few people have more than 1.00D of against-the-rule internal astigmatism. The need for a toric front surface for the correction of internal astigmatism, therefore, is relatively rare.

The action of the upper lids during blinking is such that each lens tends to rotate upward and temporally with each blink, as shown in Figure 14.4. Consequently, when a toric front surface is used, some method must be employed to stabilize the lens; otherwise, the cylinder axis will change with each blink. Two methods of lens stabilization have been found to be effective: (1) the lens can be *truncated*, or cut off at the bottom, so the lower edge of the lens will rest on the lower lid margin; or (2) a *prism ballast* lens can be used, base-down prism being lathed into the lens so the added thickness and weight of the lens will tend to keep the lens from rotating. Truncated and prism ballast lenses are illustrated in Figure 14.5. Usually, both truncation and prism ballast are used with a toric front surface lens.

The preferred procedure for fitting a truncated or prism ballast lens is to refract the patient while wearing a truncated or prism ballast trial lens (having spherical surfaces), so the axis of the required cylinder can be specified in relation to the base-apex meridian of the trial lens. Suppose a patient is refracted while wearing a −3.00D spherical prism ballast lens. The lens is found to fit well, exhibiting a good lens-cornea relationship and orienting with the base-apex meridian at 90 degrees. The refractive finding through the lens is −0.50DS − 1.00DC × 90. The total lens power required (including the power of the trial contact lens), therefore, is −3.50DS −1.00DC × 90. Because the required cylindrical correction will be in the form of a toric front surface, the lens prescription should be stated in the plus cylinder form, and the lens order should be so stated: −4.50DS + 1.00DC × 180. However, because laboratories are accustomed to receiving orders for toric front surface lenses in minus cylinder form, the order must clearly specify

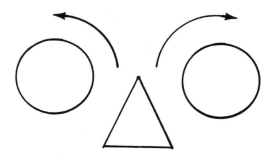

Figure 14.4 Rotation of lenses during blinking.

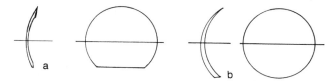

Figure 14.5 Lens designs to eliminate rotation: *(a)* truncation; *(b)* prism ballast.

a toric *front* surface. This is analogous to the situation formerly existing with ophthalmic lens laboratories: optometrists' prescriptions were written in minus cylinder form, even though the cylinder was routinely ground on the front surface of the lens.

It should be noted that the cylinder power of the lens is the same on the eye as when measured (in air) with a lensometer, because the cylinder is on the front surface only. Therefore, the lensometer should indicate the cylinder ordered (i.e., +1.00DC × 180) without the need for a conversion factor.

In the example given here, the axis of the correcting cylinder (found by refracting the patient through the trial contact lens) was 90 degrees, so it corresponded to the base-apex meridian of the prism. However, often the axis of the correcting cylinder will not be 90 degrees, so it will have to be specified at a given angle from the base-apex meridian. The method for specifying this is described in a later section on toric lens fitting.

Toric back surface lenses. When a toric back surface lens is used to obtain an adequate physical fit on a highly toric cornea, the practitioner must be aware that the toric back surface serves as a source of induced astigmatism. The amount of induced astigmatism can be determined by multiplying the difference between the keratometer values of the back surface of the lens in the two principal meridians by a constant (−0.456). This constant, as described by Sarver (1971), is the ratio of the refraction between the contact lens and the tear layer to the refraction between air and the cornea (using the index of refraction for which the keratometer is calibrated):

$$\frac{1.336 - 1.490}{1.3375 - 1} = -0.456.$$

The minus sign used for this constant (although not used by Sarver) indicates that the induced cylinder has an axis opposite to that of the original corneal cylinder.

Consider a patient with keratometer findings of 42.00D at 180 degrees and 45.00D at 90 degrees, wearing a back surface toric lens fitted parallel in all meridians (i.e., a keratometer value of 42.00DK at 180 and 45.00DK at 90). The lens required to correct the astigmatism induced by the toric back surface would be

$$-0.456(-3.00DC \times 180) = -1.37DC \times 90.$$

It should be noted that, in this example, the induced astigmatism is such as to add to any against-the-rule internal astigmatism that may be present.

When a toric back surface lens is received from the laboratory, the practitioner should know how to verify the lens using the lensometer. The power of the cylinder in air (as opposed to its power while on the cornea) can be determined by multiplying the difference between the DK values for the two principal meridians of the lens surface by the constant 1.452 (previously referred to), which compares the refraction between air and plastic to that between air and the cornea:

$$\frac{1.490 - 1}{1.3375 - 1} = 1.452.$$

Applying this constant, we find that the power of the cylinder as indicated by the lensometer should be

$$1.452(-3.00DC \times 180) = -4.36DC \times 180.$$

Bitoric lenses. Sarver (1970) suggested that, when a toric back surface lens is fitted, a toric front surface be ordered of a magnitude to neutralize the cylinder induced by the back surface. The procedure can be best demonstrated by Sarver's example, which follows.

For a given eye, a spherical contact lens (42.00DK, −2.00DS) is found to correct the refractive error, whereas a toric contact lens (42.00DK, 45.00DK) is found to provide an optimum lens-cornea relationship. The patient's refractive error is −2.00DS −3.00DC × 180 (i.e., −2.00D in the 42.00DK

meridian and −5.00D in the 45.00DK meridian). A bitoric lens for the patient would be ordered as follows:

Flat meridian: 42.00DK; − 2.00D.

Steep meridian: 45.00DK; −5.00D.

The lensometer reading for this lens will be −2.00DS −3.00DC × flat meridian.

As stated by Sarver, the power of the lens on the eye will be that of a spherical lens, and the lens can even rotate on the eye without producing a change in the cylindrical power of the system. This is because, as previously stated, the layer of tears between the contact lens and the cornea has the effect of removing the cornea from consideration— as the lens rotates through an angle of 90 degrees, the increase (or decrease) in the refracting power of the tear layer is exactly compensated by the decrease (or increase) in the refracting power of the lens.

Soft Contact Lens Optics

Refraction by the tear layer

A soft contact lens, rather than being sufficiently rigid to tend to maintain its shape while on the cornea as a hard lens does, is sufficiently flexible to tend to conform completely to the corneal curvature. To the extent that this is true, it follows that (1) when a soft lens having a spherical back surface is fitted on a toric cornea, the outer surface of the tear layer will retain its toricity, and the corneal astigmatism will not be eliminated; and (2) when a soft lens is fitted so its back surface is steeper (or flatter) than the corneal curvature, the outer surface of the tear layer will retain its original curvature, causing no change in the eye's refractive error.

Uncorrected astigmatism

A number of studies have confirmed that spherical soft contact lenses fail to correct astigmatism. Lee and Sarver (1972) found that there was a direct transfer of corneal astigmatism to the front surface of the lens for −2.50D soft lenses having center thicknesses as great as 0.68mm. In a study involving Griffin lathe-cut soft lenses in thicknesses ranging from 0.25–0.35mm, Grosvenor (1972b) found that for almost all subjects, the corneal astigmatism while wearing the lens was the same as without the lens, within the limits of keratometer accuracy. The data from this study are shown in Figure 14.6. The data points near the top of the graph are for a patient whose lenses were fitting badly, resulting in keratometer mire distortion.

It should be understood that a soft contact lens that corrects no corneal astigmatism obviously corrects no internal astigmatism, so it corrects no astigmatism at all. The author once was told about an old-timer who got into optometry by the grandfather clause and did not believe in prescribing cylinders for patients. As far as this practitioner was concerned, "cylinders were for cars," and all his patients needed were *spherical* spectacle lenses. Like this old-timer, the practitioner who fits astigmatic eyes with spherical soft contact lenses is simply failing to correct astigmatism.

As a general guide, patients having more than 1.00D of with-the-rule refractive astigmatism (i.e., spectacle astigmatism) will not be satisfied with their vision with spherical soft contact lenses. Although 20/20 refracting room acuity may be obtainable with the soft lenses in spite of the uncorrected astigmatism, and although outdoor vision may be satisfactory because of the reduction of pupil size in bright illumination, most of these patients find that their vision is uncomfortable, unclear, or both for reading and other indoor visual tasks. If the astigmatism is against-the-rule or oblique, usually no more than 0.50 or 0.75D of uncorrected astigmatism can be tolerated. On a number of occasions, the author has fitted patients having more than 1.00D of with-the-rule astigmatism with spherical soft contact lenses, but in all cases the patients complained of blurred or uncomfortable vision for near work. One patient,

who wanted soft lenses mainly for skiing, found that vision while on the ski slopes was satisfactory in spite of 1.25D of uncorrected astigmatism in one eye and 1.50D in the other; however, the patient found that reading was impossible with the lenses.

Aphakic patients are exceptions to this general rule. High plus lenses required for the correction of aphakia are often rigid enough so as much as 1.00D or more of corneal astigmatism can be eliminated, or "masked," by the lens.

Specifying power for spherical soft lenses

Soft contact lenses differ from hard lenses in that, rather than being fitted on K (or slightly steeper or flatter), the base curve is fitted considerably flatter than the curvature of the corneal apex. Therefore, the peripheral portion of the lens has about the same radius of curvature as the corneal periphery, and the central portion of the lens "drapes" itself over the corneal apex. Some of the larger, thinner soft lenses are now available in only one or two base curve radii.

Given the patient used as an example in specifying hard lens power having keratometer findings of 42.00 at 180, 43.00 at 90, and requiring a spectacle correction of −3.50DS −0.50DC × 180, the power of the soft contact lens, like the power of the hard lens for the same patient, would be specified as −3.50D sphere. However, in this case the uncorrected astigmatism would not be the internal astigmatism but the refractive astigmatism. While the lens was worn, refraction by retinoscopy or subjective examination would be expected to result in −0.50DC × 180.

Changing the base curve radius of the soft lens would have no effect on the curvature of the front surface of the tear layer and, therefore, would have no effect on the refraction of the eye. Although changing the base curve of a soft contact lens may have an effect on the fitting qualities of the lens, it will have no effect on the required power of the lens. An exception to this rule can be found, again, in the fitting of an aphakic patient. An especially thick lathe-cut aphakic soft lens may fit in such a way that a negative tear layer results. When this occurs, the required lens power will be somewhat greater than indicated by the spectacle refraction when corrected for the change in vertex distance.

Specifying power for toric soft lenses

Recall that toric hard contact lenses can be prescribed for the correction of internal astigma-

Figure 14.6 Keratometric astigmatism without and with lathe-cut soft contact lenses (Grosvenor, 1972b).

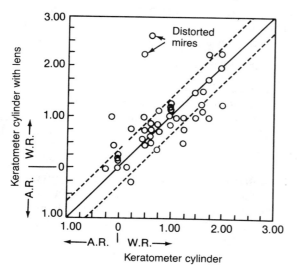

tism or to provide an adequate physical fit on a highly toric cornea. However, with soft lenses there is no problem in obtaining an adequate physical fit on a highly toric cornea with a spherical lens, so the only reason for prescribing a toric soft lens is for the correction of refractive astigmatism. As with the hard lens, a toric front surface is normally used.

Although soft contact lenses tend to rotate on the eyes much less than hard lenses do, toric front surface soft lenses must be stabilized by truncation, prism ballast, or both. The preferred procedure for fitting the lens is to refract the patient while wearing a truncated or prism ballast trial lens of the type to be prescribed, so the power and axis of the cylinder can be specified in relation to the base-apex meridian (prism ballast lens) or the vertical meridian (truncated lens). Once the power and axis of the correcting cylinder have been determined, they are specified in the manner described for a front surface toric hard lens. For example, if the patient is wearing a −3.00DS truncated prism ballast trial lens, and the refractive finding through lens is −0.75DS −1.25DC × 180, the total power required (including that of the trial contact lens) will be −3.75DS −1.25DC × 180. However, because the required toric curve will be on the front surface of the lens, the formula should be transposed to −5.00DS + 1.25DC × 90. When verifying the lens, the lensometer should indicate the cylinder ordered (+1.25D × 90) without the need for a conversion factor.

Accommodation and the Contact Lens Wearer

When a spectacle lens wearer switches to contact lenses, the demands on accommodation and convergence are altered in a number of ways. The total effect of these alterations may be negligible or great enough to constitute a major problem. In any event, the practitioner should be aware of their effects, able to predict their occurrence, and, if necessary, to take measures to minimize them.

Accommodative effort

Pascal (1947) pointed out that the diopter is an unsuitable unit to apply to accommodation for spectacle wearers. This is because the spectacle-wearing hyperope must put more accommodative effort into each diopter of accommodation than an emmetrope, whereas a spectacle-wearing myope uses less accommodative effort per diopter of accommodation. When contact lenses rather than

glasses are fitted, the hyperope loses a disadvantage and the myope loses an advantage.

The accommodative effort required by an ametrope, first while wearing glasses and then while wearing contact lenses, can be determined by considering that the refraction of the eye takes place at the corneal plane rather than at the spectacle plane.

Accommodation by a 10.00D myope

Consider a myopic patient who wears −10.00DS lenses and reads at a distance of 40cm. Referring to Figure 14.7, the vergence of the light rays coming from the object (O) is −2.50D by the time the light reaches the correcting lens. The correcting lens brings about a divergence of the rays of −10.00D, making a resulting divergence of −12.50D as the rays reach the correcting lens.

At the cornea, after having traveled 12mm more, the vergence of the light has decreased to −10.87D. The figure −10.87D was arrived at as follows:

$$-12.50D \longrightarrow 80mm.$$
$$80mm + 12mm = 92mm.$$
$$92mm \longrightarrow -10.87D.$$

The arrows ($\longrightarrow$) in these expressions indicate the conversion of diopters of vergence to millimeters of distance, or vice versa, as used routinely by Bennett (1956) and in Chapter 1 of this textbook.

Using the effective power formula, the refractive error of this patient in the corneal plane is found to be −8.93D:

$$F_C = \frac{F_S}{1 - dF_S} = \frac{-10}{1 = 0.012(-10)} = -8.93D.$$

The amount of accommodation required of this patient is the difference between the refractive error of the eye at the corneal plane and the vergence of the light rays at the same plane:

$$-8.93D - (-10.87D) = +1.94D.$$

Because the accommodation required of an emmetrope in the same situation would be 2.50D, the accommodation required by the spectacle-wearing myope is 0.56D less than that required by an emmetrope.

Accommodation by a 10.00D hyperope

As shown in Figure 14.8, for a 10.00D hyperope in the same situation, the vergence of light leaving the lens is +7.50D. On reaching the cornea, the vergence becomes 8.26D:

$$+7.50D \longrightarrow 133mm.$$

$$133mm - 12mm = 121mm.$$

$$121mm \longrightarrow 8.26D.$$

The patient's refractive error at the corneal plane is

$$F_C = \frac{+10}{1 - 0.012(10)} = +11.36D,$$

and the amount of accommodation required is

$$+11.36D - 8.26D = +3.10D,$$

or 0.60D more than that required by an emmetrope.

Clinical implications

The difference in accommodative effort has important clinical implications for spectacle-wearing patients of presbyopic or prepresbyopic ages who are to be fitted with contact lenses. The spectacle-wearing myope who is a prepresbyope may find that with contact lenses reading addition is needed that was not necessary while wearing spectacles. On the other hand, the spectacle-wearing hyperope who is an early presbyope may find that bifocals or reading glasses are not needed (at least not for another year or so) while wearing contact lenses.

Accommodative and Fusional Convergence with Contact Lenses

As a result of the differences in accommodation required with contact lenses as opposed to glasses, it follows that when a patient switches from glasses to contact lenses there will also be a change in the amount of accommodative convergence required.

Accommodative convergence

The myope will use more accommodative effort with contact lenses than with glasses, and, therefore, will use correspondingly more accommodative convergence. If the wearer happens to be exophoric at near, the increased amount of accommodative convergence will result in a decreased exophoria and, thus, will reduce the need for positive fusional vergence. However, if the wearer is esophoric at near, the resulting increase in the esophoria will require the use of more negative fusional vergence than is required with glasses, which may result in complaints of eyestrain.

Recall that for a 10.00D myope the additional amount of accommodation while wearing contact lenses is 0.56D (for a reading distance of 40cm); if we assume a 6/1 AC/A ratio, the additional amount

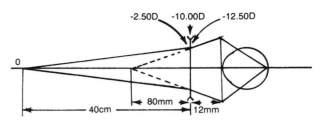

Figure 14.7 Accommodation by a 10.00D spectacle-wearing myope (Grosvenor, 1963).

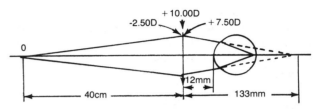

Figure 14.8 Accommodation by a 10.00D spectacle-wearing hyperope (Grosvenor, 1963).

of accommodative convergence would be 0.56(6) = 3.36Δ. If the patient's near phoria is 5Δ of esophoria with spectacles, the "new" esophoria will be about 8Δ (neglecting any change in phoria due to changes in lens centration). The required increase in the need for negative fusional vergence may bring about adaptation problems, which the practitioner may blame on the "fit" of the lenses.

The hyperope wearing contact lenses and using less accommodation will use less accommodative convergence. The patient will be expected to be more exophoric or less esophoric at near than while wearing spectacles.

Effects due to decentration

If it can be assumed that contact lenses are centered with respect to the pupils and remain centered when the eyes converge, some significant changes in phoria findings should result from the lack of prismatic effects that necessarily are present with spectacle lenses.

Most practitioners order minus lenses centered for distance rather than for near, especially if the patient is exophoric at near. This results in induced base-in prism at near, thus reducing the amount of exophoria at near.

Consider the 10.00D myope who is 7Δ exophoric at near. If the glasses are centered for distance and if the near PD is 4mm less than the distance PD, the prismatic effect at near will be 0.4(10) = 4Δ base-in.

The patient's near exophoria, therefore, will be decreased to 3Δ while wearing the glasses. However, when the patient switches to contact lenses, the prismatic effect will no longer be present, and the near exophoria will return to the originally measured value of 7Δ. This increased exophoria while wearing contact lenses will require the use of additional fusional vergence and may bring about adaptive symptoms that, again, could be blamed on the "fit" of the lenses.

On the other hand, a myope having esophoria at near and who is accustomed to the base-in prismatic effect at near while wearing glasses, may find near work more comfortable while wearing contact lenses due to the decreased demand on negative fusional vergence.

Combination of effects

Fortunately, the effects due to increased (or decreased) accommodation often combine with the effects due to the lack of induced prism by decentration to cause the fusional vergence demand to change little.

As we have seen, the exophoric myope will have to use less fusional vergence at near due to the increased accommodation with contact lenses, but will have to use more fusional vergence at near due to the lack of base-in prism power enjoyed while wearing glasses. These two effects may well cancel each other completely.

We have also found that the esophoric myope will have to use more negative fusional vergence at near due to the increased accommodation required while wearing contact lenses, but will have to use less negative fusional vergence at near due to the lack of base-in prism. Again, the two effects will tend to cancel one another.

Consideration of the combined effects for the exophoric hyperope and the esophoric hyperope also indicates that there is a strong tendency for one effect to negate the other.

Example showing combined effects

Let us return to our example of the 10.00D myope whose exophoria at near is reduced from 7 to 3Δ as a result of the base-in prism power supplied by spectacle lenses. Assuming a 5/1 AC/A ratio, the patient would be expected to use 0.56(5) = 2.8Δ more accommodative convergence with contact lenses than with glasses. The exophoria at near, therefore, would be approximately 4Δ rather than the previously stated 7Δ. These somewhat confusing changes can be tabulated as follows:

Condition	Expected near exophoria
1. With glasses, if centered for distance.	3Δ exophoria.
2. With glasses, if centered for near.	7Δ exophoria.
3. With contact lenses, neglecting the additional accommodation required.	7Δ exophoria.
4. With contact lenses, considering the additional accommodation required.	4Δ exophoria.

Low myopia with esophoria at near

Low myopes who have esophoria at near usually find that reading is more comfortable without their glasses than with them. If glasses are discarded in favor of contact lenses, the resulting esophoria at near may be a great enough problem (in terms of increased negative fusional vergence demand) that motivation for contact lens wear may be lost. The problem here is not that the contact lenses *cause* the esophoria at near but that glasses can be easily removed for prolonged near work, whereas contact lenses often cannot be easily removed for near work because of spectacle blur and the problem of loss of adaptation. This problem often can be solved by fitting soft rather than hard lenses, because the lenses can more successfully be worn on a part-time basis.

Magnification Effects with Contact Lenses

Chapter 13 pointed out that, when an ophthalmic lens is moved toward the eye, the retinal image increases in size for a minus lens but decreases in size for a plus lens. In either case, the maximum amount of change in image size will occur when contact lenses are prescribed rather than ophthalmic lenses. These effects often prove to be advantageous, as typified by the myope who is pleased to find that everything looks bigger with contact lenses and by the aphakic contact lens wearer who is pleased to find that objects have returned to nearly their normal sizes.

Induced aniseikonia occurring in anisometropia

The magnification effects just described occur as a result of *spectacle magnification*—that is, due to the magnification brought about by the lenses themselves. Of more concern in the case of the anisometropic patient is *relative spectacle magnifi-*

cation, in which the retinal image size for the eye in question is compared with that of the schematic emmetropic eye.

As discussed in Chapter 13, if the more ametropic of the two eyes is considered to have axial ametropia, the amount of induced aniseikonia is expected to be at a minimum if ophthalmic lenses are fitted. If the more ametropic of the two eyes is considered to have refractive ametropia, the amount of induced aniseikonia is expected to be at a minimum when contact lenses are fitted.

Although ametropia in excess of ± 4.00D is likely to be axial ametropia, and ametropia of less than this amount is more likely to be refractive ametropia, the one obvious situation in which refractive ametropia is present is an eye whose crystalline lens has been removed because of the presence of a cataract. A unilateral aphakic will experience a minimum of retinal image size difference for the two eyes if a contact lens rather than an ophthalmic lens is fitted for the aphakic eye.

Unilateral aphakia

Suppose that a unilateral aphakic refracted at a vertex distance of 12mm is found to require the following lenses:

Right (unoperated) eye: +1.00DS.

Left (operated) eye: +13.00DS.

Assuming that the patient is fitted with plastic spectacle lenses having an index of refraction of 1.498, that lens thickness is 2.5mm for the right lens and 7.0mm for the left lens, and that front surface power is +7.00D for the right lens and +15.00D for the left lens, the magnification brought about by each lens would be

$$\text{R.E.: } SM = \left(\cfrac{1}{1 - \cfrac{0.0025}{1.498}(7)} \right)\left(\cfrac{1}{1 - 0.015(1)} \right)$$

$$= 1.027$$

$$\%SM = 2.7\%.$$

$$\text{L.E.: } SM = \left(\cfrac{1}{1 - \cfrac{0.007}{1.498}(15)} \right)\left(\cfrac{1}{1 - 0.015(13)} \right)$$

$$= 1.336$$

$$\%SM = 33.6\%.$$

Therefore, the resulting difference in retinal image size for the two eyes is

$$33.6 - 2.7 = 30.9\%.$$

If the aphakic eye is now fitted with a contact lens rather than a spectacle lens, the required power of the contact lens will be

$$F_{CL} = \cfrac{13}{1 - 0.012(13)} = 15.40\text{D}.$$

Assuming that the contact lens has an index of refraction of 1.490, a center thickness of 0.55mm, and a front surface power of 77.50D, the magnification brought about by the contact lens will be

$$SM = \left(\cfrac{1}{1 - \cfrac{0.00055}{1.490}(77.5)} \right)\left(\cfrac{1}{1 - 0.003(15.5)} \right)$$

$$= 1.080$$

$$\%SM = 8.0\%.$$

The resulting difference in retinal image size for the two eyes is now

$$8.0 - 2.7 = 5.3\%.$$

This magnification difference would apply only if no spectacle lens were worn in front of the aphakic eye. However, the patient would typically be fitted with a plano lens in front of the aphakic eye (in addition to the contact lens) containing a bifocal addition for near work and possibly also containing any cylindrical power necessary to correct astigmatism not corrected by the contact lens. However, even a plano lens magnifies the retinal image (by virtue of the *shape factor* of the spectacle magnification formula). Assuming that the patient wears a plano lens having a center thickness of 2.0mm and a front surface power of +6.00D, the magnification brought about by this lens would be

$$SM = \left(\cfrac{1}{1 - \cfrac{0.002}{1.498}(6)} \right)\left(\cfrac{1}{1 - 0.015(0)} \right)$$

$$= 1.008$$

$$\%SM = 0.8\%.$$

The retinal image magnification for the aphakic eye, therefore, would be the product of the magnification brought about by the contact lens and by the spectacle lens, or

$$SM = (1.080)(1.008) = 1.089.$$

$$\%SM = 8.9\%.$$

Under these conditions, the difference in retinal image magnification for the two eyes becomes

$$8.9 - 2.7 = 6.2\%.$$

(Aphakic contact lenses are discussed further in a later section of this chapter.)

Field of View of the Contact Lens Wearer

To many new wearers of contact lenses, one of the main advantages is the larger field of view they provide compared with the field of view provided by glasses. This subjective awareness of a larger field of view could be due to one or a combination of the following circumstances: (1) a larger peripheral field of view, (2) a larger macular field of view, and (3) reduced lens aberration effects.

Peripheral field of view

The peripheral field of view of a correcting lens (i.e., the field of view for the steadily fixating eye) can be expressed by the following relationship:

$$\tan \phi = \frac{y(E - F)}{1000},$$

where

ϕ = one-half of the angular field of view.

y = one-half of the lens aperture (in millimeters).

E = vergence of light at the entrance pupil of the eye.

F = power of the correcting lens (see Figure 14.9).

Using this expression, the peripheral field of view can be determined for a 3.00D myope for both a spectacle lens and a contact lens, assuming the lens apertures to be 50mm for the spectacle lens and 7mm for the contact lens, and assuming the entrance pupil distance to be 15mm for the spectacle lens and 3mm for the contact lens:

$$Spectacle\ lens:\ \tan \phi = \frac{25(66.67 + 3)}{1000} = 1.7418$$

$$2\phi = 120.28°.$$

$$Contact\ lens:\ \tan \phi = \frac{3.5(333.33 + 3)}{1000} = 1.1772$$

$$2\phi = 99.31°.$$

Surprisingly, the peripheral field of view is smaller with a contact lens than with a spectacle lens.

Macular field of view

The macular field of view for a correcting lens (i.e., the field of view seen by the macula for a moving eye) can be expressed by the relationship

$$\tan \theta = \frac{y(S - F)}{1000},$$

where

S = vergence of light at center of rotation of the eye. (In determining the macular field of view, the center of rotation of the eye acts as the *stop* (for the moving eye), whereas the entrance pupil acts as the stop for the stationary eye.)

θ = one-half of the angular field of view (see Figure 14.10).

The macular field of view for the 3.00D myope (assuming a center of rotation distance of 25mm) while wearing a spectacle lens would be

$$\tan \theta = \frac{25(40 + 3)}{1000} = 1.075$$

$$2\theta = 94.14°.$$

Figure 14.9   Peripheral field of view of a lens (Grosvenor, 1976a).

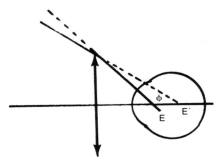

Figure 14.10   Macular field of view of a lens (Grosvenor, 1976a).

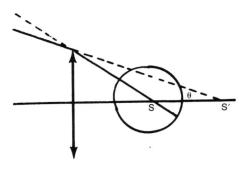

What about the macular field of view while wearing a contact lens? Because a contact lens rotates with the eye, the value of y in the equation is not limited by the aperture of the lens. Therefore, the only limit on the macular field of view while wearing a contact lens is the extent to which the wearer is able to rotate the eye. Therefore, the macular field of view through a contact lens is equal to the *field of fixation* of the eye. Thus, we can conclude that the new contact lens wearer's subjective awareness of a larger visual field is due to the fact that the macular field of view, rather than the peripheral field of view, is larger through a contact lens than a spectacle lens.

However, another important factor is that the rim surrounding a spectacle lens attracts the wearer's attention. Even with an eyesize as large as 50mm, the wearer can be aware of the presence of a rim (or even the edge of a rimless lens) while fixating steadily through the center of the lens. Contact lenses have no rims. Even through the peripheral field of view of a contact lens having a 7mm optical zone is somewhat smaller than that through a spectacle lens, the edge of the optical zone of the lens (whether a hard lens or a soft lens) gradually blends into the peripheral zone of the lens in such a way that the wearer is not aware of a boundary.

Lens aberrations

Are the effects of lens aberrations reduced with contact lenses as compared with glasses? The lens aberrations that must be taken into consideration in spectacle lens design (*oblique astigmatism* and *curvature of image*) are the aberrations that occur when the wearer turns the eyes to fixate through the periphery of the lenses. It follows, then, that because a contact lens wearer fixates only through the centers of the lenses, these peripheral aberrations should not constitute a problem.

Due to their increased curvature as compared with spectacle lenses, contact lenses are more subject to *spherical aberration* than are spectacle lenses. However, the relatively small aperture of the contact lens-eye system tends to minimize the effects of this aberration.

Optical Principles of Aphakic Contact Lenses

In Chapter 13, the disadvantages of ophthalmic lenses for aphakia are described (lens weight, lens thickness, magnified appearance of the wearer's eyes, lens aberrations, decreased field of view, and increased retinal image size), and the point is made that these disadvantages can be overcome if contact lenses rather than ophthalmic lenses are prescribed.

The advantages of contact lenses concerning lens weight and lens thickness are obvious. The magnified appearance of the wearer's eyes is eliminated with contact lenses, because the spectacle magnification is reduced to about 6 or 7 percent, (compared with 30 percent or more with ophthalmic lenses). As discussed in the previous section, the lens aberrations of oblique astigmatism and curvature of image are of little concern to the contact lens wearer, since the patient fixates only through the centers of the lenses. Further discussion is limited to the problems of field of view and retinal image magnification.

Field of view

As noted earlier, for a 3.00D myope, the peripheral field of view is smaller for a contact lens having an aperture of 7mm than for a spectacle lens having an aperture of 50mm. It is of interest to determine the extent of the peripheral field of view for an aphakic eye, first with a spectacle lens and then with a contact lens. Consider an aphakic patient who requires a +12.50D spectacle lens or a +14.50D contact lens, using the same aperture sizes as those used earlier:

$$\text{Spectacle lens:} \quad \tan \phi = \frac{25(66.67 - 12.50)}{1000}$$

$$= 1.3543$$

$$2\phi = 107.11°.$$

$$\text{Contact lens:} \quad \tan \phi = \frac{3.5(333.33 - 14.50)}{1000}$$

$$= 1.1160$$

$$2\phi = 96.27°.$$

As with the −3.00D lens, the peripheral field of view is smaller with the contact lens than with the spectacle lens.

However, for the aphakic spectacle lens wearer, the macular field of view will be greatly reduced compared with that of the myope or emmetrope. Assuming a center of rotation distance of 25mm and a 50mm aperture size, the macular field of view for an aphakic eye wearing a +12.50D lens would be

$$\tan \theta = \frac{25(40 - 12.50)}{1000} = 0.6875$$

$$2\theta = 69.02°.$$

Recall that the 3.00D myope had a macular field of

94.14 degrees. The aphakic eye is found to have a greatly restricted macular field of view through a spectacle lens as compared with the myopic eye.

This greatly restricted field of view is responsible for the roving ring scotoma and the jack-in-the-box phenomenon described in Chapter 13, and it causes the spectacle-wearing aphakic eventually to learn (as pointed out by the anonymous aphakic physician) that the world can be made to remain still only by looking through the optical centers of the lenses and by moving the head instead of the eyes. When the aphakic individual wears contact lenses, the macular field of view is limited only by the field of fixation of the eyes, and the problems of the roving ring scotoma and the jack-in-the-box phenomenon are eliminated.

Recall that the anonymous aphakic physician also commented that door jambs appear to curve inward toward the middle but gradually open up as the doorway is approached. This is due to the aberration of pincushion distortion, which can be minimized (with an ophthalmic lens) only by using lenses having absurdly steep curves. Distortion varies with the distance of the correcting lens from the stop behind the lens (the entrance pupil of the eye) and, therefore, is at a minimum when a contact lens is used.

Image magnification

It is possible for the bilateral aphakic eventually to adapt to the space distortions due to the extreme retinal image magnification caused by spectacle lenses. Although objects appear to be both larger and nearer than they really are, one can learn, with practice, to respond correctly to the new set of size and distance clues. However, the unilateral aphakic is confronted with a situation in which adaptation is not possible.

Welsh (1961) described the problems brought about by the large size difference for the retinal images of the two eyes of a spectacle-wearing aphakic. The two images are not only greatly different in size but they move back and forth at different speeds as the head is moved relative to a fixated object. Even though the patient may be able to superimpose the two retinal images (in spite of their size differences) when "aiming" the head directly at the fixated object, any movement of the head relative to the object will result in diplopia, the amount of which will vary with even slight head movements.

It was shown earlier in this chapter that the retinal image size differences could be decreased from about 30 percent if a spectacle lens is worn in front of the aphakic eye to about 6 percent if a contact lens is worn. A 6 percent image-size difference is still a large amount of aniseikonia: for example, the scale on the American Optical Space Eikonometer extends only to 4 percent magnification. However, many aphakic patients seem to be able to adapt to the amount of magnification that is present when a contact lens is worn on the aphakic eye, probably because the speed of movement of the two retinal images relative to one another is greatly decreased as compared with the situation when a spectacle lens is worn. In addition, most unilateral aphakics have a beginning (or even relatively mature) cataract in the phakic eye, and they can learn to suppress the image of this eye in the presence of the reduced aniseikonia and reduced speed of movement of the two images relative to one another when a contact lens is worn on the aphakic eye.

Enoch (1968) reported on the successful use of a reverse Galilean telescope in unilateral aphakia. The telescope consists of an overcorrection of plus power in the contact lens (for the aphakic eye), in combination with a negative spectacle lens as the objective. His report includes a table showing the amount of overcorrection and the spectacle lens powers necessary to bring about various changes in magnification. Typical values given in the table are as follows:

Magnification	Vertex distance	$F(+)$	$F(-)$
8.0%	13.9mm	5.25D	6.25D
7.4	11.9	6.25	6.75
6.9	10.2	6.75	7.25

In the table, $F(+)$ indicates the amount of overcorrection required for the contact lens, while $F(-)$ indicates the required power of the spectacle lens.

To obtain the precise vertex distance required, frames with adjustable pads and low-riding temples must be used. Enoch (1968) reports that the reverse telescope is particularly appreciated by relatively young aphakics actively engaged in occupations requiring critical vision.

Power specification

As noted earlier, soft contact lenses in the powers required for aphakic eyes are sufficiently rigid that the lens may fail to conform completely to the corneal surface. As a result, a negative "tear lens" may be formed underneath the apical portion of the lens, requiring more plus power than one would predict on the basis of objective or subjective refraction corrected for vertex distance. As an additional consequence of the failure of the lens to conform to the corneal surface, an aphakic lens may be found to eliminate a moderate amount of astigmatism.

CONTACT LENS MATERIALS AND MANUFACTURING PROCESSES

Contact lens materials can be conveniently classified into three categories: (1) conventional hard or rigid lens materials, (2) soft, flexible lens materials, and (3) oxygen-permeable hard materials. Manufacturing processes most often used are lathe cutting, used for the majority of both hard and soft lenses, and spin casting, used for some soft lenses. Some hard lenses, in particular the oxygen-permeable lenses made of silicone, are manufactured by a molding process.

Conventional Hard Lens Materials

From the time that Kevin Tuohy developed the plastic corneal lens in 1948 until the introduction of gas-permeable hard materials in the 1970s, virtually all hard contact lenses were made of PMMA. As noted by Refojo (1976), most PMMA lenses are cross-linked with a dimethacrylate comonomer.

In most respects, PMMA has been an excellent lens material. It is highly transparent, has excellent optical properties, is light in weight, is easily machined, has good dimensional stability, and is nonallergenic. A minor disadvantage of PMMA lenses is that their surfaces are relatively *hydrophobic*. A hydrophobic surface has a large wetting angle, with the result that liquid does not easily spread over the surface but tends to form droplets (as shown in the top diagram of Figure 14.11). A completely *hydrophilic* surface, as shown in the lower diagram of Figure 14.11, is one having a wetting angle of zero, allowing water to spread evenly over the surface.

The relatively hydrophobic nature of PMMA lens surfaces is not a major drawback. If a *wetting solution* is applied to the lens surfaces before the lens is put on, it renders the lens surfaces hydrophilic, so tears will spread over the lens uniformly. Once the lens has been worn for a few minutes, the mucoid layer of the tear film continues the wetting action (in the same way that it wets the corneal surface) as long as the lens is worn.

A more important disadvantage of PMMA is that lenses made of this material almost completely fail to transmit oxygen and carbon dioxide. The cornea

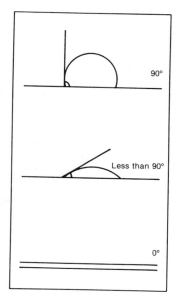

Figure 14.11 Contact angles: *(top)* hydrophobic surface; *(middle)* partially hydrophilic surface; *(bottom)* completely hydrophilic surface. Water spreads evenly over a hydrophilic surface.

has a high oxygen requirement and must constantly obtain atmospheric oxygen, dissolved in the tear film, and rid itself of carbon dioxide. As a result of PMMA's lack of ability to transmit oxygen and carbon dioxide, the lens must be fitted loosely enough so that the normal blinking action of the eyelids will constantly pump freshly oxygenated tears underneath the lens while at the same time removing the stale, carbon dioxide-saturated tears. If the tear film is not supplied with sufficient atmospheric oxygen to supply the needs of the corneal epithelium, anaerobic glycolysis takes place in the epithelium, resulting in the formation of lactic acid, which causes corneal clouding and swelling. Even relatively mild amounts of corneal swelling will cause discomfort toward the end of the wearing period and blurred vision (spectacle blur) after lens removal. Long-continued edema will cause greatly exaggerated diurnal variations in corneal curvature and thickness, and may eventually lead to lens intolerance.

Corneal edema due to the wearing of PMMA lenses can be controlled to a great extent by (1) fitting the lenses loosely enough so there is a reservoir of tears underneath the peripheral curve of the lens and so the lenses move sufficiently during the blink cycle to bring about an adequate amount of *tear pumping*; (2) giving the patient instruction in *adequate blinking*; and (3) controlling the patient's wearing time.

Long-term wearing of PMMA lenses is often accompanied by a flattening of the cornea of about 1.00D or more (as measured with the keratometer). As a result of this flattening, the lenses gradually become too steep relative to the cornea; therefore, the tear reservoir underneath the peripheral curve of the lens may be compromised, and the lenses will fail to move sufficiently during the blink cycle to bring about an adequate amount of tear pumping. A patient who has enjoyed a year or more (possibly several years) of successful lens wear may find that the lenses can no longer be worn all day long with comfort. The solution to this problem is to refit the patient with flatter lenses, reestablishing a favorable lens-cornea relationship. Unfortunately, many patients fail to seek help until the unfavorable condition has persisted so long that PMMA lenses (even if fitted correctly) can no longer be tolerated.

Another disadvantage of PMMA lenses is the tendency for some patients to develop with-the-rule corneal astigmatism after several months or years of lens wear, along with the generalized corneal flattening just described. This may occur partially as a result of long-continued corneal edema but is probably due mainly to *corneal bending*. It has been hypothesized that the constant presence of the rigid lens tends to amplify the pressure of the upper tarsal plate along the horizontal corneal meridian. It is not uncommon for a PMMA lens wearer to develop from 1.00–2.00D of with-the-rule corneal astigmatism after wearing the lenses for a year or more. It is possible that patients who develop with-the-rule astigmatism are those having low corneal rigidity and relatively stiff upper tarsal plates. Because the stiffness of the upper lid decreases markedly with age, older patients would not be expected to develop with-the-rule astigmatism due to PMMA lens wear.

Hard lens manufacturing processes

In the early days of PMMA lens manufacturing, some laboratories produced pressed or molded lenses. However, these lenses did not prove to be satisfactory, and all PMMA lenses for many years have been produced by machining on a lathe. PMMA resin is produced in the form of a long rod, which is cut into plastic buttons that can be purchased inexpensively by contact lens laboratories.

The first procedure used by the laboratory is that of lathe cutting and polishing the inner surface, or base curve, of the lens. In this manner, most laboratories acquire large inventories of semifinished lens

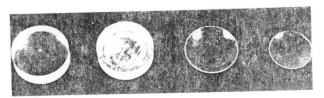

Figure 14.12   Steps in PMMA contact lens manufacture: plastic button, polished button, uncut lens, and finished lens (Grosvenor, 1963).

blanks, so when an order is received, it is necessary only to lathe and polish the front surface (to provide the ordered lens power), put on the peripheral inside curve or curves, and finish the lens edges.

Once the front surface has been lathed and polished, the lens is known as an *uncut lens* (see Figure 14.12). The parameters that can be specified for an uncut lens are base curve, power, center thickness, and diameter. Parameters that can be specified for a finished lens include base curve and secondary curve radii, peripheral curve radius and width, lens diameter, optical zone diameter, power, center thickness, and tint. (The determination of specifications for PMMA lenses is discussed in the section of this chapter on fitting procedures.)

The finishing of uncut PMMA lenses requires relatively simple and inexpensive equipment, and some practitioners stock uncut lenses and employ a technician to perform the cutdown, secondary and peripheral curve cutting and polishing, and edge-finishing processes. In this manner, the sometimes long delays in obtaining finished lenses from a laboratory can be avoided.

Soft Lens Materials

Hydrogel contact lens materials have been described in some detail by Refojo (1976). The lens originally described by Wichterle and Lim in 1960 was made from HEMA, lightly cross-linked with ethylene glycol dimethacrylate. The lens was manufactured by a spin-casting process (to be described). The Bausch & Lomb Soflens, which received FDA approval in 1971, is made of the same material and by the use of a similar spin-casting process as the original Wichterle lens.

In addition to HEMA, many soft lenses contain *vinylpyrrolidone*, either as a copolymer or as a graft polymer. By varying the content of vinylpyrrolidone in the lens, the water content can be increased from the usual HEMA water content of approximately 40 percent to as high as 80 percent or even higher. It is possible to make soft lenses that contain vinylpyrrolidone but not HEMA, and one such lens is apparently a copolymer of methyl methacrylate and vinylpyrrolidone. Other soft lenses contain neither HEMA nor vinylpyrrolidone.

The nomenclature relative to hydrogel contact lens materials is confusing. A given lens may be identified by the manufacturer's company name, by the manufacturer's trade name for the lens, by the chemical designation for the material of which the lens is made, or by the generic name for the lens material. (Generic names are nonproprietary names assigned by the United States Adopted Names [USAN] Council.) The USAN Council uses the stem *filcon* to identify all materials used in soft lenses, with the exception of the material used for the Bausch & Lomb lens and the Hydron lens named *polymacon*.

Comparison with PMMA

When the news of the development of the soft contact lens in Czechoslovakia was released, optometrists were immediately enthusiastic about these lenses because of their hydrophilic nature and because they were believed to be permeable to oxygen and carbon dioxide. However, the fact that the lenses were hydrophilic simply meant that the wearer would not have to use a wetting solution. It was reported by Hill and Fatt (1964b) that, in the lens thicknesses used at that time, the soft lens material was no more permeable to oxygen than was PMMA. It is now understood that the gas transmitted by a hydrogel lens can be increased significantly by increasing the water content of the material or by making the lens extremely thin.

As manufacturers and practitioners argued about the value of the hydrophilic nature and the gas permeability of soft lenses, wearers of the lenses were pleased with them for an entirely different reason: the lenses were comfortable. The superior comfort for the wearer, when soft lenses are compared with conventional PMMA lenses, is due to two factors: (1) the lens material is soft and flexible; and (2) the lens is large enough so its upper and lower edges are constantly underneath the lid margins, with the result that the eyelids do not have to "mount" the edges of the lens with every blink.

The almost complete lack of sensation is not the only advantage of soft lenses compared with PMMA lenses. One of the main problems with PMMA lenses is that because of the presence of numerous sensory nerve endings in the corneal epithelium and lid margins, an adaptation period of at least 2 or 3 weeks

is necessary before the lenses can be worn comfortably on a full wearing schedule. An unfortunate consequence of this adaptation period is that in the process, the corneal epithelium and the lid margins necessarily lose much of their sensitivity, with the result that a foreign body under the lens may cause little or no alarm. With soft lenses it is not necessary to build up wearing time, so less highly motivated patients may find that they can successfully wear soft lenses. In addition to the fact that it is not necessary to build up wearing time with soft lenses, it is not necessary to maintain any level of wearing time, as it is with hard lenses. This makes soft lenses ideal for part-time wear.

A further advantage of soft lenses is that the flattening of the cornea and the induced with-the-rule astigmatism that occur so often with long-term wearers of PMMA lenses are not a problem for soft lens wearers. Although soft lenses have been found to cause an increase in corneal curvature along with minor changes in corneal astigmatism for some wearers, these changes have been found to be due to the lenses being fitted too tightly, and they are to a great extent reversible when properly fitting lenses are fitted.

As for oxygen permeability, in recent years soft lenses have been made sufficiently thin to allow oxygen to be transmitted through the lens in a quantity to meet the cornea's needs, possibly with a small assist from tear pumping.

The most obvious disadvantage of soft contact lenses is that they are much more difficult to keep clean than PMMA lenses. With time, protein and other materials tend to be deposited on the lenses, so both vision and comfort are less than satisfactory, and gas permeability is compromised. (Many of the topics mentioned in these paragraphs are dealt with in more detail in later sections of this chapter.)

Soft lens manufacturing processes

The soft lens developed by Wichterle and Lim in 1960 was manufactured by a spin-casting process. A monomer solution containing the HEMA and cross-linking agent was polymerized in a rotating mold. The curvature of the mold determined the radius of curvature of the front surface of the lens, whereas the speed of rotation and other factors determined the curvature of the aspheric back surface. The Bausch & Lomb Soflens is not only made of the same materials as the original Wichterle lens, but a similar spin-casting process of manufacture is used.

All soft lenses now available in the United States, other than the Soflens, are manufactured by a lathe-cutting process. This manufacturing process is similar to that used in the cutting and polishing of PMMA lenses, with two exceptions: (1) because the material is capable of absorbing a large amount of water, polishing agents containing water cannot be used, so oil-based polishing compounds are substituted; and (2) the material is machined in the dehydrated state, after which it is allowed to hydrate in normal saline solution.

Oxygen-Permeable Hard Lenses

From the point of view of oxygen permeability, silicone is the most desirable lens material. According to Hill (1977c), the oxygen permeability of silicone is so high that there is no question that sufficient oxygen would be delivered to the cornea without the need for tear pumping. Hard contact lenses made of silicone have been under development for many years. The main problem with this material, which has been solved only recently, is poor wettability.

Lenses made of a combination of methyl methacrylate and silicone have been developed in recent years. These include the *Polycon* lens, the *Boston* lens, the *Paraperm* lens, the *Optacryl* lens, and others. These lenses achieve a significantly higher level of oxygen permeability than PMMA lenses, but additional oxygen must be supplied by the tears in the process of tear pumping.

An additional material with high oxygen permeability (although not nearly as high as that of silicone) is *cellulose acetate butyrate (CAB)*. Lenses made of this material have been developed by Danker Laboratories (the *Meso* lens), Soft Lenses, Inc. (the *Cabcurve* lens), and Rynco (the *RX–56* lens).

ANATOMICAL AND PHYSIOLOGICAL CONSIDERATIONS

Corneal Topography

More than a century ago Helmholtz formulated the concept that the cornea flattened toward the periphery and was ellipsoid in cross section, but only with the advent of corneal contact lenses has the exact nature of the corneal topography been of practical importance to vision practitioners. Bier (1957) described the cornea as having a regular central zone, an intermediate negative zone, and a more peripheral positive zone. Grosvenor (1961), reporting on a study involving 17 subjects, found

that the diameter of the optic cap of the cornea (defined as the width of the cornea through which the curvature varied by no more than 1.00D) averaged 5mm in both the vertical and horizontal meridians, and that the amount of peripheral corneal flattening averaged 6.00D nasally, 3.00D temporally, 4.00D superiorly, and 4.00D inferiorly. Mandell (1963) used a keratometer with mires of reduced size and found that the cornea begins to flatten within about 1mm of the apex. As a result, he questioned whether the optic cap of the cornea actually exists.

It is now understood that the cornea, in any one meridian, can be considered as an aspheric surface, having no spherical central portion as such. However, for diagramatic purposes it is convenient to consider the cornea as possessing a central optical portion 4–6mm in width, having the radius of curvature indicated by the keratometer finding, and having a peripheral portion whose radius of curvature is approximately 1mm flatter than that of the central portion. The cornea is shown in Figure 14.13,

Figure 14.13 *(a)* **Schematic representation of the corneal surface, having a central optical zone and a flatter peripheral zone;** *(b)* **representation of the base curve and secondary curve of a contact lens. Note that sagittal depth** *(d)* **of the cornea is greater than that of the contact lens** (Grosvenor, 1972a).

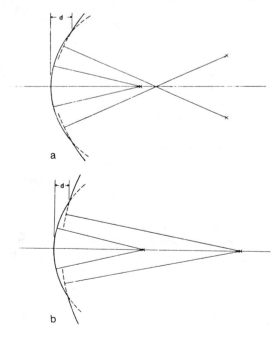

in which the center of curvature of the peripheral portion of the cornea is "offset" somewhat rather than being on the central corneal axis, in keeping with the concept of corneal topography suggested by Mandell (1962).

Figure 14.13b shows how a secondary curve or a peripheral curve is fabricated on the back surface of a hard contact lens. As pointed out by Brungardt (1962b), we fabricate a contact lens in such a way that the centers of curvature of all back surface curves fall along the same straight line, as shown in Figure 14.13b. However, we measure the peripheral cornea in such a way that the centers of curvature fail to lie along the same straight line (see Figure 14.13a). For this reason, the sagittal depth (d), as shown in the diagram, is greater for the cornea than for the contact lens having the same amount of peripheral flattening.

Corneal topography and contact lens design

Beginning with the introduction of the Tuohy lens and the microlens, it was obvious that the peripheral flattening of the cornea had to be taken into consideration in lens design. It was found that if these large, single-curve lenses were fitted parallel to the optical zone of the cornea (as measured by the keratometer), the lens would "seal off" in the periphery, leading to severe corneal edema after a few hours' wear, due to oxygen deprivation. This could be avoided by fitting the lens at least 3.00 or 4.00DK or 0.6–0.8mm flatter than the central keratometer finding. (Throughout the range of corneal radii of curvature, a change in the amount of 1.00DK—as measured by the keratometer—is approximately equal to a change of 0.2mm in the radius of curvature. This is a convenient conversion factor to keep in mind.)

The excessive movement and resulting discomfort of the large, single-curve corneal lenses led to Bier's (1957) development of the Contour lens having a central optical zone of about 6.5mm and a flatter peripheral zone to correspond to the peripheral flattening of the cornea.

All further development of PMMA lens designs necessarily took into consideration the peripheral flattening of the cornea. As lenses became smaller and thinner, they were designed to fit somewhat more tightly than the larger lenses, often having several peripheral curves, each curve progressively flatter to parallel the gradual peripheral flattening of the cornea. Two lenses are of particular interest in this regard. The *V-Contour* lens, developed by Vic

Lowe in Australia, was a 9.0mm-diameter lens having a total of six peripheral curves, each succeedingly flatter than the base curve, and a bevel 2.5mm flatter than the base curve radius. This lens was the bread-and-butter lens in Australia and New Zealand for many years. The *Con-O-Coid* lens, developed by David Volk in the late 1960s and first manufactured by Hirst Laboratories in New Zealand, was the first contact lens with a truly aspheric back surface. Whereas the base curve of the lens is specified in terms of the central keratometer findings, the back surface of the lens is also specified in terms of *eccentricity*, which varies from 0.6 (an ellipse) through 1.0 (a parabola) to 1.1 (a hyperbola). The most commonly used eccentricities are from 0.65–1.0.

With the development of soft contact lenses, in spite of the extreme flexibility of the lenses, it was necessary to take the peripheral flattening of the cornea into consideration. When the Griffin *Naturalens* was introduced in Canada in 1970, it was found that this large, relatively thick, single-curve lens had to be fitted several diopters flatter than the optical zone of the cornea, as did the Tuohy lens and the microlens. As lathe-cut soft lenses became smaller and thinner, they could be fitted somewhat steeper than the larger lenses, but they had to be fitted about 2.00 to 5.00DK (0.4 to 1.0mm) flatter than the central zone of the cornea. As noted earlier one can think of a soft lens as fitting parallel to some peripheral zone of the cornea and "draping" itself over the steeper corneal apex.

Precorneal Tear Film

As described by Wolff (cited in Last, 1968), the precorneal tear film is composed of three layers: (1) an inner, *mucoid layer* whose composition differs from that of the freely moving tears, being more like that of the corneal epithelium; (2) a middle, *watery layer*; and (3) a superficial, *oily layer*.

Jones (1973) described the mucoid layer, secreted by the goblet cells of the conjunctiva, as closely adherent to the corneal epithelium, having the function of converting the corneal surface from a hydrophobic to a hydrophilic surface and thus allowing the tear film to spread evenly over the corneal surface. He described the middle layer, secreted by the lacrimal gland and the accessory lacrimal glands, as making up approximately 90 percent of the thickness of the precorneal film and incorporating water-soluble components of the tear film, including salts, glucose, enzymes, and proteins. The outer layer, secreted mainly by the Meibomian

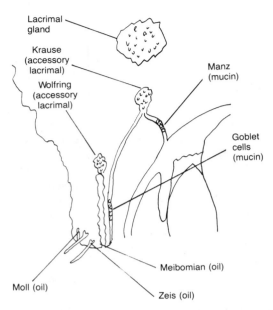

Figure 14.14 Schematic drawing showing basic and reflex secretors. The lacrimal gland is a reflex secretor; the others are basic secretors.

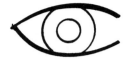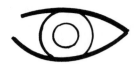

Figure 14.15 The marginal tear strips. Freshly secreted tear fluid runs around the strip from above to below without passing over the corneal or conjunctival surface.

Distribution and elimination of tears

The distribution and elimination of tears has been described by Maurice (1973). He describes the tear film as having a uniform thickness of 6μ over the corneal surface, with the thickness remaining relatively constant between blinks (indicating the absence of tear drainage during this period).

When the tears are stained with fluorescein, a black line is seen extending along the corneal surface just within the lid margins. The watery precorneal film is almost totally absent along these black lines, indicating that the black line forms a barrier between the *marginal tear strip* (see Figure 14.15) and the tear film lying within the palpebral aperture. Maurice pointed out that there is no diffusion of dye across this line and that freshly secreted tear fluid runs around the tear strip from above to below without passing over the corneal or conjunctival surface.

After reviewing a number of theories concerning the elimination of tears, Maurice (1973) proposed the following mechanisms:

1. When copious tearing occurs, the canaliculi empty immediately after a blink. However, after a brief period the canaliculi expand, causing them to fill with fluid from the marginal strip; they then act as conduits through which the nasolacrimal sac can imbibe fluid directly from the lacrimal strip. With the occurrence of a blink, the canaliculi squeeze fluid into the sac, and the sac pushes the fluid down into the nasolacrimal duct.

2. During basal lacrimation, the tear fluid is largely absorbed over the mucosa of the conjunctiva and the lacrimal drainage system. During sleep, blinking is absent and there is thus no mechanism to convey the basal tear secretion to the nasolacrimal drainage system. Maurice suggested that the freshly secreted fluid may dwell in the upper fornix, where it could be absorbed by the conjunctival mucosa.

glands, is described by Jones as being responsible for retarding the evaporation of the tear film.

The formation of the tear film has been described by Jones (1973) in terms of basic secretors and reflex secretors. The *basic secretors*, having no efferent nerve supply (see Figure 14.14), include (1) the *goblet cells* located in the tarsal conjunctiva and the *glands of Manz* located in a circumcorneal ring of limbal conjunctiva, both of which secrete *mucin*; (2) the *glands of Krause* located mainly in the upper conjunctival fornix and the *glands of Wolfring* located at the upper margin of the tarsal plate, both of which secrete *lacrimal fluid*; and (3) the large *Meibomian glands* located in the upper and lower tarsal plates, which, with the help of the glands of *Zeis* and *Moll* (located, respectively, in the palpebral margins of the upper and lower lids and in the roots of the eyelashes), secrete *oily fluid*.

The *reflex secretors* are the orbital and palpebral portions of the *lacrimal gland*, which have an efferent parasympathetic nerve supply. When the eyelids are closed, the basic secretors suffice to supply the precorneal tear film, but during waking hours the reflex secretors function to a moderate extent. Copious tearing or weeping (as when a hard contact lens is worn for the first time) is due to the stimulation of the reflex secretors.

Mucoid layer

The role of the mucoid layer in maintaining the stability of the precorneal tear film has been discussed by Lemp and Holly (1970). The corneal epithelium is a relatively hydrophobic surface, and in the absence of mucin, water does not easily spread over the surface. Mucin brings about the spreading of the tears over the surface of the cornea in two ways: (1) by lowering the surface tension of the cornea and (2) by forming an adsorbed layer of hydrated mucus, which is weakly bound to the corneal surface and thus converts the corneal surface from a hydrophobic to a hydrophilic one. The adsorbed layer of mucus is somewhat tenuous, however, and it must be periodically resurfaced by the eyelids in blinking. One important function of the eyelids, therefore, is to continually resurface the cornea with hydrated mucus.

There are two situations in which hydrated mucus is not sufficiently rubbed into portions of the corneal surface during blinking, both of which can result in the formation of corneal dry spots. When a *pinguecula* is present, it may prevent the lids from rubbing hydrated mucus into a portion of the limbal area, resulting in the formation of a dry area with corneal thinning, known as a corneal *dellen*. A PMMA lens, too, may prevent the lids from rubbing hydrated mucus into a portion of the limbal area of the cornea, also allowing the formation of dry spots. This is the mechanism responsible for the well-known *3 and 9 o'clock staining*.

Tear film breakup

If blinking is prevented for a prolonged period of time, the tear film breaks up, with the formation of dry spots. Holly (1973) suggested that in the presence of an inadequate mucin layer, the evaporation of tears occurring when blinking is prevented can allow lipids from the superficial layer to migrate onto the corneal surface. When the adsorbed mucin layer has become sufficiently contaminated by lipids, the tear film ruptures, and dry spots form (see Figure 14.16).

Tear film breakup time is defined as the interval between a complete blink and the first randomly distributed dry spot. Fluorescein is applied to the bulbar conjunctiva by means of a moistened fluorescein strip, and after blinking several times the patient is instructed to stare straight ahead without blinking. With the use of the slit lamp and the cobalt blue filter, the tear film is scanned until the first dry spot appears. With normal subjects, Lemp (1973) found that the majority of breakup times fell in the 15-to-34-second range, and that in no instance was it less

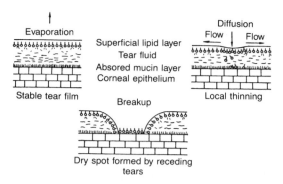

Figure 14.16 Suggested mechanism for tear film break-up, with formation of a dry spot (Holly, 1973).

than 10 seconds. A breakup time of less than 10 seconds is usually considered a negative factor in patient selection for contact lens fitting, particularly in regard to the fitting of soft lenses.

Patients with breakup times of less than 10 seconds have been found by Holly and Lemp (1971) to have abnormally low or nonexistent goblet cell populations, even though they have adequate aqueous tears. The most obvious cause of a deficient goblet cell population is vitamin A deficiency. Although this is not common in North America, it should be considered a possible cause of short tear breakup time, particularly because corneal dry spots can occur as an early sign of this condition. Other causes of loss of goblet cells (and, therefore, decreased mucin production) are ocular pemphigus, Stevens-Johnson syndrome (erythema multiforme), and chemical burns.

If a contact lens candidate is found to have a tear breakup time of less than 10 seconds, the patient can be instructed to use a *mucomimetic* tear substitute such as Adsorbotear (Burton-Parsons) or Tears Naturale (Alcon) for 1 or 2 weeks, after which the breakup test should be repeated. If improvement in breakup time is found and if the patient is subsequently fitted with contact lenses, successful lens wear may require the regular use of the tear substitute while the lenses are worn. The polymeric ingredients in Adsorbotear are polyvinylpyrrolidone, hydroxyethylcellulose, and polyethylene oxide. The ingredient in Tears Naturale is dextran.

Minute Anatomy of the Cornea

Although the cornea is normally considered as having five layers (see Figure 14.17), Feldman and

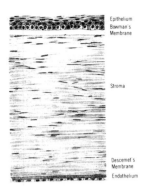

Figure 14.17   Cross section of the cornea (Wolff, 1968).

Sampson (1970) consider the *mucoid layer* of the precorneal tear film as belonging to the cornea rather than to the tear film. It is seen with the biomicroscope as the first of the bright lines in the optical section of the cornea.

The *epithelium* consists of five or six layers of epithelial cells. The deepest (germinal) layer is made up of cuboidal cells, whereas each succeeding layer becomes gradually flatter until the outer, *squamous layer* is reached. Proliferation takes place in the basal layer; a given basal cell will gradually find itself in a more and more superficial layer until, as a squamous cell, it is finally sloughed off and washed away with the tear film. Hanna and O'Brien (1960) studied the movement of the corneal epithelial cells in animals by means of radioactive labeling and found that the new basal cells moved outward at a very rapid rate, requiring only 3½–7 days to move to the superficial layer and be sloughed off.

Working with the electron microscope, Jakus (1961) found that the epithelial cells have long, fingerlike processes that fit snugly into corresponding indentations in adjacent cells. Maurice (1962) described the presence of polymorphous cellular elements, called Langerhans' cells, which send out multiple, fine processes between epithelial cells forming a syncytium with nerve fibers. Other authors have described the presence of "prickle cells," which have fine, protoplasmic fibrils that tend to join epithelial cells together.

The presence of the variously described processes and fibrils is apparently what is responsible for the fact that corneal epithelial cells are more firmly attached to one another than they are to the basement layer and are, therefore, capable of sliding action. This sliding action is demonstrated in the early stages of healing of a corneal abrasion. In the event of a corneal abrasion, healing begins to take place by the process of migration, or sliding, of cells to fill in the defect; the later stage of healing involves proliferation of new epithelial cells. A fairly extensive abrasion, thus, can heal within a 24-hour period.

Bowman's layer was once thought to be a structureless membrane but is now known to be a modification of the stroma, as described by Jakus (1964). Bowman's layer contains fibrils similar to those within the lamellae of the stroma (described in the following paragraph), but they are not regularly oriented like the stromal fibrils. This layer provides resistance to injury and infection, but it is not capable of regeneration when destroyed.

The *stroma*, which accounts for about 90 percent of the thickness of the cornea, is composed of approximately 200 layers, or *lamellae*, of collagenous tissue. All lamellae lie parallel to the corneal surface, and in any one lamella all fibrils are parallel to one another. However, alternate layers are at right angles to one another. As described by Maurice (1962), the mechanical strength of the cornea is principally a property of the stroma. He refers to the stroma as a membrane of high tensile strength that is inflated by pressure, and he compares it to a football, which is designed to take a considerable amount of punishment.

Descemet's membrane is regarded as a true elastic membrane, in that it tends to gape when cut. It offers resistance to both chemical and mechanical trauma and is the last part of the cornea to be perforated in case of a corneal ulcer or other corneal injury. It will regenerate if destroyed.

The *endothelium* is a single layer of endothelial cells lining Descemet's membrane. It is continuous with the endothelium of the iris.

The *limbus*, or transition area between the cornea and the sclera, has a width of about 1mm. At the limbus, the number of layers of epithelial cells increases to approximately ten; the stroma loses its regular arrangement, the lamellae gradually assuming the irregular pattern found in the sclera; Bowman's layer ends abruptly; and Descemet's membrane takes part in the formation of the trabecular meshwork.

The cornea is normally *avascular* except at the limbus, where small loops tend to invade the periphery. Nourishment of the cornea is due to the permeation of tissue fluid through the stroma because there are no lymphatic vessels. In some pathological conditions, blood vessels may invade the cornea. If the disease process is superficial, the blood vessels will be tortuous in pattern, whereas if the process is deep in the cornea, the vessels will be straight. After the disease process has subsided, blood may no longer be present but the vessels will remain.

The *nerve supply* to the cornea is by way of the ophthalmic division of the fifth cranial nerve. Some 60–80 nerve trunks enter the cornea radially at the limbus and branch into superficial and deep plexes, which send many fine nerve endings through Bowman's layer into the epithelium.

Physiology of the Cornea

Physiological considerations that are of importance in the design of contact lenses are corneal sensitivity, transparency, regulation of water content, and transfer of oxygen and carbon dioxide.

Sensitivity

The cornea is known to have numerous free nerve endings in the epithelium and, thus, is extremely sensitive to pain. Adler (1965) stated that more pain spots are located in the cornea and in the mucous membrane of the anus than in any other part of the body. Strughold (1953) and Bier (1957) found that corneal sensitivity is greatest at the apex and gradually falls off toward the periphery. Strughold found that the conjunctiva lining the eyelids is also sensitive to pain, and it was suggested by Dickinson (1971) that some of the discomfort associated with the old "apical touch" corneal lenses was the result of lid sensitivity rather than corneal sensitivity.

Superficial stimulation of pain in the cornea, as by a foreign body (or by a hard contact lens), is usually accompanied by marked photophobia and lacrimation—often referred to as the *foreign body reaction.*

Transparency

Because the cornea and the sclera are composed of the same general type of tissue—collagenous connective tissue—one may ask, "Why is the cornea transparent whereas the sclera is opaque?" This question can be answered by comparing the structure and the physical properties of the cornea and the sclera.

Vascularity. To be transparent, a structure must be avascular. The cornea is avascular, whereas the sclera contains numerous blood vessels.

Deturgescence. Collagenous connective tissue has the ability to hold a great deal of water. The corneal stroma is in a state of deturgescence, indicating that is does not hold all of the water that it is capable of holding. The sclera, on the other hand, is in a state of relative intumescence, containing a relatively larger proportion of water than does the cornea. If the cornea is allowed to imbibe all the water it will hold, it will become opaque, whereas the sclera will become translucent if the amount of water it holds is decreased sufficiently.

Cellular structure. The connective tissue cells in the cornea are flat and few in number compared with those in the sclera. In addition, the corneal epithelium is thin, compact, and has a smooth optical surface compared with the conjunctival epithelium, which is thicker and overlies loose episcleral tissue.

Fiber arrangement. The fibrils of the corneal stroma (the corneal lamellae) lie parallel to the surface of the cornea and are closely packed, adjacent fibers running parallel to one another. In contrast to the corneal fibrils, the scleral fibers tend to twist and turn, forming a "basket weave" network. Maurice (1960) proposed what he calls the *lattice theory of corneal transparency.* Because the diameter of the fibrils making up the corneal lattice is about one-tenth of the wavelength of light, he suggested that the stroma behaves in such a manner that all light is scattered and then recombined by interference, so the scattering is suppressed in any direction but that of the incident beam. Thus, the cornea behaves as if it had a uniform index of refraction. Maurice suggested that clouding (edema) of the cornea results from a derangement of the lamellar fibrils, or a weakening of the forces holding them in position.

Regulation of water content

If an excised cornea is placed in a container of water, it will swell and become opaque. The question now arises, "What factors prevent the cornea from imbibing water in the normal situation?"

There are three possible routes by means of which the cornea can obtain or lose water. These are the limbal vascular loops, the epithelium, and the endothelium (see Figure 14.18). Although it was formerly believed that water could readily flow across the limbus (to and from the limbal vascular loops) and likewise through the corneal stroma, Maurice (1960b) found that movement of water across the cornea takes place only by means of a slow diffusion process.

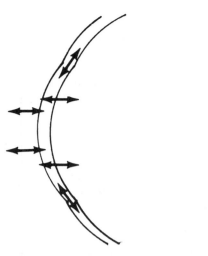

Figure 14.18 Possible routes by means of which the cornea can obtain or lose water.

Cogan and Kinsey (1942) suggested that the relative deturgescence of the cornea could be accounted for by the *osmotic pressure* of the precorneal film. They proposed that the osmotic pressure of the precorneal film is greater than that of the corneal epithelium due to the constant evaporation of tears that causes water to be removed from the cornea (the epithelium acting as a semipermeable membrane). They also proposed that the osmotic pressure of the aqueous humor is greater than that of the corneal stroma, the endothelium acting as a semipermeable membrane that allows water to move from the cornea to the aqueous.

Harris (1960) proposed that the removal of water from the cornea is due to an active pumping mechanism residing in both the epithelium and the endothelium. He proposed a *metabolic pump* requiring oxygen, and speculated that the oxygen supply normally available from the aqueous humor is sufficient to maintain a fairly effective pumping mechanism. Only when the oxygen is completely depleted does a serious handicap in the mechanism result.

Additional evidence has shown that both the osmotic theory and the metabolic pump theory are correct. The cornea's water content is regulated by both osmotic pressure and pumping. In addition to its pumping function, the endothelium is known to have an important *barrier* function. Destruction of a significant number of endothelial cells, as can occur in Fuchs' dystrophy or in cataract surgery, can interfere with the barrier function of the endothelium, so large amounts of water from the aqueous humor

can invade the corneal stroma and epithelium under the force of the intraocular pressure.

Oxygen and carbon dioxide transfer

As described by Adler (1965), the metabolic activity of the cornea involves the processes of *glycolysis* and *respiration*. Glycolysis can take place either in the presence or absence of oxygen; respiration, which takes place mainly in the epithelium, requires oxygen. Respiration results in the production of carbon dioxide and water and in the liberation of energy, which can be used for cellular activity (such as the operation of the pumping mechanism) and for maintenance of tissue temperature.

Hill and Fatt (1964a) conducted a number of experiments concerning oxygen deprivation and contact lenses. Using rabbits as subjects, they found that in the absence of blinking, the development of oxygen deprivation of the cornea (due to either lens application or lid closure) reached a maximum within 30 seconds to 1 minute of covering the cornea. Following reexposure to air, the cornea returned to its original rate of oxygen uptake within about the same period of time. From this, Hill and Fatt concluded that, at the normal blink rate (approximately 12 times per minute), replenishment of air-saturated tears by mechanical action of the lens prevents significant oxygen deprivation of the covered corneal surface.

EFFECTS OF CONTACT LENSES ON CORNEAL PHYSIOLOGY

The effects of contact lenses on the normal physiology of the cornea are discussed here in terms of inadequate blinking, corneal edema, and interference with the cornea's oxygen supply.

Inadequate Blinking

Typically, the new contact lens wearer (particularly the hard lens wearer) blinks too frequently during the first few days of lens wear and then enters a period of infrequent blinking. In addition, there is a strong tendency for contact lens wearers to become *incomplete blinkers*—the blink begins normally, but once the lid margin makes contact with the lens, the blink is completed prematurely.

Although a person who is not a contact lens wearer may experience few, if any, problems as a result of infrequent or incomplete blinking, for a contact lens wearer blinking serves a number of important functions. A correctly fitting hard lens always has a reservoir of oxygenated tears available underneath the peripheral curve, and blinking serves the important function of continually pumping these tears underneath the lens and pumping stale tears containing carbon dioxide and other waste products (including keratinized epithelial cells) out from under the lens (see Figure 14.19). Another important advantage of adequate blinking is keeping the cornea and contact lens in a hydrated condition. This occurs as a result of the continual resurfacing of the corneal epithelium and the lens surfaces with hydrated mucus. A third advantage is that blinking aids in keeping the lenses clean.

The first practitioner to emphasize the importance of blinking habits in contact lens adaptation was Stewart (1968), who defined *functional blinking* as blinking that produces (1) a natural appearance of the wearer, (2) optimum lens movement and positioning, (3) a clean anterior lens surface, and (4) observable fluid flow beneath the lens.

Blinking exercises

Stewart (1968) recommends that the contact lens practitioner teach patients to blink properly and that the emphasis to patients be on the natural appearance that will result when correct blinking habits have been established. The patient is taught to blink in three counts: "one, close; two, pause; three, open wide." After practicing in slow motion, blinking can be gradually sped up. Stewart suggests that the practitioner watch for the following signs of poor blinking: smudged lenses (a sure sign); poor tear flow under the lens, as seen with the slit lamp; and subjective symptoms such as burning, irritation, a feeling of dryness, and vague symptoms of discomfort.

Korb and Korb (1970) published a set of instructions on correct blinking to be given to new contact lens wearers. They instruct the patient to place the index fingers at the outer corners of the eyes and to make sure than no tension is felt during blinking. Patients are asked to perform this exercise 15 times per day, with each practice period consisting of ten correct blinks. The patient is instructed to blink in three counts, as recommended by Stewart.

During the prefitting examination of a contact lens candidate, the practitioner should observe both the frequency and the completeness of the patient's spontaneous blinking. Patients who have poor blinking habits in the absence of contact lenses will likely have problems once contact lens wear is begun.

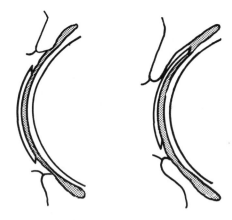

Figure 14.19 For a hard contact lens wearer, the upward lag of the lens during blinking causes fresh, oxygenated tears to be pumped underneath the lens (thickness of tear layer is exaggerated).

Blinking with soft lenses

The recommendations of Stewart (1968) and of Korb and Korb (1970) were made before soft lenses had been approved by the FDA, and, therefore, their statements applied only to PMMA lenses. However, there is no doubt that correct blinking habits are equally important for wearers of soft lenses as for wearers of hard lenses.

Even though a number of studies have shown that a certain amount of oxygen can pass through soft lens materials (and the thinner the lens, the more oxygen can pass through), a well-fitting soft lens not only makes a slight vertical translational movement over the corneal surface during a blink but also flexes, or "ripples" with each blink due to the squeezing action of the upper lid. This combination of translational movement and flexure of the lens can be assumed to serve the purpose of the well-known tear pump of the hard lens, the lens movement allowing tears containing carbon dioxide to move out from the lens with each blink to be replaced by tears containing fresh oxygen (see Figure 14.20).

Is tear pumping necessary with soft lenses?

Because PMMA lenses are almost completely impermeable to oxygen, it is agreed that tear pumping is necessary for wearers of these lenses. However, there is considerable disagreement over the necessity of tear pumping for soft lens wearers. To gain some insight into the problem, two questions

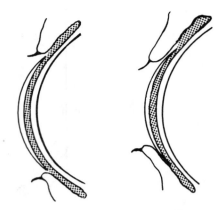

Figure 14.20   A soft contact lens exhibits less movement on the cornea during a blink than a hard lens, causing oxygenated tears to be pumped underneath the lens (thickness of tear layer is exaggerated).

can be asked: (1) Does tear exchange really occur when a soft lens wearer blinks? (2) Are soft lens materials sufficiently permeable to oxygen that tear pumping is not necessary?

Considering only the tear exchange due to the squeezing of a soft lens by the upper lid during a blink, Hayashi and Fatt (1976) developed a "lubrication theory" model of a lens-cornea system and concluded that for a normal blink, there is a 10 to 20 percent tear exchange with each blink. However, Polse (1979) fitted three subjects with soft lenses and, determining tear exchange by means of large-molecule fluorescein and fluorophotometry, concluded that only 1 percent of the tear volume was replaced with each blink. Polse calculated that the oxygen under the lens attributed to tear pumping was 15 percent or less of the total oxygen tension at the tear-lens interface. Hill and Jeppe (1975) determined oxygen permeability of Hydron and Hydrocurve material for various thicknesses and concluded that for either material within the commonly used thickness range, oxygen permeability was insufficient to meet the oxygen requirements of the corneal epithelium without a "significant assist" of a tear pump.

Even though they disagree on the amount of tear pumping necessary, all of the investigators found that some tear pumping was necessary for wearers of soft lenses.

Further advantages of adequate blinking for soft lens wearers

An additional advantage of adequate blinking with hydrogel lenses is that the movement of the lens over the corneal surface allows the removal of any sloughed-off epithelial cells, mucus, and other debris that may have collected underneath the lens. If there was no movement at all, keratinized epithelial cells (which are replaced on a daily basis) and other debris would remain underneath the lens until the end of the daily wearing period. A related advantage of adequate blinking is that by constant removal of debris from both the front and back surfaces of the lens, the lens surfaces are kept clean and "coating" of the lenses is less likely to occur.

Another problem that can be avoided if the patient learns to blink properly is drying of the lenses. Many otherwise successful lens wearers report that their lenses begin to feel dry and uncomfortable after several hours of wear. If such a patient's blinking habits are surreptitiously observed during slit-lamp examination, the patient will almost certainly be found to be a poor blinker.

In summary, correct blinking habits for wearers of soft contact lenses can have the following beneficial results:

1. Better oxygen and carbon dioxide exchange, providing increased comfort; better tolerance of the lenses by the eyes; and (in some cases) longer wearing time.
2. Removal of keratinized epithelial cells and other debris from underneath the lenses.
3. Cleaner lens surfaces, reducing the possibility of the occurrence of coating.
4. Reduced possibility of lens dehydration and the deleterious effects that may follow.
5. A good possibility of extending the useful life of the lenses as a result of the decreased tendency for lens coating and dehydration.

Corneal Edema with PMMA Lenses

From the earliest days of contact lens fitting, practitioners have been aware that contact lenses tend to cause corneal edema. The primary factor limiting the wearing time of scleral lenses is *Sattler's veil*, the appearance of rainbow halos around lights and fogginess of vision after several hours of lens wear. The first practitioner to describe the edema seen during the first few weeks of corneal lens wear was Mazow (1962), who pointed out that it usually appears as "a grayish patch several millimeters in diameter where the apex of the lens exerts the greatest influence on the cornea" and is best seen with the biomicroscope using sclerotic scatter. This edema, also called *round edema* or *central corneal clouding*, is usually accompanied by corneal steepening, a slight increase in myopia, an increase in corneal thickness, and reports of spectacle blur.

Detection of central corneal clouding

A specific method for the detection of central corneal clouding, described by Korb and Exford (1968), is introduced in Chapter 7 and is more fully described here. The method is called the *split limbal technique* and is a combination of sclerotic scatter and retroillumination. The width of the beam should be from about 1.5mm (for a blue iris) to 3mm (for a brown iris), the angle of incidence should be between 45 and 60 degrees, and observation should be made in complete darkness just after lens removal. The clouding should first be detected with the naked eye, with the patient's fixation adjusted to place the suspected area against the background of the pupil; then it should be observed under magnification. The clouded area is off-white (appearing bluish or yellowish, depending on the color of the iris), invariably corresponding in location to the centration of the lens. Corneal clouding can be graded from grade 1 through grade 4 (from barely visible to severe).

Corneal steepening

The corneal steepening that often occurs with corneal edema was described by Mazow (1962). He commented that the refracting power in the primary corneal meridian can be increased as much as 1.00D over the prefitting examination and that this gradually diminishes over a period of about 3 months. In New Zealand, Bott (1965) noted a similar increase in corneal curvature occurring with new PMMA lens wearers. In the author's experience, the usual range of corneal steepening is between 0.25 and 0.50D, and it is a rarity to find a new wearer who has no measurable increase in corneal curvature immediately after lens removal.

Increase in myopia

The steepened corneal curvature for the new lens wearer is usually accompanied by a corresponding increase in myopia or decrease in hyperopia.

Increase in corneal thickness

Many studies involving the use of electronically recorded corneal pachometry have been published by Mandell and his co-workers and by other investigators. Mandell and Polse (1969) suggested that corneal thickness changes could be used as an index for success in contact lens wearing. They reported finding a minimum corneal thickness increase in new PMMA lens wearers of 2 to 4 percent. For these patients, no corneal clouding was seen with the slit lamp, and successful contact lens wear was predicted. Mandell and Polse found that patients having a corneal thickness increase of 5 to 8 percent (accompanied by corneal clouding as seen with the slit lamp) should be watched closely for problems due to oxygen deprivation, and that patients having a corneal thickness increase of 8 percent or more would be poor wearers if they could wear lenses at all.

Spectacle blur

A further indication of corneal edema is spectacle blur, the patient's report of blurred vision with spectacles after removing the contact lenses. It appears that an important factor in spectacle blur is epithelial wrinkling—the kind of corneal change that results in distorted keratometer mire images. The duration of spectacle blur reported by a patient can be important to the practitioner in evaluating the fit of the lenses. Any spectacle blur persisting longer than 20 or 30 minutes after lens removal warrants investigation.

Corneal Edema with Soft Lenses

When soft lenses became generally available to practitioners, it was obvious that wearers of these lenses did not have the circular patch of corneal clouding seen in hard lens wearers. They usually did not show an increase in corneal curvature or myopia, or complain of spectacle blur. In a study of 30 wearers of N&N lathe-cut soft lenses, Grosvenor (1975a) found that the typical patient showed a small amount of corneal flattening during the first several weeks of lens wear that gradually returned to the prefitting curvature. It was proposed, as previously suggested by Mandell (1974), that the flattening could have been due to an overall swelling of the cornea rather than to the swelling (confined to the central area only) that one sees with PMMA lens wearers.

Further evidence that soft lenses cause an overall swelling of the cornea was presented by Sanders, Polse, Sarver, and Harris (1975), who found that corneal thickness of four Soflens wearers increased centrally, nasally, and temporally during the first 6 hours of wear. They concluded that the overall swelling of the cornea accounts for the fact that corneal edema due to soft lenses cannot easily be seen with the slit lamp, whereas corneal edema due to hard lens wear is observable because of the contrast between the central edematous portion of the cornea and the more peripheral, nonedematous portion.

Corneal striae

A more reliable indicator of the presence of corneal edema caused by soft lenses is the presence of *corneal striae*. Their existence was first noted by Sarver (1971), who reported the observation of vertical striate lines in the deep corneal layers of some wearers of soft contact lenses. He described 6–12 irregular, fine, vertical lines distributed across the cornea, apparently in the region of Descement's membrane.

Changes in corneal thickness and the observation of corneal striae were monitored for 27 wearers of Soflens lenses by Polse, Sarver, and Harris (1975). They found that 96 percent of their subjects showed an increase in corneal thickness after 4 hours of lens wear, and that there was a steady increase in corneal thickness for about the first 6 hours of lens wear, leveling off after 6–8 hours of wear. Of 18 subjects who had worn lenses for at least 3 weeks, 50 percent were found to have vertical striae (observed using a narrow parallelepiped and direct focal illumination after 8 hours) and an average increase in corneal thickness of 6.8 percent.

An investigation concerning the cause of corneal striae was conducted by Polse and Mandell (1976), who found that when the eyes were subjected to an atmosphere of pure nitrogen (by means of goggles), corneal striae were observed when the corneal thickness had increased by approximately 7 percent. These researchers concluded that corneal striae accompanying soft lens wear are caused by corneal edema, which is the result of oxygen deprivation.

Corneal edema, whether accompanying hard or soft lens wear, is an indication that the cornea is not receiving an adequate supply of oxygen. In either case, the problem can be solved by one or all of the following: (1) by instruction in correct blinking habits; (2) by reducing lens wearing time; or (3) fitting the patient with more loosely fitting lenses, allowing better access to the cornea of fresh, oxygenated tears.

How Much Oxygen Does the Cornea Need?

Studies concerning the cornea's oxygen supply deal with either the *percentage* of oxygen in the air or the *partial pressure* of oxygen. To determine the partial pressure of the oxygen in the air, the atmospheric pressure at sea level (760mmHg) is multiplied by the percentage of oxygen in air (approximately 21 percent), resulting in a partial pressure of 159mmHg.

Using a slit lamp and corneal pachometer, Polse and Mandell (1970) fitted three subjects with goggles beneath which various gases could be introduced. They found that in an atmosphere of 1.5 percent oxygen, the cornea thickened approximately 6 percent in 3 hours, whereas in an atmosphere of 2.5 percent oxygen, no corneal thickening was noted during a period of 4 hours. As a result, they concluded that the cornea requires a partial pressure of oxygen of 11 to 19mmHg (1.5 to 2.5 percent) to prevent swelling.

Several investigators have determined the level of oxygen utilization of the cornea under open eye and closed eye conditions. Fatt, Freeman, and Lin (1974) calculated the oxygen tension at the corneal epithelium to be approximately 159mmHg (21 percent) under open eye conditions and 55mmHg (7 percent) under closed eye conditions. Efron and Carney (1979) measured corneal oxygen uptake on the anesthetized corneas of 12 young adults under closed eye conditions and found the mean level of oxygen at the corneal surface to be 58mmHg, or 7.7 percent.

Hill (1977c) listed the following levels for use in comparing the equivalent oxygen performance of various oxygen-permeable contact lenses:

Oxygen in air	21 percent
Sleep (prolonged lid closure)	7 percent
To maintain glycogen levels	5 percent
To avoid corneal edema	2 percent
Transmission of PMMA	0 percent

Hill recommended that, because the oxygen levels present during sleep can result in minor corneal swelling measurable on awakening, an arbitrary level of 10 percent might be taken as an exploratory estimate of an ideal minimum.

The fact that minor corneal swelling can occur after prolonged sleep (at an oxygen level of 7 to 8 percent) (although Polse and Mandell detected no corneal swelling with an oxygen level of 2.5 percent for a period of 4 hours, may be explained at least partially by the increase in temperature of the cornea during sleep. Hill (1977a) reported an increase in temperature during lid closure of 4.5°F due to the warm capillary circulation of the palpebral conjunctiva that increases cellular metabolic activity and, thus, the demand for oxygen.

Tear Exchange Efficiency for PMMA Lens Wearers

Because the oxygen transmission of PMMA lenses is essentially zero, wearers of these lenses can obtain adequate atmospheric oxygen at the corneal surface—and thus avoid corneal edema—only through the tear exchange underneath the lens that occurs with blinking.

Fatt (1979) published a series of curves indicating the partial pressure of oxygen underneath a contact lens as a function of tear exchange efficiency. These curves indicate that for tear exchange efficiencies between *10 and 20 percent* (indicating that with each blink, fresh tears equivalent to 10 to 20 percent of the total tear volume are introduced underneath the lens), the partial pressure of oxygen underneath the PMMA lens would be between 10 and 19mmHg. These figures correspond to the Polse-Mandell range of partial pressures necessary to prevent corneal swelling. Fatt's data, therefore, reinforce the importance of sufficient tear exchange (which requires correct blinking) for PMMA lens wearers.

Oxygen Permeability of Hydrogel Lenses

As described by Refojo (1979), for a gas to permeate through a contact lens, it must dissolve into one of the surfaces of the lens and then move, or diffuse, as single-gas molecules through the lens to be released at the opposite surface. Permeability (P) is, therefore, the product of the diffusivity (D) and the solubility (k) of the gas for that particular lens material, or

$$\text{Permeability} = Dk.$$

Permeability is expressed in terms of

$$(\text{cm}^2 \times mlO_2/(\text{sec.} \times ml \times mmHg).$$

Whereas permeability is a property of the material of which the lens is made, *transmissivity* depends on both permeability and lens thickness (L):

$$\text{Transmissivity} = \frac{\text{permeability}}{\text{thickness}} = \frac{Dk}{L}$$

expressed in terms of

$$(\text{cm} \times mlO_2)/(\text{sec.} \times ml \times mmHg).$$

Because hydrogel lenses consist of interlaced macromolecules capable of absorbing large amounts of water, a gas molecule must dissolve in the water of hydration of the lens and diffuse through the water channels in the hydrogel network. As a result, a reasonably good approximation is that the gas permeability of a hydrogel lens increases exponentially with the water content of the lens (Refojo, 1979).

In summary, although soft lens materials vary from one to another in regard to oxygen permeability, for a given material the amount of oxygen transmitted through the lens to the cornea can be increased by either (1) making the lens thinner or (2) increasing the water content of the material. The ideal lens (from the point of view of oxygen transmission), therefore, would be extremely thin or would be 100 percent water!

For a hydrogel material having a water content of approximately 40 percent, Hill (1975) published data showing that oxygen performance increases slowly with decreasing lens thickness until a thickness of about 0.10mm is reached, beyond which oxygen performance increases rapidly with further decrease in thickness. For a thickness of 0.06mm (a thickness easily attained in today's lenses), approximately 6 percent oxygen would be expected to reach the cornea through the lens; this is more than enough to maintain glycogen levels and close to the amount available after prolonged lid closure. For a thickness of 0.03mm, the oxygen available to the cornea would be expected to exceed the "ideal minimum."

In a later paper, Benjamin and Hill (1979) reported that the equivalent oxygen performance of Bausch & Lomb lenses ranging from 0.055 to 0.068mm in center thickness was found to average 7 percent, compared with the predicted 6 percent. They warned, however, that such oxygen levels are critically dependent on both (1) a fit that traps a minimum stagnant tear pool underneath the lens and (2) the continuous maintenance of scrupulously clean lens surfaces.

More recently, Hill and Mauger (1980) measured the equivalent oxygen performance of lenses made of six hydrogel materials. Their results, shown in Figure 14.21, indicate that a Bausch & Lomb lens 0.06mm thick would supply sufficient oxygen to maintain glycogen levels. However, the same oxygen performance would occur with a Hydrocurve II 45 lens or Duragel 60 lens having a thickness of 0.10mm, or at even much greater thicknesses for a Duragel 75, Cooper 72–75, or Sauflon 85 lens (the numbers after each lens designate the water content of the material).

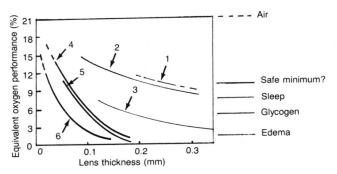

Figure 14.21 Equivalent oxygen performance of hydrogel lenses: (1) Sauflon 85 percent; (2) Cooper 72–75 percent; (3) Duragel 75 percent; (4) Duragel 60 percent; (5) Hydrocurve II 45 percent; (6) Bausch & Lomb 38.6 percent (redrawn from Hill and Mauger, 1980).

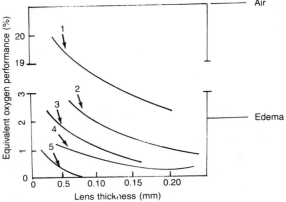

Figure 14.22 Equivalent oxygen performance of nonhydrophilic lenses: (1) Silcon (soft); (2) CAB; (3) Polycon; (4) Modified PMMA; (5) PMMA (redrawn from Hill and Mauger, 1981).

Oxygen-Permeable Hard Lens Materials

As noted earlier, the oxygen permeability of silicone is so high that there is no question that, for a 100 percent silicone lens such as the Silsoft or the Silcon lens, sufficient oxygen is delivered to the cornea without the necessity for tear pumping. However, Fitzgerald (1981) has made the point that even these lenses must be fitted loosely enough to assure adequate lens motion and tear exchange to flush corneal metabolic wastes from behind the lens and maintain wetting of the corneal surface.

Hill and Mauger (1981) published equivalent oxygen performance data for Silcon, CAB, Polycon, and PMMA materials. As shown in Figure 14.22, the Silcon lens is the only one that transmits sufficient oxygen to maintain glycogen levels, if fitted in the thicknesses ordinarily required for gas-permeable hard lenses (i.e., in the 0.10 to 0.20mm range or greater). Although CAB can transmit sufficient oxygen to avoid edema (2 percent) at a thickness of 0.08mm, and Polycon is capable of the same oxygen performance at about 0.04mm, each of these lenses must be relatively thick to maintain stability. Clinically useful thicknesses for these lenses, in minus powers, are about 0.20mm for CAB lenses and 0.13mm for Polycon. For these thicknesses, the Hill and Mauger data show that the oxygen performance of neither of these lenses exceeds 1 percent. This amount is insufficient to prevent corneal edema in the absence of tear pumping.

Corneal thickness changes of gas-permeable hard lens wearers were measured by Lowther (1981). Each of 31 patients was fitted with a Silcon lens on

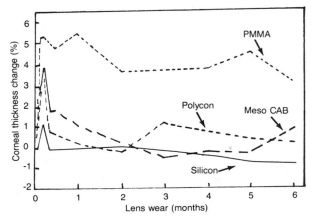

Figure 14.23 Mean corneal thickness change with months of lens wear (redrawn from Lowther, 1981a).

one eye and either a PMMA lens, a CAB lens, or a Polycon lens on the other eye. All patients were myopes of −6.00D or less, and center thicknesses averaged 0.13mm for PMMA and Polycon lenses, 0.15mm for Silcon lenses, and 0.195mm for CAB lenses. In Figure 14.23, the corneal thickness increases reported by Lowther for Silcon lenses were averaged for the three groups of patients. As shown in the diagram, PMMA lens wearers were found to have an average increase in corneal thickness of 4 percent after 6 months of lens wear, whereas CAB and Polycon wearers had less than 1 percent increase and Silcon lens wearers had no increase at all.

Clinical Implications of Oxygen-Permeable Lenses

Practitioners should not be discouraged by the fact that hydrogel lenses (in the 0.06mm range), as well as CAB and silicone/PMMA combination lenses (in the thickness range ordinarily fitted), provide sufficient oxygen to meet the cornea's needs only with the assistance of tear pumping. A high percentage of PMMA failures are failures only because the lens seals off the cornea from atmospheric oxygen. With many of these patients, the oxygen transmitted through the lens when a sufficiently oxygen-permeable lens is fitted is sufficient to turn failure into success. On the other hand, the practitioner should be aware of the importance of correct blinking habits for the wearer of any kind of lens and should remember the warning by Benjamin and Hill (1979) (regarding thin soft lenses): the fit should be such that a minimum stagnant tear pool is trapped underneath the lenses, and the lens surfaces must continually be kept scrupulously clean.

In our review of oxygen permeability, little has been said thus far about carbon dioxide. Refojo (1979) reported that the ratio of carbon dioxide permeability to oxygen permeability for plastics and rubbers is about $5:1$. Thus, if permeation of oxygen is adequate, carbon dioxide permeation also will be adequate.

FITTING PROCEDURES: HARD CONTACT LENSES

Prior to the 1970s, contact lens instruction in schools and colleges of optometry was limited to hard lenses, since these were the only lenses in existence. The new, more comfortable, soft lenses soon became so popular that in some schools the fitting of hard lenses was all but forgotten. Some readers, thinking that hard lenses will soon go the way of the horse and buggy, may wonder why anyone would bother to discuss fitting procedures for these lenses. However, there are several reasons for doing so:

1. Gas-permeable lenses, introduced in the mid-1970s, are growing rapidly in popularity and show great promise for the future. Although each manufacturer of gas-permeable hard lenses supplies its own instructions, the principles used in fitting PMMA lenses are equally applicable to gas-permeable lenses.
2. Literally millions of people have been fitted with PMMA lenses during the past 4 decades, many of

whom wear their lenses all day, every day, until problems arise. A practitioner ignorant of hard lens fitting will obviously be of little assistance to these patients.
3. Even with the ever-increasing variety of both soft and gas-permeable hard lenses available, there continue to be patients who, for one reason or another, can best be served by wearing PMMA lenses. As Lowther (1981) commented, gas-permeable lenses do not offer an adequate range of parameters involving toric lenses, bifocals, tints, and other special designs. In addition, many patients have sufficient refractive astigmatism to require toric lenses if soft lenses or gas-permeable lenses are fitted, but they will be able to wear spherical PMMA lenses.

Most of the fitting procedures discussed here are used in the fitting of PMMA lenses, but a discussion of fitting procedures specifically intended for gas-permeable hard lenses follows later in the chapter.

Patient Management

Optometric examination

When a patient requests to be fitted with contact lenses, the optometric examination is carried out in the usual manner, with emphasis being placed on the findings of particular importance in the fitting of contact lenses.

The anterior segment of the eye should be inspected carefully with the biomicroscope to make sure no condition exists to contraindicate successful contact lens wear. The cornea and conjunctiva should be studied carefully for signs of any ocular disease (past or present), and the lid margins and palpebral conjunctiva should be inspected for the presence of marginal blepharitis or conjunctivitis. The presence of a corneal scar or other indication of a preexisting condition should be noted on the record, together with an appropriate drawing or photograph. The precorneal tear film breakup test should be done, bearing in mind that anyone having a breakup time of 10 seconds or less may prove to be a poor contact lens wearer.

Careful keratometer findings should be taken, and the amount of astigmatism that will remain uncorrected with a spherical PMMA lens can be estimated by means of the formula

internal astigmatism
= refractive astigmatism − corneal astigmatism

For example, if the cornea is spherical but the subjective finding shows 1.00D of against-the-rule astigmatism, it is obvious that the 1.00D of against-the-rule astigmatism is internal astigmatism. A much better method of determining the amount of astigmatism that will remain uncorrected is refracting the patient while a PMMA lens of the appropriate base curve and power is worn.

Patient selection

During the case history, the patient should be asked why contact lenses are desired. Although the majority of patients want contact lenses for purely cosmetic reasons (i.e., to eliminate glasses), a few people have misconceptions about contact lenses that should be cleared up. These include beliefs that contact lenses will provide better vision than glasses (which may or may not be true); that contact lenses will be less bother than glasses; and that because your eyes "don't change" while wearing contact lenses, they will be cheaper in the long run than glasses.

The most highly motivated contact lens candidates are those with relatively high refractive errors (particularly myopia) who have worn glasses for a number of years and are tired of wearing them. Patients having low refractive errors (less than at least 1.00 or 2.00D of myopia or hyperopia) and those who wear glasses only on a part-time basis or not at all should be discouraged from attempting to wear contact lenses. Patients whose refractive errors are mainly astigmatism (simple myopic, simple hyperopic, or mixed astigmatism) should be discouraged unless they are particularly well motivated, because many of these patients have good visual acuity with no lenses at all.

There are several categories of patients for whom contact lenses will be optically superior to glasses. These include patients with aphakia, keratoconus, or high myopia. Contact lenses are superior to glasses for aphakia (particularly unilateral aphakia) because of the disturbing magnification effects and limited peripheral field of view provided by aphakic spectacle lenses. For all but the earliest cases of keratoconus, contact lenses are the only form of correction that will provide adequate visual acuity. In high myopia, there is a significant increase in retinal image size when contact lenses are worn rather than glasses, and this increased image size often results in improved visual acuity.

If contact lenses are to be fitted, the fitting procedures are usually carried out at a subsequent visit, or, if time permits, fitting can be done at the initial visit.

Fitting visit

It is convenient to record contact lens fitting data on a form such as the one shown in Appendix A. The patient's prefitting keratometer and subjective findings are recorded, along with the results of the biomicroscopic examination. Specifications of diagnostic lenses are recorded, together with notes concerning the fit of these lenses. The refraction through the final diagnostic lenses also is recorded, as well as the specifications for the lenses to be ordered.

Use of diagnostic lenses. One or more pairs of diagnostic lenses are inserted as required, and the position, lag, and fluorescein pattern are observed under ultraviolet light, followed by biomicroscopic examination. Because of the possibility of contamination of liquid fluorescein, only fluorescein-impregnated filter paper strips should be used. The fluorescein strip is moistened by means of saline solution or contact lens wetting solution, and while the patient looks down, a swath of fluorescein is "painted" across the superior sclera just above the limbus.

Lens placement by the practitioner. Although some practitioners prefer to place the contact lens on the patient's cornea, the author prefers to have the patient look downward and to place the lens on the superior sclera. The patient is then told to look at some object across the room (such as the acuity chart), and the lens slides down onto the cornea. After the lens is placed on the eye, the patient should be told to keep the lids relaxed and to "blink loosely." It may be best to provide a definite fixation point for the patient during lens placement. The patient can be instructed to look at one thumb, placed at about arm's length below eye level.

To remove the lens, the patient is first asked to look at a distant object. The practitioner then places one index finger on the lower lid, stretching it temporally, and places the index finger of the other hand at the center of the upper lid, rotating the finger outward and downward in an *L*-shaped movement, catching the edge of the lens under the lid and thus flipping it off the cornea.

Refraction through diagnostic lenses. Once the optimum lens fit is determined, the patient is refracted through the diagnostic lenses that provide the optimum fit. Using the retinoscope, spherocylindrical refraction is done (as is normally done in refracting spectacle patients). Any cylindrical correction found will represent the correction for internal astigmatism, because the contact lens will eliminate corneal astigmatism. For the subjective examination it is best to do a spherical equivalent, or *best sphere*, refraction, unless the patient is to be fitted with toric front surface lenses. With the best sphere refraction, the practitioner will determine what the patient's corrected acuity will be in spite of the presence of any internal astigmatism.

Specification of lens power. The diagnostic lenses used for the refraction normally will be of the base curve radii to be ordered for the patient, and the lens power will be within a few diopters of that required by the patient. Under these conditions, the lens powers in the refractor will be small enough so no vertex distance allowance will be required. For example, if −3.00D diagnostic lenses are used and if the lens powers in the refractor are −1.50D for the right eye and −1.75D for the left eye, the lens powers to be ordered for the two eyes would be −4.50 and −4.75D. If the powers of the lenses in the refractor are about ±4.50D or more, a vertex distance allowance must be made by calculation or by using a table such as the one given in Appendix C.

If the lens to be ordered will have a base curve radius steeper or flatter than that of the diagnostic lens through which the refraction was done, the lens power to be ordered must be changed accordingly. The amount of change is 1.00D more minus or less plus for each 0.2mm (or 1.00DK) that the base curve is steeper than the diagnostic lens, or 1.00D less minus or more plus for each 0.2mm (or 1.00DK) that the base curve is flatter than the diagnostic lens.

Fitting Spherical Hard Lenses

Since the introduction of the corneal lens in 1948, numerous lens "fitting philosophies" have been advocated. Recall that the original Tuohy lens and the microlens were fitted several diopters flatter than the central portion (optical zone) of the cornea. This type of fit is called the *apical touch*, or *flatter-than-K*, *fit*. The Contour lens, developed several years later, is fitted with a base curve parallel to the optical zone of the cornea and with one or more flatter (secondary or peripheral) curves. This method is called the *apical alignment*, or simply the *alignment method* or the *on-K method*.

The fact that flatter-than-K lenses tended to cause discomfort and epithelial stippling or even abrasion of the apical portion of the cornea led some practitioners to recommend an *apical clearance*, or *steeper-than-K method* of fitting. These lenses are usually fitted in such a way that the secondary curve of the lens, rather than the base curve, serves as the

bearing surface of the lens; the base curve of the lens is fitted somewhat steeper than the optical zone of the cornea.

Numerous lens diameters have been advocated, ranging from the 11.5mm Tuohy lens to the "optic cap" lens, designed to cover only the optic cap of the cornea and having a diameter of about 6.5 or 7.0mm.

In the discussion that follows, no effort is made to describe fitting procedures other than those of the *modified contour lens*. Rather than being fitted in a diameter of about 9.5mm, as originally advocated by Bier (1957), the modified form of the Contour lens discussed here has a diameter averaging about 8.8mm; has a base curve, a secondary curve, and peripheral curve; and is fitted by the apical alignment method.

PMMA diagnostic lenses

The specifications for a diagnostic lens set for PMMA lenses are given in Table 14.1. The set consists of 12 lenses, ranging in base curve radii from 8.44mm (40.00DK) to 7.42mm (45.50DK). For all lenses, secondary curve radii are 1mm flatter than base curve radii. The radius of the bevel (peripheral curve) for all lenses is 12.0mm. Overall diameter averages 8.8mm, ranging from 9.0mm for the flatter lenses to 8.6mm for the steeper lenses; and optic zone diameter ranges from 7.0 to 7.4mm. Powers of all lenses are −3.00D, and center thickness in each case is 0.13mm. This diagnostic lens set should be considered as a "starting" set. Additional sets of lenses, having the same base curve radii and secondary curve radii (in powers of −6.00D, +3.00D, and +12.00D for aphakics) would be desirable. Center thickness would be less for the −6.00D lenses than for the −3.00D lenses, but greater for the +3.00D lenses and much greater for the +12.00D lenses. Front and back radii of curvature, optic zones, and transition zones of a typical hard contact lens are shown in Figure 14.24.

Gas-permeable hard lenses

Gas-permeable hard lenses made of several different materials are available. The most successful gas-permeable hard lenses are the *silicone-acrylate* lenses, made of a co-polymer of methyl methacrylate and silicone. The presence of silicone greatly increases the gas-permeability (which is almost zero for methyl methacrylate), but causes the lenses to be more easily coated by mucus and other tear constitutents.

The hard silicone-acrylate, gas-permeable lenses available at the time of this writing are listed in Table 14.2. As noted in the table, most manufacturers have

Table 14.1 PMMA diagnostic lens set

Base curve		Secondary curve radius	Peripheral curve radius	Overall diameter	Optic zone diameter	Power	Center thickness
DK	Radius						
40.00	8.44	9.44	12.00	9.0	7.4	−3.00	0.13
40.50	8.33	9.33	12.00	9.0	7.4	−3.00	0.13
41.00	8.23	9.23	12.00	9.0	7.4	−3.00	0.13
41.50	8.13	9.13	12.00	9.0	7.4	−3.00	0.13
42.00	8.04	9.04	12.00	8.8	7.2	−3.00	0.13
42.50	7.94	8.94	12.00	8.8	7.2	−3.00	0.13
43.00	7.85	8.85	12.00	8.8	7.2	−3.00	0.13
43.50	7.76	8.76	12.00	8.8	7.2	−3.00	0.13
44.00	7.67	8.67	12.00	8.6	7.0	−3.00	0.13
44.50	7.58	8.58	12.00	8.6	7.0	−3.00	0.13
45.00	7.50	8.50	12.00	8.6	7.0	−3.00	0.13
45.50	7.42	8.42	12.00	8.6	7.0	−3.00	0.13

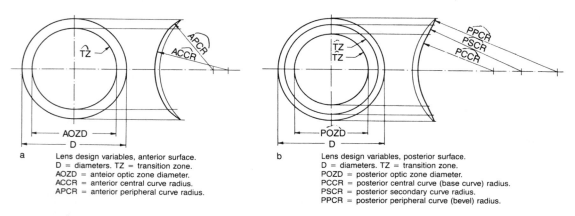

a Lens design variables, anterior surface.
D = diameters. TZ = transition zone.
AOZD = anteior optic zone diameter.
ACCR = anterior central curve radius.
APCR = anterior peripheral curve radius.

b Lens design variables, posterior surface.
D = diameters. TZ = transition zone.
POZD = posterior optic zone diameter.
PCCR = posterior central curve (base curve) radius.
PSCR = posterior secondary curve radius.
PPCR = posterior peripheral curve (bevel) radius.

Figure 14.24 PMMA lens design variables: (a) anterior surface; (b) posterior surface (Grosvenor, 1972a).

lenses available in two or three dK (permeability) values. Although those with higher dK values allow more oxygen to pass through the lens to the cornea, they tend to be more flexible and to become coated and scratched more easily than those with lower dK values. The lenses with the highest dK values (designated by *EW* in the table) have been approved by the FDA for extended wear. For some of the lenses, such as the Aquaflex HGP and Polycon II, diagnostic lens sets are available only in certain parameters. The other lenses, designated as "custom designed" in Table 14.2, may be ordered in any desired parameters.

Diagnostic lens procedure

The first step in the diagnostic lens procedure is to select a lens with a base curve radius equal to that of the flattest corneal meridian, and to place the lens

on the patient's cornea so the fluorescein pattern can be observed. It has been found that if there is 1.00D of corneal astigmatism or more, the diagnostic lens should be steeper than the flattest corneal meridian. A good rule of thumb is to select a lens with a base curve radius about one-fourth of the way between the cornea's flattest and steepest meridians. For example, if the keratometer finding is 42.00D at 180 and 44.00D at 90, a 42.50DK lens (having a base curve radius of 7.94mm) should be selected.

Because the placement of the lenses causes a certain amount of tearing (particularly if the patient has never worn contact lenses before), it will be necessary to wait until tearing has subsided before evaluating the fit of the lenses. When tearing has subsided, fluorescein is instilled by means of a fluorescein-impregnated filter paper strip (as already described), and the tear layer underneath the lens is

Table 14.2   Silicone-acrylate, gas-permeable hard contact lenses (Tyler's Quarterly, 1987)

Manufacturer	Trade name	dK	Diameter (mm)	Base curve radii (mm)
Cooper-Vision	Aquaflex HGP	14.6	8.9mm	7.0–8.3mm
			9.3	7.0–8.9
Danker Labs	Dura-Sil	18	(Custom-designed)	
Optocryl, Inc.	Optacryl 60	18	(Custom-designed)	
	Optacryl K	32	(Custom-designed)	
Paragon	Paraperm O$_2$	15	(Custom-designed)	
	Paraperm O$_2^+$	39	(Custom-designed)	
	Paraperm EW	56	(Custom-designed)	
PDC	Oxyflow 39	39	(Custom-designed)	
	Oxyflow EW	56	(Custom-designed)	
Polymer Technology	Boston II	14	(Custom-designed)	
	Boston IV	28	(Custom-designed)	
Sola-Syntex	Polycon II	12	8.5	7.1–8.6
			9.0	7.1–8.6
			9.5	7.1–8.6
			10.0	7.4–8.6
Permeable Contact Lens	SGP	19	(Custom-designed)	

inspected with the aid of a source of ultraviolet light, such as the *Burton lamp.*

Fluorescein patterns. Using the alignment, or "on-K," method of fitting, the optical zone of the lens constitutes the bearing surface, and the fluorescein pattern (see Figure 14.25a) indicates a very thin, even layer of tears underneath the optical zone, with an increasingly green layer under the secondary curve and particularly under the bevel. If the lens is fitted steeper than the flattest meridian of the optical zone of the cornea, an apical clearance fit results, and the fluorescein pattern would be similar to that shown in Figure 14.25b, having a black layer of touch (where there is no fluorescein) under the secondary curve, with a bright green area of apical pooling under the optical zone of the lens. If a lens is fitted flatter than the flattest meridian of the cornea, an apical touch fit will result, and the fluorescein pattern (see Figure 14.25c) will have a wide area of staining under the secondary and peripheral curves and a relatively small central area of apical touch.

In with-the-rule astigmatism of about 1.00D or more, the area of touch tends to have a *dog bone* or *dumbbell* shape (see Figure 14.25d), with fluorescein pooling appearing above and below the horizontal meridian of the cornea.

The accurate evaluation of fluorescein patterns requires a certain amount of experience. One

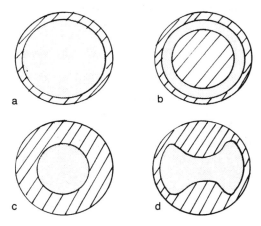

Figure 14.25 Fluorescein patterns: (a) alignment, or "on-K," fit; (b) apical clearance, or "steeper-than-K," fit; (c) apical touch, or "flatter-than-K," fit; (d) dumbbell-shaped area of touch in with-the-rule astigmatism. The cross-hatched areas indicate pooling of fluorescein, and the shaded areas indicate a lack of fluorescein, or "touch." However, even in the areas of touch, there is an extremely thin layer of fluorescein-stained tears.

method of gaining this experience quickly is to select, for each patient fitted, a lens for one eye that you think will give you the typical alignment pattern and to select a lens for the other eye that is about 1.00D steeper than the flattest corneal meridian. The steeper lens should be found to have an apical clearance fluorescein pattern, in contrast to the "on-K" lens having the alignment pattern.

Lens position and lag. In evaluating the fluorescein pattern, the examiner also observes the position and blink lag of the lens. The lens should position centrally on the cornea, with its upper edge just underneath the margin of the upper lid, and it should lag downward approximately 3mm after each blink (see Figure 14.26). A lens that lags excessively or fails to center on the cornea (locating upward, downward, nasalward, or temporalward) is considered to be a *loose lens*, whereas a lens that centers well but has insufficient lag is said to be a *tight lens*. If a lens "rides high," it may do so because the lens is too loose or because the upper lid is holding the lens up. The examiner should gently hold the patient's upper lid up (away from the lens). If the lens drops downward, this means the lid was holding it up; if not, it means that the lens is too loose.

If a lens is found, on the basis of the position, lag, or fluorescein pattern, to be too loose, a diagnostic lens having a steeper base curve or a larger diameter should be tried. If a lens is found to be too tight, a lens having a flatter base curve or a smaller diameter should be tried.

Selection of lens parameters

In many cases, a pair of diagnostic lenses (possibly even the first pair tried) will be satisfactory in terms of fluorescein pattern, position, and lag. If so, the parameters of these lenses can be used in ordering the patient's lenses. There are situations, however, in which one or more parameters may be specified differently than the parameters of the diagnostic lenses.

Base curve radius. Usually a diagnostic lens having the correct base radius will be found. However, if the diagnostic lenses are available in steps of 0.50DK (0.10mm), as in the set described in Table 14.1, it often may be necessary to specify a base curve radius halfway between the radii of two diagnostic lenses. For example, if the flattest meridian of the patient's cornea is 42.25D, and if the 42.00 and 42.50DK lenses fit equally well, a decision may be made to order a 42.25DK (8.96mm radius) base curve.

Secondary and peripheral curve radii. Using the method of fitting described here, the

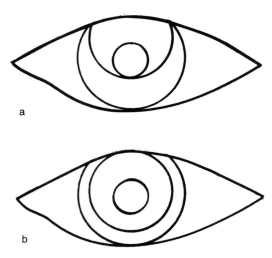

Figure 14.26   A PMMA lens fitted by the on-K, or alignment, method: *(a)* just after a blink; *(b)* after the blink lag has taken place. Normally the lens will stay in the position shown in *(b)* until the next blink.

secondary curve radius is specified 1.00mm flatter than the base curve radius, and the peripheral curve radius is a standard 12.0mm. Occasionally a diagnostic lens whose base curve appears to be correct, as judged by the fluorescein pattern, will appear to be too tight (insufficient depth of fluorescein) or too loose (excessive depth of fluorescein) in the area under the secondary curve. This problem can be solved by flattening or steepening the secondary curve radius. However, the recommended procedure is to try a lens with a flatter base curve or smaller diameter (and a smaller optic zone diameter), or one with a steeper base curve or larger diameter (and a larger optic zone diameter).

Overall diameter. If the diagnostic lens centers well, has an adequate amount of lag, and provides a good apical alignment fluorescein pattern, the overall diameter of the diagnostic lens can be considered to be correct. If the patient has a large palpebral aperture or an exophthalmic eye, the lens may fit too loosely, failing to center and having an excessive amount of blink lag. In such a case, a lens having a larger overall diameter should be tried. (The fluorescein pattern of a too-small or a too-large lens may— but not necessarily—aid in the evaluation of the fit, resembling a flat fit in the first case and a steep fit in the second.) If the diagnostic lens set does not include a large lens of the correct base curve radius, a good system is to order a larger lens to use as a diagnostic lens. In general, diameter increments should be specified in 0.2mm steps: if an 8.8mm lens appears to be too small, a 9.0mm lens should be tried.

If a patient has a small palpebral fissure or an enophthalmic eye, the lens may fit too tightly, centering well but having an inadequate amount of lag. In such a case, a lens having a smaller overall diameter (0.2mm smaller) should be tried or should be ordered as a trial lens.

Optic zone diameter. In the method of fitting described here, the optic zone diameter is varied with the overall diameter. As indicated in the diagnostic lens specifications given in Table 14.1, in each case the optic zone diameter is 1.6mm smaller than the overall diameter. This results in a total peripheral curve width of 0.8mm (on each side of the optic zone), 0.5mm of which is the width of the secondary curve and 0.3mm of which is the width of the bevel (see Figure 14.27).

Power. As noted earlier, the power of the lens is specified as the power of the diagnostic lens together with any additional lens power found to be required in the best sphere subjective refraction. If the lens power used in the refraction is ±4.50D or more, an allowance for change in vertex distance must be made. If the lens to be ordered will have a base curve steeper or flatter than that of the diagnostic lens, the lens power will have to be made 1.00D more minus or less plus for each 0.2mm of steepening of the base curve radius, or 1.00D more plus or less minus for each 0.2mm of flattening of the base curve radius.

Figure 14.27 Typical relationships between overall diameter, posterior optic zone diameter, and widths of secondary and peripheral curves for a PMMA lens designed for an alignment fit. All parameters are specified in millimeters.

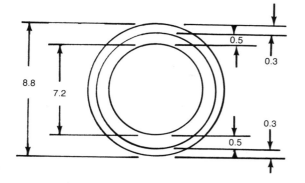

Center thickness. In most cases, the center thickness of the lens will be specified as that of the diagnostic lens. If the lens to be ordered will have a power different from that of the diagnostic lens, as a general rule, for each diopter of increase (or decrease) in minus power, the center thickness decreases (or increases) 0.01mm. However, for lenses in excess of −6.00D, center thickness should be no less than 0.10 or 0.09mm, to keep the lens from flexing excessively. (Very thin PMMA lenses have been known to turn inside out.)

For plus lenses, center thickness increases at a rate higher than 0.01mm for each diopter of power, and for lenses of about +3.00D or more, a lenticular front surface should be used to minimize central thickness. Center thickness of plus lenses, as well as details concerning lenticular front surfaces, can be determined by means of thickness tables or can be left to the laboratory.

Tint. Because a contact lens is extremely thin compared with an ophthalmic lens, the incorporation of a tint is of little value in preventing glare or in absorbing radiation in the visible spectrum. Many new PMMA lens wearers will complain of photophobia due to the lens acting as a foreign body, and they will benefit from the use of plano sunglasses for outdoor wear.

Some patients will request a tint for cosmetic reasons (to alter the color of their eyes). Tints are available in many colors, usually in three shades. However, Moreland (1972) has shown that a no. 2 blue lens can cause a protan color vision anomaly, so such lenses should be used with caution. It is unlikely that a no. 1 tint, in any color, would interfere with color vision. Because colorless contact lenses are easy to lose and hard to find, it is best to specify a no. 1 tint, in whatever color the patient desires, for all PMMA lenses.

Lens order

The parameters normally specified in an order for a spherical PMMA lens include:

1. Posterior central curve (base curve) radius. (The adjective *posterior* need not be used in a lens order when specifying posterior central curve radius, secondary curve radius or width, or peripheral curve radius or width.)
2. Posterior secondary curve radius.
3. Posterior peripheral curve (bevel) radius and width.
4. Overall diameter.
5. Posterior optic zone diameter.

6. Power.

7. Center thickness.

8. Tint.

If a front surface lenticular design is to be used, the anterior peripheral curve radius and anterior optic zone diameter may be specified in the order or determined by the laboratory. The radii and "zones" for a typical contact lens are shown in Figure 14.24.

Verification of finished lenses

When the finished lenses are received from the laboratory, the following lens parameters should be verified:

1. *Base curve radius*, using the Radiuscope or keratometer.

2. *Power*, using the lensometer (always placing the back surface of the lens against the lens stop).

3. *Overall diameter, optic zone diameter, secondary curve width*, and *peripheral curve width*, using the measuring magnifier.

4. *Center thickness*, using the dial thickness gauge.

It is impossible to verify the radii of secondary and peripheral curves. Lens surfaces and edges should be inspected for optical imperfections and for edge form, using a low-powered binocular microscope or the slit-lamp microscope. (Contact lens standards and tolerances proposed by the American National Standards Institute (ANSI) are shown in Appendix B.)

Delivery of lenses

When the finished lenses are delivered to the patient, a recommended procedure is for the practitioner to place the lenses on the patient's eyes, check visual acuity and subjective best sphere overrefraction, verify the fluorescein pattern, and then instruct the patient in the procedures for placement and removal of the lenses. Observe the patient while he or she practices placement and removal until you are satisfied that these procedures are performed correctly. During the remainder of this visit, the patient is given instruction concerning hygienic care of the lenses and is provided with a wearing schedule to be followed until the first progress visit.

In many practices, instruction in lens placement and removal and in hygienic care of the lenses is done by a trained assistant or an optometric technician.

Placement and removal of lenses by patient

Before the lenses are delivered to the patient, they should be removed from the mailing case, cleaned with a contact lens cleaning solution, thoroughly rinsed, and placed in a contact lens storage case filled with fresh soaking solution. They should be hydrated in the case for at least 24 hours before delivery.

The patient is first asked to wash the hands and is then seated at a table with the contact lenses, solutions, mirror, and tissues all conveniently located. The patient takes the right lens out of the container and places it in the palm of one hand; places a drop of wetting solution on the lens, and gently rubs the lens with the index finger of the other hand. The patient then places the lens on the tip of the index finger of the right hand, holds the lower lid downward with the second finger of the right hand, and holds the upper lid upward with the index finger of the left hand. The patient then places the lens on the cornea, being careful not to blink until the lens is actually on the cornea. The left lens is then taken out of the container and placed on the eye in the same manner. The patient is instructed never to have both lenses out of the container at the same time (except when one lens is on the eye), so the lenses cannot possibly become switched, right for left.

To remove the lens, the patient should bend the head over the table, fixing a gaze straight ahead. While the patient opens the eyes wide, he or she is asked to place the tip of the index finger at the outer corner of the eye so pressure is applied to both the upper and lower lid margins, then press back slightly to the bone, pull towards the ear, blink, and catch the lens in the other hand held close to the eye. The lid margins should clear the top and bottom of the lens until the blink, and in blinking the patient should flick the lid only, not screw up the eye. The patient should be required to place and remove both lenses twice, without assistance, before being allowed to take them home.

Patient instructions

The patient must be instructed concerning hygienic care of the lenses. This involves the use of three solutions: the cleaning, storage, and wetting solutions. After removing each lens at night, the patient places the lens in the palm of the left hand (if right-handed) or on the tip of the left index finger, places a drop of cleaning solution on the lens, and rubs the lens (using the index finger of the right hand) to remove the film of material accumulated during the day's wear. The lens is then rinsed thoroughly with water and placed in the storage case, and the case is filled with fresh storage solution. In the morning, the lens is removed from the storage case; the lens is rinsed with tap water; a drop of wetting solution is placed on the lens and rubbed onto the lens surfaces; and the lens is ready to be placed on the eye.

The importance of cleaning the lenses *at night* should be impressed on the patient. If lenses are not cleaned until the next morning, mucus and other material deposited on the lens during the day will remain on the lens during the night (in spite of the fact that the lens is immersed in the storage solution), and it will gradually be adsorbed onto the surface of the lens, causing the accumulation of a coating on the lens surfaces.

Wearing schedules. A recommended procedure is to instruct the patient to wear the lenses 4 hours the first day and to increase wearing time 1 hour each day for the first week, then maintain wearing time at 8 or 10 hours until the first progress visit. The patient is told that if, for any reason, the lenses are not worn the full number of hours on a given day, they should only be worn (on the next day) an hour more than on the previous day. At the first progress visit, a decision is made concerning further increases in wearing time.

Although optometrists formerly considered the patient to be a failure if the lenses could not be worn during all waking hours, it is now realized that most patients get along better if the corneas are exposed to atmospheric oxygen at least a few hours each day. One way to accomplish this is to instruct the patient not to put the lenses on in the morning until an hour or so after rising, and to remove the lenses about 1 hour before going to bed. Another way is to have the patient take a break of 1 or 2 hours in the middle of the day.

All contact lens wearers should have a backup pair of glasses in a current prescription. If backup glasses are not available, many patients will overwear their lenses or wear the lenses when suffering from an abrasion or other problem.

Blinking instructions. The patient should be told of the importance of correct blinking with contact lenses and should be instructed in the performance of blinking exercises (described in the corneal physiology section earlier in the chapter). The amount of emphasis to be placed on blinking exercises will depend to a great extent on the patient's blinking habits, as observed surreptitiously during slit-lamp examination both without and with lenses.

Progress visits

Several progress visits are ordinarily scheduled during the first several weeks of lens wear. The author usually finds it satisfactory to schedule the first progress check within 1 or 2 weeks after lens delivery, and to schedule two or three additional progress visits, as needed, at intervals of about 2 weeks.

A convenient record form for use in progress visits is shown in Appendix A. It is not necessary to perform all of the tests listed on the form at every progress visit. It is suggested, however, that the following tests be done at the first progress visit:

1. Visual acuity with lenses on.
2. Subjective refraction (best sphere) with lenses on.
3. Fluorescein pattern interpretation.
4. Biomicroscopic examination with lenses on.
5. Biomicroscopic examination after lens removal.
6. Keratometry.

In subsequent progress visits, the findings taken after lens removal assume increased importance. The biomicroscopic examination will reveal the presence of corneal edema or staining; the keratometer findings will indicate whether the cornea has steepened or flattened, or whether astigmatism has been induced as a result of contact lens wear; and the subjective refraction will reveal any refractive changes due to lens wear.

Criteria for a successful fit

To consider a patient successfully fitted, Mazow (1962) stated that at least 8 hours of daily wear should be achieved, the lenses must have the desired visual effect, they must be comfortable, there must be no damage to the corneas or the adnexa, and there should be no more than 0.50D of change in corneal curvature and no distortion of the keratometer mire images after 3 months of lens wear.

Somewhat similar criteria were proposed by Sarver and Harris (1971), but with the addition of "normal appearance of the patient." They evaluated 122 consecutive patients according to their criteria and found that the following percentages of patients were rated as successful on each criterion:

Wearing time (minimum of 8 hours per day)	87% successful
Comfort (only a slight lens awareness)	91% successful
Vision (no significant blur)	86% successful
Absence of ocular tissue changes	87% successful
Normal appearance of patient	93% successful
All criteria	73% successful

Yearly progress examinations

During the fitting visit, every patient should be told to return for a progress examination once each year as long as contact lenses are worn. The yearly progress examination should include not only an evaluation of the fit of the lenses but also a shortened version of the original data base examination, including tests of refraction, binocular vision, and eye health (including biomicroscopy, ophthalmoscopy, and tonometry). In addition, the lenses themselves should be inspected for the presence of scratches, cracks, pits, warpage, or other signs of wear.

Fitting Toric Hard Lenses

The optical considerations involved in the fitting of toric front surface lenses, toric back surface lenses, and bitoric lenses are discussed in the "Optical Principles of Contact Lenses" section earlier in the chapter. Recall that because a spherical hard lens tends to maintain its curvature while on the cornea, corneal astigmatism is greatly reduced or eliminated while the lens is worn, and only internal astigmatism remains. Experience indicates that a toric front surface is seldom required unless the patient's internal astigmatism is 0.75D or more.

For a patient having a large amount of corneal astigmatism, a toric back surface lens is sometimes fitted to provide a comfortable physical fit. However, a toric back surface serves as a source of uncorrected astigmatism. This astigmatism can be eliminated by the use of a toric front surface in addition to the toric back surface, resulting in a bitoric lens.

Fitting toric front surface lenses

If a comparison of a prospective contact lens wearer's keratometric and refractive astigmatism indicates the presence of 0.75D or more internal astigmatism (which is almost always against-the-rule), the patient should be refracted while wearing a spherical hard lens. Both a spherocylindrical and a best sphere refraction should be done. The spherocylindrical refraction will determine the amount of uncorrected astigmatism present while wearing the lens, and the best sphere refraction will indicate the corrected acuity with a spherical contact lens in spite of the astigmatism.

If the amount of uncorrected astigmatism is found to be no more than 0.75 or 1.00D while the patient is wearing the spherical contact lens, and if the best acuity while wearing the lens is about 20/20, consideration should be given to fitting a spherical lens. However, if the uncorrected astigmatism while wearing the lens is more than 1.00D, or if the best acuity with the spherical lens is poor (20/30 or worse), the patient is not likely to have acceptable visual acuity and visual comfort unless a toric front surface is used.

One of the most commonly used methods of stabilizing a toric front surface lens on the eye involves the use of a truncation together with prism ballast (Figure 14.5). Another common method involves the use of prism ballast with a round lens (i.e., without truncation); a less commonly used method involves truncation without prism ballast. Whichever method is used, the axis of the correcting cylinder should be determined while the patient wears a *spherical* lens of the type that is to be ordered.

If a prism ballast lens is to be fitted, the axis of the correcting cylinder will be specified in relation to the base-apex meridian of the prism (the base-apex meridian being in the 90-degree meridian). If the prism ballast lens is to be truncated, the base-apex meridian will be perpendicular to the truncation. The truncation, therefore, provides the practitioner with a convenient method of specifying cylinder axis. For example, if the required cylindrical correction is to be -1.00×90, and if the lens orients itself on the patient's eye so the truncation is at 180 degrees, the cylinder to be ordered is -1.00×90.

If a round prism ballast lens is to be used, the manufacturer usually marks the base-apex meridian by means of a dot or a vertical line near the lower edge of the lens. If the lens is not marked, the practitioner should locate the base-apex meridian while the lens is mounted in a lensometer and mark it by means of a felt-tipped pen. If a truncated lens without prism ballast is used, the minus cylinder axis will be specified in relation to the vertical meridian of the lens (which will be perpendicular to the truncation).

Locating the axis meridian. It is imperative that the practitioner have available a method of locating the position of the axis meridian of a front surface toric lens. The most convenient and effective method involves the use of a protractor reticule mounted in the telescope of the slit lamp. Although few slit lamps are equipped with reticules, they are available as an extra-cost item with some slit lamps; for others it is possible to obtain a reticule from a scientific supply company and have it mounted in the telescope. A second method of locating the position of the axis meridian involves the use of a slit lamp of the Haag-Streit design. Some of these slit lamps are equipped with a protractor scale on the lamp housing, and the practitioner simply rotates the lamp housing (with the slit as dim as possible) until

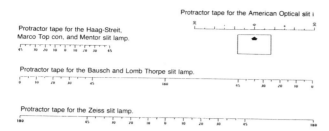

Figure 14.28 **Protractor tapes (*not* drawn to size) for slit lamps, designed by Malin and Kohler** (from Malin and Kohler, 1981).

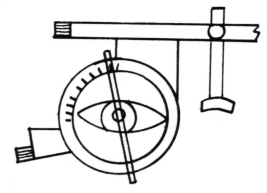

Figure 14.29 **Use of a trial frame and streak retinoscope beam to determine the orientation of the base-apex meridian of a prism-ballasted toric lens. The base-apex meridian of this lens is located at 100 degrees** (based on a suggestion by Boltz, 1982).

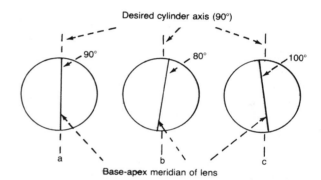

Figure 14.30 **Specifying orientation of the cylinder axis on the basis of orientation of a diagnostic lens: (*a*) cylinder axis for patient's lens is specified as 90 degrees; (*b*) cylinder axis is specified as 100 degrees; (*c*) cylinder axis is specified as 80 degrees. For either eye, the procedure is to add to the cylinder axis if the base-apex is displaced clockwise and to subtract if counterclockwise.**

the slit beam is parallel to either the truncation or the base-apex meridian and reads the angle of rotation on the protractor scale. Malin and Kohler (1981) have designed protractor tapes for use with four commonly used types of slit lamps (see Figure 14.28). In reference to using one of these tapes to locate the meridional orientation of a prism ballast lens whose base-apex meridian is marked at the bottom of the lens, Malin and Kohler note that if the mark indicates that the prism base rotates toward the *subject's right*, you *add* (remembering "SRA") the quantity to the axis of the patient's spectacle prescription; if it rotates to the left, you subtract the amount from the spectacle cylinder axis. (Although Malin and Kohler designed the tapes for use with toric soft lenses, they are equally applicable for toric hard lenses.)

A third method of locating the position of the axis meridian involves the use of a trial frame and either the slit-lamp beam or the beam of a streak retinoscope. Using the slit-lamp beam, the patient is seated in the slit lamp wearing a trial frame, and the slit-lamp beam is oriented either parallel to the truncation or parallel to the base-apex meridian of the lens. Boltz (1982) has suggested that a streak retinoscope be used to locate the meridian parallel to the truncation or to the base-apex meridian, as the patient is seated in the ophthalmic chair (see Figure 14.29).

Once the base-apex meridian of the lens has been located, the axis meridian for the correcting cylinder can be determined with the help of the diagrams shown in Figure 14.30. Consider a patient who requires the cylinder −1.00 × 90. If the base-apex meridian is located at 90 degrees, as shown in Figure 14.30a, the cylinder to be ordered is obviously −1.00 × 90. If the base-apex meridian is located at 80 degrees, as shown in Figure 14.30b, for the cylinder axis to be located at 90 degrees with respect to the eye, it will have to be ordered as −1.00 × 100.

Inspection of Figure 14.30c shows that if the base-apex meridian is located at 100 degrees, the cylinder will have to be specified as −1.00 × 80. These diagrams illustrate Malin and Kohler's suggestion that you add to the cylinder axis if the prism base has rotated to the subject's right (SRA). Another rule of thumb is to add to the cylinder axis if the base-apex meridian is displaced clockwise and to subtract if it is displaced counterclockwise. Each of these rules applies to either the right or left eye.

Patient management. After tearing has subsided and the lens has settled down, a truncated prism ballast lens should orient in such a way that the lower, truncated edge of the lens remains parallel or nearly parallel to the lower lid margin between blinks. If the lens rotates more than a few degrees between blinks it is too loose, and a lens with a steeper base curve should be tried. If the lens fails to drop all the way down and rides high (and with the lower edge not parallel to the lower lid margin), it is probably due to the upper lid margin holding the lens up and can easily be determined by holding the upper lid upward and seeing if the lens drops downward. If this is the case, the upper edge of the lens should be made thinner to allow the lens to drop down.

The patient should be observed several times during a period of at least an hour to make sure the lens remains in a relatively constant position. It is not absolutely necessary that the lower edge of a truncated lens be parallel to the lower lid margin, but it is essential that it maintain a constant position with the passing of time. For a nontruncated prism ballast lens, the base-apex meridian should maintain a constant position in relation to the vertical meridian of the eye. Each time the patient is observed, the location of the truncation or the base-apex meridian should be noted, using one of the methods that has been described.

It is not advisable to order toric lenses for a patient if a lens cannot be found that will maintain its meridional orientation while on the eye. For moderate amounts of astigmatism, a toric lens that will be off axis by as much as 20 degrees or more will usually provide much less satisfactory visual acuity than a spherical lens.

If the diagnostic lens is found to meet all of the requirements of an adequate fit, including good centration, an on-K fluorescein pattern, adequate lag, and patient comfort, and is also found to maintain its meridional orientation on the eye, the patient should be refracted while the lens is worn to determine the spherical power and cylindrical power and axis. When the patient's lenses have been received and dispensed, the lens fit and orientation should be similar to the fit and orientation of the diagnostic lens, as should be the visual acuity through the lens. If satisfactory acuity is not obtained, a spherical (not a spherocylindrical) overrefraction should be done. If a spherocylindrical refraction is done, the result would be two lens formulas involving obliquely crossed cylinders, and mathematically resolving obliquely crossed cylinders are not practical in a busy practice unless a programmable calculator or microcomputer is available.

A common cause of poor acuity is malorientation of the lens. If this is found to be the problem, and if it is concluded that the original orientation was measured correctly, the practitioner may consider ordering a new lens at the new axis. However, before this is done, the spherical power, cylindrical power, and cylinder axis should be verified by means of a lensometer. Because the cylinder is on the front surface, the cylinder power and axis determined by the lensometer should be the same as that indicated in the lens order. The lens should, of course, be oriented in the lensometer so that the base-apex meridian (or the meridian perpendicular to the truncation) is located at 90 degrees.

Fitting toric back surface lenses

As noted earlier, a toric back surface lens is used not for the correction of astigmatism but for the purpose of providing a *comfortable physical fit* on a highly toric cornea. Due to the relative flexibility of gas-permeable materials, spherical lenses made of these materials will tend to flex (bend) more on a toric cornea than will a PMMA lens. The amount of flexure can be easily determined by taking a keratometer finding while the patient wears a spherical lens: if there is no flexure, the "over-K" finding will be spherical (in spite of the presence of corneal astigmatism), but if astigmatism that is found, it will be due to flexure. For example, if the over-K finding shows 43.00 at 180/44.00 at 90, this can be interpreted as meaning that lens flexure is creating (or "undercorrecting") 1D of with-the-rule astigmatism. Because high corneal astigmatism (more than 2.50 or 3.00D) is almost always with-the-rule astigmatism, any flexure of a spherical lens on such a cornea will leave a part of the corneal astigmatism uncorrected—which will tend to compensate for any internal astigmatism (almost always against-the-rule). If the uncorrected corneal astigmatism is from 0.50 to 1.00D in the with-the-rule direction, no significant refractive astigmatism is likely to result. However, larger amounts of astigmatism may be sufficient to make the fitting of a bitoric lens advisable.

Working with PMMA lenses, Harris and Chu (1972) found that a lens having a central thickness less than 0.13mm will tend to flex significantly on a highly toric cornea. In a recent study, Harris, Gale, Gansel, and Slette (1987) fitted 12 eyes having corneal toricities ranging from 1.75 to 3.25D with Paraperm O_2 and Boston II lenses having center thicknesses of 0.10 to 0.20 mm. They found that in all cases there was lens flexure, and induced residual astigmatism, which increased as center thickness of the lens decreased, and that the flexure tended to result in residual astigmatism of 0.50D or more for center thicknesses less than 0.15mm. Harris et al. noted that, because flexure differed somewhat for the two lens types, the practitioner should use the same "brand" of lens for fitting that will be ordered for the patient. The results of Harris et al. confirm the practice of increasing the *thickness* of a spherical gas-permeable hard lens (to 0.15 or 0.16mm) to avoid fitting a bitoric lens.

It should be understood that a toric back surface lens does not require the use of prism ballast or truncation to provide lens orientation. Meridional orientation will be determined by the toric back surface of the lens riding on the toric cornea—this has been compared to the way a saddle "orients" on a horse's back.

When toric back surface lenses are fitted, a toric diagnostic lens set should be used. The usual starting point is to fit each principal meridian approximately parallel to the curvature in that meridian. For example, if the keratometer finding is 42.00 at 180 and 45.00 at 90, a lens having keratometric values of 42.00 and 45.00D should tried. Often, the lens will fit too tightly on the cornea unless some of the corneal toricity is left uncorrected. For example, for the eye just described, a 42.00/44.00 lens may be found to have better movement on the eye than a 42.00/45.00 lens. In any case, when such a patient is fitted, the practitioner should watch carefully for signs of corneal edema and be prepared to loosen the lens by modification, if necessary.

Sarver's (1970) method of fitting a bitoric lens, having a front surface cylinder designed to compensate for the astigmatism induced at the back surface of the lens, is described earlier. Using Sarver's example of an eye having the refractive error −2.00DS −3.00DC × 180, if a spherical lens (42.00DK, −2.00D) is found to correct the refractive error and a back surface toric lens (42.00DK, 45.00DK) is found to provide an optimum lens-cornea relationship, a bitoric lens having the following parameters may be ordered:

Flat meridian: 42.00DK, −2.00D.
Steep meridian: 45.00DK, −5.00D.

The lensometer reading for this lens will be −2.00DS −3.00DC, axis flat meridian. The lens will have the effect of a *spherical lens* on the eye, and even can rotate on the eye without inducing astigmatism. A Polycon II gas-permeable bitoric lens making use of

this "spherical power effect" principle is now available.

Sarver, Kame, and Williams (1985) reported on a study in which 50 patients were fitted with Polycon II spherical power-effect bitoric lenses. These lenses are available in a 36-lens set consisting of three sets of 12 lenses (varying in base curve), the lenses in one set having a toricity of 2.00DK, those in the second having a toricity of 3.00DK, and those in the third set having a toricity of 4.00DK. After successful fitting was completed, Sarver et al. found that the mean base curve in the flattest meridian was 0.45DK flatter than the flattest corneal meridian, and that the mean toricity was 0.50DK less than the toricity of the cornea. However, there was a considerable amount of variation in the lens-cornea bearing relationship, many eyes being fitted with lenses having toricities as much as 1.00–2.00DK less than that of the cornea, with a few eyes being fitted with lenses having toricities greater than that of the cornea. Sarver et al. reported that 36 of the patients were fitted with spherical, power-effect lenses, whereas 14 were fitted with "cylindrical power-effect" lenses (i.e., lenses having an additional cylindrical component for the correction of residual astigmatism).

The results of Sarver et al. (1985) emphasize the importance of using bitoric diagnostic lenses in such fittings. Sarver et al. recommend that, if the spherical power-effect lens that provides the best fit results in more than 0.50D of uncorrected refractive astigmatism, a cylindrical power-effect lens should be ordered. In such a case, the amount of cylinder to be ordered would be that found in retinoscopy or subjective overrefraction. Further, the order should specify the spherical power-effect lens used for the fitting and overrefraction, with the addition of the necessary spherical and cylindrical components found in the overrefraction.

FITTING PROCEDURES: SOFT CONTACT LENSES

Fitting procedures for soft contact lenses differ from those for hard contact lenses in a number of ways. One of the most important differences is that fluorescein is not used in the fitting of soft lenses. The "pore size" of soft lens materials is large enough that sodium fluorescein will be absorbed by the lens and will be retained permanently. Experiments have been done with large-molecule fluorescein, having molecules large enough that they are not absorbed by the lens. Unfortunately, the level of fluorescence is insufficient to be of any use in evaluating the thickness of the tear layer underneath the lens.

Fluorescein can, however, be used in the prefitting examination (for the precorneal film breakup test) or for slit-lamp examination after lens removal, as long as the dye is completely removed from the tear film before a soft lens is inserted. In the author's experience, the most effective way to remove the dye is to instill 1 or 2 drops of a mucomitetic solution such as *Adapettes* or *Adsorbotear* into the conjunctival sac of each eye, instruct the patient to blink several times, and then remove any remaining dye from the lid margins with a tissue. Using the Burton lamp (the ultraviolent light source used to inspect fluorescein patterns), the examiner then inspects the cornea, conjunctiva, and lid margins to make sure no fluorescein remains.

Another important difference between soft and hard lenses is that, due to their flexible nature, soft lenses (as already indicated) fail to conform to the corneal surface and, thus, fail to eliminate corneal astigmatism. An additional difference, also due to the flexibility of the lenses, is that it is impossible to measure the base curve of a soft contact lens on a Radiuscope or a keratometer. Various methods of base curve measurement have been developed but none has been generally accepted for routine clinical use.

Still another result of the extreme flexibility of soft lenses is the fact that far fewer diagnostic lenses are required. Whereas hard lens base curves are available (and required) in steps of 0.05mm (0.25DK), soft lenses are available in base curve steps no smaller than 0.10, 0.20, or even 0.30mm. Some of the newer, thinner, soft-lens designs are available in only a single base curve.

Patient Management

Optometric examination

As is the case when a patient is to be fitted with hard contact lenses, emphasis should be placed on the findings that are of particular importance in the fitting of the contact lenses. A careful slit-lamp examination, including the precorneal film breakup test, should be done. As far as astigmatism is concerned, it is the refractive astigmatism with which the practitioner must be concerned, because soft lenses fail to correct either corneal or internal astigmatism (unless a toric front surface is used). If refractive astigmatism is found to be in excess of 1.00D with-the-rule or 0.75D against-the-rule or

oblique, the use of a toric front surface should be considered.

Patient selection

The main advantage of soft lenses for the new wearer is that the lenses cause little, if any, discomfort and do not require an adaptation period as hard lenses do. For this reason, many patients who would not be considered as candidates for hard contact lenses may be considered as soft lens candidates. This applies particularly to patients who would like to wear their lenses only on a part-time basis (i.e., for work, social wear, or sports only). With soft lenses it is not necessary to maintain wearing time, as it is for hard lenses.

Fitting visit

The fitting data record form recommended for PMMA lenses, shown in Appendix A, is also appropriate for recording fitting data for soft lenses. Specifications of diagnostic lenses are recorded, together with notes concerning the fit of the lenses, the refraction through the lenses to be fitted, and information concerning the lenses to be ordered.

Use of diagnostic lenses. Diagnostic lenses are inserted, and the fit of the lenses is assessed by means of the slit lamp. As with hard lenses, the position and lag of each lens following a blink is evaluated.

Lens placement by the practitioner. The author uses a placement procedure similar to that described for hard lenses, except the patient is instructed to look (at the thumb) *downward and inward*, so the lens can be placed on the superior temporal sclera. The larger size of soft lenses requires a larger area on which to place the lens, and sufficient area is available on the superior temporal sclera. For lens removal, the author elevates the patient's upper lid slightly with the index finger of one hand and places the index finger of the other hand firmly against the lower part of the lens. The patient is then instructed to look upward, and the lens is gently pinched off the cornea with the thumb and forefinger as the patient looks upward.

Refraction through diagnostic lenses. When the optimally fitting lenses have been selected, retinoscopy, and subjective refraction are done while the lenses are worn. Retinoscopy is done with both spheres and cylinders, in the usual manner, to determine the amount of astigmatism that will remain uncorrected when the lenses are worn. With rare exceptions, this will be within about ±0.25D of the subjectively determined cylinder without the lens. Unless toric front surface lenses are to be fitted, subjective refraction is normally done with spheres only (best sphere refraction).

Specification of lens power. The power of the trial lens will normally be close enough to the required lens power that the power of the lenses in the refractor will be relatively small. However, if the power of the lenses in the refractor should be as great as ±4.50D or more, the change in power due to the change in vertex distance should be determined by calculation or by use of a table. Because there is no tear lens underneath a well-fitting soft contact lens, it is not necessary to make a change in the lens power to be ordered if the lens will have a different base curve than the diagnostic lens through which the refraction was done.

Fitting Spherical Soft Lenses

Soft contact lenses are presently available in both spin-cast and lathe-cut designs. Until recently, the only spin-cast lens manufactured in the United States was the Bausch & Lomb Soflens. Today, spin-cast lenses are also manufactured by American Hydron and Ocular Sciences. Soflens spin-cast lenses in the past have been available in a number of *series* of lenses, each lens series having its own base curve, diameter, and center thickness. However, with these lenses the base curve is on the front surface of the lens rather than the back (due to the method of manufacture), so the base curve of the lens bears no particular relationship to the curvature of the wearer's cornea. Further, for each lens series, what distinguishes a lens of one power from one of another power is not the front surface curvature (as is the case with lathe-cut lenses) but the curvature of the back surface. The result of this method of manufacture is that for a given lens series, the higher the minus power of a given lens, the steeper the back surface.

Lathe-cut lenses made by more than two dozen manufacturers have now been approved by the FDA. As with lathe-cut hard lenses, the base curve is on the back surface. Each lathe-cut lens manufacturer's lenses typically are available in only one or two diameters and in a small number of base curve radii. The paucity of base curve radii can be accounted for by the fact that if a lens is sufficiently thin and is fitted sufficiently flat, it will drape itself over corneas having a wide range of radii of curvature.

Diagnostic lenses

For the fitting of lathe-cut lenses, diagnostic lens sets need to include only a relatively small number of lenses, because these lenses are typically available in only one or two overall diameters and in only two or three base radii. On the other hand, spin-cast lenses, typically having a different base curve radius for every lens in the series, tend to require a larger diagnostic lens set, consisting of lenses of various powers. A representative selection of daily-wear, lathe-cut spherical soft lenses is given in Table 14.3, and daily-wear, spin-cast spherical soft lenses are listed in Table 14.4.

Evaluation of lens fit

Because fluorescein cannot be used to evaluate the fit of a soft contact lens, the most convenient method of evaluating the fit involves the use of the biomicroscope. The keratometer and the retinoscope are also of value in evaluating the fit.

Biomicroscope. After waiting a few minutes for the lenses to "settle," the lens fit is evaluated by means of the biomicroscope. The lens should be well centered on the cornea. Because most soft lenses have a diameter in excess of 13 or 14mm, the lens should extend from 0.5–1mm or more beyond the limbus, extending onto the sclera. (The corneal diameter, or "visible iris diameter," averages about 12mm horizontally and 11mm vertically.) The lens may tend to decenter upward or outward slightly. This is no problem as long as the lens covers the entire surface of the cornea. If the lens does *not* cover the entire surface of the cornea, the portion of the cornea not covered will tend to become desiccated, because the epithelium will not be resurfaced with hydrated mucus during blinking.

The lag that occurs following each blink can best be observed by placing the narrow slit-lamp beam at the lower nasal portion of the eye and asking the patient to blink. The amount of blink lag can be estimated by comparing it with the amount the lens overlaps the limbus. For a 14mm lens, overlapping the limbus by about 1mm on either side, a lens that lags 1mm would lag by an amount just equal to the overlap of the lens. After evaluating the blink lag, the patient should be asked to look upward, and the downward lag should be noted.

The amount of blink lag expected varies from one lens design to another. The "standard thickness" lenses (which have now been largely replaced by ultrathin lenses) transmit a relatively small amount of oxygen, so most of the cornea's oxygen must be

Table 14.3   Representative lathe-cut, spherical soft lenses for daily wear (*Tyler's Quarterly*, 1987)

Manufacturer	Trade name	Water content (percent)	Diameter (mm)	Base curve radii (mm)	Center thickness (mm)[a]
American Hydron	Zero-6	38%	14.0mm	8.4, 8.7, 9.0mm	0.06mm
	Z-plus	38	14.0	8.4, 8.7, 9.0	0.10
	Mini-lens	38	13.0	8.1–9.1	0.10
Barnes-Hind	SoftMate B	45	14.3	8.7	0.07
		45	14.8	9.0	0.07
	SoftMate DW	45	14.8	8.5, 8.8	0.05
	Hydrocurve II	45	13.5	8.3, 8.6	0.05
		45	14.5	8.9	0.05
		45	15.5, 16.0	9.2–10.18	
Ciba Vision Care	CibaSoft	37.5	13.8	8.3, 8.6, 8.9	0.06
		37.5	14.5	8.6, 8.9, 9.2	0.04–0.09
	CibaThin	37.5	13.8	8.6, 8.9	0.035
Cooper-Vision	Aquaflex Superthin	42.5	13.8	8.2–9.1	0.05–0.10
	Aquaflex Standard	42.5	13.2	7.8–8.9	0.10–0.18
N&N	Tresoft Standard	46	13.5–14.5	8.2–8.8	0.15–0.20
	Tresoft Thin	46	13.7	8.2, 8.5, 8.8	0.07–0.09
Sola-Syntex	CSI	38.5	13.8	8.0, 8.3, 8.6	0.06
		38.5	14.8	8.6, 8.9, 9.35	0.06
Vistakon	Hydromarc	43	14.0, 14.5	8.15–9.05	0.11
Wesley-Jessen	DuroSoft 2 (D2–T3)	38	13.5	8.2, 8.5, 8.9	0.06
	DuroSoft 2 (D2–T4)	38	14.5	8.3, 8.6, 9.0	0.06

[a]For minus lenses.

Table 14.4   Representative spin-cast, spherical soft lenses for daily wear (*Tyler's Quarterly*, March, 1987)

Manufacturer	Trade name	Water content (percent)	Diameter (mm)	Center thickness (mm)[a]
American Hydron	Hydron Spin-cast	38%	14.5mm	0.07mm
Bausch & Lomb	SofSpin	38	14.0	0.05–0.09
	U-3	38	13.5	0.07
	U-4	38	14.5	0.07
	L-3	38	13.5	0.06
	L-4	38	14.5	0.06
	O-3	38	13.5	0.035
	O-4	38	14.5	0.035
Ocular Sciences	CQ4	38.6	14.5	0.07

[a]For minus lenses.

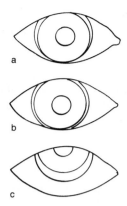

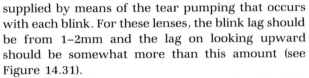

Figure 14.31 A well-fitting hydrogel lens: *(a)* **just after a blink;** *(b)* **after blink lag has taken place;** *(c)* **downward lag on looking upward. The lens normally rides in the position shown in** *(b)* **until the next blink.**

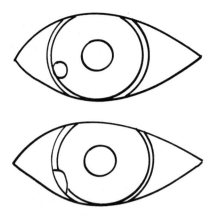

Figure 14.32 Air bubbles under a soft lens: *(a)* **indicates lens may be too steep or too large;** *(b)* **indicates lens may be fitting too flat.**

supplied by means of the tear pumping that occurs with each blink. For these lenses, the blink lag should be from 1–2mm and the lag on looking upward should be somewhat more than this amount (see Figure 14.31).

The amount of blink lag necessary for ultrathin lenses (lenses thinner than 0.10mm) is a matter of controversy. Some practitioners believe that because these lenses transmit oxygen, it is not necessary for oxygen to be supplied by tear pumping and, therefore, the lenses need not lag at all. Others believe that because the lenses transmit insufficient oxygen to serve the cornea's full requirements, at least a small amount of blink lag is necessary. Another factor to be considered is that, if there were no lens movement at all, desquamated epithelial cells and other debris that constantly accumulate underneath a lens would have no method of escape until the lens was removed at night. Even a small amount of lens movement (approximately 0.5 to 1mm) appears to be sufficient.

If a lens appears to have insufficient lag, the practitioner should attempt to displace the lens upward with the fingertip. If the lens does not move easily on the cornea it is too tight, and a flatter or smaller lens should be tried.

Occasionally an air bubble will be found to be trapped underneath the lens. If the patient is asked to close the eye and gently massage the upper lid, the bubble will often disperse. However, if the bubble persists, it may indicate a problem in the fit of the lens. An air bubble underneath the lens that does not extend to the edge of the lens may indicate

that the lens is too steep or too large; an air bubble extending to the edge of the lens may indicate that the base curve or the peripheral curve of the lens is too flat or the lens is too small (see Figure 14.32.)

Keratometry. A keratometer finding taken with the lenses on will often supply the optometrist with useful information. The keratometer finding should indicate (1) clear mire images, (2) the same amount (and axis) of corneal astigmatism as without the lens, and (3) no change in the appearance of the mire images between blinks. A "waterfall" appearance usually indicates that the lens is too loose; if the mires are clear at first but then begin to blur after a blink, this, too, is an indication that the lens is too loose. If the mires are distorted just after a blink but then begin to clear up, it may be an indication that the lens is too tight. A tight lens, however, may often give a clear mire image with no change between blinks; fortunately, the presence of a tight lens can be determined by slit-lamp examination.

Retinoscopy. Retinoscopy is an alternative procedure for determining lens fit on the basis of optical clarity. If the retinoscope reflex is distorted, it may indicate that the lens is not conforming to the corneal contour.

Patient symptoms. If a lens is fitting excessively loosely, being too small in diameter or having too flat a base curve, it may result in extreme discomfort accompanied by conjunctival injection and lacrimation. An additional cause of discomfort is the presence of a foreign body under the lens. It will not be flushed out by the tears, as it would be with a hard lens, so the lens must be taken off, rinsed well, and put back on the eye. A lens that fits too tightly will be just as comfortable as one that is an optimum fit. A helpful criterion in hydrogel lens fitting is to fit the loosest lens that will not cause discomfort.

Lens order

Although the lens specifications of PMMA lenses are universally applied, making it unnecessary to specify a trade name when ordering these lenses, this unfortunately is not the case with soft lenses. The rapidly growing number of lenses that have received FDA approval are all trade name lenses, each lens being made of a material somewhat different than the next and with slightly different specifications for the fitting parameters.

In addition to the trade name of the lens being ordered, an order for a soft contact lens should include the following parameters: base curve radius, overall diameter, and power. Radii of secondary curves (not always used on soft lenses) and of peripheral curves, peripheral curve width, optic zone diameter, and central thickness are all "standard" for a given lens and, therefore, cannot be specified by the practitioner.

Verification of finished lenses

When the finished lenses have been received from the laboratory, the only specifications that can be verified are lens power, overall diameter, and center thickness. To verify lens power, the lens is rinsed well with saline solution to remove all excess storage solution (which in some cases contains a liquid polymer), dried gently with a lintfree towel, and placed on the lensometer stop so the power can be read. For hard as well as soft contact lenses, a projection lensometer is preferred, as the lens can be placed in a horizontal position, as opposed to the almost-vertical position required with the ordinary lensometer. The diameter is verified by a measuring magnifier while the lens is in the hydrated state. Although not specified by the practitioner, the optic zone of the lens can also be measured. The lens thickness is verified by a dial thickness gauge. To avoid puncturing or tearing the lens, a dial gauge with a rounded (rather than sharp) pin should be used.

Contact lens standards and tolerances developed by the American National Standards Institute are given in Appendix B.

Delivery of lenses

When the finished lenses are delivered to the patient, the practitioner should place the lenses on the patient's eyes, check visual acuity and best sphere subjective refraction, and then verify the fit of the lenses with the slit lamp. Following this, the patient is instructed concerning procedures for lens placement, removal, and hygienic care. In many practices, this instruction will be given by a trained assistant or an optometric technician.

Placement and removal of lenses by the patient

The patient is instructed to wash the hands and is seated at a table with a mirror and other required paraphernalia close at hand. The practitioner removes the right lens from the container, rinses it with fresh saline, and places it on the patient's index finger. The patient is instructed to place the lens on the cornea, using exactly the same method described for hard lens placement. Assuming that the patient is right-handed, the middle finger of the right hand is used to hold the lower lid down, and the index finger of the left hand is used to hold the upper lid up. Due to the large size of the soft lens, the patient must hold the eyes open widely. The left lens is then placed on the eye in the same manner. If there is much of a delay in the patient's putting on the lens, it should be remoistened with saline solution.

To remove the lens, the patient uses the method already described for removal by the practitioner. As the patient looks straight ahead, the upper lid is held up with the index finger of the left hand, while the index finger of the right hand is placed firmly on the lower part of the lens. The patient then looks upward, and during the upward movement the lens is gently pinched off the cornea with the thumb and index finger. The lens is then rinsed in saline and placed in the container before the second lens is removed.

Patient instructions

Patient instructions concerning hygienic care of soft lenses will depend on the disinfection system to be used.

Chemical system. If a chemical system is to be used, three solutions will be dispensed to the patient along with the lenses and the lens container: a surfactant (surface-acting) cleaning solution, a storage solution, and a saline solution. After removing each lens at night, the patient places the lens in the palm of the left hand (if right-handed) or on the tip of the left index finger, places 1 or 2 drops of cleaning solution on the lens, and then rubs the lens using the index finger of the right hand to remove any mucus or other material that may have accumulated on the lens during the day. The lens is then rinsed well with saline and placed in the storage case, and the case is filled with fresh storage solution. In the morning the patient simply takes the lens out of the case, rinses it with saline solution, and places it on the eye.

Heat disinfection. If a heat disinfection system is to be used, a heating unit and two solutions (a cleaning solution and a saline solution) will be dispensed to the patient along with the lenses. After removing each lens at night, the patient cleans the lens (as described above) with the cleaning solution, and rinses it with saline solution, prior to heat disinfection. The next morning the patient removes the lens case from the disinfecting unit, removes each lens (rinsing it with saline from the storage case), and puts it on.

It is even more important for wearers of soft lenses than hard lenses to emphasize the importance of cleaning the lenses *at night*. Patients who clean their lenses in the morning or not at all will eventually find that the lenses are unwearable due to deposits of proteins and other materials.

Hydrogen peroxide. Disinfection systems involving the use of hydrogen peroxide have been increasingly popular in recent years. After the lenses are cleaned, using a surfactant cleaner, they are rinsed with saline and stored overnight in the hydrogen peroxide solution. With some hydrogen peroxide systems this procedure must be followed by the use of a neutralizing solution (such as sodium bicarbonate or sodium pyrovate), whereas other systems make use of a catalytic disc for neutralization.

Enzyme cleaner. Even though a surfactant cleaner is used nightly prior to disinfection, soft lenses tend to become coated with protein materials originating in the tear film. Periodic use of a papain enzyme cleaner is usually effective in removing these coatings. Most practitioners instruct patients to use the enzyme cleaner weekly. Because papain enzyme acts by reducing the size of protein molecules adhering to the lens, it is necessary to mechanically rub the lens to remove both the enzyme cleaner itself and the tear film proteins. This should be followed by thorough rinsing with saline and disinfection of the lenses. Enzyme cleaner is not recommended for use with a chemical system in which chlorhexidine is used, since the chlorhexidine in the storage solution tends to bind strongly to proteins. According to Gold and Orenstein (1980), papain will bind, attract, and increase the concentration of chlorhexidine in the lens.

Wearing schedules. Because soft contact lenses require little or no adaptation, the author instructs the patient to wear the lenses 8 hours each day starting with the first day, until the first progress visit, which is usually at the end of 1 or 2 weeks at the most.

Progress visits

It may be a good idea to stretch progress visits out over a greater period of time for soft lens wearers than for hard lens wearers. This is because soft lens wearers do not have to go through the adaptation period required of hard lens wearers, and also because when problems occur with soft lens wearers, they tend to occur later than the problems with hard lens wearers. The first progress visit could be at the end of 2 weeks, the second at the end of 4 weeks, the third at the end of 2 months, and the fourth at the end of 3 months.

The record form for progress visits, shown in Appendix A, is suitable for both hard and soft lens wearers. As is the case with hard lens wearers, the findings with lenses on are of the greatest importance during the first few progress visits. For the later progress visits, however, the findings after lens removal assume increased importance.

Yearly progress examination

The yearly progress examination should include a repetition of the portions of the optometric data base dealing with refraction and with ocular health, in addition to an evaluation of the fit of the lenses and the physical condition of the lenses themselves. Using a low-power binocular microscope or the slit-lamp biomicroscope, the lenses should be inspected carefully for the presence of coating, tears, pits, scratches, and other signs of damage.

Blinking. The patient should be told of the importance of correct blinking and should be instructed to perform blinking exercises regularly (as described earlier in this chapter). If soft contact lenses require any adaptation on the part of the patient, it is learning correct blinking habits.

Fitting Toric Soft Lenses

The optical considerations involved in the fitting of toric soft lenses are discussed in the "Optical Principles of Contact Lenses" section earlier in the chapter. Recall that spherical soft lenses conform to the corneal surface to the extent that there is a direct transfer of corneal toricity to the lens, so these lenses fail to eliminate corneal astigmatism as hard lenses do.

Clinical experience has indicated that patients with no more than 0.75 to 1.00D of with-the-rule refractive astigmatism can obtain adequate visual acuity with spherical soft contact lenses, in spite of the presence of the astigmatism. This applies also to patients having no more than 0.50 or 0.75D of against-the-rule or oblique refractive astigmatism. Many patients having refractive astigmatism greater than these amounts will have unsatisfactory visual acuity, visual comfort, or both with spherical soft contact lenses. However, for patients having refractive astigmatism as great as 1.25D, a diagnostic lens trial with spherical soft lenses is advisable before proceeding with toric fitting. A spherical lens that provides 20/20- or 20/25 acuity will often be more satisfactory than a toric lens that orients at an incorrect axis.

Methods of determining cylinder axis location (the use of a reticule in the telescope of the slit lamp, a protractor mounted on the slit-lamp housing, and a trial frame) are described in the discussion of toric hard lens fitting. The principles of toric lens fitting discussed for toric hard lenses have equal application for toric soft lenses. The patient should wear the lenses for 20 minutes or more before a decision is made on lens orientation, following which the position of the lens should be observed on a number of occasions during a period of 1 hour or more.

Fitting should be done by the use of a diagnostic lens set available from the manufacturer. The diagnostic lens having the spherical power, cylindrical power, and cylinder axis closest to the required parameters should be used. If the lens is found to orient at an incorrect axis, a diagnostic lens with the correct axis should be tried before the patient's lens is ordered.

Diagnostic lens procedures

Most "inventory" lenses—lenses that laboratories have available on a regular basis—achieve meridional orientation by the provision of prism ballast, either with or without truncation (see Figure 14.33). Most "custom" lenses—lenses that are available only on special order—achieve meridional orientation by the provision of both a lower truncation and prism ballast (see Figure 14.34). The parameters of representative toric soft lenses, available on inventory, are listed in Table 14.5. Of the lenses listed in the table, the *Hydrocurve* II, *Bausch & Lomb Optima*, and *Hydromarc* are prism-ballasted; the Hydron *Zero–T* and the Wesley-Jessen *DuroSoft 2* are prism-ballasted with a lower truncation; and the Ciba *ToriSoft* lens achieves meridional orientation by a "double slab-off" contruction (see Figure 14.35) designed to provide meridional orientation by the

Figure 14.34 A truncated and prism-ballasted toric soft contact lens.

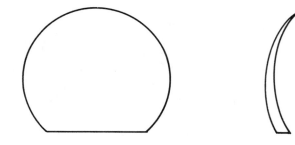

Figure 14.33 A prism-ballasted toric soft contact lens.

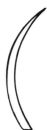

Figure 14.35 Ciba ToriSoft lens, having double slab-off construction.

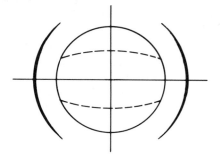

Table 14.5   Representative toric soft lenses for daily wear, available on inventory (*Tyler's Quarterly*, March, 1987)

Manufacturer	Trade name	Diameter (mm)	Base curve radii (mm)	Stabilization
American Hydron	Zero–T	13.0, 14.3mm	8.3mm	Ballasted, truncation
Barnes-Hind	Hydrocurve II	13.5	8.6	Ballasted
		14.5	8.9	Ballasted
Bausch & Lomb	Optima Toric	14.0	8.3, 8.6, 8.9	Ballasted
Ciba Vision Care	ToriSoft	14.5	8.6, 8.9, 9.2	Double slab-off
Vistakon	Hydromarc Toric	14.5	8.3, 8.7, 9.0	Ballasted, lower slab-off
Wesley-Jessen	DuroSoft 2 Toric	13.5	8.3, 8.5	Ballasted, truncation
		14.5	8.3, 8.6	

presence of "thin zones" at the upper and lower portions of the lens. Inventory lenses are available in rather narrow ranges of cylinder powers and axis: they are typically available in cyclinder powers in the −1.00 to −2.00D range, with cylinder axes within 20 degrees of 180 and 90 degrees, in 5-degree steps. If a lens has parameters outside those available in inventory lenses, a custom lens will have to be ordered. Unfortunately, there is often a long delay in receiving a custom lens from a laboratory, and, in any case, the lens must be considered as a diagnostic lens until proven otherwise.

When the diagnostic lens has been placed on the eye and has been allowed to settle, slit-lamp examination should indicate that the lens moves freely in the primary position and during upgaze, as would be expected for a spherical lens. The lens should be worn for a long enough time so that the position of the base-apex meridian can be monitored several times at intervals of about 5 minutes. The base-apex meridian can be identified, as shown in Figure 14.36, by a dot at the 6 o'clock position (Hydromarc), three "laser-trace" marks at the bottom of the lens (Bausch & Lomb Optima and Hydrocurve II), horizontal lines in the 180 meridian (Ciba), or by the truncation itself (Hydron and Wesley-Jessen), which, of course, is 90 degrees from the base-apex meridian.

In evaluating the fit of a toric soft lens, the examiner should look for evidence of both *malorientation* and *excessive rotation*. A well-fitting lens should locate with the base-apex meridian oriented vertically (or as much as 5–10 degrees nasalward at the bottom, due to the lid action), should rotate slightly upward and nasally with each blink, and then immediately return to the vertical or near-vertical position. If the lens does not rotate excessively but consistently orients at a position other than vertical (the orientation being *measured* by one of the methods previously described rather than being "guesstimated"), the axis for the lens to be ordered is determined by the rule, "If the base-apex meridian is oriented in the clockwise direction (as compared to the vertical meridian), you *add*, but if it is oriented in the counterclockwise direction, you *subtract*." However, if the lens rotates excessively, the base-apex meridian being in a different position every

Figure 14.36   Methods of identifying the base-apex meridian of a toric soft contact lens: *(a)* dot at 6 o'clock; *(b)* laser marks at bottom of lens; *(c)* horizontal lines in the 180 meridian; *(d)* the truncation which is 90 degrees from the base-apex meridian.

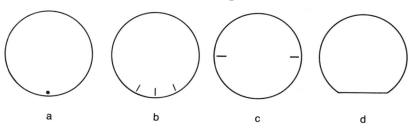

time the lens is evaluated, the lens may be fitting too tightly or too loosely, and a flatter or a steeper lens should be tried. Unfortunately, some inventory lenses are available only in a restricted range of base curve radii.

In a discussion of toric lens fitting, Boltz (1982) suggested that, because toric soft lenses are prism ballasted and are therefore thicker and stiffer in the lower part of the lens, they should be fitted more loosely than spherical soft lenses to avoid corneal edema. Boltz recommended that the lens have from 1.5 to 2mm movement in the straight-ahead position with no limbal compression or conjunctival depression. In addition, he suggested that the orientation of the lens be determined after several blinks and after eye movements upward, downward, and laterally. Problems noted by Boltz include poor distance vision due to residual refractive error, poor near vision due to lens rotation with downward gaze, and edema due to the thicker lower portion of the lens.

Experience has shown that patients having *oblique* corneal astigmatism are difficult to fit with toric soft lenses, because the meridional variation in edge thickness is such that the thickest portion of the lens may not correspond with the position of the prism base. In such a case, torsional forces exerted by the upper lid during blinking may result in the lens not returning to the same meridional orientation after each blink. If a patient having oblique corneal astigmatism wants to be fitted with contact lenses, a higher degree of success may be obtained by fitting spherical, gas-permeable hard lenses.

Once the lens having the optimum base curve radius, spherical and cylinder power, and cylinder axis has been chosen, visual acuity should be measured and a spherical overrefraction should be done. In the event that visual acuity through a well-fitting lens is poor, the overrefraction will determine whether the problem is due to the spherical power or to the cylinder power and axis. It is usually not helpful to do a spherocylindrical subjective refraction, because the required cylinder power and axis can be determined only by resolving obliquely crossed cylinders. However, if satisfactory acuity is not obtained with an apparently well-fitting lens, the lens can be *rotated* slightly in both the clockwise and counterclockwise directions in an effort to improve visual acuity.

Lens ordering. In the order for a toric soft lens, the cylinder axis is specified in relation to the *base-apex meridian*. Although most toric soft lenses have front surface cylinders, some have back surface cylinders—this is not a problem because the lens is sufficiently thin and flexible to allow the toricity of the back surface to be transferred to the front surface of the lens. In either case, it is convenient for the practitioner to specify the order in minus cylinder form, and the manufacturer will transpose the prescription, if necessary.

Verification. Sometimes practitioners neglect to verify the power of a toric soft lens before dispensing it to the patient because of an assumed difficulty in doing so. However, if a projection lensometer is used, the procedure is not as difficult as one might imagine. As with a spherical lens, the lens is first rinsed with saline and is allowed to dry for several seconds. It is then placed on the lens stop of the projection lensometer, with the base-apex meridian located at 90 degrees. The sphere power, cylinder power, and cylinder axis determined by the lensometer should be exactly as ordered, no conversion factor being necessary. Because the power and axis will vary somewhat with the state of hydration, several readings should be taken, and the readings averaged. Garnett and Wells (1983) investigated the accuracy of measurement of toric soft lenses as compared to toric hard lenses and spectacle lenses, and found the standard deviation of the readings to be $\pm0.09D$ for toric soft lenses as compared to $\pm0.06D$ for hard lenses and $\pm0.03D$ for spectacle lenses. They found that if three readings are taken in each principal meridian, the power of a toric soft lens will be accurate within $\pm0.33D$, and that if five readings are taken, the power will be accurate within $\pm0.25D$.

Dispensing and follow-up care. When the lenses are dispensed, the fit should be reevaluated in terms of position, movement, and position of the base-apex meridian; and visual acuity and spherical overrefraction should be verified. If, after the lenses have been allowed to settle, meridional orientation and/or visual acuity are not satisfactory, it may be necessary to reorder the lens or lenses. If so, the lens prescription, as determined by the lensometer, assumes an important role: if the cylinder power and/or axis of the lens received from the laboratory are incorrect, the practitioner should expect the laboratory to replace the lens at no charge. However, if the lens is correct in both cylinder power and axis but is not orienting correctly or providing satisfactory acuity, the practitioner will have to decide whether to reorder the lens immediately or to have the patient wear the lenses for a week or so before deciding on a reorder.

Experience has shown that toric soft lenses are more sensitive to the accumulation of lens coatings and other problems than are soft spherical lenses. Although a spherical lens that is moderately coated or has lost some of its flexibility may be worn satisfactorily for a period of several months, a moderately coated toric lens in a similar condition may fail to achieve meridional orientation consistently and may have to be replaced. Therefore, the useful life of a toric soft lens may be somewhat shorter than that of a spherical lens.

CONTACT LENSES FOR PRESBYOPIA

When a presbyopic patient is fitted with contact lenses, the practitioner has a number of alternatives available to provide near vision for the patient: (1) the patient can be fitted with contact lenses for distance vision use and with reading glasses or bifocals (with plano uppers), to be worn with the contact lenses for near work; (2) a contact lens for distance vision can be fitted on one eye and a contact lens for near vision fitted on the other eye (the *monovision* system); or (3) bifocal contact lenses can be fitted.

Contact Lenses and Reading Glasses

Many patients who desire contact lenses for cosmetic reasons have no objection to wearing either hard or soft contact lenses for full-time wear and wearing reading glasses or bifocals for near work. By wearing glasses for near work only, the patient is doing what must be done by emmetropic members of his or her age group. Many of these patients are pleased with "half-eye" reading glasses, since it is obvious that a person who wears such glasses needs them for reading only. An advantage of wearing reading glasses or bifocals for near work is that a correction for residual astigmatism, or even a prism correction, in the case of a binocular vision problem, can be incorporated into the lenses.

Monovision Fitting

For a patient who is not willing to wear reading glasses along with contact lenses, the *monovision system* often presents an attractive alternative to bifocal contact lenses. There are two categories of

patients for whom only *one* contact lens will be needed: the low myope (no more than about 2.00 to 3.00D), who may be fitted with a distance lens for one eye and with no lens for the eye to be used for reading; and the emmetrope or very low hyperope, requiring a reading lens for one eye and no lens for the eye used for distance vision. However, in the majority of cases, contact lenses must be fitted for both eyes. In any case, the decision must be made as to which eye is fitted with the distance lens and which with the near lens. Normally, the distance lens is fitted on the dominant eye. Another approach suggested by Brungardt (1971) is to allow the patient to decide. If both eyes require the same lens power, the patient is instructed to wear the distance lens on the right eye and the near lens on the left eye for a period of about 2 weeks, and then to wear the lenses on the opposite eyes for an equal period of time.

For monovision fitting to succeed, the patient must have equally good visual acuity in both eyes. For a person who is not yet a presbyope and is fitted with lenses for all distances, the presence of uncorrected astigmatism in one eye, resulting in slightly lowered acuity, may cause no problem, because "one eye sees what the other eye does not see." However, with monovision fitting, one eye is unable to "help" the other, so a small amount of uncorrected astigmatism, resulting in an acuity loss of one line of letters or less, will often be sufficient for the system to result in failure. For this reason, gas-permeable hard lenses are often the lenses of choice for monovision fitting. If a patient has even as much as 0.75D of refractive astigmatism, spherical soft lenses may not provide sufficiently sharp visual acuity with each eye. Although toric soft lenses could be fitted, experience shows that if one lens occasionally rotates "off axis"—which may not be a problem for a nonpresbyope—either distance or near vision can be annoyingly blurred.

Does monovision fitting sacrifice binocular vision?

Although the optometrist may feel uneasy about allowing a patient to engage in tasks such as automobile driving with one eye purposely blurred, Koetting (1966) tested the stereopsis of a number of patients who had been fitted with monovision lenses and found that 94 percent exhibited stereopsis within the norms established for their age group. More recently, McGill and Erickson (1987) compared near-point stereopsis with monovision fitting and four trade name "simultaneous vision," bifocal contact lenses, using ten presbyopic patients as subjects.

They found that monovision generally produced the least reduction in stereopsis as compared to baseline stereopsis with near-point spectacle lenses.

Even though these studies show the presence of stereopsis for monovision wearers, it is possible that success with monovision requires a smooth transition of vision from one distance to another. In this regard, the combined roles of *accommodation* and *depth of field* should not be overlooked. The monovision wearer who is an early presbyope (requiring only about a +1.00D add) may have relatively large pupils with the result that the depth of field is limited, but may have a sufficient range of accommodation so that *both* eyes will have acceptably clear retinal images for intermediate distances, allowing a smooth transition for distance-to-near or near-to-distance vision. The older monovision wearer (requiring about a +2.00D add) will have smaller pupils and, therefore, a larger depth of field in spite of a smaller range of accommodation.

In a theoretical study, Erickson (1987) addressed the possible limitation that an intermediate correction cannot be incorporated into a monovision correction without compromising distance and/or near vision. On the basis of a prescription strategy that involved leaving half the amplitude of accommodation in reserve and assuming a 0.50D depth of focus, Erickson concluded that for adds as high as 2.00D, little or no compromise in resolution is created for any gaze position or viewing distance. In a study involving six monovision wearers, Schor and Erickson (1987) compared the binocular depth of field for each subject to the sum of the two monocularly determined depths of field. They found that two of the subjects lacked a preference for a sighting eye and demonstrated complete binocular summation of their monocular ranges. The remaining subjects preferred to sight with one eye, some of whom showed partial binocular summation of the monocular ranges whereas others tended to suppress information from the nondominant eye regardless of clarity. On the basis of these results, it can be inferred that greater success in monovision fitting should be expected for patients whose sighting dominance is not pronounced.

Clinical procedures

In monovision fitting a convenient method used to determine the amount of add involves the crossed-cylinder finding at near, together with the plus-and-minus-to-blur findings. The power of the add through a correct-fitting diagnostic lens can be verified by having the patient "trombone" a magazine or newspaper back and forth while wearing the lenses to be ordered. While becoming adapted to monovision lenses, the patient will find that visual acuity at arms-length distance is about equally good (or equally poor) for the two eyes. Beyond that distance, vision will be poorer with the "near" eye, whereas for closer distances, vision will be poorer with the "distance" eye. Therefore, for successful adaptation, each eye must "learn" to suppress vision at the distance for which it is out of focus. The writer's experience is that few patients have difficulty learning to suppress distance vision while reading. However, some patients do have difficulty in some distance vision tasks, particularly night driving, when light sources can cause an annoying diplopia. A solution to this problem is to provide the patient distance lenses for both eyes and a near lens for one eye; an alternate solution is for the patient to wear glasses for night driving.

Bifocal Contact Lenses

Bifocal contact lenses have been available in PMMA and soft contact lens constructions for some time. At the time of this writing, however, only one gas-permeable bifocal, the *Tangent-Streak* (a one-piece bifocal having a horizontal dividing line), has received FDA approval.

Hard bifocals

The first bifocal contact lenses to be developed were one-piece concentric bifocals, having the distance portion in the center of the lens and the near portion in the periphery. The concentric front surface bifocal (see Figure 14.37a) has a distance portion about 4mm in diameter and an annular near portion having a width of about 3mm. This lens must be fitted loosely, so that it lags upward (with relation to the cornea) by about 2mm when the eyes are depressed for near vision. The concentric front surface bifocal is called an *alternating vision lens*, in contrast to the concentric back surface bifocal, called a *simultaneous vision bifocal*, which retains its central position during reading. The concentric back surface bifocal (see Figure 14.37b) has a small (2–3mm) distance portion and a relatively wide annular near portion, and is fitted so that there is little or no lag. The wearer's pupil must be sufficiently large so that approximately 50 percent of the pupillary area is covered by the distance portion of the lens and 50 percent is covered by the near portion. Although, in theory, the lens does not lag upward for near vision, it is likely that some upward lag will be present if

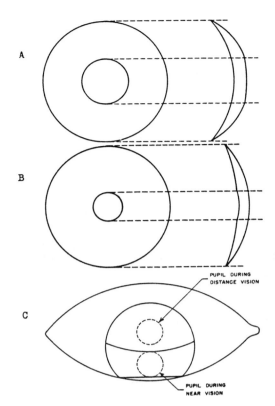

Figure 14.37 *(a)* Concentric front surface bifocal; *(b)* concentric back surface bifocal; *(c)* one-piece lower segment bifocal stabilized by both truncation and prism ballast.

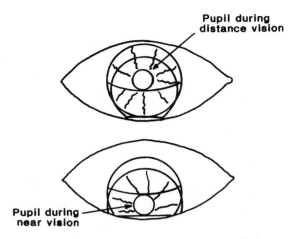

Figure 14.38 Position of pupil during distance vision and during near vision while wearing a bifocal contact lens.

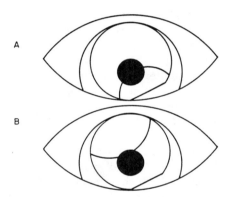

Figure 14.39 For an upcurve, or crescent-shaped, bifocal, the segment will tend to remain in front of the pupil when the lens rotates.

the lens is to be successful in providing distance and near vision.

Hard bifocal contact lenses having the segment located in the lower part of the lens (rather than in the center) are available in both one-piece and fused constructions. Such a lens must be stabilized by truncation or by prism-ballast, as with a toric lens. The first one-piece lower segment bifocal lenses to become available were stabilized by *both* truncation and prism-ballast (see Figure 14.37c). Borish (1985) has pointed out that if a prism-ballasted minus lens is truncated, the truncation removes the thickest portion of the lens, therefore reducing the effect of the truncation. Borish recommends truncation of prism-ballested lenses only for plus lenses. As shown in Figure 14.38, such a lens must lag upward sufficiently, for reading, for the pupil to be within the segment area.

Fused bifocal contact lenses are available with segments of various shapes. The upcurve, or cresent-shaped, segment has been one of the more successful

of these lenses: when the eyes are lowered for reading they also converge, with the result that the lens rotates upward and nasally. As shown in Figure 14.39, for an upcurve or cresent-shaped bifocal the segment will tend to remain in front of the pupil when the lens rotates.

Borish (1985) has described what he has found to be the most successful method of fitting hard bifocal contact lenses. The patient is first fitted with prism-ballasted *single-vision* lenses in the same parameters envisioned for the bifocal lenses, and near vision is provided by means of reading glasses. The practioner uses a red felt-tipped pen to color-in the area where the segment will be placed, and the patient is instructed to look in a mirror several times each day to ascertain whether the pupil is above the colored area for distance vision and within the colored area for near vision. Once the patient has become adapted and the lenses are orienting correctly, the bifocal lenses can be ordered. On the other hand, some patients are satisfied with single-vision contact lenses and reading glasses, and decide against ordering the bifocals.

Gas-permeable hard bifocals

Remba (1987) described a clinical study in which 24 presbyopic patients were fitted with the Tangent-Streak bifocal, 22 of whom had no adverse ocular responses. He reported a success rate of 85 percent, with 1.8 lenses per eye needed to attain success, without advanced physiological responses.

In ordering bifocal lenses (for a patient who has adapted to prism-ballast, single-vision lenses), it will be necessary for the lenses to orient themselves when the patient looks downward so the lower portion of the lens remains in front of the pupil rather than swinging nasally. If the lens swings nasally or otherwise shows signs of fitting too loosely, a slightly tighter single-vision lens should be ordered (steeper base curve, steeper secondary curve, or larger optic zone and overall diameter). If the lens fits so tightly that it fails to lag upward during downward gaze, a somewhat looser lens (flatter base curve, flatter secondary curve, or smaller optic zone and overall diameter) should be ordered. Due to the high cost of bifocal lenses, it is essential that all fitting problems be solved at the single-vision stage.

Segment height is specified so the segment will infringe slightly on the lower portion of the pupil while the patient looks straight ahead. This can be determined by measuring the distance from the lower edge of the prism ballast or truncated single-vision lens to the lower edge of the pupil, to the nearest 0.5mm (as the patient looks straight ahead in normal room illumination), and adding from 0.5–1mm. If the segment height proves to be too great, it can be reduced, if necessary, by increasing the truncation (assuming that a truncated lens is used). However, if the segment height proves to be too small, a new lens will need to be ordered.

One of the main problems in fitting bifocal contact lenses is making sure the lens drops down for distance vision and lags upward adequately for near vision, without excessive nasalward rotation. The probability of success in bifocal contact lens fitting is acknowledged to be rather low. Those practitioners who claim 90–95 percent success in fitting single-vision contact lenses seldom claim more than 40–50 percent success in bifocal contact lens fitting.

Nonbifocal contact lenses for presbyopia

It has been shown by Brungardt (1962a) that if a PMMA lens is provided with an optically perfect secondary curve of sufficient width, the secondary zone of the lens can function as a bifocal segment. With this design it is necessary that the lens remain centered for distance, while fitting loosely enough so the lens lags upward when the patient looks downward for near vision. Brungardt showed that, for a lens with a 42.75DK (7.90mm) base curve radius, the increase in plus power through the secondary curve will be 0.75D for each 0.1mm of flattening of the secondary curve relative to the base curve.

More recently, a number of lens constructions involving aspheric surfaces have been designed as substitutes for bifocal lenses. With these lenses, the minus power gradually decreases (or plus power gradually increases) from the center toward the periphery of the lens. None of these lenses has achieved a high level of popularity.

Soft bifocals

Although several manufacturers of soft contact lenses have introduced bifocal lenses, none has achieved a high degree of success. In 1981, Bausch & Lomb introduced the *PAI*, which was actually a reintroduction of an older spin-cast lens series. The PAI lens, like all spin-cast lenses, is an aspheric back surface lens which, as in the case of the "nonbifocal" hard lenses just described, provides a certain amount of added plus power when the wearer views through a point near the periphery of the lens. According to the manufacturer, the PAI lens has a "nominal" addition of +1.50D. Some practitioners have recommended the fitting of this lens in a "modified mono-vision" system, in which the distance power of the lens to be used for near vision is a compromise between the power required for distance and that required for near.

Representative soft bifocals currently available are summarized in Table 14.6. Four types of bifocal construction are represented in the table:

1. Lenses of aspheric, back surface bifocal construction include the Bausch & Lomb PAI and the Hydrocurve II. These lenses must move upward ("translate") when the eyes are lowered for reading, so a relatively loose fit should be obtained. Like the Bausch & Lomb lens, the

Table 14.6   Representative soft bifocal contact lenses for daily wear (*Tyler's Quarterly*, March, 1987)

Manufacturer	Trade name	Diameter (mm)	Base curve radii (mm)	Segment style	Mode of action
Barnes-Hind	Hydrocurve II	14.8mm	9.0mm	Aspheric	Translating
Bausch & Lomb	PA1	13.5	(spin-cast)	Aspheric	Translating
	Cresent	14.0	8.6, 8.9	Crescent segment, truncated	Translating
Ciba Vision Care	BiSoft	13.8	8.3, 8.6, 8.9	Concentric	Simultaneous
University Optical Products	Alges	14.0	8.6, 8.9	Concentric, center-add	Simultaneous
Wesley-Jessen	DuroSoft	13.5	8.5	Crescent segment, truncated, prism-ballant	Translating

maximum addition in the periphery of the Hydrocurve II is +1.50D.

2. Lenses having crescentic segments include the Bausch & Lomb Crescent bifocal and the Wesley-Jessen DuroSoft bifocal, the former being a truncated lens and the latter having both truncation and prism ballast.

3. The Ciba BiSoft lens is a simultaneous-vision lens having the distance portion at the center.

4. The Alges bifocal is a simultaneous-vision lens having the near portion at the center.

A basic problem in the fitting of soft bifocal lenses is the difficulty in getting a soft lens to translate sufficiently for the near area to be centered in front of the wearer's pupil. Although a hard lens can be made to translate as much as 3–4mm when the eyes turn downward for reading, it is often difficult to provide even half that much translation for a soft lens. As for the simultaneous-vision soft lenses, Borish (1985) has concluded that simultaneous vision is not a tenable concept, and that these lenses are successful in providing near vision only if they *translate*.

In a discussion of patient selection for soft bifocals, Josephson and Caffery (1986) note their difficulty in switching successful monovision wearers to bifocals; because these patients are well adapted, the monovision arrangement satisfies these authors' requirements. Josephson and Caffery also note that low myopes are not motivated to wear bifocal contacts because they can more easily remove their glasses for reading, but that motivation for bifocal contacts may increase as the presbyopia

progresses. In addition, low hyperopes often are not successful because they may fail to attain high-contrast acuity for distance vision, and patients who wear their lenses only for social occasions may not be as well motivated as those who wear them daily. Other patient selection factors discussed by Josephson and Caffery include extremes of pupil size, flaccidity of eyelids, and astigmatism. They note that pupils smaller than 3mm or larger than 5mm may present visual problems with any kind of bifocal; that flaccid lids can inhibit lens movement, making translation of the lenses difficult; and that even small amounts of astigmatism can further complicate the visual compromise imposed by a bifocal contact lens.

Two soft bifocal contact lens constructions were evaluated by Molinari and Caplan (1986). A concentric translating bifocal, the *Soft-form* bifocal, was fitted on 42 patients, only 20 of whom were still wearing the lenses after a period of 5 months. Complaints voiced by some of these patients included photophobia, vertical diplopia, and poorer quality of vision than with glasses. The authors noted that among the less-successful wearers were patients who were emmtropic or had low refractive errors, young presbyopes, patients with large pupils, and patients with significant anisometropia. In the same study, Molinari and Caplan also reported on 18 patients fitted with the Hydrocurve II aspheric bifocal, 8 of whom were still wearing the lenses at the end of one year. Disadvantages noted were complaints of "tremendous" flare at night, reduced sharpness in distance vision compared to glasses, and some difficulty in reading, particularly for patients who required the higher adds. Molinari and Caplan concluded that, although neither of the bifocal designs was a panacea for fitting presbyopic patients, there are some patients who, with careful screening and selective prescribing, will do exceedingly well with these bifocal soft lenses.

CONTACT LENSES FOR KERATOCONUS

Keratoconus is a form of corneal dystrophy in which the apical portion of the cornea becomes very thin and very steep, and sags downward slightly. The condition becomes evident at puberty and gradually progresses throughout life, often with long periods of remission. In later life, some keratoconus patients experience corneal *perforation*, followed by scarring. Others will have *corneal hydrops*, a condition in which an excessive amount of water passes into the cornea from the aqueous due to a break in Descemet's membrane. In either of these conditions, a corneal transplant will have to be done. Fortunately, the prognosis is very good for keratoconus patients after transplant surgery.

The optical correction of keratoconus has been an important stimulus in the evolution of contact lenses since the earliest beginnings of contact lens technology. Dickinson and Hall (1946) called attention to the writings of the astronomer Sir John Herschel who, in 1827, suggested that an optical correction should be provided for an irregular cornea by adapting a spherical lens to the eye, having its surface in contact with the cornea. Graham (1959) reported that E. Kalt experimented with contact lenses having no scleral flange for the correction of keratoconus in 1888, and that A. E. Fick discussed the possible use of contact lenses for the correction of keratoconus in 1887.

Although the etiology of keratoconus is not well understood, Sabiston (1965) has pointed out an association among keratoconus, dermatitis, and asthma. He reported having seen 12 patients with Keratoconus. All patients were between the ages of 8 and 36 years; all had dermatitis; and some had asthma. Sabiston suggested that a common factor of the eye condition and the dermatitis is that the tissues involved arise from *ectoderm*, and the primary lesion appears to commence in the basal epithelial cells. In all three disease processes, the lesion primarily affects epithelial surfaces (including the constantly regenerating bronchial linings), and the underlying mesodermally derived tissues are secondarily involved in the process. Sabiston found a strong hereditary influence, as many members of a single family often exhibit various phases of asthma, hay fever, eczema, exaggerated reaction to various forms of physical and emotional stress, and a high degree of allergic hypersensitivity.

Patients and practitioners alike are enthusiastic about contact lenses for keratoconus, and for good reason. Contact lenses are the *only* optical means of providing good visual acuity for patients with keratoconus. Many practitioners believe that contact lenses tend to retard the rate of progression of keratoconus, due to the gentle pressure of the lens on the corneal apex. However, this contention has been difficult to prove because keratoconus patients typically enjoy long periods of remission (lasting as long as many years) even when contact lenses have not been fitted. Further, Hartstein and Becker (1970) have reported that a number of patients have developed keratoconus while wearing hard contact lenses.

Symptoms and Signs of Keratoconus

The most important clinical indications of keratoconus are the following: (1) complaints of unsatisfactory vision in spite of reasonably good visual acuity; (2) very steep keratometer readings, perhaps off the scale, with a large amount of astigmatism and distortion of mires; (3) a swirling reflex may be found on retinoscopy, appearing as a bright red spot having no true with or against motion and, therefore, impossible to neutralize; (4) distorted rings will be seen Placido's disc; (5) Munson's sign, an indentation of the lower lid when vision is directed downward, may be noted; and (6) biomicroscopic examination reveals a thinning and steepening of the corneal apex, and possibly vertical striae, opacities, and other appearances that have been described by Doggart (1948).

Hard Lenses

Although keratoconus is normally a bilateral condition, the process is usually found to begin in one eye before the other. In the early stages, the keratoconic cornea may be highly sensitive, but as the condition progresses, the corneal sensitivity decreases significantly. For this reason, if one eye of a keratoconic patient is at an early stage and the other is at a later stage, it may be desirable to begin the procedure by fitting only the more severely affected eye with a contact lens, providing a spectacle correction for the other eye.

Except in the early stages, an eye having kerato-conus requires an extremely steep contact lens, having a small optic zone and a moderate-to-large amount of minus power. As shown in Figure 8.14 (see Chapter 8), a keratoconic cornea is steep only in the apical portion, and may have as much as 8–10D of peripheral flattening. The fitting of a keratoconic eye should not be attempted without a fitting set of such lenses. Most contact lens laboratories are able to lend the practitioner a set of three or four steep lenses. If the keratometer readings are off the scale, the upper end of the range of the instrument can be extended from the normal 52.00D to 63.00D by taping a +1.25D trial lens to the keratometer mire plate. When this is done, the practitioner simply adds 9D to the finding in each principal meridian. However, it is often possible to make a fairly intelligent estimate of the keratometer finding even when it is off the scale. In any event, the keratometer finding will provide only a starting point; base curve determination can be carried out only with the careful application of diagnostic lenses.

Fitting procedures

Because the optic cap of the cornea tends to be small in keratoconus, an optic zone diameter of 5–6mm is usually required, along with a smaller than normal overall diameter. The base curve will have to be somewhat flatter than the corneal apex, along with considerably more flattening in the peripheral area than would be the case with a normal cornea. The resulting fluorescein pattern, as shown in Figure

Figure 14.40 Typical fluorescein pattern in keratoconus (fluorescein pooling is shown by cross-hatched areas and touch is shown by shading). The area of central touch is shown in the lower part of the lens because most cones point downward slightly.

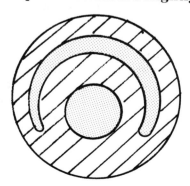

14.40, will have a definite area of apical touch and an incomplete ring-touch in the periphery. If the area of touch is too small, the peripheral ring-touch will not be present, and a steeper lens should be tried. On the other hand, a too-large area of touch will tend to result in the peripheral touch being exaggerated, in which case a flatter lens should be tried. Lenses for keratoconus must be truly "custom fitted." It is probably unwise for the practitioner to attempt to fit a patient having this condition unless he or she possesses (and can effectively use) lens modification equipment.

Prognosis

As in the case of other pathological conditions, the practitioner fitting a keratoconus patient should maintain contact with the ophthalmologist. Although long remissions tend to occur, the condition can progress, and in severe cases a corneal graft may be necessary. Any retrograde changes, such as corneal hydrops or perforation should immediately be called to the attention of the ophthalmological consultant. Progress visits should be scheduled at regular intervals, for as long as the patient continues to wear contact lenses. Lens changes may be required as the condition progresses, and occasionally it will be found that a well-fitting lens will no longer provide optimum visual acuity because of slight changes in the refraction. In such a case, one alternative is to prescribe glasses (usually low-power sphero cylinders) to be worn in addition to the contact lenses.

Soft Lenses

Although some practitioners have recommended the use of soft contact lenses for keratoconus, the large amount of corneal astigmatism present in this condition makes their use impractical. Toric soft lenses can be fitted, but the necessity to fit "custom lenses"—because of the small size of the corneal apex and the extreme amount of astigmatism usually encountered—together with the frequent lens changes that are sometimes needed, tend to make the fitting of these lenses unduly expensive and, therefore, impractical.

To provide the patient with the comfort of a soft lens and the vision available with a hard lens, some practitioners recommend the use of a "piggy back" lens. The eye is first fitted with a soft lens in the usual manner, and a hard lens is fitted on top of it so that it lags upward during a blink just as it would on the cornea. This method of fitting, however, has seen relatively little use.

CONTACT LENSES FOR APHAKIA

During the 6 years since the First Edition of this text was written, the popularity of intraocular lenses for aphakia has increased rapidly. Although lens implant surgery was then considered by some ophthalmologists to be an experimental procedure, at the time of this writing the safety of the procedure has been demonstrated to the point that it is not only embraced by the ophthalmological community, but for the majority of surgeons it is the procedure of choice for the treatment of aphakia. However, there will remain a continuing need for the fitting of contact lenses for aphakia, both for the many thousands of aphakic patients who have been fitted with glasses or contact lenses in the past and will need to be refitted, and for the minority of newly aphakic patients who will have undergone nonimplant surgery.

Hard Lenses

Prior to the advent of contact lenses, cataract surgery often resulted in a keyhole pupil and a large amount of against-the-rule corneal astigmatism (due to postoperative sagging of the cornea). Welsh (1961) pointed out that if the aphakic has a keyhole pupil as a result of the operation, a lenticular lens cannot be used, and the heavier and less successful single-cut lens must be used. He suggests that round pupil surgery be done on patients who are to be fitted with contact lenses, and that surgical procedures be designed to minimize postoperative corneal astigmatism.

The patient is normally fitted with postoperative spectacles, and contact lens fitting is done when the eye has completely healed and the corneal astigmatism has stabilized. Koetting (1966) recommended that patients be fitted with contact lenses within about 12 weeks after surgery. Enoch (1971) concluded that 3 months is a safe time to fit contact lenses for older patients when a section has been performed (as is necessary for senile cataracts), but a period of 2 months is sufficient for older children when needling has been performed.

Aphakic contact lenses differ from those fitted for myopes or low hyperopes not only in their increased thickness and weight but in the shape of the edge. A minus lens edge has prism with a "base-toward-the-edge" orientation and is usually held up nicely by the upper lid (sometimes riding excessively high); a high plus lens edge has a prism with an "apex-

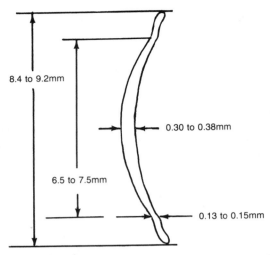

Figure 14.41 Dimensions for an aphakic lens recommended by Polse (1969).

toward-the-edge" orientation and tends to be pushed downward by the upper lid. This problem can be solved by providing the aphakic lens with an edge shaped like a minus lens, in the form of a lenticular lens. A cross-section diagram of such a lens is shown in Figure 14.41.

Polse (1969) presented a clinical procedure that he used successfully in fitting 75 aphakic patients. He recommended lens dimensions as follows:

Lens diameter: 8.4–9.2mm.
Optic zone diameter: 6.5–7.5mm.
Minimum center thickness: 0.30–0.38mm.
Minimum junction thickness: 0.13–0.15mm.
Edge thickness of minus carrier: approximately 0.22mm.
Radius of front lenticular curve: 1.0–2.0mm flatter than radius of base curve.

Polse recommended a set of ten diagnostic lenses, all having a power of +13.00D, base curves ranging from 8.33 to 7.50mm, and other specifications similar to those given.

Enoch (1971) made the following suggestions concerning management of the aphakic patient. (1) Because an aphakic has poor uncorrected vision, Enoch recommends the use of a light tint to enable the patient to keep track of the lenses. (2) If the patient is a bilateral aphakic, it is a good idea to provide a pair of aphakic spectacles with one lens removed. The patient inserts the first lens through the opening in the frame and uses the spectacle lens in front of the other eye to see while doing so. Then the patient uses the first contact lens to see what he or she is doing while inserting the second contact lens. (3) In the initial stages, corneal sensitivity is low because many nerves have been cut. This makes early adaptation somewhat easier but requires that the patient be watched more closely. At some point in time, the innervation returns, and the patient may experience a period of discomfort.

Soft Lenses

Soft contact lenses provide a good alternative to hard lenses for the correction of aphakia. The flexibility of soft lenses is not a disadvantage in aphakia, because the high plus lenses need for aphakics are sufficiently thick and rigid to eliminate well over 1.00D of corneal astigmatism. Aphakic soft lens fitting differs little from the fitting of other spherical soft lenses. However, because high plus lenses have markedly different fitting qualities than minus lenses or plus lenses of low power, aphakic fitting should not be attempted without the use of an aphakic diagnostic lens set.

An interesting problem that sometimes arises in the fitting of aphakic lenses is that a higher-power lens may be required than is predicted on the basis of the subjective refraction as corrected for the change in vertex distance. This is apparently because the lens fits on the eye in such a way as to cause a minus-powered tear lens. (The fitting of aphakic patients is considered further in the following discussion of extended-wear lenses.)

EXTENDED-WEAR LENSES

Since hydrogel lenses were first introduced in Czechoslovakia in the early 1960s, many contact lens practitioners have looked forward to the day when wearers of these lenses can wear them continuously with no need for daily lens insertion and removal. However, when lenses specifically designed for continuous wear became available, many problems occurred:

1. After several weeks or months of wear, many lenses became badly coated with materials originating from the tear film, so both vision and comfort were unacceptably poor.
2. Severe corneal edema, neovascularization, and even corneal decompensation occurred with some wearers.
3. Because the idea of continuous wear did not necessitate the wearer being instructed in procedures for lens insertion and removal, some wearers were unable to remove the offending lenses when serious problems occurred.
4. Some lenses of high water content were so frail that attempts at removal often resulted in the lens being removed in pieces.

Because of these and other problems, the concept of *continuous wear* eventually gave way to the concept of *extended wear*. Patients fitted with lenses for extended wear are taught to insert and remove their lenses and are instructed to wear their lenses on a 24-hour basis for specific periods of time and to remove them periodically for cleaning and disinfection. One recommended procedure is for the patient to wear the lenses continuously for a 7-day period, removing them for cleaning and disinfection on weekends.

Corneal-Bandage Lenses

Extended-wear lenses have been found to be particularly suitable for use as a "corneal bandage" and for the optical correction of aphakia. Few optometrists are currently involved in the fitting of corneal bandage lenses. This is not surprising, since most, if not all, wearers are under the care of an ophthalmologist for the condition for which the bandage lens is prescribed. However, optometrists should be aware of the conditions for which corneal bandage lenses can be used and of some of the problems involved in the fitting of these lenses.

Conditions for which bandage lenses are indicated include keratoconjunctivitis sicca and other dry-eye conditions, bullous keratopathy, Fuchs's dystrophy, anterior membrane dystrophies (including recurrent corneal erosion, Meesmann's epithelial dystrophy, fingerprint dystrophy, and Reis-Bückler's dystrophy), some kinds of corneal ulcers, and some conditions resulting from corneal trauma (Feldman, 1979). As described by Feldman, the mechanisms of action of bandage lenses are (1) protecting the eye from the environment, (2) keeping the eye from desiccating, (3) providing the eye with an adequate refracting surface, and (4) prolonging drug exposure.

One of the main problems involved in the fitting of bandage lenses is drying of the lenses (as well as the eyes). Most bandage lens wearers must make continual use of artificial tears. Another problem is coating of the lenses. The lenses quickly become coated with mucus and proteins from the wearer's tear film, so lens life tends to be short. A third problem is the possibility of infection. With 24-hour-a-day lens wear, the constant increase in corneal temperature encourages the growth of microorganisms. As Feldman (1979) commented, one who fits extended-wear lenses becomes well acquainted with his or her patients!

Extended-Wear Lenses for Aphakia

Patients most likely to benefit from extended-wear aphakic lenses are older aphakics who, because of arthritis, unsteady hands, or senility, are unable to handle daily-wear lenses. For many of these wearers a family member must assume the responsibility for periodic lens removal, cleaning, disinfection, and reinsertion. .

Availability of oxygen to the closed eye

When the eyes are open, the corneas are exposed to air containing approximately 21 percent oxygen. In studies by Fatt, Freeman, and Lin (1964) and by Efron and Carney (1979), it was found that the oxygen available to the closed eye is approximately 7–8 percent. Hill (1979) has shown that when the eyes are closed, there is not only less oxygen available to the cornea, but also (1) an increase in corneal temperature of 4.5°F, causing additional oxygen consumption; (2) a decrease in tear osmolarity (0.89 percent compared with 0.97 percent for the open eye), favoring corneal swelling; and (3) an increase in the acidity of the tears (pH of 7.28 compared with 7.46 for the open eye), also favoring corneal swelling. With all of these problems, how does the closed eye succeed in tolerating a contact lens?

The ability of the closed aphakic eye to tolerate a contact lens has been investigated by Korb, Richmond, and Herman (1980), who fitted three patients with extended-wear lenses of various thicknesses both before and after cataract surgery. They found that before surgery, a lens of 0.35mm thickness produced a corneal thickening of 30 percent with massive edema, epithelial bullae, corneal staining, and epithelial folds. After surgery, however, the 0.35mm lens caused a corneal thickening of 10 percent with no other significant changes. Korb et al. suggested three possible explanations for the apparently decreased oxygen demand of the cornea after lens extraction: (1) the absence of the lens may allow an increase in the amount of aqueous humor in the eye; (2) the removal of the lens eliminates a source of oxygen demand for the aqueous humor, making more oxygen available for the cornea; or (3) the corneal denervation as a result of the surgical incision brings about a decreased oxygen demand for the cornea.

Oxygen transmission of extended-wear lenses

It has been shown that lenses made for myopes of 0.06mm or less in center thickness and of materials having a water content of approximately 40 percent can supply the cornea with sufficient oxygen for the closed-eye conditions. However, for lenses in the high plus powers needed in aphakia, such thicknesses are unattainable. This has encouraged manufacturers to increase the water content of their materials so to increase the oxygen transmission.

Lens fitting and maintenance

As noted earlier, with the advent of oxygen-permeable materials there has been a tendency to minimize the importance of correct lens fitting procedures, particularly in regard to fitting the lenses loosely enough so tears can be pumped underneath the lenses during blinking. Feldman (1980) emphasized that ultrathin lenses *do* pump tears if fitted loosely enough and that dirty lenses lose their oxygen permeability rapidly (studies of oxygen transmissions of extended-wear lenses are always done with brand new lenses).

In discussing ultrathin lenses made of a material having a water content of 55 percent and diameters of 15–16mm (the Hydrocurve II lens), Feldman (1977) warned that there is a tendency on the part of some fitters to fit these lenses in a marginally steep fashion. He pointed out that a properly fitted extended-wear lens "looks to be a little sloppy," moving freely with blinking and displacing downward as much as 3 or 4mm on upward gaze. He suggested that the fitting procedure start with the flattest lens in the diagnostic set, and that the correct lens to fit is the flattest lens that is stable on the eye. Because lens parameters tend to change with time, a patient whose lenses are marginally steep when first fitted may, after a few weeks, begin to experience discomfort, loss of acuity, and perilimbal injection, which can lead to corneal vascularization. The parameters of representative extended-wear lenses for aphakia are given in Table 14.7.

Gas-permeable hard lenses for aphakic extended-wear

In the first study making use of gas-permeable hard lenses for extended-wear, Benjamin and Simons (1984) fitted 22 aphakic patients (31 aphakic eyes) with Polycon II lenses. The patients wore the lenses for a 3-month period, removing them for cleaning about once every 4 or 5 days. The success rate

Table 14.7   Representative aphakic extended-wear lenses (*Tyler's Quarterly*, March, 1987)

Manufacturer	Trade name	Water content (percent)	Diameter (mm)	Base curve radii (mm)	Central thickness (mm)
Breger Muller Welt	EW Aphakic	45%	14.0mm	8.6, 8.9mm	0.26–0.42mm
Barnes-Hind	Hydrocurve High Plus	55	14.0	8.5	0.10 (minimum)
			14.5	8.8	0.10 (minimum)
Ciba Vision Care	Sofcon EW Aphakic	55	14.0	7.8, 8.1 8.4, 8.7	0.10–0.44
			14.5	8.1, 8.4	0.10–0.44
Cooper-Vision	Aphakic Permalens	71	14.0	8.1, 8.3	0.40 (minimum)
			14.5	8.3, 8.6, 8.9	0.40 (minimum)
Bausch & Lomb	CW 79	79	14.4	8.1, 8.4, 8.7	0.49–0.79

(success being determined on the basis of a lack of complications) was reported as 95 percent. The authors commented that one advantage of hard (as opposed to soft) extended-wear lenses for these patients was that the rigid lens material masked corneal astigmatism normally present after cataract surgery, with the result that an overrefractive spectacle correction for distance vision was not needed for the 22 patients. Several patients were fitted by means of the monovision system.

Benjamin and Simons (1984) reported mean changes in spherical refraction of −0.14D on the fourth day of lens wear, decreasing to −0.06D at 90 days, and a mean corneal flattening of 0.18D on the fourth day, increasing to 0.46D at 90 days. However, both refractive changes and corneal flattening varied widely from one subject to another. Three of the patients were reported to have complications: (1) one patient developed an epithelial defect (grade 4 staining), occurring after the first night of extended wear and gradually receding over a 2-week period; (2) a second patient developed a central keratitis during the first week of extended-wear, which was successfully treated by an ophthalmologist; and (3) a third patient developed a single branch of neovascularization in one eye during the first week of extended-wear, which had developed from the surgical incision, and which was resolved by having the patient wear the lenses alternately on daily-wear and extended-wear schedules. Benjamin and Simons noted that, although these lenses possess lower oxygen transmissivities than many extended-wear hydrogel materials, they have the advantage of also supplying oxygen to the cornea by means of the "tear pump." They also suggested that corneal oxygena-

tion could occur by tear pumping from rapid eye movement during sleep, which accounts for 20 percent of adult sleeping time.

Extended-Wear Cosmetic Lenses

The adjective *cosmetic* embraces all uses of extended-wear lenses other than the correction of aphakia. The motivating factors for extended-wear fitting in aphakia, as already discussed, are (1) many aphakic patients are unable to handle and care for contact lenses on a daily basis, and (2) the aphakic eye has a greater tolerance for a contact lens in the closed-eye condition because of its lower oxygen requirement. However, once it was found that aphakics could successfully wear contact lenses overnight, there was a clamor for extended-wear lenses for people other than aphakics.

One of the chief aims in the design of extended-wear lenses has been to provide as much oxygen for the cornea as possible. As noted earlier in this chapter, for the wearer of a soft contact lens, oxygen can reach the cornea (1) from the tears, by means of the tear pumping that occurs with each blink; and (2) through the lens, the amount of oxygen depending on the oxygen permeability of the material and the thickness of the lens. Therefore, the amount of oxygen available to the cornea can be increased by (1) fitting the lens in such a way as to allow it to move freely, (2) increasing the water content of the lens material, or (3) making the lens thinner. Although for several years only *soft* (hydrogel) lenses were available for extended-wear, the FDA has now begun to approve gas-permeable hard lenses for extended-wear.

Soft Lenses for Extended-Wear

Patient selection

When fitting extended-wear lenses, patient selection is of great importance. Slit-lamp examination should show a clear, white eye with no indications of marginal blepharitis or conjunctivitis, and an absence of follicles, papillae, or other signs of allergic reaction or hypersensitivity. The precorneal film should show an absence of mucus strands and other debris, and tear break-up time should be adequate—at least 10–12 seconds. When a diagnostic lens is in place, it should remain clean and wet while on the eye. Stewart (1982) has warned that patients having a history of allergies, abnormal Meibomian secretion (resulting in a frothy or soapy appearance of the tear film), or excessive mucous secretion may not be good candidates for extended-wear lenses. He also has noted that the practitioner should resist the temptation to fit extended-wear lenses on a patient who has failed to follow instructions with daily-wear lenses, commenting that these patients are usually even poorer candidates for extended-wear than for daily-wear of lenses.

The patient may have unwarranted expectations and should be advised realistically of the advantages and disadvantages of extended-wear lenses. The advantages will, of course, already be apparent to the patient—the fact that the lenses won't have to be put on and taken off daily, and the (much overblown) idea that it will be possible "to see clearly, if I have to get up during the night, without putting on glasses or contacts." He or she should be told that (1) the long-term cost will be greater than for daily-wear lenses, because without daily cleaning the lenses tend to become coated more quickly and, therefore, tend to have a shorter useful life; and (2) there is a greater possibility of adverse effects such as infection, corneal ulceration, or corneal vascularization than with daily-wear lenses. It has been the author's experience at the University of Houston that many patients request extended-wear lenses because of magazine advertisements or advertisements by commercial practitioners; but once they have a better understanding of the problems that may occur, they are often happy to be fitted with daily-wear lenses.

Fitting and follow-up procedures

The fitting procedures differ little from those for the fitting of daily-wear lenses, with the exception that the lenses must move very freely, showing downward movement (lag) of 1 to 2mm after a blink in the primary position and 2mm or more when looking upward. This movement is necessary not only to provide adequate oxygen to the cornea by tear pumping—in addition to the oxygen that permeates through the lens—but to flush out the potentially toxic debris (such as dried mucus and oily secretions, and desquamated epithelial cells) that would otherwise accumulate underneath the lens.

Although *extended-wear* has been defined by at least one manufacturer as "30-day wear," most patients are much more successful if they are instructed to remove the lenses every 7 days. Usually, this is done on a weekend; after removal, the lenses are cleaned and disinfected, and are stored overnight and inserted the next morning. Some patients find that the lenses become sufficiently coated during the 7-day period to cause discomfort and poor vision; for these patients, twice-weekly removal will often solve the problem.

Extended-wear lenses are available in a variety of water contents and thicknesses, as shown in Table 14.8. In general, the lower water content lenses are very thin, while the thickness increases with increasing water content. When only high water content lenses were available for extended wear, the lenses were usually fitted for overnight wear from the first day, because the material was not sturdy enough to survive daily handling. With the availability of extended-wear lenses having water contents of 38–55 percent, the practitioner has the option (for a patient who has not previously worn contact lenses) of having the patient wear the lenses on a daily-wear basis for the first 2–3 weeks—long enough to learn how to handle the lenses and to gain experience in cleaning and disinfecting procedures—before beginning overnight wear.

Before the lenses are worn for extended-wear, the patient should be instructed to discontinue lens wear and contact the practitioner if any of the following symptoms occur: (1) blurring of vision, (2) discomfort, or (3) the presence of a "red eye," as these symptoms may indicate an eye infection or other complication. The patient should also be told that the crucial time of day is *just after arising* in the morning: if at that time the lenses fail to move sufficiently, the debris in the tears underneath the lens can become toxic, eventually causing an infection, corneal vascularization, or other problems. The patient should be given a bottle of a "rewetting solution," and instructed to put a drop or two of the solution in each eye on arising and to "blink and move the eyes around" to make sure the lenses are mobile.

A patient who has not previously worn contact

lenses (and who is being fitted with low or medium water content lenses) should be put on a wearing schedule, just as for a daily-wear patient, and scheduled for a progress visit after about 2 weeks. If all is well at that time, an early morning appointment is made, and the patient is instructed to wear the lenses overnight (for the first time) on the night before the appointment. This will allow the practitioner to evaluate the lens fit and the eyes for any effects of overnight wear.

Frequent office visits are necessary during the first month of wear and particularly during the first week. O'Hara (1982) has commented that 90 percent of the problems occurring with extended wear will occur during the first month and recommends that the patient be seen at the end of the first 24 hours of wear and again after 3 days, 1 week, 2 weeks, 1 month, and 3 months. Patients are scheduled for an office visit at intervals of no longer than 6 months as long as they wear extended-wear lenses.

If routine office visits for extended-wear patients are scheduled late in the day, the practitioner may not be aware of corneal striae or other signs of corneal edema, that may be present in the early morning hours. Schock (1982) reported that in a study of extended-wear patients conducted at the Cornea and Contact Lens Research Unit in Australia, wearers' corneas were found to have an increase in thickness of from 10 to 15 percent on awakening, with deswelling occurring during the day. An accumulation of debris was often found underneath the lens in the morning, consisting of mucus, remnants of squamous epithelial cells, and inflammatory cells. If the lenses moved sufficiently during the day, the debris eventually would be gotten rid of. However, if the lenses failed to have sufficient movement for this to occur, the patient would experience a red-eye reaction. The occurrence of this reaction reinforces the importance of fitting the lenses loosely enough so they will move on the eyes during normal blinking and eye movements.

Clinical studies

A large number of clinical studies of extended-wear soft lenses have been published. In one of the first of these, DeCarle (1979) reported fitting 177 patients with the *Permalens*, in which 136 patients (77 percent) were still wearing the lenses after 6 months. The greatest problem was coating of the lenses with protein and calcium deposits. All but 41 patients required at least one lens change during the 6-month period. In another early study, Davis (1980) reported on 97 aphakic patients who had been fitted with the *CSI* lens, 80 of whom were still wearing the lenses at the end of 6 months. The most common reasons for discontinuing lens wear were edema and related changes (five patients), and corneal staining related to inadequate ocular secretions (five patients).

A clinical study in which 114 myopic patients

Table 14.8   Representative cosmetic extended-wear lenses (*Tyler's Quarterly*, March, 1987)

Manufacturer	Trade name	Water content (percent)	Diameter (mm)	Base curve radii (mm)	Central thickness (mm)
American Hydron	Zero-4	38%	13.8mm	8.6mm	0.04mm
Bausch & Lomb	03	38	13.5	(spin-cast)	0.035 (−3)
	04	38	14.5	(spin-cast)	0.035 (−3)
Sola-Syntex	CSI T	38.5	13.8	8.0, 8.3	0.035
				8.6, 8.9	
		38.5	14.8	8.6, 8.9, 9.35	0.035
Barnes-Hind	Hydrocurve II	55	14.0	8.5	0.05 (minimum)
			14.5	8.8, 9.1	0.05 (minimum)
Wesley-Jessen	DuroSoft 3 (D3.X4)	55	14.5	8.3, 8.6, 9.0	0.06
Vistakon	Vistamarc	58	14.0	8.0, 8.3, 8.6	0.06 (−3)
American Hydron	X-70	70	14.3	8.4, 8.7, 9.0	0.14–0.17
Cooper-Vision	Permalens	71	13.5	7.7, 8.0, 8.3	0.23 (−3)
		71	14.2	8.6	0.23 (−3)
Bausch & Lomb	CW 79	79	14.4	8.1, 8.4, 8.7	0.49–0.79

were fitted with Bausch & Lomb 03 and 04 lenses was reported by Klein (1983). The lenses were removed every 7 days for cleaning and disinfection. Of the 114 patients, 84 (74 percent) were able to wear the lenses successfully for a period of 6 months. The most common causes of dropping out of the study were what Klien called "corneal decompensation" (seven patients), inadequate vision (seven patients), difficulty in handling the lenses (five patients), lens drying (five patients), discomfort (three patients), lens awarenesses (two patients), and noncomplience (one patient).

Weissman, Remba, and Fugedy (1987) reported on the results of a survey designed to compare the daily-wear (DW) and extended-wear (EW) fittings of 2,926 members of the AOA Contact Lens Section. Replies were received from 759 optometrists, 440 of which were sufficiently complete to be included in the data base. The following mean incidences of complications were reported: severe red eyes, 5 percent for DW and 12 percent for EW; corneal neovascularization greater than 2mm, 0.6 percent for DW and 3 percent for EW; corneal infection, 0.5 percent for DW and 3 percent for EW. The respondents' preferences were as follows: 61 percent of respondents preferred "thin" lenses having a medium water content (55–60 percent) and 23 percent preferred "ultra-thin" lenses having a low water content (38 percent); 70 percent currently used overnight removal and cleaning every 7–14 days; and 60 percent favored hydrogen peroxide cleaning regimens.

Regular lens replacement

With the increasing use of extended-wear lenses, it has become obvious that many of the problems that occur with these lenses—problems due to lens coatings and other changes in the lenses themselves—tend to occur mainly after the lenses have been worn for several weeks or months, and that these problems are resolved when replacement lenses are fitted. For this reason, some practitioners have arranged with their extended-wear patients to have the lenses replaced at the end of each 6 months. The results of this arrangement have been encouraging, since the practitioner is freed from spending an inordinate amount of time dealing with problems that occur as a result of patients wearing "worn-out" (and badly fitting) lenses. This idea has been carried to the extreme by those who have recommended the fitting of inexpensive "throw-away" lenses, designed to be purchased in "six-packs" and worn for only a few weeks before being replaced.

The value of regular replacement of low water content extended-wear lenses was investigated by Kotow, Holden, and Grant (1987). Their subjects included 48 myopic patients who were fitted with Bausch & Lomb 03 and 04 lenses, having a water content of 38 percent and a center thickness of 0.035mm. The patients were randomly assigned to one of four groups, having the lens for one eye replaced (1) once a week, (2) once every 2 weeks, (3) once every 4 weeks, and (4) once every 12 weeks. The fellow eye of each subject served as a control, having the lens replaced at the end of one year or sooner if needed. Subjects removed their lenses for a period of 16 hours at the end of each 2 weeks. After 48 weeks of extended wear, 18 of the original 48 subjects had been discontinued from the study: 7 for noncompliance and 11 because of papillary hypertrophy or other problems.

For the 30 subjects who completed the study (Kotow et al., 1987), the most noteworthy finding was the almost complete absence of *acute red-eye response* for eyes wearing regularly replaced lenses. Acute red-eye response was thought to be caused by the accumulation of debris beneath or on the surface of a lens that had become immobile, and during this study no significant build-up was observed on the regularly replaced lenses. Papillary hypertrophy, on the other hand, was *not* related to regular replacement, occurring about equally for replaced and nonreplaced lenses (worn on control eyes). Kotow et al. concluded that "regular replacement of lenses does help to avoid one of the main adverse effects of extended wear—the acute red-eye response—but there is no justification at this stage for replacing low water content extended-wear lenses more frequently than every 3 months."

Gas-Permeable Hard Lenses for Extended-Wear

Many laboratory and clinical studies of gas-permeable hard lenses for extended-wear have been reported, and the FDA has thus far approved one gas-permeable hard lens for extended wear—the Paraperm EW, having a Dk value of 56.

Clinical studies

Using lenses intended only for daily-wear, Levy (1985) reported that 15 subjects were fitted with Polycon II lenses and 15 with the Boston IV lens, worn on an extended-wear basis for a period of 1 year. All subjects removed the lenses for a period of

12 hours every 7 days. At the end of 1 year, 22 of the original 30 subjects were still wearing their lenses; seven Polycon II wearers and one Boston IV wearer were discontinued because of biomicroscopic findings and subjective complaints that appeared to be due to lens wear. Levy noted that the major problem experienced in the study was corneal molding due to lens compression after sleeping with the lenses on, manifested as a fluorescein-staining "ring" corresponding to the position of the lens edge. This compression led to corneal ulceration in one subject, which resolved with treatment. Levy concluded that in the longer term, the success of these lenses for extended-wear appeared to be related to the oxygen permeability of the lenses, since only 8 of the 15 wearers of the Polycon II lens (Dk = 10–12) completed the 1-year study whereas 14 of the 15 wearers of the Boston IV (Dk = 24–26) completed the study.

A clinical study in which 18 myopic patients were fitted with the Paraperm EW lens was reported by Henry, Bennett and Forrest (1987). At the end of 1 year, 15 patients (83 percent) were still wearing the lenses. One of the three patients who discontinued had lost interest in extended-wear. The other two drop-outs were the only two patients who had entered the study with a tear break-up time of less than 10 seconds: one of these patients had difficulty due to the lens adhering to the cornea, and the other experienced persistent dryness and moderate discomfort. The most common adverse clinical sign was desiccation (3 and 9 o'clock staining), found in 53 percent of the routine assessments. Other adverse signs included central corneal clouding (16 percent of assessments), conjunctival injection (13 percent), deposits and/or film (11 percent), and decreased visual acuity (9 percent). The symptoms most commonly reported by the patients were redness (10 percent of assessments), deposits of film (8 percent), blurred vision (7 percent), discomfort (4 percent), and dryness (2 percent). Henry et al. concluded that the success of the study was due to the high oxygen permeability of the lenses (Dk = 56) together with "tear pumping", and that the ocular complications occurring during the course of the study were "mild and not vision threatening."

In a 6-month extended-wear study, Polse, Sarver, Rivera, and Bonanno (1986) fitted 45 myopic subjects with the Boston *Equalens* (Dk = 40). They reported the following complications: lens-adherence syndrome (10 percent), superficial limbal keratitis (10 percent), epithelial microcysts (5 percent), endothelial polymegathism (5 percent), and giant papillary

conjunctivitis (5 percent). Schnider, Zabkiewicz, Terry, LaHood, and Holden (1986) found the following complications among 125 patients wearing gas-permeable, extended-wear hard lenses for periods ranging from 6 months to 2 years: a peripheral corneal ulcer resulting from moderate to severe 3 and 9 o'clock staining; an acute red-eye reaction following an episode of overnight lens binding; and several cases of papillary hypertrophy.

Corneal flattening has been reported as a result of both extended-wear and daily-wear of gas-permeable hard lenses. Henry, Bennett, and Forrest (1987) reported a mean corneal flattening at the end of 1 year of 0.33D in the vertical meridian and 0.43D in the horizontal meridian. Corneal flattening was accompanied by a mean change in spherical equivalent refraction of 0.30D *less myopia*, and by a mean change in refractive astigmatism of 0.37D less with-the-rule astigmatism. In a study of daily-wear, gas-permeable lenses for the control of myopia, Perrigin, Quintero, Perrigin, and Grosvenor (1987) found that, after wearing Paraperm O_2^+ lenses (Dk = 39) for 1 year, mean corneal flattening for 58 myopic children was 0.20D. Further, the mean increase in myopia was 0.06D per year as compared to 0.60D per year for a group of subjects who wore their lenses on an irregular basis.

Lens binding, or adhesion to the cornea after all-night wear, is a frequent complication of gas-permeable extended-wear hard lenses. As noted earlier, this problem has been reported by Levy (1985), who referred to it as compression resulting in a fluorescein-staining ring, by Polse et al. (1986), and by Schnider et al. (1986). Stevenson (1986) reported that, in a study in which 20 subjects were fitted with the Equalens, the most significant slit-lamp finding was the adhesion of the lens to the cornea on awakening, occurring in 10 percent of subjects and resulting in corneal moulding and staining. Swarbrick and Holden (1986) reported a 22 percent incidence of lens binding, on awakening, for 179 extended-wear patients. In the majority of cases, the lens bound nasally, moved spontaneously in less than an hour, and produced staining of the central cornea and the inferior conjunctiva. On the basis of an analysis of both lens factors and fitting factors, the authors concluded that lens binding occurs more frequently when a large, slightly steep-fitting lens with little edge lift is worn overnight on a flat cornea.

Using broader criteria for the definition of binding, Zabkiewicz, Terry, Holden, and Schnider (1987) found that 80 percent of patients who had worn gas-permeable, extended-wear hard lenses from 4–15 months regularly presented with clinically observable signs of lens binding. Zabkiewicz et al. suspected binding whenever corneal indentation, arcuate staining, abundant back surface debris, and peripheral corneal distortion were noted. They found that a significant increase in the frequency of binding with the time the lenses were worn.

How important is Dk?

In an *AOA Journal* editorial, Goldberg (1986) questioned the importance of an excessively high Dk for gas-permeable, extended-wear hard lenses. He pointed out that Dk (gas-permeability) is an indirect unit of measurement that fails to take into consideration the thickness of the material (recall that the amount of oxygen actually getting through the lens, called the *transmissivity*, is given by the permeability divided by the thickness, L, of the lens, or Dk/L).

> Regardless of the material's Dk value, the lens-cornea fitting relationship must allow the tear pumping mechanism to flush tears easily under a lens and to remove all corneal metabolites. This mechanism furnishes a fresh supply of oxygen with each blink. Consequently, the ability of a contact lens material to transmit oxygen is secondary to a good lens-cornea relationship. The primary considerations of a good lens-cornea relationship encompass a good tear pumping mechanism and adequate lens movement. . . . There is no conclusive data which confirm that a high Dk rigid gas permeable material will assure a successful fit at the exclusion of other related factors. The factors that affect the oxygen performance of a corneal lens on the eye are center thickness, oxygen flux and oxygen tension under a lens worn for daily or overnight wear. . . . (Goldberg, 1986, p. 172)

Practitioners who have been involved in the fitting of PMMA lenses (having a gas-permeability of *zero*) know the importance of fitting lenses loosely enough so that the cornea receives adequate oxygen by tear pumping. Unfortunately, in the design of inventory gas-permeable lenses, most manufacturers have "squandered" the oxygen-permeability of their lens material by making both the overall diameter and optic zone diameter so large that tear pumping is far less than optimum. Although a popular design for a PMMA lens—to be fitted by the "parallel, or alignment," method—involves an overall diameter of 8.8mm and an optic zone of 7.2 mm (ranging from about 9.0/7.4 for a very flat cornea to 8.6/7.0 for a very steep cornea, as shown in Table 14.1), gas-permeable lenses available on inventory, also intended to be fitted by the alignment method, have overall diameters of 9.0 or 9.2mm and optic zone

diameters of 7.8 or 8.2mm. Although these larger lenses may be more comfortable than smaller lenses and allow faster adaptation, in many cases they provide insufficient tear pumping even for daily-wear, much less for extended-wear.

Two additional observations should be made: (1) Goldberg's (1986) conclusion concerning the importance of tear pumping is supported by the finding of Swarbrick and Holden (1986), who found that lens binding occurs more frequently when a large, slightly steep-fitting lens with little edge lift is worn overnight on a flat cornea; and (2) Levy's (1985) conclusion—that in the longer term, the success of gas-permeable lenses for extended-wear appears to be related to the oxygen permeability of the lenses; only 8 of the 15 wearers of the Polycon II lens (Dk = 10–12) but 14 of the 15 wearers of the Boston IV (Dk = 24–26) completed the study.

CORNEAL CHANGES DUE TO CONTACT LENS WEAR

PMMA Lenses

Some of the problems that can occur as a result of wearing PMMA lenses are briefly discussed in the section on contact lens materials earlier in the chapter. The problems include the early changes of corneal edema and spectacle blur, largely due to the inability of the lenses to transmit oxygen and carbon dioxide, and the long-term changes of corneal flattening and with-the-rule astigmatism. As pointed out earlier, corneal edema can be controlled to a great extent by (1) fitting the lenses loosely enough so there is a reservoir of tears underneath the peripherery of the lenses and so the lenses move sufficiently during the blink cycle to bring about an adequate amount of tear pumping; (2) giving the patient instructions in adequate blinking; and (3) controlling the patient's wearing time.

Adaptation to contact lenses

Since the earliest days of hard lens fitting, practitioners and patients have been aware that some kind of adaptation must take place during the early stages of contact lens wear. Wearing time had to be built up slowly or the wearer would find the lenses uncomfortable due to edema, abrasions, and other forms of corneal insult. It was found that a lens that was fitted too loosely could not be tolerated for long because of prolonged tearing, photophobia, and mechanical trauma to the cornea and lid margins; whereas a lens fitted too tightly would cause corneal and lid edema after several hours of wear, leading to lens intolerance due to subjective symptoms such as burning, stinging, headaches, and visual disturbances.

There evolved what can be called the "classical" theory of contact lens adaptation, which has two parts:

1. When a contact lens is first placed on the cornea, it acts as a foreign body; causing pain, photophobia, and lacrimation. It is necessary, therefore, for the sensory nerve endings in the corneal epithelium and lid margins, supplied by the ophthalmic division of the fifth cranial nerve, to adapt to the presence of the lenses. Such adaptation was assumed to be complete when the patient reached the stage at which he or she was no longer aware of the lenses.

2. The presence of a contact lens on the cornea tends to cause edema and other forms of insult to the epithelium, apparently because of interference with the normal metabolic processes. If wearing time is built up gradually, the cornea will eventually be able to tolerate the lens with little or no pathological response. Therefore, it must be true that the corneal metabolism somehow adapts to the presence of the lens.

The first part of this theory has never been questioned. A number of studies have correlated corneal and lid margin pain thresholds with lens adaptation and have shown that the neural receptors do, in fact, undergo adaptation. Shirmer (1963) used an aesthesiometer to measure pain thresholds in both adapted and unadapted contact lens wearers and found that the adapted wearers had significantly lower corneal sensitivity. Pain thresholds on the lower lid margins of four subject were measured by Lowther and Hill (1968) during the first 3 weeks of lens wear. They found that adaptation of the lower lid margins took place within 7–14 days, and that adaptation occurred earliest on the portion of the lid margin most often contacted by the lens.

The second part of the theory—involving some form of adaptation of the corneal metabolic processes—is based on the writings of Smelser and his co-workers and has been discussed by Mazow (1962) and other authors. Smelser and Ozanics (1952) fitted subjects with steep contact lenses and found that halos (due to the presence of severe corneal edema) were reported by the subjects within 2 hours. However, when oxygen was added to the tear fluid, they found that the halos were not seen until 7 hours' wear and that the oxygen bubble beneath the lens gradually diminished in size, indicating that the oxygen was being used by the cornea. Fitting fluid-

containing scleral lenses to the eyes of guinea pigs, Smelser and Chen (1955) found a marked increase in the amount of lactic acid in the cornea during the first 6 hours of wear, indicating that the lenses were causing a slowing down of the metabolic processes of the cornea.

As a result of these and other investigations, Smelser (1955) proposed the existence of a metabolic pumping mechanism, working at the cellular level, which would aid in removing excess water from the cornea. As noted earlier in the discussion of corneal physiology, Harris (1960) also proposed the presence of a metabolic pumping mechanism residing in both the epithelium and the endothelium. Such a pump would require the presence of oxygen, and Harris proposed that the oxygen supply normally available from the aqueous humor is sufficient to maintain an effective pumping mechanism under normal circumstances.

The possibility that *tearing* is an important factor in causing corneal edema was suggested by Harris and Mandell (1969), who used a corneal pachometer to measure the corneal thickness of two new contact lens wearers. They found an increase in corneal thickness of 8 percent during the first 3 hours of lens wear and concluded that this corneal edema was caused by the fact that the excessive tearing brought about by the contact lens has a *low tonicity* and, therefore, causes the movement of water into the cornea by the process of osmosis. They found that the amount of corneal thickening decreased with repeated daily contact lens wear, and they proposed that the adaptation process can be accounted for on the basis of the decrease in tearing that accompanies adaptation of the neural receptors in the lid margins to stimulation by the contact lens. If contact lens adaptation can be accounted for entirely on the basis of adaptation of neural receptors, as Harris and Mandell suggested, the second part of the classical adaptation theory (having to do with adaptation of corneal metabolism) would appear to be unnecessary.

The idea that there is a metabolic change that enables the cornea to adapt to a contact lens has been rejected by Feldman (1970) on the basis that if the concept of metabolic adaptation is correct, the cornea should become more tolerant of hypoxia after adaptation. Because his laboratory studies indicated that this did not occur, Feldman concluded that the more likely explanation for the cessation of edema is the gradual development of *good blinking habits* by the wearer. He believes that the cause of corneal swelling in new contact lens wearers is interference with tear exchange brought about by insufficient blinking. This causes hypoxia of the epithelium, so the epithelial cells no longer have the oxygen necessary to operate the metabolic pump, thus allowing water to accumulate. Feldman further proposed that the stroma is not involved in contact lens edema; this would occur only if the endothelial pump is interfered with.

As already noted, it has been observed that new contact lens wearers typically blink too frequently during the first few days of lens wear and then enter a period during which blinking occurs too infrequently and often with incomplete lid closure. On the basis of the findings of Harris and Mandell (1969) and of Feldman (1970), we can conclude that, in addition to adaptation of the sensory nerve endings in the corneal epithelium and lid margins, adaptation to PMMA lenses requires the establishment of correct blinking habits. Too frequent blinking can cause corneal edema due to the hypotonicity of the tears (Harris and Mandell), whereas too infrequent blinking can cause corneal edema due to insufficient tear exchange leading to hypoxia (Feldman).

Detection of corneal edema

As described earlier in the section on corneal physiology, the presence of corneal edema can be detected by a number of methods, including (1) detection of central corneal clouding by means of the slit lamp, (2) corneal steepening as determined by keratometry, (3) an increase in myopia as determined by refraction, or (4) a report of blurring when glasses are worn after contact lens removal (spectacle blur). An additional method involves measurement of corneal thickness by means of pachometry. However, this procedure, to be accurate, requires the use of elaborate instrumentation, which is not practical for routine clinical use.

Slit-lamp examination for corneal clouding should be a routine procedure in progress visits for PMMA lens wearers. Because the clouding persists for only a short time after lens removal, the examination should take place immediately after the lenses are removed. Using the split-limbal method of illumination described by Korb and Exford (1968), the examination should be conducted in complete darkness with the examiner partially dark adapted; the naked eye should first be used, followed by the use of low power magnification; the patient's fixation should be adjusted so the suspected area (usually the corneal apex) is seen against the background of the pupil; and the slit width should vary from 1.5mm (blue iris) to 3mm (brown iris) with the beam at an angle of 45–60 degrees. With practice, the examiner will be able to grade central corneal clouding from grade 1 (barely visible) to grade 4 (severe).

At the first progress visit, central corneal clouding of grade 1 or possibly grade 2 is an expected finding, whereas more severe clouding is an indication that either the lenses are fitting too tightly, the patient has been increasing wearing time too rapidly, or correct blinking habits have not been established. The presence of grade 3 or 4 corneal clouding can often be correlated with the appearance of the fluorescein pattern, as observed with the aid of the Burton lamp. The failure of the bright green ring (indicating fluorescein pooling under the peripheral curve) to extend all the way around the circumference of the lens is an indication that the tears may not be supplying a sufficient amount of oxygen to the cornea. This problem can be solved easily by either flattening or increasing the width of the peripheral curve. If the bright green ring is found to extend all the way around the circumference of the lens, the problem may be that the lens is fitting too tightly and, thus, not lagging sufficiently with each blink. With each blink, each lens should move upward and, after the blink, quickly lag downward at least 2 or 3mm. However, too much lag can also be a problem, as this will cause excessive tearing, which can also cause corneal edema. Excessive blink lag and excessive tearing will usually result in complaints of irritation and discomfort, whereas insufficient blink lag will tend to affect comfort only after several hours of lens wear, when the patient will find that the lenses feel hot and dry. If both the fluorescein pattern and the blink lag are found to be within normal limits for a patient who has excessive corneal clouding, the clouding can be due either to too rapid an increase in wearing time or to poor blinking.

Because corneal swelling due to hard contact lens wearing typically is confined to the apical portion of the cornea, one would expect that the presence of central corneal clouding would be well correlated with corneal steepening as found by keratometry and with an increase in myopia as found by retinoscopy or subjective refraction. However, such a correlation is not always found. For example, Mandell and Polse (1971) fitted two subjects with tightly fitting contact lenses and made corneal thickness measurements at 5-degree intervals across the horizontal meridian of each subject's cornea, prior to lens insertion and after 2 hours of lens wearing. They found that swelling of up to 6 percent occurred in the central area, with little or no swelling in the periphery. Slit-lamp examination revealed central corneal clouding corresponding to the area of increased thickness, whereas keratometer findings taken before and after the lens was worn showed little or no change. From this they concluded that the keratometer mire reflection points, approximately 3mm apart, nearly corresponded to the limits of the edematous area.

Prediction of successful lens wear

Before ordering lenses for a patient, it is helpful if the practitioner is able to predict the patient's success at lens wear. Corneal edema occurs within the first 2 or 3 hours of lens wear. Therefore, to determine if the patient will be a successful wearer, all that is necessary is to determine how much edema occurs during the first 2 or 3 hours of lens wear, using as a criterion central corneal clouding as observed by the slit lamp, corneal steepening, increase in myopia, or the patient's report of spectacle blur.

Brungardt and Potter (1972) made a strong case for the prediction of successful lens wear on the basis of the increase in myopia occurring during the early hours of lens wear. These investigators monitored 53 contact lens patients for a 90-day period, completing a series of testing procedures on day 1 (after 2½ or 3 hours of wear), day 5, day 30, and day 90. The testing procedures involved the following: (1) keratometer findings, (2) subjective refraction, (3) visual-acuity testing, and (4) slit-lamp inspection for central corneal clouding. Brungardt and Potter found that changes in refraction and visual-acuity loss were good predictors of success or failure in contact lens wear, whereas corneal steepening and the presence of central corneal clouding were less valuable as predictors. On day 1, after 2½ or 3 hours of lens wear, 75 percent of the patients were found to have little change in refractive error and were subsequently found to adapt to their lenses quickly, whereas those showing larger increases in myopia were found to be slow adaptors.

In another report, Brungardt (1972) stated that after the first 3 hours of contact lens wear, the practitoner should expect a steepening of the cornea of 0.37D or less, an increase in myopia of 0.37D or less, and no loss in visual acuity with the subjective refraction in place. For the 25 percent of patients who will have an increase in myopia of 0.50D or more, the fault may be in the lens design, or possibly the patient should not wear contact lenses. In such a case, Brungardt recommends that a definite change in lens design be made (usually a loosening) before the patient is dismissed as a poor contact lens risk. On the fifth day's testing, a few of the original 75 percent (the fast-adapting group) will be identified

as problem wearers, but their problems will be less severe than those that were evident on the first day. The problems may be solved in some cases by encouraging the patient to blink more often and in other cases by loosening the lenses slightly. The exact loosening procedure should be determined by fluorescein pattern analysis.

Spectacle blur

Spectacle blur can occur either in the early or the later stages of contact lens wear. It is apparently caused by one or a combination of the following factors: (1) irregularity of the corneal surface (the kind of irregularity that distorts the keratometer mire image); (2) corneal edema or other insult; and (3) steepening or flattening of the cornea, usually involving changes in the axis and power of the corneal astigmatism.

Studies reported by Rengstorff (1966a) and by Sarver and Harris (1967) indicate that lens diameter is one factor of importance in spectacle blur. Rengstorff investigated visual-acuity loss of 83 soldiers who had worn contact lenses for varying periods of time. The subjects gave up their contact lenses for a period of several weeks, during which refractions were done at intervals of from 1 day to 3 weeks after lens removal. It should be noted that *visual-acuity loss* refers to loss of acuity with the best refractive correction. Comparing subjects wearing large lenses with those wearing small lenses, Rengstorff found that 70 percent of those wearing small (8.6 to 9.3mm) lenses attained 20/20 acuity after lens removal, whereas only 35 percent of those wearing large (10.3 to 11.0mm) lenses had 20/20 acuity. Sarver and Harris (1967) studied the incidence of spectacle blur for a group of 42 wearers on the basis of the patients' subjective reports, and they found that spectacle blur was reported by 11 of 12 patients wearing large (9.0 to 9.9mm) lenses but by only 16 of 24 patients wearing small (8.0–9.0mm) lenses.

When spectacle blur occurs during the first several weeks of contact lens wear, steps taken to minimize corneal edema (lens modification, reduction in wearing time, or improvement of blinking habits) will usually also serve to minimize spectacle blur. When spectacle blur occurs after months or years of lens wear, it may be related to edema or corneal flattening, changes in astigmatism, or other corneal changes.

Fluorescein staining

In the typical progress examination routine, fluorescein is instilled while the lenses are being worn to evaluate the fluorescein pattern, after which the lenses are removed and the eyes are inspected for corneal clouding and other changes, including fluorescein staining. At this point, there is usually sufficient fluorescein in the tear fluid so an additional application is not necessary.

Patterns of staining vary with the type of lenses being worn. In former years, when lenses were fitted relatively large and flat, staining of the corneal apex often occurred due to the mechanical pressure exerted by the lens. With smaller, steeper lenses, the occurrence of apical staining (although rare) indicates a physiological rather than a mechanical cause: anoxia results from a lack of tear exchange under a tightly fitting lens. The most commonly seen form of staining with today's smaller lenses is the so-called limbal, or 3 and 9 o'clock, staining. This form of staining is often found in otherwise well-adapted and satisfied lens wearers, often after several months of lens wear. The patient's only complaint, if any, may be that the eyes appear to be bloodshot. Lemp and Holly (1970) concluded that the cause of 3 and 9 o'clock staining is localized drying of the cornea due to inadequate resurfacing of the mucoid layer of the precorneal film because of lack of lid-corneal congruity just beyond the edge of the lens. They believe that poor blinking and excessive rigidity of the tarsal plate may also be involved. Although many suggestions have been made concerning methods of refitting the patient's lenses to eliminate limbal staining, experience indicates that other than loosening the lens fit to provide more lens movement, the only effective method is to aggressively instruct the patient in correct blinking habits.

It was found by Korb and Korb (1970) that fluorescein staining was present in 111 of 300 corneas of patients who had never worn contact lenses. Of the 111 staining corneas, 39 had "lid closure" staining, 33 had "lid margin" staining, 2 had "diffuse" staining, and 37 had more than one of the three types of staining. The authors concluded that lid closure staining was accompanied by an obviously incomplete blink; lid margin staining was due to lid pressure; and diffuse staining was due to poor wetting, poor blinking, or both. In an addendum to their paper, Korb and Korb reported that 71 of the subjects had been fitted with contact lenses and had worn them for 3 months, and that there was a trend toward a *lower* incidence of corneal staining than was found prior to contact lens wearing.

Long-term corneal changes

The most obvious long-term corneal changes, occurring with many PMMA lens wearers after a year or more of lens wear, are corneal flattening and the occurrence of with-the-rule corneal astigmatism. A number of studies have shown that the original corneal steepening, due to edema, gradually decreases and is eventually replaced by corneal flattening, which tends to be permanent. This reversal (from steepening to flattening) can occur after as little as 8 weeks or as much as a year or more of lens wear. For example, Hazlett (1969) found that for 40 patients fitted with lenses averaging 8.7mm in diameter and 0.11mm in thickness, corneal curvature in both the flatter and the steeper meridians had flattened to an average of 0.50D flatter than the prefitting curvature by the end of 8 weeks. On the other hand, Rengstorff (1969b) combined the data of a number of investigators and found that mean corneal curvature (1) steepened by 0.75D at the end of 1 week of lens wear, (2) flattened by 0.50D by the end of 6 months of lens wear, and (3) flattened a further 0.50D by the end of 1 year, resulting in a curvature 0.25D flatter than the prefitting curvature (see Figure 14.42). He found that by the end of 2 years, the average curvature was 0.62D flatter than the prefitting curvature, and this was true for patients who had worn their lenses for as long as 9½ years.

The occurrence of with-the-rule astigmatism in long-term wearers of PMMA lenses is typified by reports by Janoff (1976) and by Hartstein and Becker (1970). Janoff reported on a patient whose corneal astigmatism increased in the with-the-rule direction, 2.50D in one eye and 3.25D in the other, over a 12-year period of lens wear. Hartstein and Becker reported that some of their patients developed not only with-the-rule astigmatism but also keratoconus while wearing contact lenses. In an earlier paper,

Figure 14.42 Mean corneal curvature immediately after lens removal as compared to corneal curvature prior to lens wear (redrawn from Rengstorff, 1969b).

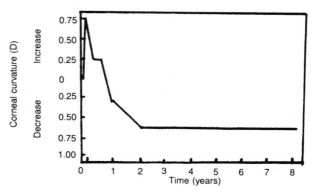

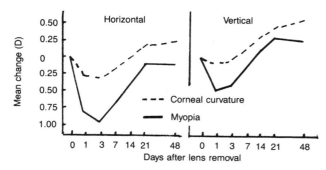

Figure 14.43 Mean corneal curvature and myopia changes occurring after removal of contact lenses (redrawn from Rengstorff, 1969a).

Hartstein (1965) reported that 12 patients—all satisfied lens wearers—had developed from 2.50 to 6.00D of with-the-rule astigmatism but had only 0.00 to 1.00D of astigmatism before wearing contact lenses. These patients had worn their lenses for 2–6 years.

Many long-term wearers who develop corneal flattening or with-the-rule astigmatism will be asymptomatic but others will consult the optometrist (usually after many years of successful all-day wear) with complaints involving vision, comfort, or both. Unfortunately, many of these patients have no backup glasses or their eyes have changed so much since being fitted with contact lenses that their precontact lens glasses are useless. As a general rule, any corneal flattening will be accompanied by a corresponding decrease in myopia, and any increase in with-the-rule corneal astigmatism will be accompanied by a corresponding increase in with-the-rule refractive astigmatism. Therefore, the "old" glasses will correct for too much myopia, for insufficient astigmatism, or both. However, one of the most bothersome problems from the patient's point of view is the change in cylinder axis that accompanies the change in astigmatism. The patient, therefore, is likely to not be able to obtain satisfactory vision with either the contact lenses or the glasses.

To understand how to effectively care for a problem patient who has experienced corneal and refractive changes, it is necessary to have an understanding of the possible diurnal changes in corneal curvature and refraction, as well as the possible changes on lens removal.

Diurnal corneal and refractive changes

When a long-term contact lens wearer has a complaint associated with corneal flattening or with-the-rule astigmatism, pronounced diurnal changes in corneal and refractive findings will often be found. In such cases, the corneas will be at their flattest (and refraction the least myopic) in the early morning hours, before the lenses are worn; they will be at their steepest (and refraction the most myopic) after the lenses have been worn for a period of 8 hours or more. In addition, large changes in both corneal and refractive astigmatism will often be found between morning and night. Therefore, refraction of such patients both early in the morning and late in the afternoon will usually assist the practitioner in arriving at a solution to the patient's problem.

Corneal and refractive changes after lens removal

Many patients (and apparently even some practitioners) mistakenly believe that if contact lenses are causing trouble, the best thing to do is to remove the lenses 3 or 4 days prior to the optometrist's examination. Nothing could be farther from the truth! Rengstorff (1969a) has shown that a decrease in myopia as great at 1.00D can occur during the first 3 days after lens removal, after which it gradually increases to a stable level within 21 days or more. In addition to the changes in myopia, unpredictable changes in astigmatism often occur during the first several days after lens removal (see Figure 14.43). Therefore, when an appointment is made for a patient who is having problems, the patient should be instructed to continue to wear the lenses until the day of the appointment. If possible, the appointment should be made either early in the morning prior to the patient's putting on the lenses or late in the afternoon after all-day wear.

Prescribing glasses for the contact lens wearer

The problem of prescribing glasses for the contact lens wearer arises in a number of situations, ranging from the asymptomatic college student who wishes to remove the contact lenses in the evening to study with glasses to the symptomatic patient who has poor vision with both contact lenses and glasses. The latter patient may ultimately require both new glasses and new contact lenses, but often the provision of new glasses will be the first priority, because they will make it possible for the patient to gradually reduce contact lens wearing time.

For the student who wants to wear glasses in the evening, the decision is an easy one: a refraction is done in the late afternoon or in the evening, after at least 8 hours of lens wear. If spectacle blur, corneal clouding, or distorted keratometer mire images are present, it is advisable to wait 30–45 minutes after lens removal before doing the refraction. Alternately, the refraction can be done soon after lens removal and repeated 30–45 minutes later (the patient waiting while the practitioner examines another patient).

For the symptomatic patient who will ultimately need both new glasses and new contact lenses, the practitioner should strongly consider refracting the patient both early in the morning before lens wear and late in the afternoon or in the evening after at least 8 hours of lens wear. If the diurnal variation in refraction is great (i.e., more than 1.00D spherical equivalent), the practitioner may decide on a compromise prescription on the basis of the ultimate prescription being probably somewhere between the two extremes. In writing such a prescription, astigmatism becomes a problem. Because having a cylinder at the incorrect axis is usually worse than having no cylinder at all, small cylinders (up to 0.75 or 1.00D) are often best neglected.

An additional approach to the problem patient, although requiring more time, is to perform two or more refractions in the late afternoon or evening, after lens removal, at intervals of from 30 minutes to 1 hour. Still another approach, if the patient's vision without either contact lenses or glasses (or with the old glasses) is sufficient, is to instruct the patient to gradually reduce wearing time, leveling off at 8 hours per day. If a refraction is then done at the end of the 8-hour wearing period, the chances are good that the resulting lenses will provide good vision. In any case, the patient should be made to understand that it is impossible to promise that the first prescription will be the final one, because the eyes are constantly changing after lens removal. Most patients will accept this, and some will feel somewhat responsible for having neglected their eyes for a long period of time.

Prescribing new contact lenses for the problem patient

As noted earlier, the typical problem patient has worn lenses successfully, all day long, for a number of years. Because there have been so few problems, the patient may not have returned to the practitioner for routine progress examinations. The patient may find it necessary to wear the contact lenses all day long to have acceptable vision, because the corneal changes that have taken place have resulted in intolerable spectacle blur.

The complaint that finally brings the patient to the practitioner may be either discomfort or poor vision, but it is more likely to be discomfort. Even though the cornea may have flattened and increased in with-the-rule astigmatism, the tear layer will generally compensate for these changes to the extent that 20/20 acuity will be possible when the lenses are worn. However, the fact that the lenses are now too steep for the corneas (the corneas having flattened and the lenses having stayed about the same) means that the patient should be expected to have tight symptoms: a feeling of dryness or burning, often accompanied by a headache or general fatigue toward the end of the wearing period. The obvious solution to the problem is to refit the patient with flatter lenses based on the current keratometer findings.

Noting that Rengstorff and others have shown that corneal curvature and refraction tend to stabilize during a period of from 3–6 weeks after lens removal, the practitioner may be tempted to have the patient discontinue lens wear until stabilization has taken place and then refit the contact lenses. However, such a procedure is not only inconvenient and potentially dangerous for the patient because of the need for good vision for work or for driving a car, but sudden long-term withdrawal of lenses may result in severe corneal distortion and irreversible corneal damage (Rengstorff, 1975).

Although "cold turkey" withdrawal of lenses is both inconvenient and dangerous, experience indicates that gradual lens withdrawal tends to result in stabilization of the cornea (e.g., in reduced diurnal variation in keratometer findings and in subjective refraction) together with a reduction in the severity of the patient's symptoms. A recommended procedure is to advise the patient to reduce wearing time, by no more than ½ or 1 hour per day, to no more than 8 or 9 hours per day prior to ordering new lenses. This will mean that until the new lenses are delivered, the patient will be able to wear the contact lenses during the working or school day and will have to get along as best as possible during the evening hours.

For a patient who has no glasses (or no usable glasses) and is not willing or able to go without contact lenses or glasses during the evening, the practitioner's first priority may be to order an up-to-date pair of spectacle lenses for the patient (as described in the previous section) with full knowledge that the lenses may have to be changed once the patient has adapted to the new contact lenses.

Lens-related problems

In some cases, problems that bring a PMMA lens wearer back to the optometrist are due not to ocular changes but to changes in the lenses themselves. These may be roughly classified as either changes in lens curvature or changes in lens surfaces.

Although PMMA is a relatively stable material, lenses made of it are sometimes found to flatten or steepen significantly (0.10mm or more) or to warp over a period of months or years. Warping may occur due to extreme heat, as when the lenses are left in the glove compartment of an automobile on a hot day. It is impossible to detect warping of a lens by means of the lensometer, because both the front and back surfaces will have toric curvatures that will cancel each other out. However, warping can be detected by measuring the radius of curvature of the back surface of the lens, using either a Radiuscope or a keratometer. Although immersing a lens in boiling water for several minutes may sometimes reduce or eliminate the warpage, usually it will be necessary to order a new lens.

Changes in lens surfaces are usually the result of careless or nonexistent lens care procedures on the part of the patient. Although all contact lens practitioners instruct (or should instruct) their patients to clean their lenses at night before placing them in the storage container, a surprising number of patients report that they clean their lenses in the morning, if they clean them at all. An important part of the history for any problem contact lens wearer is to innocently ask how he or she cares for the lenses.

Unless lipids and other materials arising from the tear film are removed from the lenses each night before storage, the lenses will gradually become coated with these materials. This coating will eventually interfere with both vision and comfort and can lead to complete intolerance of the lenses. Fortunately, the coating can usually be removed by the diligent use of a surfactant cleaner and, if not, by repolishing the lenses.

Surface and edge inspection can be done most readily by the use of either the slit-lamp microscope or other low-power binocular microscope. Additional surface changes that are often found are scratches and roughened edges. Although even relatively large scratches may have little or no effect on vision because they are filled in by tears, they do have an effect on comfort: repolishing of scratched lenses almost always results in a report that the lenses "feel like new."

If the practitioner does not possess modification equipment, the alternative is to send the patient's lenses to a laboratory for repolishing. This will usually result in a delay of a week or more, and because many patients will have neither an extra pair of contact lenses nor a wearable pair of glasses,

they naturally will resist giving up their lenses for this period of time. Therefore, any practitioner who is serious about contact lens fitting is advised to purchase lens modification equipment and to learn how to use it. Relatively little skill and experience states that oxygen is transmitted through the *flange* of the Polycon aphakic lens.

The manner in which an oxygen-permeable lens is fitted can play an important role in determining the total amount of oxygen reaching the cornea, because a significant amount of oxygen reaches the cornea via the tear layer if the lens moves sufficiently during the blink cycle. In general, gas-permeable lenses should be fitted no more tightly than PMMA lenses. This is particularly true for plus lenses: it is conceivable that a tightly fitting gas-are required to master the techniques of reducing diameter, applying secondary and peripheral curves, blending transition zones, and polishing lens surfaces and edges. Even though lens modification can ultimately be assigned to a trained technician, the practitioner will understand these procedures only if he first learns to do them himself.

Gas-Permeable Hard Lenses

Gas-permeable hard lenses were developed to prevent the problem of corneal edema that is so prevalent with wearers of PMMA lenses. The extent to which a gas-permeable lens prevents corneal edema depends on a number of factors, including (1) the oxygen permeability of the material from which the lens is made, (2) the thickness of the lens, (3) the manner in which the lens is fitted, and (4) the condition of the lens surfaces.

Recall that, although oxygen permeability is a function of the material, the amount of oxygen passing through the lens to the cornea, or the *oxygen transmissivity*, depends on lens thickness as well as permeability:

$$\text{Transmissivity} = \frac{\text{permeability}}{\text{thickness}}.$$

In thicknesses ordinarily used for minus lenses, oxygen permeability of FDA-approved materials is sufficiently high to diminish greatly the possibility of the occurrence of corneal edema. For plus lenses, the increased center thickness significantly reduces the amount of oxygen reaching the cornea through the lens. However, even for plus lenses, if any oxygen is transmitted through the lens to the cornea, it will be more than would reach the cornea through a PMMA lens having zero oxygen permeability. It is of interest that Syntex, in its promotional material, permeable plus lens could allow less oxygen to reach the cornea than would a correctly fitting PMMA lens.

In any discussion of oxygen permeability, the condition of the lens surfaces cannot be ignored. All measurements of oxygen permeability are made with new lenses, and there is no doubt that the presence of a coating of lipids and other materials on the lens surfaces will have a significant effect on the amount of oxygen reaching the cornea.

Lens stability

As noted earlier, one of the main problems with oxygen-permeable lenses, as compared with PMMA lenses, is lens stability. A lack of stability has two major consequences in fitting contact lenses: (1) the lens will fail to mask, or eliminate, corneal astigmatism; and (2) the curvature of the lens may tend to change with time. As for change in lens curvature with time, this is particularly true of CAB material because the lens curvature and other parameters change as the state of hydration changes.

An additional consequence of the instability of CAB material is that the lenses will deform if not handled properly or if exposed to excessive heat. Stranch (1981) has suggested that the use of a mechanical cleaning system such as Hydro-Mat, Swirl Clean, or a small ultrasonic unit can reduce the amount of lens handling that may tend to warp or flatten the lenses, and the patients should be warned not to leave the lenses (in the case) in a parked car in the sun.

Stranch (1981) also made the point that, when CAB lenses are fitted on a patient whose corneas have been flattened as a result of PMMA lens wear, the corneal steepening that will occur may result in originally well-fitted CAB lenses fitting too loosely. Although this is a desired effect, it may mean that steeper lenses will have to be ordered.

Problems relating to lens surfaces

Experience with silicone-acrylate lenses indicates that they become coated more quickly than PMMA lenses with proteinaceous material from the precorneal film. Harris (1981) recommends the use of Lobob, D-film, or GelClean for cleaning the lenses and a combination solution such as Soaklens or Soak-and-Wet for lens storage. As with PMMA lenses, it is imperative that patients clean the lenses at night prior to overnight storage.

A lens-surface problem regarding CAB lenses, described by Stranch (1981), is the formation of dry spots on the lenses, which apparently occurs due to the migration of the plasticizer to the surface of the lens. He notes that, when these spots occur, it is usually within a week or two after dispensing the lenses; the only solution to the problem is to return the lens to the manufacturer for replacement.

Problems relating to long-term wear

Few, if any, reports of corneal changes associated with long-term daily-wear of these lenses are available. Inasmuch as the changes resulting from long-term wear of PMMA lenses have been a result of the presence of corneal edema and the pressure exerted on the cornea by the relatively rigid lenses, it is hoped that reports of long-term changes resulting from gas-permeable lens wear will continue to be conspicuous in their absence.

The most common problems resulting from *extended-wear* of gas-permeable hard lenses, as described earlier, are lens adherence and corneal flattening.

Soft Contact Lenses

When soft contact lenses first became available in the United States in the early 1970s, it was believed that, because of their hydrophilic nature, high water content, and oxygen permeability (which for the thick lenses then in use was more imaginary than real), the lenses would cause few, if any, adverse ocular changes. One by one, however, reports of adverse effects began to appear in the literature.

These adverse effects were different from those due to hard lenses and varied from innocuous to threatening. For example, corneal edema and fluorescein staining were found to occur with soft lenses, but they differed from the corneal edema and staining that occurred with hard lenses. After the adaptation period, some patients' corneas became steeper rather than flatter as with hard lenses, and they had a consequent increase in myopia rather than a decrease as with hard lenses. Problems relating to lens-care systems became apparent in the form of red-eye syndromes, contamination of lenses, sensitivity to preservatives in lens care solutions, and more severe lens coating than had ever occurred with hard lenses. This coating appeared to be the cause of giant papillary conjunctivitis, a continuing problem for some soft lens wearers.

Adaptation to soft contact lenses

As noted earlier in the section on contact lens materials, the almost complete lack of sensation caused by a soft contact lens (even when worn for the first time) is due to a combination of two factors:

(1) the lens is soft and flexible, and (2) the lens is large enough so its upper and lower edges are both constantly underneath the lid margins.

In our earlier discussion of adaptation to hard contact lenses, we concluded that this adaptation involved the adaptation of the sensory nerve endings in the corneal epithelium and lid margins, as well as the establishment of correct blinking habits. Because soft lenses require little or no adaptation of neural receptors, adaptation is mainly a matter of establishing correct blinking habits.

Corneal edema

Corneal edema is less likely to occur with wearers of hydrogel lenses than with PMMA lens wearers, particularly when the lenses are fitted in thicknesses of approximately 0.06mm or less. When edema does occur, it is in the form of an overall swelling that cannot be seen with the slit lamp, rather than the familiar central corneal clouding seen with PMMA lens wearers. However, the presence of edema due to soft lens wear is revealed by the appearance of corneal striae—multiple vertical striate lines in the region of Descemet's membrane, seen with the slit lamp, using a narrow parallelopiped under direct illumination and with high magnification. As already indicated, Polse and Mandell (1976) found that corneal striae occur when the corneal thickness

increases by 7 percent. To obtain this amount of corneal swelling, the cornea must be submitted to less than 1.5 percent oxygen for a period of 3 hours.

As noted by Benjamin and Hill (1979), who found that the equivalent oxygen performance of HEMA lenses averaging 0.06mm in thickness was 7 percent, the presence of corneal striae indicates that (for lenses of this thickness) the cornea is not receiving the amount of oxygen that the lens is capable of supplying. When striae are found in a soft lens progress examination, the practitioner should consider the following possible causes: (1) the lenses may be fitting so tightly that metabolic wastes are forming a stagnant pool underneath the lens; (2) the lenses may be sufficiently coated with material originating from the tear film to interfere with their gas permeability; or (3) the patient may not be blinking often enough or may be a partial blinker. The cause of the problem can be determined by carefully evaluating the fit of the lenses, inspecting the lenses under a low-power binocular microscope, and observing the patient's blinking habits. A positive result often will be found in two or sometimes three of these tests.

Corneal curvature and refractive changes

Although early reports stated or implied that corneal curvature and refractive changes were absent or minimal with soft contact lenses, it soon became apparent that corneal steepening and an increase in myopia could occur with these lenses. These changes, rather than occurring after months or years of lens wear, were found to occur in a matter of days or weeks. One of the earliest reports was that of Hill (1974), who fitted five patients with Bausch & Lomb spin-cast lenses; one patient was found to have pronounced corneal steepening accompanied with microcystic edema.

In a study involving 30 patients fitted with N&N lathe-cut lenses, Grosvenor (1975a) reported a tendency for some patients' corneas to flatten during the first few weeks of lens wear and then gradually begin to steepen. Data for two of the most extreme cases are shown in Figure 14.44. Subject J.D.'s corneal curvature flattened slightly during the first 3 weeks of the lens wear, accompanied by a decrease in myopia, but by the end of 17 weeks the curvature had steepened to 0.50D more than the original keratometer readings, with a consequent increase in myopia of 0.50D.

Subject M.I., who admitted to wearing contact lenses 20 hours per day while studying for final exams, was found to have an increase in corneal

Figure 14.44   Changes in corneal curvature and subjective refraction of soft lens wearers (redrawn from Grosvenor 1975a).

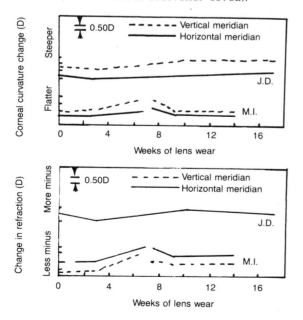

refracting power of almost 1.00D and an increase in myopia of more than 1.00D after only 7 weeks of lens wear. After going without lenses for 3 days and agreeing to a greatly reduced wearing schedule, subject M.I.'s keratometer findings and subjective refraction stabilized by the end of an additional 7 weeks. An additional finding was that a few patients in the study were found to have increases in astigmatism of as much as 0.50 or 0.75D after several weeks of lens wear. In all cases, keratometric and refractive findings (both spherical and cylindrical) returned to prefitting levels with the fitting of looser lenses, a reduction in wearing time, instruction in correct blinking habits, or a combination of these procedures.

Grosvenor (1975a) concluded that the original corneal flattening was due to edema of the entire extent of the cornea (rather than the central circular clouding seen in hard lens wearers) and that the later steepening was due to a mechanical pressure effect exerted by the lenses. The lenses used in this study were very thick (0.20 to 0.25mm) by today's standards. Fortunately, with the ultrathin lenses in use today, corneal steepening is a much less common finding. It does, however, occur occasionally, so postwearing keratometer findings and subjective refraction constitute important steps in soft lens progressive examinations.

Corneal vascularization

The cornea is normally avascular. Cogan (1948) attributed this avascularity to the compactness of the corneal tissue (a property shared by cartilage and nails) and suggested that when the cornea becomes swollen and, therefore, less compact, spaces are opened up through which vessels can grow. It has been suggested by Collin (1970) that enzymes such as collagenase, fibrinolysin, and hyaluronidase may cause degeneration of the stroma, leading to vascularization. Whatever the cause, the fact remains that long-continued anoxia and the resulting edema can lead to vascularization of the limbal area of the cornea. Ruben (1981) suggested that, whereas the normal limbal arcades extend about 1mm into the cornea, the presence of superficial vessels extending as much as 2 or 3mm into the cornea must be considered as abnormal.

The presence of corneal vascularization (often called *neovascularization*) accompanying soft lens wear usually indicates that the affected area has been anoxic and edematous for a long time. It is most likely to occur when the patient has been wearing very thick lenses; for example, for the correction of

aphakia (particularly if lenses are worn on an extended-wear basis). Otherwise, the practitioner should suspect the presence of one or more of the causes of edema listed in the previous discussion (tightly fitting lenses, coated lenses, or poor blinking habits). The most immediate method of controlling the vascularization is to have the patient discontinue lens wear. Once the most likely cause of the vascularization has been determined and corrected, lens wear can be resumed; however, the patient should be kept under careful observation.

In a comprehensive discussion of corneal vascularization, Ruben (1981) made the point that anti-inflammatory drugs such as prednisolone have been used in the treatment of neovascularization, but that their long-term use may induce glaucoma in susceptible patients; in extreme cases, diathermy, galvanic electrolysis, and laser or microcautery occlusion of the vessels are possible forms of treatment.

Corneal infiltrates

Occasionally, a soft lens wearer is found to have one or more areas of corneal infiltration. These infiltrates are gray to white in appearance, usually occur near the limbus, and are seen with an optical section or a narrow parallelopiped. They have ill-defined borders and can sometimes be mistaken for arcus senilis, except that they occur in young patients. The patient may be asymptomatic or may complain of redness of the eyes. As with giant papillary conjunctivitis and other conditions induced by the wearing of contact lenses, the infiltrates eventually go away when contact lens wear is discontinued.

Falasca and Panariello (1981) reported on four contact lens wearers found to have corneal infiltrates. All four patients complained of redness of the eyes. Only one of the patients was a hard lens wearer: the patient's problem was believed to be a result of poor lens wettability and was solved by repolishing the lenses and instructing the patient in the regular use of a rewetting solution (Blink-n-Clean). The other three patients were soft lens wearers, one of whom was found to have inferior vascularization approximately 1.5mm into the cornea. Two of the three patients were fitted with hard lenses with apparent success; infiltrates were found to recur for the third patient when successively fitted with PMMA, BP-Flex, CAB, and Polycon lenses, so contact lens wearing was ultimately discontinued. The authors speculated that corneal infiltrates occur as a result of an antigen-antibody reaction, and that the contact lens or something adherent to it plays the role of antigenic stimulus.

In an addendum to the report by Falasca and Panariello (1981), Josephson (1981) emphasized that patients should not rewear hydrogel lenses as long as the infiltrates are present. If the infiltrates are found to no longer be present after a period of 2 or 3 weeks, he suggests that the patient be instructed to wait an additional 2 or 3 weeks as a safety period before lens wear is resumed.

Fluorescein staining

One of the last procedures conducted during a soft contact lens progress visit is inspection of the eyes with the slit lamp, after lens removal, with the aid of fluorescein. This procedure is particularly important for a patient reporting symptoms of discomfort. In the author's experience, the most common forms of corneal staining are (1) desiccated areas where the lens fails to cover the cornea and (2) a generalized epithelial stippling due to sensitivity to an ingredient (such as thimerosal) of a lens-care solution or excessive coating of the lens. A less common cause of epithelial stippling is viral kerato-conjunctivitis, which is discussed later in the chapter.

Desiccated areas are most likely to occur with smaller lenses, such as the original 12.3mm Bausch & Lomb lens, when the lens decenters temporally. When this occurs, the stained, desiccated area is typically in the lower nasal portion of the cornea, just inside the limbus. This problem can usually be solved by fitting a larger lens that, even though it, too, may decenter temporally, is large enough to cover the entire cornea.

An important step in the practitioner's search for the cause of epithelial stippling is inspection of the lenses with a low-power binocular microscope (like the slit-lamp microscope) for the presence of lens coating. Lens coating is less likely to occur if a chemical disinfection system is used than if a thermal system is used. If lenses covered with lipids, mucus, and other protein materials originating from the tears are boiled, these materials are precipitated on the lenses during boiling. Most of this lens coating can be avoided by the daily use of a surfactant cleaner, but if the coating is allowed to accumulate, it can usually be removed by periodic use of a papain enzyme cleaner. However, for extensively coated lenses, even this procedure may not be effective.

Problems relating to preservatives in lens-care solutions

Some of the most perplexing problems associated with hydrogel lens wear have been those associated with preservatives used in solutions formulated for use with these lenses. Because HEMA and other hydrogel lens materials contain a high percentage of water and have a relatively large "pore size," they tend to absorb materials with which they come into contact, including components of the precorneal film and chemical preservatives in lens-care solutions. Some substances tend to adsorb onto (adhere to) the lens surfaces.

The development of hygienic care systems for PMMA lenses presented few, if any, problems. Originally, the only solution used was a wetting solution, developed by Barnes-Hind, which was used for wetting the lenses prior to insertion and also for cleaning. Lenses were originally stored dry, but when it was found that the lenses were more comfortable when kept in a hydrated condition, practitioners began to advise their patients to store their lenses overnight in water. Eventually, storage solutions were developed. Prior to the availability of cleaning solutions, some practitioners instructed their patients to periodically clean their lenses with a liquid household detergent such as Joy (and to rinse the lenses well before putting them back on).

The development of hygienic lens-care systems for hydrogel lenses, however, was an entirely different matter. Some of the preservatives routinely used in hard lens solutions, including benzalkonium chloride and chlorobutanal, were found to be absorbed and concentrated by the lenses and so could not be used. In the United States, the first hygienic lens-care system to be approved for use with hydrogel lenses, which involved unpreserved saline solution and boiling, used no chemical preservatives. However, it was soon found that the lenses became coated with proteins originating from the tears and other substances; prior to the development of surfactant cleaners and the papain enzyme cleaner, many soft lens wearers had to replace their lenses within a year or even within 6 months. Meanwhile, chemical systems were developed for use in Canada and other countries, and were eventually approved by the FDA for use in the United States. These systems use thimerosal and chlorhexidine as preservatives, but these products have been found to cause persistent problems for some lens wearers.

On the basis of experience with solutions containing thimerosal and chlorhexidine in Canada, the author's estimate is that about 5 percent of potential lens wearers are unable to use these solutions and an additional 5 percent are likely to have problems.

For the practitioner who would like to identify

those patients who may be sensitive to thimerosal, chlorhexidine, or both, a trial of several days' wear using lenses that have been stored in Flexsol is recommended. If symptoms of itching or hyperemia do not develop within the first few days or weeks of lens wear, a severe reaction in the future can be considered unlikely.

Problems with surfactant and enzyme cleaners

Surfactant cleaners are designed for nightly cleaning of lenses before storage or thermal disinfections. As described by Gold and Orenstein (1980), these cleaners remove proteins, protein-bound chlorhexidine, mucin, lipids, oils, creams, and other materials, and their use must be followed by an adequate rinsing prior to disinfection.

The papain enzyme is intended for the periodic removal of protein deposits remaining in spite of the daily use of the surfactant cleaner. Gold and Orenstein (1980) compared the action of papain enzyme when used to clean contact lenses to its action as a "tenderizing agent" in meat tenderizers. It acts by reducing the size of the protein molecules that adhere to the lens surfaces. The enzyme cleaner does not "remove" protein materials from the lens surface, so a crucial step in the use of this cleaner is to physically rub the lens to remove both the tear proteins and the papain enzyme. Otherwise, a film made up of tear protein molecules and the papain vegetable protein will remain on the lenses.

In discussing the use of the enzyme cleaner, Krezanoski (1977) advised that when papain cleaning is employed, it is most important to remove the enzyme carefully with the prophylactic detergent (surfactant) cleaner followed by thorough rinsing, and that any residual enzyme on the lens surface should be inactivated or denatured by a thermal treatment.

The compatibility of the enzyme cleaner with chemical disinfection was studied by Fichman, Baker, and Horton (1978), who selected 25 hydrogel lens wearers who had developed palpebral and bulbar conjunctival injection that was thought to be due to the fact that these patients used both the enzyme cleaner and chemical disinfection. Each of the patients was supplied with a new pair of lenses similar to the present pair and was instructed to use the chemical disinfection system but to use the enzyme cleaner once each week on the right lens only. By the end of 3 months, 20 of the 25 patients developed red right eyes (but apparently none developed red left eyes).

In an addendum to the report by Fichman et al. (1978), White pointed out that in the United States the directions for the use of the enzyme cleaner were written specifically for the Bausch & Lomb Soflens and for thermal disinfection. In other countries (where chemical disinfection is likely to be used), the directions specify that the lenses be soaked for 2 hours in the enzyme cleaner, be manually cleaned and rinsed, and then be soaked overnight in the disinfecting solution. For practitioners who would like to have their patients use the enzyme cleaner while using chemical disinfection (involving chlorhexidine as a preservative), the method described by White is recommended.

Methods of lens inspection

Numerous methods have been recommended to inspect hydrogel lenses for surface coatings or deposits. Reference has already been made to the use of the slit lamp for this procedure, as well as the method described by Remba using a 5 to 7× hand magnifier. Inexpensive, low-power binocular microscopes also are available from a number of contact lens equipment suppliers.

Bailey (1975a) recommended the use of a water cell (previously described by Poster, 1971) for inspection of the lens in the hydrated state. Such a holder is essentially a "sandwich" having a ¼-inch piece of plastic in the center and two thin plates of glass (35mm film holders or microscope slides) on the outside. To hold the lens, a hole can be drilled in the piece of plastic or a slot can be cut in the plastic. The two glass plates are cemented to the plastic (Bailey recommends silicone rubber bathtub caulk cement), and the cell is filled with distilled water. The wet cell described by Poster (1971) is shown in Figure 14.45.

To inspect the lens for surface defects and inhomogeneities in the lens material, the lens cell is held at a distance of 12–15 inches from the viewer's eye and

Figure 14.45 Water cell for inspecting soft contact lenses (redrawn from Poster, 1971).

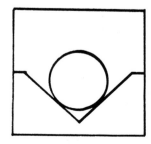

a horizontal fluorescent tube is used as a background. The cell is moved up and down to detect surface defects and deposits. For more critical inspection, Bailey (1975a) recommends the use of a $25\times$ stereomicroscope with a white cloth or other mat white material covering the stage. The microscope light is directed onto the stage behind the cell so the cell and the lens are illuminated from below by diffused light. Surface irregularities are detected by slowly moving the light back and forth so that light and dark portions are alternately seen.

Types of surface deposits

An almost endless list of inorganic and organic substances has been found to be deposited on (and in) hydrogel lenses. Krezanoski (1977) has commented that the debris found in each lens reflects each patient's tear makeup, method of handling, disinfection regimen, hygienic habits, environment, and other variables. Some of the most often identified substances include iron, mercury, calcium, proteins and lipids, and mucus.

Iron. Deposits of iron were identified on hydrogel lenses by Tsuda, Tanaka, Anan, and Yoshida (1981). These authors commented that deposits of iron particles come from the air and are often seen in lenses of patients who live or work in factory districts or near railroads. These particles sometimes can be removed by rubbing the lens surface with the fingers. The area surrounding the iron particle is stained a reddish brown.

Mercury. Deposits of mercury on the lenses of four soft lens wearers were described by Riley, Doyle, and Felty (1981). Six lenses were involved (one lens each for two patients, and two lenses each for the other two), and all lenses were badly discolored, ranging from light gray to black. The lenses were analyzed for mercury content using instrumental neutron activation analysis, and the amount of mercury in each sample was extrapolated by computer. All four patients used a lens-care routine that included saline preserved with thimerosal, and the authors suggested that mercuric sulphide may have been formed by precipitation of sulfur from rubber gaskets used in the lens containers during thermal disinfection. Riley et al. also submitted eight hydrogel lenses to 395 disinfection cycles each, using a Bausch & Lomb boiling unit and preserved saline (Boil 'n Soak). No surfactant cleaner was used, and the lenses were not handled. However, they were exposed to air to change or check saline and to inspect the lenses for color changes. After the 395 cycles, both of two Hydrocurve II lenses were found to develop gray-black mottle spots, but no such spots were found on WJ Durasoft lenses, Bausch & Lomb Soflens lenses, or Aosoft lenses (two lenses of each type were used).

Calcium. Patient-worn Bausch & Lomb Soflens lenses were inspected by Lowther, Hilbert, and King (1975), who found the lenses to have small, white spots having a crystalline appearance and a dense, lobular structure (under high magnification). These deposits developed on lenses of patients who used nondistilled water containing calcium carbonate and other materials. When new lenses were subjected to a heating cycle with nondistilled water, a crystal formation was found to develop, but the dense bulbar structure (apparently due to a component in the tear film) did not appear. The deposits on the patient-worn lenses were found to extend into the lens material almost halfway through the lens and were found to contain mucopolysaccharides and proteins originating from the tears. Freiberg (1977) found calcium deposits on new, unworn Soflens lenses that were boiled in solutions containing calcium carbonate and calcium phosphate. He stressed the importance of using only normal saline solution prepared from distilled water. He suggested that an inorganic salt on a patient-worn lens could become coated with a hydrophobic organic protein or lipid substance from the tears.

Proteins and lipids. In the reports just cited, organic proteins, lipids, and mucopolysaccharides originating from the wearer's tears were identified in hydrogel lens deposits. These deposits were thought to be deposited on preexisting calcium deposits or other inorganic salts and, therefore, were apparently "deposits on deposits" or "coatings on coatings," which would be expected to occur when patients use nondistilled water for heat disinfection of their lenses. However, Rofojo and Holly (1977) exposed hydrogel lenses to each of three protein solutions, in the absence of calcium or other inorganic salts. On the basis of the resulting deposits, they concluded that tear proteins (serum albumin, gamma globulin, and lysozyme) readily adsorb onto the surfaces of hydrogel lenses and that the adsorbed proteins are in a somewhat denatured state (especially if the patient's lenses are boiled regularly).

Mucus. Coatings on previously unworn lenses, worn for specific periods of time, were studied by

Fowler and Allansmith (1980). Lenses worn for only 30 minutes were found to have one-layer deposits over approximately 50 percent of the anterior surfaces, whereas lenses worn on a long-term basis (and routinely cleaned) were found, after a day's wear, to be covered by a thicker coating, which may have indicated that a new coating had been deposited on top of the old coating each day the lens had been worn. It was concluded that these coatings consisted of mucouslike material, which may have derived from the secretory cells of the conjunctiva and the lacrimal gland.

Giant papillary conjunctivitis

Many otherwise successful wearers of hydrogel lenses have been found to develop a syndrome consisting of mucous deposits on the lenses, mild itching, and ultimately decreased lens tolerance. Eversion of the upper lid of a patient with this syndrome reveals the presence of giant papillae similar to those seen in vernal conjunctivitis. Patients with this condition have been studied by Allansmith, Korb, Greiner, Henriquez, Simon, and Finnemore (1977), who described the following clinical stages: (1) minimal symptomatology, including increased mucus at the nasal corner of the eye on awakening; (2) mild blurring of vision and increased lens awareness; (3) increased mucous discharge, more severe itching, and excessive lens movement on blinking; and (4) a total loss of lens tolerance. On eversion of the upper lid, they found giant papillae on the tarsal conjunctiva similar to those found in vernal conjunctivitis.

Once a contact lens practitioner first sees giant papillary conjunctivitis in a hydrogel lens wearer, he or she usually incorporates eversion of both upper lids into the prefitting and progress examination routines. Fortunately, the condition clears up quickly (at least as far as symptoms are concerned) by simply discontinuing lens wear.

Both Allansmith et al. (1977) and Refojo and Holly (1977) concluded that tear proteins that adsorb onto the surface of hydrogel lenses, being in a somewhat denatured state (especially if the lenses are regularly boiled), may desorb onto the tear film and/or contact the tarsal conjunctiva. They act as an antigen in predisposed patients, thus resulting in the development of allergic conjunctivitis.

In a later study, Fowler, Greiner, and Allansmith (1979) found that mucous deposits on hydrogel lenses worn by asymptomatic wearers were similar to the deposits on lenses of wearers who had giant papillary conjunctivitis. They concluded that the development of giant papillary conjunctivitis is influenced more by individual differences in patients than by difference in lens deposits.

It has been the author's experience that giant papillary conjunctivitis occurs much more frequently with some manufacturers' hydrogel lenses than with others. This may be due to differences in lens materials or in lens finishing. The patient's original complaint often involves only one eye, and the condition tends to occur after several weeks of uneventful lens wear. By the time the patient is seen, the condition has usually reached stage 2 or 3 (as described by Allansmith et al., 1979), with the patient complaining of itching and the presence of mucus. Increased lens lag after a blink is a sure sign and is not easily missed by the practitioner, in that the blink lag of a well-fitting hydrogel lens is usually minimal. The increased lag is a result of the increased wettability of the lens (to the point of feeling slimy) as well as of the tarsal conjunctiva.

The patient should be questioned concerning lens-care procedures, particularly in regard to the daily use of a surfactant cleaner. Consideration should be given to fitting the patient with a different manufacturer's soft lenses or even with hard lenses. In many cases, the lens or lenses will be so badly coated that they will not be salvageable.

Lens contamination

When lathe-cut soft lenses first became available in Canada, some patients were found to develop a red-eye syndrome involving pronounced injection of the bulbar conjunctiva after several weeks of lens wear. When the storge solutions in these patients' lens containers were cultured, they were found to be contaminated with *Pseudomonas aeruginosa*. Fortunately, it was later concluded that even though the lenses were contaminated (apparently due to inadequate hygienic procedures on the part of the manufacturer), the red-eye syndrome was caused not by bacterial infection but by a steepening of the lenses. The problem was solved, for most patients, by refitting with flatter lenses.

These reports of contamination led to an investigation conducted at the University of Waterloo in which 107 clinic patients were fitted with soft contact lenses. The patients' tear samples and lens storage cases were cultured at regular intervals for a period of several weeks (Charles, Callender, and Grosvenor, 1973). Patients were fitted with Griffin, Bausch & Lomb, or N&N lenses, and all patients used Flexsol for lens cleaning and storage and Normol for lens rinsing. Microbial contamination of tear samples was found to decrease during soft lens wear, apparently because of the presence of residual solution preservatives (thimerosal and chlorhexidine) in the lenses.

Each wearer's lens storage case was cultured an average of four times, and microbial contamination was found in only 9 of 392 samplings (Charles et al., 1973). The wearers whose storage cases were found to be contaminated were questioned, and it was found that without exception they had not followed instructions concerning hygienic care of their lenses. Whenever contamination was found, the microbiologist filled the lens storage case with fresh Flexsol, and the microorganisms were killed in minutes. The authors concluded that when properly utilized by the wearer, the Flexsol/Normol system was a safe and effective method of hygienic lens care.

More recently, Myrowitz, Pearlman, and Goldberg (1981) reported on a patient who developed pseudomonas keratitis as a result of a contaminated lens disinfecting solution. This patient, who was a successful but intermittent wearer of soft lenses, visited a hospital emergency room complaining of a sharp, knifelike pain and photophobia in the right eye. Bacteriologic studies indicated the presence of *Pseudomonas aeruginosa* in the patient's lens solution. Treatment with Gentamycin resulted in a quiet eye after several weeks, but with 20/50+ vision and a 5mm circular corneal opacity.

An important lesson to be learned from the Myrowitz et al. (1981) case is that no matter how effective a disinfecting system is, patients can get into trouble if the system is not used correctly. In addition to being an intermittent lens wearer, this patient was reported to have rinsed the lenses with tap water. When lenses are worn only intermittently, patients often fail to think of redisinfecting lenses before wearing them after a period of several days or weeks of storage. Any residual bacteria that may be in the storage case (particularly if the patient is careless in handling the lenses) will have had an opportunity to multiply sufficiently to cause an infection.

Viral keratoconjunctivitis

Viral keratoconjunctivitis occurs in a wide variety of forms and may be due to any of several viruses. It is typically characterized by the presence of follicles in the lower tarsal conjunctiva, superficial punctate lesions in the corneal epithelium that stain with fluorescein, a watery discharge, and complaints of a foreign body sensation and photophobia. Additional findings will depend on the causative

agent. For example, pharyngoconjunctival fever ("swimming pool conjunctivitis"), usually caused by adenovirus 3, can be accompanied by a sore throat and a mild fever but usually runs its course by the end of 2 weeks. In epidemic keratoconjunctivitis, usually caused by adenovirus 8, subepithelial opacities occur beneath some of the punctate lesions and can persist for as long as a year or even longer.

Riley and Pressburger (1981) reported on a patient who was apparently free of ocular disease prior to being fitted with soft contact lenses but developed viral keratoconjunctivitis when contact lens wear was attempted. On each of four attempts to wear soft contact lenses, over a period of more than a year, the patient experienced irritation after a few hours' wear, and slit-lamp examination disclosed conjunctival injection, punctate epithelial staining, small epithelial opacities, and large follicles in the inferior fornix. The patient was referred for ophthalmological consultation, and the condition was diagnosed as a subclinical case of adenoviral involvement exacerbated by soft lens wear. The authors concluded that the disease was either pharyngoconjunctival fever or epidemic keratoconjunctivitis.

A somewhat similar case was seen by the author at the University of Houston. An otherwise successful soft lens wearer developed lens intolerance and was found to have follicles in the lower conjunctival sac and punctate epithelial staining with subepithelial opacities. Subjective symptoms were a foreign body sensation and pronounced photophobia. The staff ophthalmologist diagnosed the condition as epidemic keratoconjunctivitis and advised the patient not to wear contact lenses again until the condition had completely cleared up. The patient was monitored for a period of several months, and although lens wear was attempted on two occasions, the condition recurred each time the lenses were worn.

The highly contagious nature of epidemic keratoconjunctivitis has been stressed by Dawson (1979). He described a well-documented outbreak in which an eye, ear, nose, and throat physician developed a florid case of epidemic keratoconjunctivitis. During the physician's illness, 21 of 90 patients who visited the office for eye problems were infected with the disease. The infections were found to be associated with Schiötz tonometry, the application of eye drops, slit-lamp examination, and minor surgery. This demonstrates how important it is for practitioners to wash their hands before and after examining each patient.

The management of epidemic keratoconjunctivitis, as described by Dawson (1979), involves only supportive treatment (cold compresses and astringent drops) in the early stages. If marked subepithelial opacities occur, steroid drops may be administered three or four times a day until the opacities disappear. However, Dawson emphasized that such therapy is justified only for the rare patient whose visual acuity is so markedly reduced by the opacities that daily tasks cannot be performed.

Study Questions

1. Ignoring any effects of the contact lens on the tear layer, what power contact lens would be required for a patient whose refraction at a vertex distance of 15mm were (a) −6.00D? (b) +6.00D?

2. Why would a practitioner consider fitting a patient with hard contact lenses having (a) a toric front surface? (b) a toric back surface?

3. (a) What is the effect on the visual field of the large amount of plus lens power required in an aphakic spectacle lens? (b) Is this problem solved when a contact lens is worn instead of a spectacle lens? How?

4. How much time is required for a corneal epithelial cell to work its way outward from the germinal layer to the superficial squamous layer and be sloughed off?

5. (a) What two properties determine the gas permeability of a contact lens material? (b) How does the water content of a contact lens material affect gas permeability? (c) What factors determine the transmissivity of a contact lens?

6. List five criteria for a successful contact lens fit.

7. Briefly describe the procedures that can be used in evaluating the fit of a soft contact lens using the slit lamp.

8. What problems are aphakic patients likely to have when wearing extended-wear hydrogel lenses?

9. For wearers of PMMA lenses, what changes in corneal curvature and subjective refraction would you expect to find (a) during the first few weeks of lens wear? (b) by the end of 1 or 2 years of lens wear? (c) during the first 3 or 4 days after the abrupt discontinuation of lens wear?

10. If a contact lens has a back surface radius of curvature of 8mm, (a) what is the keratometer value of the surface? (b) what is the refracting power of the surface?

11. What effect does a hard contact lens have on corneal astigmatism, assuming that the lens is rigid enough to maintain its curvature while on the cornea?

12. What advantage does a contact lens have as compared with a spectacle lens in regard to the wearer's field of vision?

13. A patient's keratometer finding is 42.50 at 180 and 43.50 at 90, and refraction at a vertex distance of 14mm is −6.50D. If a spherical hard lens is to be fitted, its back surface having a radius of curvature 0.20mm flatter than that of the horizontal meridian of the cornea, what power should be specified for the lens?

14. If the oxygen transmission of PMMA is virtually zero, how can the cornea be supplied with adequate oxygen while wearing such a lens? What implications does this have in the fitting procedures and patient instructions for PMMA lens wearers?

15. List the advantages of correct blinking (a) for hard contact lens wearers; (b) for soft lens wearers.

16. What percentage of oxygen must be available to the cornea (a) to avoid corneal edema? (b) to maintain glycogen levels? (c) to achieve Hill's "ideal minimum"?

17. For what categories of patients are contact lenses optically superior to glasses?

18. List the parameters that are specified in an order for PMMA lenses.

19. List the various methods of determining the meridional orientation of a toric front surface hard or soft contact lens.

20. As used in hard lens fitting, describe the appearance of a fluorescein pattern indicating (a) an alignment, or "on-K," fit; (b) a "flatter-than-K" fit; (c) a "steeper-than-K" fit; (d) a satisfactory fit on a cornea having with-the-rule astigmatism.

21. List a number of methods for providing a presbyopic contact lens wearer with vision for close work.

22. Briefly describe the procedures used to evaluate the fit of a soft contact lens by means of the keratometer.

23. For what corneal disease conditions are extended-wear "bandage" lenses indicated?

24. How may (a) excessive tearing and (b) inadequate blinking be responsible for corneal edema in a contact lens wearer?

25. If new contact lenses (either hard or soft) are to be prescribed for a PMMA lens wearer who wears the lenses all day long but is having problems, what is the recommended procedure for refitting?

26. According to Cogan, to what is the avascularity of the cornea due? How can the wearing of a contact lens cause blood vessels to grow into the cornea?

27. What effect does a soft contact lens have on corneal astigmatism, assuming that the lens is flexible enough to conform to the curvature of the tear layer?

28. (a) Does a myope have to use more or less accommodation while wearing contact lenses than while wearing glasses? (b) Of what importance is this for the myopic presbyope?

29. For an aphakic patient, how does a contact lens differ from a spectacle lens in regard to the aberration of distortion? Explain your answer.

30. If a contact lens candidate is found to have a precorneal film breakup time of less than 10 seconds, what might be done in an attempt to improve the breakup time prior to making a decision on fitting contact lenses?

31. How does corneal edema for hydrogel lens wearers differ from that occurring for hard lens wearers?

32. When determining the contact lens power to be ordered for a patient by refracting the patient while wearing the best-fitting contact lens, should a spherocylindrical refraction or an equivalent sphere refracton be done? Why?

33. List the procedures that may be carried out to predict whether a prospective hard lens wearer will be a successful wearer.

34. In general, how do the fitting procedures for gas-permeable hard lenses differ from the fitting procedures used for PMMA lenses?

35. When corneal edema is found to occur with a hard lens or soft lens wearer, what steps may be taken to solve the problem?

36. What criterion is recommended for determining the base curve radius of a soft contact lens to be ordered for a given patient?

37. When considering whether to fit a patient with a spherical or a toric hydrogel lens, should the practitioner be concerned with the amount of corneal astigmatism or the amount of refractive astigmatism? Why?

38. (a) Why might it be desirable for an extended-wear patient to be examined early in the morning? (b) Why is it important for extended-wear lenses to be fitted so there is some lens movement with blinking?

39. In what way(s) do the eyes adapt, during the first few days or first few weeks of lens wear, (a) when fitted with PMMA lenses? (b) when fitted with hydrogel lenses?

40. What procedures may be used when a long-term hard lens wearer is to be fitted with spectacles for part-time (e.g., evening) wear?

41. Corneal striae are found to occur, with soft lens wearers, when the increase in corneal thickness has reached what percentage?

42. In regard to giant papillary conjunctivitis occurring as a result of hydrogel lens wear, (a) what are the patient's symptoms? (b) what are the clinical signs? (c) what is the probable mechanism responsible for the condition?

43. How does the fitting of soft contact lenses for extended wear compare to the fitting of soft contact lenses for daily wear in terms of (a) patient selection? (b) the lenses themselves? (c) the lens fit?

44. List the considerations that are of importance in patient selection for soft bifocal contact lenses, including both positive and negative factors.

45. Discuss monovision fitting in terms of (a) patient selection; (b) fitting procedures; (c) possible adaptation problems.

46. What are the advantages and disadvantages of gas-permeable hard lenses for extended wear as compared to soft lenses for extended wear?

CHAPTER 15

Prescribing Optical Aids for Low Vision

Low vision, also referred to as *partial sight* or *subnormal vision*, has been defined by Mehr and Freid (1975) as "reduced central acuity or visual field loss which even with the best optical correction provided by regular lenses still results in visual impairment from a performance standpoint" (p. 1). According to these authors, this definition assumes that (1) the vision loss is bilateral, (2) some form vision remains, and (3) "regular lenses" do not include reading additions over +4.00D, telescopes, pinholes, visors, or other unusual devices that would be categorized as low-vision aids.

The level of visual acuity necessary to impair visual performance varies to some extent from one person to another. Although corrected acuity of 20/70 or worse is usually considered to put an individual in the low-vision category, someone whose occupation or avocation requires the perception of fine detail (e.g., an accountant or machinist) may be at a serious disadvantage with corrected acuity of 20/30 or 20/40, whereas an individual whose visual requirements are not as exacting may have relatively little difficulty with acuity of 20/70 or 20/80.

Even when central acuity is reasonably good, a visual field loss can cause a significant impairment in visual performance. For example, in retinitis pigmentosa it is not uncommon for a patient to have 20/30 or 20/40 acuity in spite of the fact that the total extent of the visual field may be no more than 10 degrees. Both central acuity and the extent of the visual field are considered in the definition of *legal blindness* in the United States. To qualify for an income tax deduction as legally blind, an individual must have central acuity (with the best corrective lenses) of 20/200 or worse, or a total visual field of 20 degrees or less.

WHO ARE THE LOW-VISION PATIENTS?

The population of low-vision patients is made up mainly of two groups of people: (1) those having congenital eye diseases and diseases occurring early in life, such as retrolental fibroplasia, retinoblastoma, congenital cataracts, optic nerve disease, and retinitis pigmentosa; and (2) those having degenerative diseases occurring later in life, such as diabetic retinopathy, macular disease, senile cataracts, glaucoma, and retinal vascular disease. In terms of the total number of low-vision patients, the older patients are clearly in the majority. However, those whose visual impairment occurs early in life are at a more serious disadvantage, because the handicap will not only be present for a great number of years but also during the school years and the individual's productive, income-producing years. Nevertheless, because the great majority of low-vision patients seen by the primary care optometrist are older people whose visual impairment is due to degenerative conditions, the following discussion is directed mainly toward the care of this group of patients.

PRIMARY VERSUS SECONDARY CARE

Although the care of patients having severe low-vision problems may require a secondary care practitioner who specializes in visual rehabilitation, it is fortunate that the primary care optometrist can easily acquire the knowledge and skill necessary for the care of a high percentage of the low-vision population.

The basic knowledge of visual and optometric science already possessed by the primary care optometrist provides a firm background for an understanding of the problems in the diagnosis and treatment of the visually impaired patient. This applies particularly to the visually normal patient already under the practitioner's care who becomes a member of the low-vision population as a result of the progression of a preexisting condition or the occurrence of a degenerative disease such as macular degeneration or diabetic retinopathy. In such cases, the provision of appropriate optical aids at an early stage may enable the patient to continue in his or her usual occupation and leisure activities with little or no interruption. As the condition progresses, routine progress examinations will enable the practitioner to prescribe additional (or stronger) aids when their need is apparent. In contrast to this, the patient who has had a severe visual handicap for an extended period of time may have given up all hope of ever again living as a sighted individual, and the patient may require the sophisticated visual aids, counseling, and mobility instruction available only in practices specializing in visual rehabilitation.

EXAMINATION OF THE LOW-VISION PATIENT

Low-Vision History

The approach taken during the low-vision history will depend on whether the patient's vision problem is recently acquired or long-standing. For the patient whose problem is recently acquired, the history taking may differ little from the routine procedure. This is particularly true for a patient who has been under the practitioner's care as a normally sighted individual. In most of these cases, the nature of the preexisting ocular or systemic disease will already have been known, and the patient will already have been referred for any appropriate medical or surgical care. The procedure, therefore, differs from the routine history mainly in that the practitioner should determine (1) to what extent the reduced vision constitutes a handicap in the patient's everyday life and (2) what the patient would like to be able to do, visually, that he or she is now unable to do.

The patient having a long-standing vision problem is usually referred by a friend or acquaintance or has been brought to the practitioner by a family member. With this patient, a large number of questions will have to be asked. If the patient is senile or hard of hearing, it may be necessary to ask at least some of the questions of the family member (usually a son, daughter, or spouse) accompanying the patient.

The following questions usually will be necessary: How long has the vision problem been present? Does the patient or family member know what disease condition caused it? What forms of medical or surgical treatment have been undertaken? Is the patient now under the treatment of an ophthalmologist? What is the patient's occupation (if presently working), or if not employed, what are his or her usual daily activities? Is the patient able to read or engage in other visually oriented activities, such as watching television, sewing, other handwork, hobbies, or avocations? Is vision better in bright light or in dim light? Have vision aids other than ordinary glasses or contact lenses been prescribed? If so, have they been used successfully, and are they now being used routinely? From the patient's point of view, what is the purpose of today's examination? And finally, the universal question. What is it that the patient would like to be able to do visually that he or she is now unable to do?

The exact questions, as well as the order in which they are asked, will necessarily vary from one patient to another. The answer to a given question may make the asking of another question unnecessary or may suggest other questions that should be asked. In any case, the use of 8 or 10 appropriately phrased questions should enable the practitioner to get to the heart of the problem quickly enough to avoid unduly tiring the patient. As a final question, it is sometimes a good idea to ask, Is there anything else that you think I should know about your (or the patient's) vision problem? [For additional suggestions concerning the low-vision history, readers are referred to Mehr and Freid (1975, pp. 81–83) and Bailey (1978d).] A record form for the low-vision examination can be found in Appendix A.

Examination

Although the specific procedures and the order in which they are performed may differ to some extent from one low-vision patient to another, the following sequence of procedures is recommended as a general guide:

1. Visual acuity examination.
2. Visual field examination.
3. Ocular health examination.

4. Refraction.

5. Trial with near-vision aids.

6. Trial with distance-vision aids.

Trial with near-vision aids is usually done before trial with distance aids, because most low-vision patients are more concerned with being helped for near vision than for distance vision.

Visual acuity examination

The projected chart used for patients having normal vision is of little use in measuring the visual acuity of low-vision patients for three reasons: (1) the angular size of the largest letter (usually 20/200 or 20/400) is much too small for many low-vision patients; (2) the steps between letter sizes for the larger letters are much too large (i.e., 20/400 to 20/200–20/100); and (3) the projected chart does not allow the flexibility of testing distance that is necessary for acuity testing of the low-vision patient.

Several cardboard distance visual-acuity charts have been designed for use with low-vision patients. Among these are the Feinbloom number and letter charts and the Bailey-Lovie acuity chart. Both the Feinbloom and the Bailey-Lovie charts have been designed for use at any testing distance.

The Feinbloom charts (see Figure 15.1) are in the form of loose-leaf cards containing numbers ranging from 700–20 feet in size (designating 20/700 to 20/20 acuity if used at a distance of 20 feet), as well as cards containing letters ranging from 600–60 feet in size (for 20/600 to 20/60 acuity at 20 feet). If the Feinbloom number charts are used at a 10-foot testing distance, the range of acuities available is from 10/700 (equal to 20/1400) to 10/20 (equal to 20/40); if they are used at a 5-foot distance, the range of acuities extends from 5/700 (or 20/2800) to 5/20 (or 20/80).

The Bailey-Lovie chart (see Figure 15.2) is designed so there is a constant size progression ratio (5/4) through the chart, each row having the same number of symbols and a constant spacing being used between rows and between letters. The chart is designed on a logarithmic basis, and visual acuity is designated in terms of the logarithm of the minimum angle of resolution, or logMAR. For example, an acuity of 20/200 represents a minimum angle of resolution of 10 minutes of arc; because the logarithm of 10 is 1.0, visual acuity of 20/200 can be expressed as a logMAR of 1.0. If follows that an acuity of 20/20, representing a minimum angle of resolution of 1 minute of arc whose logarithm is 0.0, has a logMAR of 0.0. On the chart shown in Figure

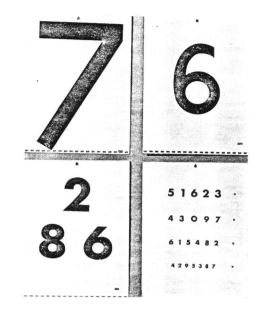

Figure 15.1 Feinbloom acuity charts for low-vision patients (Mehr and Freid, 1975).

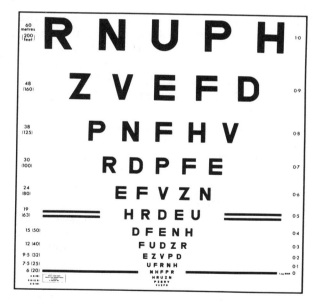

Figure 15.2 The Bailey-Lovie acuity chart. Snellen acuities are designated to the left of the chart, and logMAR acuities are designated to the right (Bailey, 1980b).

15.2, there are 10 steps between 20/200 (logMAR 1.0) and 20/20 (logMAR 0.0).

When the Bailey-Lovie chart is used at a distance other than 20 feet (or 6m), a correction factor must be applied. For example, at a distance of 16 feet (4/5 of 20 feet), the patient will be able to see an

Table 15.1 Snellen and logMAR acuity for various testing distances

20 feet		10 feet		5 feet		2.5 feet	
20/200	1.0	10/200	1.3	5/200	1.6	2.5/200	1.9
20/160	0.9	10/160	1.2	5/160	1.5	2.5/160	1.8
20/125	0.8	10/125	1.1	5/125	1.4	2.5/125	1.7
20/100	0.7	10/100	1.0	5/100	1.3	2.5/100	1.6
20/80	0.6	10/80	0.9	5/80	1.2	2.5/80	1.5
20/63	0.5	10/63	0.8	5/63	1.1	2.5/63	1.4
20/50	0.4	10/50	0.7	5/50	1.0	2.5/50	1.3
20/40	0.3	10/40	0.6	5/40	0.9	2.5/40	1.2
20/32	0.2	10/32	0.5	5/32	0.8	2.5/32	1.1
20/25	0.1	10/25	0.4	5/25	0.7	2.5/25	1.0
20/20	0.0	10/20	0.3	5/20	0.6	2.5/20	0.9

additional row of letters as compared with the 20-foot distance, because the chart is 0.1 log unit closer than the standard 20-foot distance. Therefore, a correction factor of 0.1 must be added to the patient's logMAR score at the 16-foot distance. It follows that at 12.8 feet, (4/5 of 16 feet), the patient will be able to see still another row of letters, and 0.2 (instead of 0.1) must be added for acuities taken at this distance. For any testing distance, the patient's true logMAR acuity score is determined by adding the distance correction factor to the logMAR chart score. In Table 15.1, logMAR values are shown for 20-, 10-, 5-, and 2.5-foot testing distances.

Procedure. Whether the Feinbloom, Bailey-Lovie, or other visual-acuity charts are used, it is important for the examiner to begin the visual acuity testing at a sufficiently close distance so the patient can read several symbols, or rows of symbols, on the chart. This gives the patient a feeling of accomplishment; starting the acuity test at a distance of 20 feet will discourage the patient if few letters can be seen. It is convenient to have the acuity chart mounted on a movable stand. Each position of the chart can be marked on the floor by pieces of tape or other markers, and for each distance, the refracting unit light or other light source can be adjusted to provide an adequate level of illumination.

Bailey (1980b) suggests that for a patient with very poor acuity, the clinician may decide to begin the acuity testing at a distance of 2.5 feet. If the patient is successful in reading several rows of letters at this distance, the chart is moved to 5 feet and the test repeated. The chart is next moved to 10 feet, and the patient is again asked to read as many letters or numbers as possible.

Acuity for each eye, of course, is tested separately; even if the patient claims to be blind in one eye, acuity for that eye is tested. When there is an obvious difference in acuity for the two eyes, it is preferable to determine the acuity of the better eye first at each distance. The patient should be given the opportunity to move the head so to view the symbols on the chart eccentrically, which will be necessary if there is a central scotoma. As suggested by Jose, Browning, and Brilliant (1982), if the patient has obvious difficulty reading the chart at a given distance, the examiner should not urge the patient to continue trying but to casually end the test and go on to something else.

Visual acuity should be recorded in terms of the testing distance and the letter size (e.g., 5/100, 10/40, and so forth). If the Bailey-Lovie chart is used, acuity should be recorded in terms of both Snellen and logMAR units.

Visual field examination

Whereas visual field testing for the normally sighted person is done to detect any disease condition affecting the visual fields, for a low-vision patient the main purpose of visual field testing is to determine the extent of intact retina that is available for magnification (Jose et al., 1982). An appropriate starting point for the visual field examination is the Amsler chart test, described earlier in this chapter. The examiner should use chart no. 1 initially and follow the instructions accompanying the test. If the patient has difficulty seeing the fixation dot, chart no. 2 (with diagonal lines crossing at the center) should be used. In any case, any missing lines (representing scotomatous areas) or irregularties in the line pattern should be plotted on a recording chart by the examiner.

For tangent screen testing, Jose et al. (1982) recommend the use of 6 and 20mm targets. A large *X* can be taped to the tangent screen, using masking tape, for a patient who has a central scotoma. The patient should be watched carefully during the examination for changes in fixation and for eccentric viewing. For peripheral field testing, Smith (tape no. 3) recommends that the patient be instructed to watch his or her own finger (even a totally blind person can fixate a finger). Again, large test targets should be used. Peripheral field testing will often provide additional information concerning any reported mobility problems.

Ocular health examination

Biomicroscopy, ophthalmoscopy, and tonometry should be performed in the same manner as for a normally sighted patient. Like visual field findings, the results of the ocular health examination will tend to confirm problems in fixation or mobility reported by the patient. The results of field testing and ocular health testing will enable the practitioner to confirm the previously diagnosed cause of the patient's visual loss. If there is any doubt concerning the stability of the condition responsible for the visual loss (i.e., whether medical or surgical treatment is indicated), ophthalmological consultation should be provided.

Refraction

Keratometry. Unless keratometry findings are included in the patient's previous record, the refractive examination should begin with keratometry. Because many low-vision patients will have opaque media (making retinoscopy difficult), information concerning astigmatism obtained by keratometry can be of great importance. For patients of any age, the application of Javal's rule will predict refractive astigmatism with reasonable accuracy. Neither nystagmus nor the presence of a central scotoma makes keratometry impossible. If the patient is asked to "look down the center of the tube," fixation often will be accurate enough so a usable keratometry finding can be obtained.

Retinoscopy. Retinoscopy and subjective testing should be done with a trial frame and trial lenses. With trial lenses, it will be possible for the examiner to watch the patient's eyes and determine whether central or eccentric fixation is used. If there are opacities in the media, radical retinoscopy should be done. The examiner moves in to whatever distance is necessary (i.e., 33, 25, or 20cm) to obtain a retinoscope reflex and subtracts the appropriate working distance lens power (i.e., 3.00, 4.00, or 5.00D) from the finding. Care should be taken to stay as close as possible to the patient's visual axis.

Subjective refraction. For subjective refraction, the chart should be placed at the 10-foot distance if visual acuity was found to be adequate at that distance. Otherwise, a closer distance may have to be used. If retinoscopy was not possible, the subjective testing should begin with large lens changes. Bailey (1978b) suggests that subjective testing begin with +6.00D, plano, and −6.00D lenses, with succeeding lens powers being used to "bracket" the patient's refractive end-point. In all cases, large, abrupt lens changes should be made. It is not reasonable to expect a patient who has reduced visual acuity to be able to respond subjec-

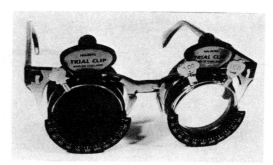

Figure 15.3   Halberg clips for use in overrefraction (Bailey, 1978d).

tively to lens changes as low as 0.25D or even 0.50D.

If the patient has a previous spectacle correction, Bailey (1978d) recommends that an overrefraction be done using Halberg clips. As shown in Figure 15.3, Halberg clips are placed over the patient's existing spectacle correction, each clip having two cells for trial lenses. If the overrefraction involves cylindrical lenses, the examiner simply takes the spectacles—with Halberg clips and trial lenses—to the lensometer and reads the back vertex power of the combination.

Binocular vision testing. For a low-vision patient, binocular vision testing is usually limited to the cover tests at distance and near, using test objects sufficiently large to be seen by the patient. In interpreting the results of the cover tests, the possibility of a central scotoma and, therefore, eccentric fixation in one or both eyes must be kept in mind.

Trial with near-vision aids

The simplest form of near-vision aid for a low-vision patient is a *high addition*, either in the form of a bifocal addition or a lens intended strictly for near vision. Magnification brought about by a high addition, as specified by lens manufacturers, is based on the concept of a 25cm reading distance being the least distance of distinct vision. The magnification existing when an individual looks at an object located 25cm from the spectacle plane is considered to be 1 ×; magnification increases proportionately as the object is placed at distances closer than 25cm. The effect of object distance on retinal image size is shown in Figure 15.4. The retinal image for a distance of 12.5cm will be twice as large (2×) as for a distance of 25cm; the retinal image for a distance of 5cm will be five times as large (5×) as for a distance of 25cm.

Using this system, the lens power required to

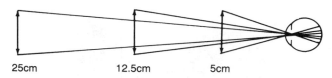

25cm   12.5cm   5cm

Figure 15.4   The effect of object distance on retinal image size (relative distance magnification). At 5cm the retinal image is five times as large as when the same object is placed at 25cm.

bring about a given level of magnification will depend on whether the patient is considered to make use of accommodation while using the high addition. For example, a child who has a large amplitude of accommodation may be able to read at a distance of 25cm without the need for an addition, but an elderly patient who is an absolute presbyope would require a +4.00D addition for a 25cm reading distance. The addition would have to be increased to +8.00D for a 12.5cm reading distance (for 2× magnification) and to +20.00D for a 5cm reading distance (for 5× magnification).

Unfortunately, many systems of specifying magnification of low-vision aids are currently in use. In the system just described, the magnification and the power of a bifocal addition to bring about that magnification (assuming that no accommodation is being used) are related by the simple formula:

$$\text{Magnification} = \frac{F_e}{4},$$

where

F_e = the equivalent power of the bifocal addition or reading lens.

Although this system is favored by lens manufacturers, practitioners usually favor a system based on a normal reading distance of 40cm (rather than 25cm). Rosenberg (1981) has recommended that magnification be specified in terms of equivalent power of the lens. This system has the advantage that it does not presuppose a particular reading distance, and therefore it can be applied to any aid for near vision without regard to the intended reading distance.

Specification of print size

Bailey (1978c) reviewed a number of systems for specifying print size for near vision and recommended the use of the *M system* because it is compatible with the traditional Snellen method of

denoting visual acuity. Using the M system, the size of the print is indicated by the distance in meters at which lowercase letters (without ascenders or descenders) subtend 5 minutes of arc. For 1M print, letters such as *x*, *o*, *a*, or *c* subtend 5 minutes of arc at a distance of 1m. When used at a distance of 40cm, a 1M letter subtends an angle of 2.5(5), or 12.5 minutes of arc, and is therefore the equivalent of a 20/50 reduced Snellen letter. This acuity is recorded, using the M system, as 0.40/1M.

As long as only the 40cm reading distance is considered, the numerator of the *M* fraction remains the same, and the denominator increases with increasing print size. For example, 0.40/2M would indicate that the patient can read 2M print (twice as large as 1M print) at 40cm; 0.40/4M would indicate that the patient can read print four times as large as 1M print at 40cm. For a 20cm distance, the fraction 0.20/1M indicates that the patient can read 1M print at that distance.

Near acuity charts. In *Clinical Low Vision*, Faye (1976) recommends the use of both single letter charts and continuous text reading charts for determining near acuity of a low-vision patient. The single letter chart is used only for rapid screening of acuity prior to the use of the continuous text chart. Faye recommends the Lighthouse near acuity chart with sans serif letters (see Figure 15.5) for single letter acuity and the Sloan-Lighthouse reading acuity cards (see Figure 15.6) for continuous text acuity. Both the Lighthouse cards and the Sloan-Lighthouse cards are designated in M-system acuity.

Determining power of the reading addition

In general, a person having a 20/50 reduced Snellen acuity at a distance of 40cm is able to read normal newspaper, book, or magazine print. Because 20/50 print at 40cm is the equivalent of 1M print, the practitioner can estimate the reading addition that will be required for a patient on the basis of the size of the print that can be read, using the M system, at a distance of 40cm (or, if necessary, at a closer distance). For example, if a presbyopic patient can read 4M print at a distance of 40cm with a +2.50D addition, it will be necessary to make the angular size of the print four times as large if 1M print is to be read. This can be done by moving the print to a distance of one-fourth the 40cm distance, or 10cm. At 10cm, a +10.00D addition will be required. To take another example, a presbyopic patient who can read only 8M print at 40cm would require print having an angular size eight times as large as it is at 40cm. This would require moving the 1M print to one-eighth of the 40cm distance, or 5cm, therefore requiring a +20.00D addition.

It should be understood that the system described here provides the practitioner with only a tentative addition. The addition should be placed in the trial frame, and the patient, seated at a table or desk,

Figure 15.5 Lighthouse near acuity chart (Faye, 1976).

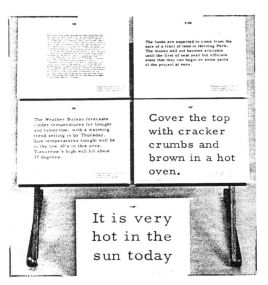

Figure 15.6 Sloan-Lighthouse reading acuity card (Faye, 1976).

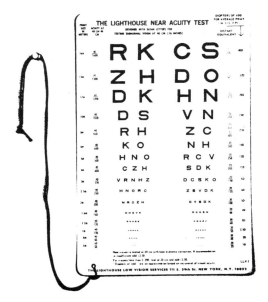

should be given the opportunity to read a magazine or newspaper with the lens. Subsequently, stronger or weaker additions at correspondingly closer or farther distances can be tried. For lenses of greater than about +10.00D in power, trial case lenses (being biconvex in form) introduce large amounts of distortion, oblique astigmatism, and curvature of image. Therefore, for additions of high power, lenses of the kind to be prescribed (e.g., American Optical aspheric lenses or Feinbloom microscopic lenses) should be used rather than trial case lenses; tentative additions (based on both reduced Snellen and M-system acuity) for various levels of visual acuity at 40cm are shown in Table 15.2

Trial with distance-vision aids

Distance-vision aids for low-vision patients are usually *afocal telescopes*. An afocal telescope is designed in such a way that if parallel rays of light enter the objective, parallel rays will emerge from the eyepiece. However, if an afocal telescope is used at a distance closer than infinity, the divergence of the rays of light entering the objective will be greatly increased when the rays emerge from the eyepiece. This increase in the divergence of light that occurs when an afocal telescope is used to view an object at a finite distance has been referred to by Bailey (1978e) as the vergence amplification effect. The value of the vergence amplification effect is the square of the magnification brought about by the telescope in question. For a $3\times$ telescope, the vergence amplification effect is equal to 3^2, or 9. As shown by Bailey, if a $3\times$ afocal telescope is used to view an object at a distance of 4m, the vergence of light rays entering the objective (0.25D) is increased by a factor of 9, so light emerging from the eyepiece has a vergence of 9(0.25), or 2.25D, thus requiring 2.25D of accommodation on the part of the wearer.

When afocal telescopes are used as trial aids with

Table 15.2 Tentative high additions and reading distance based on Snellen and M-system acuity (assuming no patient accommodation).

Snellen	M system	Addition	Distance
20/50	0.40/1M	+2.50D	40cm
20/100	0.40/2M	+5.00D	20
20/150	0.40/3M	+7.50D	13.3
20/200	0.40/4M	+10.00D	10
20/300	0.40/6M	+15.00D	6.7
20/400	0.40/8M	+20.00D	5

low-vision patients, the vergence amplification effect can be avoided by holding in front of the afocal telescope a lens of the power indicated by the object distance (i.e., +0.25D for a 4m distance, +0.50D for a 2m distance, and so forth). However, if the telescope being tried has a knurled focusing ring, the use of a plus lens in front of the objective lens will not be necessary.

Jose et al. (1982) have suggested that only two telescopes are needed to assess a low-vision patient's prognosis for successful telescope use: a 2.5× monocular telescope and a combination 6×/8× moncular telescope. They suggest that the appropriate telescope can be determined on the basis of the following guide:

Best corrected distance acuity	Magnification
20/100	2.5×
20/100–20/300	6.0×
20/300–20/600	8.0×

If the best corrected distance acuity is poorer than 20/600, Jose et al. state that the prognosis is poor for the use of a telescope without extended training. These authors have suggested the following procedures for the use of trial telescopes:

1. The doctor should focus the telescope initially for a 10-foot viewing distance.
2. The patient first should be asked to locate a large object at the end of the examination room. Having the patient find the doctor's white coat while standing next to the chart is a useful way to orient the patient concerning the location of the chart.
3. The test should be discontinued if the patient cannot find the chart within a few minutes.
4. For the 6× telescope, the successful patient is the one who quickly finds the chart at an acuity level six times that of the best corrected distance acuity (e.g., from 20/300 to 20/50). (Jose et al., 1982.)

Types of afocal telescopes

Ophthalmic telescopes are available in either Galilean or Keplerian designs. A Galilean telescope has a convex objective and a concave ocular, and its use is confined to telescopes having a magnification in the range of 1× to 3× or 4×. A Keplerian telescope has a convex objective and a convex ocular, and it requires an erecting prism to erect the otherwise inverted image. While Galilean telescopes can be used for head-borne telescopes of low power, Keplerian telescopes (because of the need for an erecting prism) are bulky and, therefore, are used mainly as hand-held telescopes for specific tasks such as identifying the number on a bus or the name of a street. Keplerian telescopes are available in powers ranging from 3× to as high as 15×.

Telescopes for near vision

Due to the vergence amplification effect, when a telescope is used for near vision, a convex lens in the form of a "reading cap" must be mounted in front of the objective. The reading cap has a power equal to the reciprocal of the reading distance (e.g., a +5.00D lens for a 20cm reading distance). The advantage of a telescope with a reading cap, as compared with a high addition for near work, is that for equal magnification, a greater working distance can be obtained. However, this greater working distance is obtained at the expense of a smaller field of view.

PRESCRIBING FOR THE LOW-VISION PATIENT

Visual tasks for the low-vision patient, like those for the normally sighted patient, can be categorized as either distance-vision or near-vision tasks. Distance-vision tasks tend to be related to mobility, whereas near-vision tasks are related to sedentary activities such as reading and various kinds of handwork. An elderly patient who is in poor health and is not physically fit may not wish to be mobile and, therefore, may benefit mainly from the use of near-vision aids. In contrast, a healthy, alert individual will want to take advantage of aids that will increase mobility as well as those that will make reading and other near-vision tasks possible.

Aids for distance vision are in the form of *afocal telescopes*. The Galilean telescope, having a convex objective and a concave eyepiece, is limited in magnifying power to no more than 2 or 3× when used as an aid for low vision, but it is sufficiently compact to be used as a head-borne (worn in a spectacle frame) visual aid. The Keplerian telescope, having a convex objective and a convex eyepiece, can be obtained in magnifying powers as high as 15×. However, because of the need for an erecting prism, this form of telescope is bulky and is used mainly as a hand-held (rather than a head-borne) aid.

Most aids for near vision, including high-addition bifocals and high plus reading glasses, are classified as *microscopes*. The term *microscope* used here infers no specific appearance of the aid or number of lenses involved: a microscope may involve only a single lens or two or more lenses. Another form of near-vision aid is a telescope with a reading cap. Additional near-vision aids include many varieties of hand-held magnifiers and stand magnifiers.

In recent decades, many sophisticated (and expensive) aids for low vision have been introduced. These include projection magnifiers, closed-circuit television, and aids making use of fiber optics. Because such aids are not likely to be used by the primary care optometrist, they are not discussed here.

AIDS FOR DISTANCE VISION

For a discussion of the optical principles of afocal telescopes, the reader is referred to any standard optics textbook or to Bailey (1981). For either the Galilean telescope (see Figure 15.7a) or the Keplerian telescope (see Figure 15.7b), both the object and the image are located at infinity ("parallel rays in, parallel rays out"). For either form of telescope, the magnification is equal to the refracting power of the eyepiece divided by the refracting power of the objective,

$$M = -\frac{F_2}{F_1},$$

and the separation of the objective and the eyepiece, or the thickness (t) of the telescope, is equal to the secondary focal length of the objective minus the primary focal length of the eyepiece,

$$t = f'_1 - f_2 = \frac{1}{F_1} + \frac{1}{F_2}.$$

Head-Borne Telescopes

With few exceptions, head-borne aids for distance vision are Galilean telescopes. Among the most popular head-borne telescopes are those designed by William Feinbloom and marketed under the name Designs for Vision. These are available as full-diameter telescopes and as Bioptic telescopes. The full-diameter telescope (see Figure 15.8a) as the name implies, extends over the entire aperture of the spectacle lens, whereas the Bioptic telescope (see Figure 15.8b) is a smaller-diameter telescope confined to the upper portion of a carrier lens. Lenses correcting the patient's refractive error can be incorporated into the telescope and the carrier lens. Full-diameter telescopes are available in magnifying powers of 1.3, 1.7, and 2.2×, whereas Bioptic telescopes are available in powers of 2.2, 3, and 4×.

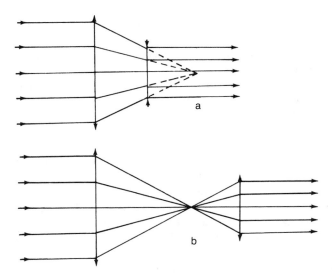

Figure 15.7 Afocal telescopes: *(a)* Galilean; *(b)* Keplerian.

Bailey (1978a) commented that the most useful of the Bioptic telescopes in his experience has been the 2.2×.

Bipotic telescopes are also available in Keplerian form. These are referred to as expanded field telescopes, having magnifying powers of 3, 4, and 6×. As described by Bailey (1978a), these telescopes have a wider field of view than the Galilean Bioptic telescopes but are longer, heavier, and cost about three times as much.

When a telescopic system is used for distance vision, the practitioner can expect distance acuity to improve by the amount indicated by the magnifying power of the telescope. For example, if a patient's best corrected distance acuity is 20/200, it should be improved to 20/100 with a 2× telescope, to 20/70 with a 3× telescope, or to 20/50 with a 4× telescope. However, in the presence of an extremely constricted visual field, as may occur in the later stages of retinitis pigmentosa, a higher power

Figure 15.8 Designs for Vision telescopes: *(a)* 2.2× full-diameter; *(b)* 2.2× Bioptic telescopes.

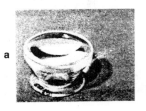
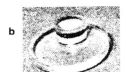

telescope may have the effect of extending the image of the fixated object onto the nonseeing portion of retina and thus hinder visual acuity rather than helping it.

Nonprescription head-borne telescopes known as *sportscopes* are available from a number of manufacturers. Because these telescopes are made in quantity (not being intended only for low-vision patients), they are relatively inexpensive. They have the additional advantages that (1) either of the two telescopes can be individually focused to provide a spherical equivalent correction, (2) they can be adjusted for interpupillary distance, and (3) either telescope can be removed from the frame and used as a monocular. The Selsi 2.8× sportscope is shown in Figure 15.9a.

Another popular form of nonprescription head-borne telescope is the monocular clip-on telescopic unit. These are intended to be worn, when needed, over the patient's distance correction. Clip-on units are available from Albert Aloe and from Selsi. Each unit has a magnifying power of 2.5× and can be focused. The Selsi model (see Figure 15.9b) also has an adapter ring in which a near addition can be mounted.

Hand-Held Telescopes

Although head-borne telescopes are available in magnifying powers as high as 6×, such high magnifying powers are not practical for constant wear. Even in Bioptic form, Bailey (as already noted) considers the 2.2× the most useful magnifying power. The sportscopes and clip-on units, designed so they do not have to be worn for constant wear, have magnifying powers of only 2.5 and 2.8×.

Higher magnifying powers in the form of hand-held telescopes are useful for patients whose best

Figure 15.9 Nonprescription telescopes: *(a)* Selsi 2.8× sportscope: *(b)* Selsi 2.5× clip-on telescope with ring for reading addition; *(c)* Selsi 6×/8× hand-held telescope.

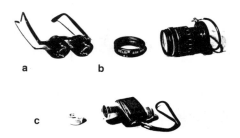

corrected distance acuity is about 20/200 to 20/600; they are used for such momentary visual tasks as identifying a street sign or the route number of a bus. Examples of these aids are the Selsi Miniscope (see Figure 15.9c), which is provided with two interchangeable objective lenses, one providing 6× and the other providing 8× magnification; and the Selsi Miniature Monocular, available in both 6 and 10× magnifying powers.

Jose et al. (1982) advise that if a patient's best corrected visual acuity is poorer than 20/600 (10/300), prognosis is poor for the use of a telescope without extended training. However, even with this low level of visual acuity, aids for near vision can often be used successfully.

AIDS FOR NEAR VISION

Although magnification for head-borne distance-vision aids is limited for all practical purposes to no more than about 3×, much higher magnifying powers can be achieved for near vision by virtue of the increase in retinal image size that occurs when reading material is held closer than the normal reading distance. As shown in Figure 15.4, if 25cm is considered to be the "normal" reading distance, placing reading material at a distance of 5cm provides a retinal image five times the size of that for the 25cm distance. Using the magnification system used by lens manufacturers (and assuming that the patient is a complete presbyope), 5× magnification would be produced by a +20.00D addition, and 10× magnification would be produced by a +40.00D addition. It should be understood that this magnification is not produced by the lens itself but by virtue of the fact that the lens makes a much closer reading distance possible, thereby increasing the retinal image size. This form of magnification is sometimes called *relative distance magnification*.

Most vision practitioners favor a 40cm reading distance rather than the 25cm distance; because of the confusion concerning reading distance, and it has been recommended that microscopic lenses be designated in terms of equivalent refracting power rather than magnifying power. If the practitioner uses a chart in which acuity is designated according to the M system (such as the Lighthouse near acuity chart or the Sloan-Lighthouse reading acuity cards) at a distance of 40cm, the required reading addition can be estimated on the basis of the smallest print the patient is able to read. If the patient can read 1M print at 40cm, only a +2.50D addition is required;

however, if the smallest print the patient can read at 40cm is 4M print, a +10.00D addition, or 4(+2.50), is required, along with a reading distance of 10cm.

Head-Borne Microscopic or High-Addition Lenses

For a practitioner who is just beginning to be involved in low-vision care, one of the main obstacles will be to abolish the idea that "you never prescribe an addition stronger than +2.50D." Many patients with recently developed low-vision problems will require additions no higher than +3.00 or +4.00D to read 1M print at the distance indicated by the addition (33 or 25cm). In these cases, no "special" lenses are required: ordinary bifocals or reading glasses can be used, as long as the lenses are properly centered for the closer reading distance.

A wide variety of microscopic aids are available. The patient's distance prescription can be incorporated in some, but not all, of these aids. For simplicity, only some of the more commonly used aids are described here.

The American Optical Corporation has available both glass and plastic microscopic lenses (see Figure 15.10). The glass microscopic lenses are available in magnifying powers of 2, 4, 6, and 8× and are in bifocal form. The patient's distance prescription can be incorporated in the carrier lens. AOlite plastic aspheric lenses are available in magnifying powers of 6, 8, 10, and 12×. These are single-vision lenses rather than bifocals, and it is not possible to incorporate the distance correction. AOlite lenses are also available as half-eye lenses mounted in frames, in back vertex powers of +6.00, +8.00, and +10.00D. (Note that these are relatively low powers, corresponding to magnifying powers of 1.5, 2, and 2.5×.)

Volk Conoid lenses are glass aspheric lenses available from the American Bifocal Company. They are full-diameter (not bifocal) lenses, allowing the incorporation of a cylindrical correction, and are available in refracting powers of +15.00 to +50.00D. Stronger lenses (in powers as high as +100.00D) are available but without the possibility of including a cylindrical correction (Mehr and Freid, 1975).

Both full-diameter and bifocal microscopes are available from Designs for Vision (Figure 15.11). The full-diameter microscopes are available in magnifying powers from 2 through 20×, and the patient's distance prescription can be included. The bifocal microscopes are available in magnifications ranging from 2 through 10×, and the distance prescription can be ground into the carrier lens.

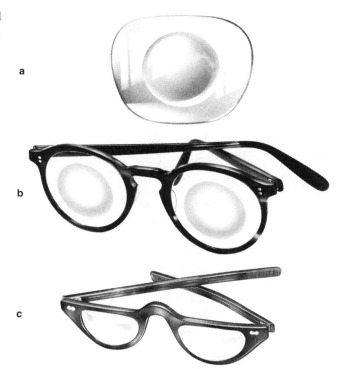

Figure 15.10 American Optical microscopic lenses: (a) glass; (b) AOLite plastic aspheric; (c) AOLite plastic aspheric half eyes.

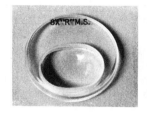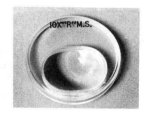

Figure 15.11 Designs for Vision bifocal microscopes: (left) 8× and (right) 10×.

Centration of High-Addition Lenses

When microscopic or high-addition lenses are prescribed for both eyes, centration becomes an important factor because of the unusually close reading distances required. The decision to prescribe high-addition lenses for both eyes or for just one eye depends on a number of factors. If the visual acuity of one eye is much poorer than the other eye (e.g., 20/400 versus 20/50 with the required reading addition), it is preferable to prescribe a high addition only for the better eye and provide a "dummy" lens for the poorer eye. However, if acuity is about the same for the two eyes, it is usually advisable to prescribe for both eyes.

Bailey (1979) suggested that a patient's binocularity at near can be tested quickly and easily by the bar reading test. If a pencil is held vertically about halfway between the eyes and the printed page, it will block out a vertical strip of print if the patient is reading monocularly but not if the patient is reading binocularly. In the same article, Bailey made the point that binocularity becomes impractical for working distances closer than 10cm, and that the amount of decentration required when high additions are prescribed binocularly can be determined by the use of the following rule of thumb: for each diopter of working distance, give 1.5mm of decentration (total for both eyes); if the distance PD is more than 65mm, give an additional 1mm of decentration.

Rather than using the rule of thumb, the decentration can be calculated by use of a simple formula:

$$\text{Total decentration} = \frac{27\,(\text{distance PD})}{\text{working distance} + 27}.$$

Referring to Figure 15.12, *27* represents the 27mm distance from the spectacle plane to the imaginary line joining the centers of rotation of the eyes; all

Figure 15.12 Method of calculating decentration for high additions. The formula,
$$\textbf{Total decentration} = \frac{\textbf{27\,(distance PD)}}{\textbf{working distance} + \textbf{27}},$$
is derived on the basis of the similar triangles, ABC and A′B′C. In this example, for a 64mm distance PD and a working distance of 100mm, or 10cm, each lens must be decentered in 7mm.

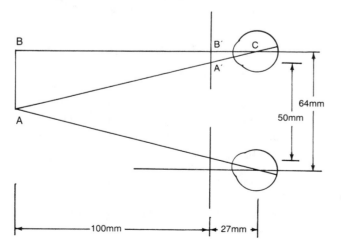

distances are specified in millimeters. For example, if the patient's distance PD is 64mm and the working distance is to be 10cm (using a +10.00D addition), the total decentration (for both lenses) will be

$$\text{Total decentration} = \frac{27(64)}{127}$$

$$= 14\text{mm; or 7mm per lens.}$$

The 27mm distance is only an approximate distance based on an average vertex distance of 13mm and an average center of rotation distance of 14mm. In individual cases (e.g., where there is a particularly short or particularly long vertex distance), a lower or higher value can be used.

Telescopes with Reading Caps

When an afocal telescope is prescribed for distance vision, it can be adapted for near vision by placing a reading cap on the front of the telescope. For a given reading distance, the power of the reading cap must be the same as it would be in the absence of the telescope. For example, a +8.00D reading cap would be required for a 12.5cm reading distance. However, the total magnification will be the product of that brought about by the telescope and that due to the object distance. If in the previous example the telescope had a magnifying power of 2×, the total magnifying power of the combination would be

$$(2\times)(2\times) = 4\times.$$

Most ophthalmic telescopes, such as those made by Designs for Vision, have reading caps available in a range of powers.

The combination of a distance telescope and a reading cap, often referred to as a *telemicroscope*, has the advantage of providing a greater working distance for a given amount of magnification but with a somewhat reduced field of view. In our example, the combination provides a magnification of 4× at a working distance of 12.5cm, whereas with a high addition and no telescope, a magnification of 4× would require a working distance of 6.25cm. Telemicroscopes, therefore, are advantageous for individuals who must be able to work at as great a distance as possible. Individuals in this category include a typist who must place the copy to be typed at a distance no closer than 10 or 12 inches or a pianist who must be able to see the music at about the same distance. Designs for Vision makes a combination bifocal microscope and Bioptic telescope with a reading cap, called the *Trioptic* (see Figure 15.13).

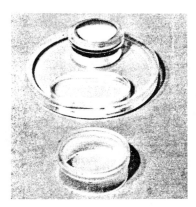

Figure 15.13   Designs for Vision Trioptic: a combination of a Bioptic telescope and a bifocal microscope. A reading cap for the telescope is shown below. The wearer has four components to choose from: the distance correction in the unmagnified carrier portion, the afocal telescope, the telescope with the reading cap, and the microscope.

Hand Magnifiers

Hand magnifiers are particularly useful for specific short-term tasks, such as reading a menu or looking up a telephone number, but they can also be used for extended reading. If a hand magnifier is held at a distance from the printed page equal to its focal length, the patient will see an enlarged, erect image of the print. The image will be formed at infinity, so it will be seen clearly through the patient's distance correction without the need to accommodate. However, if the patient looks through an ordinary bifocal while holding the magnifier in the same position, the print will become blurred and will clear up only if the magnifier is moved closer to the page.

Bailey (1980a) discussed the optical principles involved when a hand magnifier is used in combination with a bifocal addition by a completely presbyopic patient. If the magnifier and the bifocal addition are each considered thin lenses, the equivalent power (F_e) of the system is indicated by the formula

$$F_e = F_1 + F_2 - zF_1F_2,$$

where

F_1 = the power of the magnifier

F_2 = the power of the bifocal addition

z = the separation between the two lenses.

Inspection of this formula indicates that if the two lenses are in contact (in which case $z = 0$), the third term drops out, and the effective power of the system is equal to the combined power of the lenses ($F_1 + F_2$). In his discussion, Bailey (1980a) pointed out that when the lenses are separated by a distance equal to the focal length of either the magnifier or the bifocal addition, both the second and third (or first and third) terms drop out, with the result that the refracting power of the system is equal to the power of just one of the lenses. For example, if the lenses are separated by a distance equal to the focal length of the magnifier so that $z = f_1$, the equivalent power of the system becomes

$$F_e = F_1 + F_2 - f_1F_1F_2 = F_1.$$

If the lenses are separated by a distance equal to the focal length of the reading addition so that $z = f_2$, the equivalent power becomes

$$F_e = F_1 + F_2 - f_2F_1F_2 = F_2.$$

Further, when the patient holds the magnifier so it is farther than one focal length from the spectacle lens, the power of the bifocal addition makes a negative contribution to the total equivalent power of the system. Therefore, it can be concluded that when a hand magnifier is to be held at a distance from the reading material greater than its focal length, the patient should use distance correction to have the maximum magnifying power. By using the bifocal rather than the distance correction, the total equivalent power would be less than that due to the magnifier, and the greater the power of the addition, the less will be the total power (Bailey, 1980a).

An additional method of using a hand magnifier is for the patient to hold the magnifier in contact with distance correction—using it, in effect, as a high addition. This requires that the patient move in close to the print, as with a high addition. Faye (1976) pointed out that some patients resist a high addition in spectacle form but are willing to use a hand magnifier. For these patients, a hand magnifier held against the spectacle correction serves as a simple and inexpensive method for the patient to gain experience with a high addition. After practicing with a hand magnifier in this manner, the patient may eventually request or accept a high addition in spectacle form.

Faye (1976) suggests that when a patient begins to use a hand magnifier, while wearing the distance correction the patient should first place the magnifier close to the page and then raise is slowly until

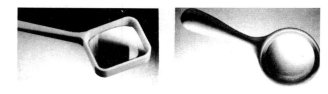

Figure 15.14   COIL aspheric hand magnifiers.

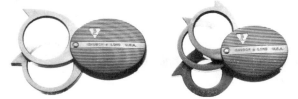

Figure 15.15   Bausch   &   Lomb   pocket magnifiers.

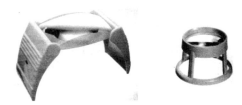

Figure 15.16   COIL stand magnifiers.

the image is increased to its maximum size without distortion.

Combined Optical Instruments Limited (COIL) markets a series of plastic aspheric hand magnifiers in various powers (see Figure 15.14). A number of companies manufacture pocket magnifiers. Bausch & Lomb has available a series of pocket magnifiers in a wide range of magnifying powers (see Figure 15.15). These magnifiers have one, two, or three lenses.

Stand Magnifiers

A stand magnifier (see Figure 15.16) is similar to a hand magnifier but is provided with a support so that a constant distance from the page can be maintained. To reduce the effects of peripheral aberrations, the page-to-magnifier distance is usually set at slightly less than the magnifier's focal length. Faye (1976) made the point that the image is intended to be viewed from a normal reading distance (40cm with a +2.50D addition). She also suggested that patients be instructed to look directly into the lens

because aberrations are accentuated by viewing the image from an angle.

An interesting variation of the stand magnifier is what is sometimes called a *paperweight magnifier*. This is a thick, planoconvex lens that the patient slides along the page. One such magnifier is called the Visolett. Although their magnifying power is relatively small, paperweight magnifiers are popular with low-vision patients. An advantage of this form of magnifier is that, unlike most other stand magnifiers, it is not necessary for the light to be perpendicular to the lens surface at the pole. This magnifier also has good light-gathering properties.

Training in the Use of Near-Vision Aids

When high-addition lenses are first prescribed for a recent visual loss, many patients expect that the new lenses will enable them to read at their accustomed distance. Even after the situation is carefully explained to them, patients have a tendency to resist holding reading material sufficiently close.

Training should begin during the original examination, when the patient is first introduced to near-vision aids, and it should be continued when the aid is dispensed. The patient must be able to demonstrate ability in using the aid successfully before it is taken home. Additional training sessions should be scheduled as needed.

During training sessions, the patient should be seated at a table, with adequate illumination in the form of a goose-neck lamp or other adjustable reading lamp. Magazines, newspapers, and books should be available in various sizes of print. For aids requiring very close reading distances, a recommended method is to have the patient begin with the nose touching the print and to gradually back away until the print is in focus. Due to the small depth of focus of high plus lenses, the patient will have to maintain the reading distance very precisely for the print to remain in focus.

Because the field of view for most near-vision aids is very small, the patient may have difficulty proceeding along the correct line of print and will almost certainly have trouble finding where the next line of print begins. These problems can be solved by having the patient move the finger along the print or by having him or her move a card (such as a 3 × 5 index card) along underneath the print. Another good method of keeping the print in view is to have the patient use a typoscope (see Figure 15.17). This aid not only helps the patient stay on the correct line

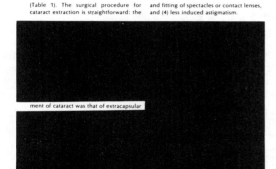

(Table 1). The surgical procedure for cataract extraction is straightforward: the

ment of cataract was that of extracapsular

and fitting of spectacles or contact lenses, and (4) less induced astigmatism.

leaves the lens capsule in place and therefore is a modification of earlier extracapsular techniques.[2]

The controversy surrounding phako-emulsification is whether the advantages of the technique outweigh its disadvantages.[3] The advantages are: (1) smaller incision compared with more conventional procedures (about 25 vs. 160 degrees); (2) reduced complications of wound healing; (3) faster patient rehabilitation with respect to hospitalization time

debated among ophthalmologists. The debate focuses on whether the phako-emulsification technique reduces the risk of retinal tears or increases the risk of macular edema. Epidemiological studies are needed to resolve this question. Most likely the technique will be a supplemental one added to the routine intracapsular procedures.

If the phakoemulsification technique is to be used, the ophthalmologist should be asked about his rate of success and the

Figure 15.17   A typoscope assists the reader in staying on the correct line and also reduces glare. Typoscopes are available from Designs for Vision and other suppliers or can be made using cardboard or plastic.

of letters but reduces the glare from the page surrounding the line of print being read.

It is usually helpful to have the patient begin by reading print (with the newly prescribed aid) that is somewhat larger than normal print. Have a large-print book or a large-print copy of *Reader's Digest* available, or have the patient begin by reading newspaper headlines. Goodlaw has designed a reading chart that includes print varying in size from 36-point newspaper headline type through book, newspaper, and telephone directory type (Mehr and Freid, 1975, p. 158).

It is important for patients to understand that, because the image of the print will be spread out over a larger-than-normal area of the retina, more than the normal amount of illumination may be required. The patient or a family member should be instructed to obtain an adjustable reading lamp of the kind used for the training.

Accessory Items

A number of helpful items are available, and all low-vision patients should be told about them. Because short reading distances require the patient to hold the book or other reading material upward at an angle or tilt the head downward almost to the surface of the table or desk, many patients find that reading is more convenient if a reading stand is used. The patient should be encouraged to write with a black, felt-tipped pen on lined paper having large spaces between lines. Family members and others who write letters to the patient should be encouraged to do the same. Other items that can be helpful are needle threaders, music stands for piano music, large-number dials for telephones, and large-sized playing cards. Many of these items can be obtained from the American Printing House for the Blind.

Large-Print Books

Many books have been printed in large print for use by low-vision patients (including many Agatha Christied mysteries and the *Reader's Digest*). These books are usually printed in 18- or 24-point type (from two to three times the size of normal print). They are expensive, but collections of them can be found in many libraries. A patient who must depend on large-print books obviously will have a rather limited choice of reading material. Large-print books have rather limited use, because the majority of low-vision patients can read ordinary print with microscopic lenses of adequate power. However, for patients requiring such high magnification that normal print cannot be read even with mircoscopic lenses, large-print books can be used in combination with the microscopic lenses.

Study Questions

1. What advantages does the Bailey-Lovie visual-acuity chart have as compared to an ordinary Snellen chart for testing the visual acuity of a low-vision patient?

2. At what distance should the examiner begin visual acuity testing with a low-vision patient? Why?

3. (a) What is the purpose of visual field testing for a low-vision patient? (b) What modification can be made in the tangent screen if a low-vision patient is found to have a central scotoma?

4. What is meant by the "vergence amplification effect"?

5. (a) In what way is the M system of specifying print size, for low-vision patients, comparable to the traditional Snellen method of designating visual acuity? (b) What is meant by the designation 0.40/1M? (c) by the designation 0.40/3M? (d) by the designation 0.20/2M?

6. Why do large-print books have rather limited use?

7. What is the practical limit of magnification provided by a head-borne visual aid for (a) distance vision? (b) near vision?

8. How can a hand-held magnifier be used (on a temporary basis) by a low-vision patient to gain experience with a high addition?

9. (a) Using the M system, how can the required power of a low-vision patient's reading addition be estimated? (b) What would be the estimated addition for a patient who could read 2M print at 40cm? (c) for a patient who could read 5M print at 40cm?

10. What advantage and disadvantage does a tele-microscope (telescope with a reading cap) have for near vision as compared to a microscope (high add)?

CHAPTER 16

Implementing the Concept of Primary Care Optometry

WHAT IS PRIMARY CARE OPTOMETRY?

The term *primary care practitioner* is defined as a practitioner who serves as a patient's point of entry into the health-care system. Having once entered the health-care system, the patient may be found to require the services of a secondary or tertiary care practitioner. Although the great majority of optometric services are performed on a primary care basis, occasionally a patient requires the services of a secondary or tertiary care optometrist. Areas of secondary and tertiary optometric care include the care of pediatric patients, the care of patients having unusual binocular vision problems, the rehabilitative care of patients having low-vision problems, geriatric patient care, and some of the more sophisticated diagnostic procedures such as electrodiagnosis.

In implementing the concept of primary care optometry, there appears to be a difference of opinion in the profession concerning whether the primary optometrist serves as a point of entry into the overall *health-care system* or serves in a more limited sense as a point of entry into the *eye-care system*. The problem here is partly one of semantics: the eye-care system is obviously a part of the health-care system, so entry into the eye-care system is, in effect, entry into the health-care system.

However, the problem is, in fact, more than just a matter of semantics. Some authors use the term *primary care optometry* to indicate that the optometrist shares the role of the general medical practitioner as a point of entry into the health-care system (not just by virtue of the fact that the patient enters the eye-care portion of the health-care system). This concept, if carried to the extreme, would imply that the optometrist's background should include the same kinds of preclinical and clinical training as that received by the general medical practitioner, prior to entering optometric practice. Because this training would have to be provided in addition to the present preprofessional and professional optometric curriculum, the resulting training program would have to be a very long one indeed.

Those who suggest that the primary care optometrist should share (with the general medical practitioner) the responsibility of serving as an entry point into the health-care system often make the point that if a patient is not currently under the care of a medical practitioner, and if in the optometrist's routine health screening procedures find that the patient has a general health-care problem, the responsibility for getting the patient into the health-care system is the optometrist's.

Herein lies the controversy: given that an optometric patient who has no general medical practitioner is well served if the optometrist discovers high blood pressure or diabetes and refers the patient to a medical practitioner for treatment, are we correct in stating that the primary care optometrist should undertake the responsibility of detecting and diagnosing *any and all health-care problems?* This predicament can be avoided by simply concluding that *for those health-care problems that the primary care optometrist can uncover in routine health screening procedures*, he or she does act as a point of entry into the health-care system. However, we cannot conclude that the optometrist acts as a point of entry into the health-care system for *all* health-care problems.

SCREENING FOR GENERAL HEALTH PROBLEMS

In addition to optometrists' obvious role in evaluating their patients' refractive, binocular vision, and ocular health status, optometrists are in a position (as already indicated) to screen for many of the more commonly occurring general health problems. In an article entitled "Optometry: The Profession's Role in Primary Health Care" (*AOA Reference Materials on Primary Care Optometry*, 1977), Wright, Bucar, Clason, and Miller described a study conducted in 1961 that found that for a group of 306 optometrists, 2.19 percent of all optometric patient visits resulted in referral of a patient to another health-care practitioner. On the basis of the results of this study, these authors concluded that it was not unlikely that the number of referrals at that time (1977) exceeded 1 million annually.

In the same article, Wright et al. (1977) defined *primary care* as "that level of care at which entry into the health care system occurs and at which the basic services that most of the people need most of the time are received." They suggested that optometrists assume the following responsibilities: (1) to provide an entry, screening, and referral point for the rest of the health-care system; (2) to seek not only to cure or alleviate specific complaints but to assume some responsibility for health maintenance; (3) to concern themselves with human support services that are necessary for the effective and efficient utilization of the health-care system; and (4) to serve as a focal point for coordinating and monitoring the continuity of care that patients require.

Wright et al. (1977) discussed the primary care optometrist's role in screening and referral for the following high-incidence health problems (although they warned that the list was not an exhaustive one): hypertension, diabetes, nutritional deficiencies, neurological problems, and dermatological problems.

Hypertension

Many of the reasons for optometric screening for hypertension by means of routine sphygmomanometry are discussed in Chapter 5: (1) a large proportion of the population visits a medical practitioner only rarely, but many of these same people visit an optometrist on a regular basis; (2) hypertension is not only the greatest single causative factor

in death, but it is responsible for a considerable amount of ocular morbidity; (3) although generalized hypertension can be detected by means of the ophthalmoscope, it can be detected at a much earlier stage by measuring the patient's blood pressure; (4) hypertension is accompanied by relatively few subjective symptoms, but one of the most prominent symptoms is headache (which may cause the patient to visit an optometrist, believing the headaches are due to eyestrain); and (5) sphygmomanometry can easily become a part of every optometrist's examination routine.

Wright et al. (1977) made the additional points that (1) the delivery of optometric services is a nonthreatening form of health care for the patient who is reluctant to seek general or preventative medical care, so optometry becomes a natural primary health-care source for a large patient population; and (2) optometrists provide over two-thirds of the primary eye care services delivered in the United States, and thus they can be an effective resource in identifying many of the nation's estimated 12 million unknown hypertensives and in directing these patients into proper health-care channels.

Screening for hypertension is particularly appropriate in an optometric practice in which many of the routine preliminary tests (including visual acuity, tonometry, and visual field screening) are already performed by a trained assistant or technician. A convenient time to perform sphygmomanometry is just after completion of the history, when the patient is relaxed.

Information concerning the instrumentation and procedures for hypertension screening can be found in Chapter 6. As described in that chapter, referral criteria recommended as a result of the Framingham study are (1) *normal range*, systolic pressure below 140mmHg and diastolic pressure below 90mmHg; (2) *hypertensive range*, systolic pressure 160mmHg or more or diastolic pressure of 95mmHg or more; and (3) *borderline range*, systolic pressure between 140 and 160mmHg or diastolic pressure between 90 and 95mmHg.

Patients whose pressures are found to be in the hypertensive range should be referred for further evaluation and possible treatment. Patients whose pressures are in the borderline range should be rescreened at a later date. If on rescreening the pressures are still in the borderline range, the practitioner may elect to refer the patient or to schedule an additional rescreening.

Diabetes

Diabetes, like hypertension, is a major cause of death. More important, it is a much greater threat to vision than is hypertension, diabetic retinopathy being one of the major causes of blindness. Diabetes occurs in two forms: *juvenile-onset diabetes*, which has a strong hereditary component and is due to a deficiency in the amount of insulin; and *adult-onset diabetes*, which occurs mainly in middle-aged and older obese individuals and is thought to be due to fat cells interfering with the utilization of insulin. There are a great many ocular manifestations of diabetes, including (1) changes in refraction, (2) snowflake cataracts, (3) senile cataracts, (4) loss of accommodation, (5) diabetic retinopathy, (6) rubeosis iridis, and (7) lipemia retinalis.

Changes in refraction are in the direction of more myopia (or less hyperopia) occurring when blood glucose levels are high, and reversing when glucose levels have returned to normal. *Snowflake cataracts* occur in youth-onset diabetes in the form of multiple white dots located just beneath the anterior and posterior lens capsules. *Senile cataracts* occur in adult diabetics and are often present at an earlier age and progress more rapidly than in nondiabetics. *Loss of accommodation* tends to occur at an earlier-than-normal age and is thought to be associated with an earlier occurrence of senile cataracts. *Diabetic retinopathy* occurs in two stages. (1) *Background retinopathy* begins with the presence of microaneurysms of the retinal vessels at the posterior pole of the fundus, most of which are beyond the resolving power of the direct ophthalmoscope, and progresses to small blot hemorrhages, dilation of the retinal veins, and both waxy appearing and cotton-wool exudates. (2) *Proliferative retinopathy* begins with the presence of newly formed blood vessels on the surface of the optic disk and retina, some of which may hemorrhage into the vitreous and lead to the formation of a vitreous membrane and, ultimately, to retinal detachment. *Rubeosis iridis* is defined as the growth of newly formed blood vessels on the surface of the iris, which may invade the anterior chamber angle and result in secondary glaucoma. *Lipemia retinalis* may occur in a diabetic coma, the blood column in the retinal arteries and veins having a uniform, salmon pink color.

Of all of the possible ocular manifestations of diabetes, a *change in refraction* is the one most likely to enable the optometrist to detect a previously undiagnosed case of diabetes. This is because a change in refraction tends to occur at a relatively early stage. As noted in the discussion of patient history in Chapter 5, any middle-aged patient who complains of blurred distance vision should be suspected of having diabetes (if an increase in myopia is found to occur in both eyes) or nuclear cataracts (if myopia is found to occur in only one eye or is further advanced in one eye than in the other). Unfortunately, further changes in refraction may occur if the blood glucose level varies with time, so the lens prescription determined at the original examination may no longer be suitable when the glasses are dispensed. Once the patient understands the problem, he or she may be willing to forgo a change in lens prescription until the blood sugar level is under control.

The most severe ocular manifestations of diabetes are diabetic retinopathy (which may eventually lead to blindness as a result of retinal detachment) and rubeosis iridis (which may lead to blindness as a result of secondary glaucoma). Because diabetic retinopathy seldom occurs unless the patient has had diabetes for many years, the discovery of retinal changes will lead to the detection of a previously undetected case of diabetes only if the patient has grossly neglected his or her health care.

Diagnosis of diabetes is made, by the medical practitioner, on the basis of any of a number of tests, including blood glucose testing and the glucose tolerance test. While the treatment of juvenile onset diabetes often requires the subcutaneous injection of insulin, the treatment of adult-onset diabetes may require only strict attention to diet or a combination of diet and one of the oral hypoglycemic drugs. [For additional information on diabetes, standard textbooks on general pathology, ocular pathology, and pharmacology should be consulted.]

Nutritional Deficiencies

Although we tend to think of nutritional deficiencies as occurring only in impoverished countries, many people in the United States and other developed countries are malnourished. This can be a result of poor economic status, a lack of knowledge of nutrition, or both.

The nutritional disorders occurring in impoverished countries have been described by Robbins and Angell (1976). These disorders include marasmus, kwashiorkor, and nutritional growth failure. *Marasmus* is an extreme state of malnutrition, usually occurring during the first year of life, due to a deficiency in the intake of calories. *Kwashiorkor* is a generalized edema, possibly complicated by skin pigmentation, hepatomegaly, and anemia, due to a dietary deficiency of protein in spite of an adequate calorie intake. *Nutritional growth failure* is defined as a retardation of normal growth and development due to inadequacies in the diet.

Even though few people in the United States and other developed countries are afflicted with these severe nutritional disorders, *vitamin deficiencies* may occur either as *primary* deficiencies (due to inadequate dietary intake) or as *secondary* deficiencies (due to factors such as malabsorption by the intestine, interference with storage, increased losses, increased requirements, or inhibition of utilization).

The vitamin deficiency having the greatest effect on the eyes is vitamin A deficiency. The best-known result of vitamin A deficiency is night blindness, due to a deficiency in carotines, which are present in yellow vegetables, liver, and animal fats such as butter and cod liver oil. Vitamin A has been found to be necessary for the maintenance of epithelial tissue, and additional ocular conditions resulting from a deficiency of this vitamin include mucin deficiency, xerophthalmia, and keratomalacia. As described in Chapters 7 and 14, a *mucin deficiency* results in an unusually short precorneal film breakup time and is considered a negative factor in predicting successful contact lens wear. A severe deficiency of vitamin A may cause *xerophthalmia*, a keratinization of the epithelium of the conjunctiva that often occurs in the form of *Bitot's spots* (accumulations of keratin debris); and *keratomalacia*, which involves ulceration, softening, and opacification of the cornea.

An additional vitamin deficiency (although a controversial one, according to Robbins and Angell) is *ariboflavinosis*, due to a deficiency of vitamin B_2, which can include lesions of the lips and tongue, a scaly dermatitis extending from the nasolabial folds onto the cheeks, and corneal vascularization.

Robbins and Angell consider *obesity* a form of nutritional disease, pointing out that excessive fat stores clearly play a causal role in diabetes mellitus, hypertension, cardiovascular disease, and respiratory insufficiency.

Neurological Problems

The optometrist's examination routine includes a number of procedures that are normally included in a neurological examination. The integrity of the second cranial nerve is investigated in visual acuity and visual field testing. The nerve fibers making up the visual pathway pass through (or adjacent to) numerous intracranial structures, including the cavernous sinus, the pituitary body, and many structures within the temporal, parietal, and occipital lobes, with the result that the combination of the visual field findings and associated symptoms may permit a precise localization of a neurological lesion.

The integrity of the third, fourth, and sixth cranial nerves (and a portion of the seventh) is investigated in the tests of ocular motility; the parasympathetic and sympathetic innervation of the eye are investigated during tests of accommodation and pupillary function.

Many of the specific neurological entities that the optometrist may be able to detect in the course of the patient history and preliminary examination are discussed in Chapters 5 and 6. For example, the practitioner may be able to tentatively diagnose many of these entities on the basis of history alone, including migraine, muscular contraction headache, cluster headache, trigeminal neuralgia, multiple sclerosis, hypertension, and temporal arteritis. (However, a definitive diagnosis of many of these conditions can be made only after referral for appropriate diagnostic procedures.) As stated in the previous discussions, classical migraine is diagnosed *solely* on the basis of the triad of symptoms that includes a visual aura, a hemicranial headache, and nausea; a tentative diagnosis of common migraine is indicated if the patient reports a protracted, severe "sick headache." Muscular contraction headaches tend to occur after a period of tension and may occur in the frontal, vertical, or occipital areas. Cluster headache is a severe, boring, unilateral headache occurring in the temporal region and often accompanied by ipsilateral lacrimation and nasal congestion. Pain due to trigeminal neuralgia is unique in that it occurs in the facial area and is usually brought about by the inadvertent touching of a "trigger zone."

A patient who has multiple sclerosis may describe a "shadow" (scotoma) in the visual field that "comes and goes." The scotoma typically involves the central field, and careful questioning is necessary to differentiate this form of transient loss of vision from that occurring in migraine, temporal arteritis, or carotid artery occlusive disease. A tentative diagnosis of temporal arteritis is strengthened when an older patient (usually over the age of 60) who complains of transient loss of vision also has a history of pain in the temporal region, particularly when combing the hair. A complaint of headaches in the morning, relieved by drinking a cup of black coffee, should suggest the possibility of hypertension and the need for performing sphygmomanometry.

It should be understood that all of the neurological conditions referred to above are those that cause headaches, visual symptoms, or both, so the patient may well believe that the problem is caused by his or her *vision*; it is clearly the optometrist's responsibility to direct the patient to the appropriate practitioner.

Unfortunately, most conditions involving visual field defects do not result in a *positive* scotoma (a scotoma that the patient is aware of), as multiple sclerosis does. Therefore, the patient with a bitemporal hemianopsia due to a pituitary tumor, or with a homonymous hemianopsia or quadrantanopsia resulting from a cerebral vascular accident, often has no idea of a visual field loss until told by the optometrist after visual field testing.

Even though lesions of the sympathetic, parasympathetic, or pupillomotor pathways are relatively rare in a healthy, ambulatory population, the optometrist is often in a position to detect and tentatively diagnose pupillary abnormalities as a result of tests of pupil function. One of the most threatening pupillary abnormalities is Horner's syndrome, or sympathetic paralysis (manifested as a unilateral miosis, ptosis, and apparent enophthalmos); among the possible causes of this abnormality are a malignant tumor of the lungs and (in an older individual) an insufficiency in the vetebral-basilar circulation. Another important abnormality is the Marcus Gunn pupil, detected by the swinging flashlight test and indicating the presence of a conduction defect of the optic nerve of the affected eye.

When a patient is found to have lowered visual acuity in one eye, even with the best spectacle correction, the neurodiagnostic tests described in Chapter 7—which require little, if any, specialized equipment and little time—should be performed. These include the light stress test, the brightness comparison test, color vision testing, and the use of the Amsler charts.

Dermatological Problems

Many dermatological problems manifest themselves on the eyelids or on the face near the eyes. Not surprisingly, patients often expect the optometrist to be able to help them with such problems. Dermatological lesions involving the eyelids or the face can vary greatly in severity, from relatively innocuous

styes or warts on the lid margins to malignant tumors such as basal cell and squamous cell carcinomas.

Although a thorough discussion of these dermatological conditions is beyond the scope of this text, the practitioner should be aware that the basal cell carcinoma is the most common malignancy of the ocular adnexa, expressing itself in the early stages as a small elevation on or near the eyelid with rolled edges, or even as a notch or furrow in the lid margin. Although not likely to spread to a distance by metastasis, it has a prediliction for spreading directly through the facial tissues and invading the orbit: early detection and surgery are of great importance.

REFERRALS AND FOLLOW-UP CARE

For primary care optometry to be practiced to its fullest extent, the practitioner must establish a network of consultants in all health care areas. In all cases, such a referral network begins with the *general medical practitioner*. Just as the optometrist considers him or herself a primary care practitioner in the eye-care field, the general medical practitioner is considered a primary care practitioner in the health-care field.

Although the optometrist sometimes plays the role of entry for a patient into the health-care field (and not just the *eye-care* field), he or she plays this role by default for a patient who is not under the care of a medical practitioner. Even though this state of affairs does exist for some patients, it is equally true that many patients who seek out the services of an optometrist *are* under the care of a general medical practitioner. For these patients, one would expect general medical referrals (as opposed to ophthalmological referrals) to be "brokered" through the general medical practitioner unless either the patient or the medical practitioner requests the optometrist to take on this role.

General Health Problems

The action taken by the optometrist when a previously undiagnosed health problem is discovered depends not only on whether the patient is already under the care of a medical practitioner but on the nature of the problem. For example, it is likely that a patient's general medical practitioner would want to personally manage the patient's hypertension or nutritional deficiency, but one would expect that the responsibility for the diagnosis and treatment of

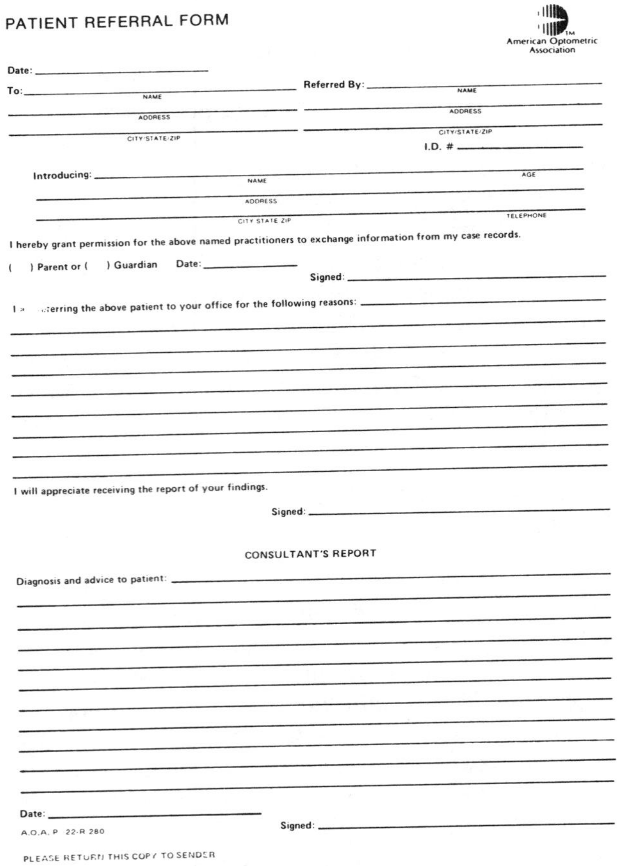

PATIENT REFERRAL FORM

American Optometric Association

Date: _____

To: _____   Referred By: _____
         NAME   NAME
_____   _____
         ADDRESS   ADDRESS
_____   _____
         CITY·STATE·ZIP   CITY/STATE·ZIP
                                                 I.D. # _____

Introducing: _____   AGE
                        NAME
_____
         ADDRESS
_____
         CITY·STATE·ZIP   TELEPHONE

I hereby grant permission for the above named practitioners to exchange information from my case records.

(   ) Parent or (   ) Guardian   Date: _____

                                          Signed: _____

I am referring the above patient to your office for the following reasons: _____
_____
_____
_____
_____
_____
_____
_____
_____

I will appreciate receiving the report of your findings.

                                          Signed: _____

CONSULTANT'S REPORT

Diagnosis and advice to patient: _____
_____
_____
_____
_____
_____
_____
_____
_____
_____

Date: _____   Signed: _____

A.O.A. P 22·R·280

PLEASE RETURN THIS COPY TO SENDER

Figure 16.1   The AOA patient referral form.

diabetes, a neurological problem, or a threatening dermatological problem might be turned over to another practitioner.

Further complicating the situation is that in many urban communities the general practitioner or "family doctor" has been to a great extent replaced by the internal medicine specialist, or *internist*. Internists tend to vary widely in their backgrounds: the optometrist may find that one internist has a strong background in endocrinology and will consider him or herself capable of managing a patient's diabetes, whereas another, having taken residency under a neurologist, will consider him or herself well qualified to diagnose neurological problems (although referring the patient to a neurosurgeon if surgical treatment is needed).

For convenience in making referrals for general health problems, the optometrist should have the name, address, and telephone number of the patient's general medical practitioner (or whatever practitioner serves the function of a general practitioner) on file in the patient's record. Then, when a

general health problem is found to exist, the optometrist can (after discussing the matter with the patient) contact the practitioner by telephone or letter regarding the problem.

Experience has indicated that communication with the medical practitioner is far more effective if the optometrist contacts the practitioner *both* by telephone and by letter. By telephoning the medical practitioner, the optometrist can quickly describe the findings to the other doctor, who can just as quickly indicate whether he or she would like to manage the patient's problem, would like to refer the patient to another practitioner, or, as a third alternative, would prefer the optometrist to handle the referral. If the medical practitioner chooses to manage the problem, a referral letter (either on a form like the American Optometric Association form shown in Figure 16.1 or a typed letter) may be sent with the patient or by mail prior to the patient's visit. If it is mutually agreed that a third practitioner is to be asked to manage the patient's problem, it will be worth the optometrist's time and effort to telephone this practitioner to briefly discuss the problem and then to follow up the telephone conversation with a letter.

As has been indicated, if the patient is not already under the care of a medical practitioner, the optometrist serves as an entry point for the patient into the health-care system, and has the responsibility of referring the patient to a practitioner who can effectively manage the problem. The optometrist, therefore, should be reasonably well acquainted not only with the general medical practitioners in the geographical area but with practitioners in a variety of areas of specialization, including internal medicine, cardiology, neurology, and dermatology.

Ocular Health Problems

When an optometrist enters practice, one of the first tasks will be to obtain as much information as possible concerning each of the eye care practitioners in the geographical area. Not only will it be necessary that the optometrist refer patients to ophthalmologists from time to time, but often it will be necessary to refer a patient to an optometrist who practices in a secondary care area such as pediatric optometry or rehabilitative optometry. Obtaining information about ophthalmologists will be easy if the optometrist joins an already existing practice, as senior associates or partners will be able to supply this information. The optometrist who opens an office or purchases an existing practice must first become acquainted with the other optometrists in the community and then find out to whom *they* refer patients who have ocular health problems.

Ophthalmologists vary greatly in their interests, abilities, and the types of practices they conduct. Newly licensed optometrists may be surprised to learn that many ophthalmologists run their practices much like optometrists run theirs, spending most of their time refracting, and operating an optical dispensary on the premises or directing patients to a dispensary at another location. These ophthalmologists provide medical treatment for ocular health problems, but they may do relatively little ocular surgery: even some well-known ophthalmic surgeons limit their surgery to one or two mornings per week. What has just been described is the ophthalmologist who practices essentially on a primary care basis, perhaps receiving an occasional referral from a general practitioner or an optometrist, but mainly seeing patients who come in "off the street," as an optometrist does. The reason these ophthalmologists do relatively little surgery is that their surgical practices are limited to the "surgical cases" screened from their daily refractions. For example, if in a given patient population only 1 patient out of every 200 had cataracts in need of surgery, the ophthalmologist would have to do (on the average) 200 refractions to find a patient in need of cataract surgery.

Ophthalmologists practicing on a secondary care basis are those who receive sufficient numbers of referrals from other practitioners so they can spend a reasonable amount of their time managing patients who have medical or surgical problems. Other than minor surgical procedures such as opening styes, or removing chalazia or pterygia, the most often-performed operation in ophthalmology is *cataract surgery*. Therefore, ophthalmologists who are secondary care practitioners usually perform a sufficient number of cataract operations to become highly skilled in this procedure. Another important area of surgery for the secondary care ophthalmologist is *ocular muscle surgery*.

Tertiary care ophthalmologists are those engaged in forms of treatment needed by relatively small numbers of people. A rapidly developing area of tertiary care ophthalmology is *retinal surgery*. With the development of diagnostic procedures such as binocular indirect ophthalmoscopy with scleral depression and fundus fluorescing angiography, and the development of surgical procedures such as vitrectomy and photocoagulation, treatment is now available for retinal problems that previously would have gone untreated or even undiscovered.

Once the optometrist is aware of the interests and abilities of each of the ophthalmologists in the geographical area, he or she can refer any patient having an ocular health problem to the ophthalmologist who is best equipped to manage that problem. As already discussed in regard to referrals of patients having general health problems, the optometrist should telephone the other doctor to briefly discuss the patient's problem and should then send a referral letter, either with the patient or in the mail. Telephoning the ophthalmologist in the patient's presence has the advantage that an appointment can be set up for the patient during the conversation.

Referral Letters

When a form such as the AOA referral form (see Figure 16.1) is used, the message must be short and to the point. There is space for little more than the optometrist's pertinent examination findings and an indication of what is expected of the practitioner to whom the patient is being referred. However, the use of such a form has two important advantages over the more formal, typed letter: (1) since completing the form requires only a few minutes' time, bypassing the more time-consuming processes of dictating and typing, it is convenient for use with patients who are referred for urgent conditions or emergencies and must see the practitioner within just a day or two (or even the same day); and (2) the use of such a form makes writing a report so easy for the doctor to whom the patient is referred that the optometrist almost always receives a reply. Even when there is no urgency or emergency, this referral form is a good one to use when only a brief message is required.

When time is not a problem and when the situation requires a relatively detailed message, a typed letter is often preferable. In most cases the letter need include only four paragraphs, and each paragraph will require no more than two or three sentences. The heading of the letter should include the patient's name, just above the greeting, in the form "re: John R. Jones." The following outline is suggested.

Paragraph 1. This paragraph identifies the patient, usually in terms of name, age, and sex, and indicates when the patient was examined and the nature of the patient's chief complaint or the reason for the examination.

Paragraph 2. This paragraph relates the pertinent optometric findings. Usually the refractive findings, corrected visual acuity, and any significant binocular vision problem will be sufficient.

Paragraph 3. This paragraph relates the pertinent ocular health findings. Normally these will be summarized in terms of the findings resulting from the external examination, internal examination, tonometry, and visual fields or other pertinent findings.

Paragraph 4. This paragraph may or may not give the optometrist's tentative diagnosis (or *clinical impression,* as it is often called). It will usually indicate what the optometrist expects the other practitioner to do, and it requests a report of the practitioner's findings.

When appropriate, the optometrist may wish to enclose a copy of visual field charts or any other recorded findings.

Although the information concerning refractive findings and visual acuity may not seem important, in many instances this information (particularly corrected visual acuity) is crucial; if the optometrist fails to provide it, the ophthalmologist will have to take the extra time to do a refraction.

Referral Versus Consultation

The term *referral* can have either of two meanings: it can be used to indicate that the patient is being "sent off" to another practitioner, who will then take complete charge, or it can be used to indicate that the patient is being referred for *consultation,* after which the patient will return to the referring practitioner. In this discussion the term *referral* always has the latter meaning—referral for the purpose of consultation—and is never used to mean that the practitioner to whom the patient is sent will take complete charge of the patient's care.

In discussing referral with a patient, the optometrist should make it clear that the other doctor will give an opinion or diagnosis concerning the problem at hand. Even though the second doctor may institute treatment (e.g., treatment for hypertension or cataract surgery), the patient should understand that the optometrist will continue to manage his or her vision care.

Occasionally, an optometrist will find that an ophthalmologist will be unwilling to have the patient return for continuing vision care. For example, after

cataract surgery the ophthalmologist may refract the patient and prescribe aphakic lenses, to be dispensed by the practitioner's dispensary. Fortunately, this now seldom occurs. When it does occur, it is either because (1) a particular ophthalmologist considers optometrists to be competitors, and is more interested in refraction than in surgery; or (2) the optometrist has failed to make the referral in such a way that the ophthalmologist is unmistakenly aware of the source of the patient. Unfortunately, there are a few optometrists who fail to understand the importance of making a direct referral to a specific practitioner, simply leaving it to the patient to find an ophthalmologist who will take care of the problem.

The concept of referral for consultation rather than "sending off" the patient is of equal importance when a primary care optometrist refers a patient to a secondary care optometrist. If, for example, a secondary care optometrist practices pediatric optometry, he or she will return a patient to the referring practitioner once the initial evaluation has been completed, leaving the prescribing of glasses to the referring optometrist. If a program of vision therapy is carried out, the patient will be referred back to the original optometrist once the vision therapy is completed. If a secondary care optometrist fails to return the patient to the original optometrist, he or she will never receive a second referral from that optometrist.

Another important concept of primary care is that the primary care practitioner considers him or herself a *family* practitioner, expecting to care for all members of a patient's family. If the pediatric or rehabilitative optometrist to whom he or she refers a patient takes over the vision care of other members of a referred patient's family, again the practitioner should not expect to receive a second referral from that optometrist.

No more than a generation ago, optometry was almost entirely a profession of individual practitioners, each of whom provided complete vision care to all of his patients, and (with some exceptions) each of whom was extremely reluctant to refer a patient to a fellow optometrist. Even with the development of secondary areas of optometric practice, the reluctance to refer patients for secondary care still persists. Fortunately, during recent years increasing numbers of optometrists have pooled their resources and talents, forming group practices. Many of these group practices cater to all the major areas of primary and secondary care optometry. In a typical two-optometrist practice, one practitioner may specialize in the areas of pediatric optometry and binocular vision, while the other specializes in contact lens fitting, rehabilitative optometry, and geriatric optometry. Usually all members of a joint practice examine primary care patients, referring from one practitioner to another whenever it is in the best interests of the patient to do so.

Patient Monitoring

Many patients are found to have borderline ocular health problems requiring monitoring on a continuing basis. For example, a patient who has borderline intraocular pressure in the absence of glaucomatous cupping of the optic nerve head or glaucomatous field defects (a condition sometimes referred to as *ocular hypertension*) is usually considered not to require treatment, but the patient's intraocular pressure, optic nerve head appearance, and central fields should be monitored on a routine basis. Although in the past this monitoring was usually done by an ophthalmologist, there is no reason that it cannot be done by an optometrist. In many cases this monitoring is done with the knowledge and agreement of the ophthalmologist to whom the patient will ultimately be referred. The concept of monitoring rather than referring for a borderline or incipient condition applies to many progressive conditions including cataracts, keratoconus, and inactive cases of uveitis. In states where dilation is allowed (which are now in the majority), monitoring may often include photodocumentation. When the optometrist has a good working relationship with the ophthalmological consultants, there will often be advance agreement concerning the particular stage at which a patient is referred to the ophthalmologist.

PATIENT COUNSELING

Implicit in the role of the optometrist as a primary care practitioner is the concept that the optometrist not only examines patients and provides treatment (occasionally arranging for treatment provided by other practitioners), but also *counsels* and *educates* patients. Recall that in the problem-oriented system of medical records developed by Dr. Lawrence Weed, *patient education* is an important aspect of any treatment plan.

Counseling and patient education are necessary in all aspects of optometric care. Patients whose only problem is myopia, hyperopia, or astigmatism naturally expect the optometrist to be able to provide information concerning these refractive anomalies. They often want to know how the conditon came about, whether it will progress with the passage of time, if wearing glasses will help the condition or will make their eyes "weaker," and even if they might eventually go blind.

Patients who are to be fitted with types of vision aids to which they are unaccustomed (bifocal or trifocal lenses, aphakic lenses, contact lenses, and low-vision aids) have a right to expect the optometrist to fully inform them about the use of these "new" (to them) forms of visual correction.

Patients who are being referred to other practitioners, whether for problems of ocular health or general health, are particularly in need of counseling. A patient being referred because of cataracts will want to know whether (or when) surgery will be necessary, what kind of anesthetic will be used, how long he or she will have to stay in the hospital, and whether glasses, contact lenses, or intraocular lenses should be fitted after surgery. A patient being referred for a general health problem may want to know how the optometrist arrived at the diagnosis or at the decision to refer, what may be expected in the way of medical or surgical treatment, and what the outcome (prognosis) may be. In many cases the optometrist will have to tread a fine line between unduly alarming the patient and making the patient feel that the referral is unnecessary.

Patients expect the optometrist to be able and willing to provide information not only concerning their particular problems, but a wide variety of topics concerning vision. The family optometrist is expected to be well informed on topics ranging from optics and color vision to learning disorders and the latest procedures for retinal surgery. The desirability for the practicing optometrist to possess a strong background in visual science was emphasized by Hofstetter (1950), who referred to the optometrist as the "general practitioner in the field of vision" (p. 270). Hofstetter made the point that the public is more aware of this role than the optometrist, commenting that "Newspapermen who interview speakers at optometric conventions do not ask for opinions on refraction or spectacles. They want advice on television viewing, on the effect of atomic radiation on vision, on the visual status of humans today as compared to 100 years ago, on the relationship of vision to autombile driving, in fact even on the possibility that we can predict sex pre-natally by inspecting the ocular fundus! In short, they are seeking *the general practitioner in the field of vision*" (1950, p. 270).

Pamphlets and Audiovisual Aids

The amount of information that can be imparted verbally is limited not only by the constraints of time but by the capacity of a patient to remember specific details concerning a heretofore unfamiliar subject. Usually the practitioner's explanations can be supplemented, but not supplanted, by the use of well-chosen pamphlets or audiovisual aids. The American Optometric Association has available pamphlets on an unusually wide variety of subjects concerning vision, and a large variety of audiovisual presentations are also available.

APPENDIX A

Problem-Oriented Optometric Records

Appendix A.1   Patient Information Form

PATIENT INFORMATION FORM [*]

Patient's name	Address	Date
City State Zip Tel Home		Work
Date of birth Parent's name (if patient is a minor)		
Occupation of patient or parent Employed by		
Were you referred by a patient? If so, by whom?		
Do you wear glasses? If so, how long have you worn them?		
Do you wear contact lenses? If so, how long have you worn them?		
Have you ever had an eye injury, disease or operation? If so, please describe:		

What is the reason for today's examination?

_____ Routine examination: no problems or complaints

_____ Blurred distance vision   _____ Blurred near vision

_____ Feeling of eyestrain   _____ Headaches

_____ Double vision   _____ One eye turns in or out

_____ Eyes burn or itch   _____ Eyes water

_____ Other: _____

Do you have any of the following conditions?

_____ Hypertension (high blood pressure)

_____ Arteriosclerosis (hardening of the arteries)

_____ Diabetes

_____ Kidney ailment

_____ Difficulty with hearing

_____ Other: _____

Are you currently taking any medications, either prescribed by a doctor or purchased without a prescription? If so, please indicate:

Do you have any drug allergies or sensitivities? If so, please indicate:

Is there anything else you think the doctor should know about your eyes or about your state of health?

[*] To be completed by patient (or parent) prior to examination.

Appendix A.2 Optometric Data Base Form

OPTOMETRIC DATA BASE

<table>
<tr><td rowspan="5">PAT PROFILE</td><td colspan="6">Name   Address   Date</td></tr>
<tr><td colspan="6">City   State   Zip   Tel Home   Work</td></tr>
<tr><td colspan="6">Date of birth   Age   Sex   Race   Referred by</td></tr>
<tr><td colspan="6">Occupation   Hobbies</td></tr>
</table>

HISTORY	Present Rx #1 R _____ #2 R _____
	L L
	Ocular history
	Health history
	Medications Drug allergies
	Family ocular and health history
	Chief complaint

PRELIMINARY EXAM	Vis acuity Unaided Dist R 20/ L 20/ OU 20/ Near R 20/ L 20/ OU 20/
	Pres Rx Dist R 20/ L 20/ OU 20/ Near R 20/ L 20/ OU 20/
	Cover test Unilateral Alternating
	Corneal reflex test NPA NPC
	Pupils Size Direct Consensual Near
	Motility Stereopsis Color vision
	Confrontations Central fields
	IOP R L Instr Time BP

EXTERNAL EXAM	Tear film
	Break-up time
	Cornea
	Lids/conjunct
	Angle width
	Ant ch/iris R L
	Lens

INTERNAL EXAM	Lens
	Vitreous
	Disc
	C/D ratio
	Vessels
	V/A ratio
	Ven pulsation
	Macula
	Macular reflex
	Background R L
	Periphery

Appendix A.2   *(continued)*

PD   /   Optometric Data Base, page 2

REFRACTION	Keratometry R _____ L _____	Javal Expected R _____ L _____	
	Static Retinoscopy R _____ L _____	Dynamic Retinoscopy R _____ L _____	
	BVA Subjective R _____ L _____	Other Subjective R _____ L _____	
	Acuity R 20/ L 20/ OU 20/ R 20/ L 20/ OU 20/		

BINOCULAR VISION

6M Phorias   Diss Lat _____ Vert _____   Assoc Lat _____ Vert _____

Vergences BI ___ / ___ / ___   BO ___ / ___ / ___   Vert R ___ / ___   L ___ / ___

40cm Phorias   Diss Lat _____ Vert _____   Assoc Lat _____ Vert _____

Vergences BI ___ / ___ / ___   BO ___ / ___ / ___   Vert R ___ / ___   L ___ / ___

Cross cyl Mon R _____ L _____   Bin R _____ L _____   Acuity R 20/ _____ L 20/ _____

Ampl accom R _____ L _____   Rel accom Neg _____ Pos _____

Gradient phoria +1.00 _____   −1.00 _____   Range from _____ to _____

ADDITIONAL TESTS

INITIAL PROBLEM LIST

No _____ Problem _____ Resolved _____

INITIAL TREATMENT PLANS

Problem No _____ Treatment Plan _____

PRESCRIPTION

	Sphere	Cyl	Axis	Prism	Base		Sphere	Cyl	Axis	Prism	Base
R						R					
L						L					

Add _____ Bifocal _____   Add _____ Bifocal _____

Next appointment _____

Appendix A.3   Record of Patient Visits Form

RECORD OF PATIENT VISITS

Date	Reason for Visit

PROBLEM LIST

No	Date Entered	Problem	Date Resolved
1			
2			
3			
4			
5			
6			
7			
8			
9			
10			
11			
12			
13			
14			
15			

Appendix A.4   Progress Notes Form

PROGRESS NOTES

Patient	Date

Reason for visit

Major problem(s)

SYMPTOMATIC

OBJECTIVE

ASSESSMENT

PLAN

Next appointment

Appendix A.5   Contact Lens Fitting Data Form

CONTACT LENS FITTING DATA

Patient	Date
Reason for wanting contact lenses	
Allergies, chronic diseases or other possible contraindications	

Keratometer R _____   Subjective R _____ 20/

L _____   L _____ 20/

Estimated   Hard lenses R _____   Soft lenses R _____
residual
astigmatism   L _____   : _____

Corneal diameter   Palpebral fissure   Pupil size

Trial lenses #1

R _____

L

Trial lenses #2

R _____

L

Trial lenses #3

R _____

L

Final trial lenses   Over-refraction through final trial lenses

R _____   R _____

L _____   L _____

Lenses to be ordered: Type of lens _____ Laboratory_____

	BC	SC	Diam	OZ	PC	CT	Power	Tint	Other Specifications
R									
L									

Next appointment

Appendix A.6   Contact Lens Progress Examination Form

CONTACT LENS PROGRESS EXAMINATION

Patient	Date

Lens type	Wearing time	Time worn today

SYMPTOMATIC

   Patient's
   symptoms

OBJECTIVE   WITH LENSES ON   WITH LENSES OFF

Visual acuity R   L   Slit lamp

Retinoscopy   R

             L

Subjective   R   20/   Keratometer R

            L   20/   L

Fluorescein   Retinoscopy R
pattern

                                 L

                     Subjective   R   20/

Slit lamp   L   20/

ASSESSMENT

PLAN

New lenses ordered R

                L

Instructions to patient

Next appointment

Appendix A.7   Low-Vision Evaluation Form

LOW VISION EVALUATION

PA PROFILE	Name Address Date
	City State Zip Tel Home Work
	Date of birth Age Sex Race Referred by
	Occupation Hobbies
HISTORY	Duration and cause of visual problem Present Rx R
	L
	Previous surgical or medical treatment
	Presently under ophthalmological treatment?
	Visually-oriented activities
	Patient's visual needs
	Health history
	Chief complaint
PRELIMINARY EXAM	Vis acuity Unaided Dist R / L / Near R / L /
	Pres Rx Dist R / L / Near R / L /
	Cover test Unilateral Alternating
	Motility Color vision
	IOP R L Instr Time BP
	Visual field evaluation
EXTERNAL EXAM	Tear film
	Break-up time
	Cornea
	Lids/conjunct
	Angle width
	Ant ch/iris
	Lens
INTERNAL EXAM	Lens
	Vitreous
	Disc
	C/D ratio
	Vessels
	V/A ratio
	Ven pulsation
	Macula
	Macular reflex
	Background
	Periphery

R   L

R   L

Appendix A.7   *(continued)*

PD	/	Low Vision Evaluation, page 2				
REFRACTION	Keratometry	R_____		Javal Expected	R_____	
		L			L	
	Retinoscopy	R_____	Subjective	R_____		
		L		L		
	Acuity	R ____ / ____ L ____ / ____				
DISTANCE VISION AIDS	Instrument		Power		Acuity R_____	
					L_____	
	Instrument		Power		Acuity R_____	
					L	
	Instrument		Power		Acuity R_____	
					L	
NEAR VISION AIDS	Instrument		Power	Dist	Acuity R_____	
					L	
	Instrument		Power	Dist	Acuity R_____	
					L	
	Instrument		Power	Dist	Acuity R_____	
					L	
ADDITIONAL TESTS						
ASSESSMENT						
PLAN AND PRESCRIPTION						

APPENDIX B

American National Standards Institute Prescription Requirements

Appendix B.1 American National Standards Institute Requirements for First-Quality Prescription Ophthalmic Lenses (ANSI Z80.1–1972 Revision of Z80.1–1964).

Inspection routine of prescription lenses	Tolerance	Provisions and testing procedures
Physical quality and appearance Surface imperfections	No pits, scratches, grayness, or water marks shall be acceptable. Minute hairline scratches should not be a cause of rejection.	Lenses shall be inspected against a dark background in light from an open-shaded 40-watt incandescent clear lamp with the lens 12 inches from the light source.
Internal defects	No bubbles, striae, and inclusions shall be acceptable.	
Localized power errors	Waves (see provisions).	Waves found by visual inspection shall be passable if no deterioration in image quality is found when the localized area is examined with a standard lens-measuring instrument.[a]
Refractive power (diopters) Untreated crown or flint glass lenses	0.00 to 6.00 ± 0.06 6.25 to 12.00 ± 1 percent Above 12.00 ± 0.12	Power in each principal meridian shall be measured on a standard lens-measuring instrument[a] at the optical center as specified. Maximum cylinder power variation ±0.12.
Impact resistant lenses	0.00 to 6.00 ± 0.12 6.25 to 12.00 ± 2 percent Above 12.00 ± 0.25 The difference in the refractive power errors of the two lenses of a pair shall not exceed the tolerance as specified above for a single lens, for example:	

Error		Difference
O.D.	O.S.	
+0.06	−0.06	0.12
+0.12	+0.06	0.06
−0.12	−0.12	0.00

Inspection routine of prescription lenses	Tolerance	Provisions and testing procedures
Refractive power addition	±0.09D The curves for the reading and distance portions of a one piece bifocal shall meet sharply and both of these curves, immediately adjacent to the line, shall be free from surface irregularities.	Power of additions must be measured in accordance with instructions below.[b]

Appendix B.1   (*continued*)

Inspection routine of prescription lenses	Tolerance	Provisions and testing procedures
Cylinder axis		Axis should be determined in relation to the cutting or mounting line.
Untreated crown or flint glass lenses	0.12 to 0.37 ± 3 degrees 0.50 to 1.00 ± 2 degrees 1.12 on up ± 1 degree	
Impact resistant lenses	0.12 to 0.37 ± 5 degrees 0.50 to 1.00 ± 3 degrees 1.12 on up ± 2 degrees	
Prism power and location of specified optical center	Vertical ± 0.25Δ for each lens or 0.25Δ imbalance. Horizontal ±0.25Δ for each lens or 0.50Δ imbalance.	The lens should be measured at the specified reference point, formerly referred to as optical center. A lens specified without prism shall be treated as a 0Δ lens.
Segment size	±0.5mm. Pair must be symmetrical on visual inspection. Trifocal intermediate vertical dimension shall be ±0.25mm singly or within ±0.25mm paired.	Segment size shall be measured on segment side of lens.
Segment location	As specified within ± 0.5mm.	Measured from the apex of the bevel to the highest portion of the segment on the concave side of lens.
Thickness	As specified within ± 0.2mm.	To provide best cosmetic effect.
Lens size		Lens shapes must match. Edges must be straight and smooth and sharp edges must be removed.
Rimless	±0.5mm	
Bevel, for plastic frames	±0.5mm	
Bevel, for metal frames	To fit standard specified frame.	
Impact resistant occupational protective lenses	Tolerance for power, size, etc., shall be as above, except minimum thickness edge or center 3.0mm.	Shall meet the requirements of American National Standard Z87.1–1968.
Impact resistant dress eyewear lenses	All impact-resistant treated glass, dress eyewear lenses must be of not less than 2mm optical center thickness, with average thickness between the center and the thinnest edge not less than 1.7mm and an edge thickness of not less than 1mm at the thinnest point of the edged lens.	Before they are mounted in frames, all plastic and impact-resistant treated glass lenses shall be capable of withstanding an impact test of a ⁵⁄₈ in. steel ball dropped fifty inches. This test is to be conducted at room temperature, with the lens supported by a plastic tube (1 in. ID 1¼ in. OD) with a ⅛ in. × ⅛ in. neoprene gasket on the top edge.
Warpage	The curves in the principal meridians of the mounted lens must be within a tolerance of ±1.00 diopter of the design specifications of the lens. The present level of the art dictates that this requirement not apply to plastic lenses mounted in metal frames.	The curves shall be measured with an ophthalmic lens clock.

[a]Standard lens-measuring instruments include the recognized type, such as a vertometer or lensometer that measures the vertex power.
[b]A generalized set of instructions for measuring the power of additions is as follows: (1) place the lens in the instrument with the segment surface against the lens positioning tube; (2) measure the power through the reading portion, focusing on the vertical lines of the target image; (3) focusing on the vertical lines of the target image, measure the power through the distance portion. The measurement through the distance portion must be made as far above the optical center of the distance portion as the measurement through the segment is below the optical center of the distance portion; (4) the true reading addition is the difference between the distance and reading portions as measured in steps (2) and (3); (5) because of prisms encountered when measuring a strong bifocal through the reading portion, the target may be blurred. To eliminate this, place on the prism holder an auxiliary prism of sufficient power to center the target image.

Appendix B.2   American National Standards Institute Prescription Requirements for First-Quality Contact Lenses (ANSI Z80.2–1972).

Prescription Requirements for Corneal Lenses
(all measurements are made in air with lenses in an air-dried state.)

Parameter		Tolerance
Diameter		±0.05mm
Posterior optic zone diameter	Light blend	±0.1mm
	Medium or heavy blend	±0.2mm
Posterior central curve (base curve) radius		±0.025mm
Posterior secondary, intermediate, or peripheral curve width	Light blend	±0.05mm
	Medium or heavy blend	±0.10mm
Posterior secondary, intermediate, or peripheral curve radius		±0.1mm
Refractive power	+10.00D to −10.00D	±0.12D[a,b,c]
	More than ±10.00D	±0.25D
Prism power (measured from the geometric center)		
If lens power is:	+10.00D to −10.00D	±0.25Δ
	More than ±10.00D	±0.50Δ
Cylinder power	Less than 2.00D	±0.25Δ
	2.00D to 4.00D	±0.37Δ
	Greater than 4.00D	±0.50D
Cylinder axis		±5°
Toric base curve radii	Δ r 0 to 0.20mm	±0.02mm[c]
	Δ r 0.21 to 0.40mm	±0.03mm
	Δ r 0.41 to 0.60mm	±0.05mm
	Δ r > 0.60mm	±0.07mm
Bifocal refractive power addition		±0.25D[b]
Bifocal segment height		−0.1mm to +0.2mm
Center thickness		Less than ±0.02mm[d]
Edges		As specified.
Anterior peripheral curve radius		±0.2mm
Anterior optic zone diameter		±0.1mm
Optical quality and surface quality		No bubbles, striae, waves, inhomogeneities, crazing, pits, scratches, chips, lathe marks, or stone marks.
Color		Pigment inert and uniformly distributed.

[a]If the lens base curve and power errors are cumulative (i.e., base curve and lens power errors both add plus power or both add minus power to the refractive correction), the cumulative error shall not exceed 0.25D.
[b]The cumulative errors in power between the right and left lenses shall not exceed 0.25D.
[c]Symbols used are as follows: D—diopters; Δ—prism diopters; Δ r—difference between radii of principal meridians.
[d]The algebraic differences in thickness error between right and left lenses shall not exceed 0.02mm.

APPENDIX C

Contact Lens Tables

Appendix C.1   Conversion from Spectacle Refraction to Contact Lens Refraction (Calculated for a spectacle vertex distance of 12mm. For minus, read left to right; for plus, read right to left).

5.00	4.75	7.12	6.62	10.00	9.00	14.25	12.25
5.12	4.87	7.37	6.75	10.25	9.12	14.75	12.50
5.37	5.00	7.50	6.87	10.50	9.25	15.00	12.75
5.50	5.12	7.62	7.00	10.75	9.37	15.50	13.00
5.62	5.25	7.75	7.12	11.00	9.62	15.75	13.25
5.75	5.37	7.87	7.25	11.25	9.75	16.25	13.50
5.87	5.50	8.00	7.37	11.50	10.00	16.75	13.75
6.00	5.62	8.12	7.50	11.75	10.25	17.00	14.00
6.12	5.75	8.25	7.62	12.00	10.37	17.25	14.25
6.37	5.87	8.50	7.75	12.50	10.75	17.62	14.37
6.50	6.00	8.75	8.00	12.75	11.00	18.00	14.50
6.62	6.12	9.00	8.25	13.00	11.25	18.12	14.75
6.75	6.25	9.25	8.37	13.50	11.50	18.50	15.00
6.87	6.37	9.50	8.62	13.75	11.75	18.75	15.25
7.00	6.50	9.75	8.75	14.00	12.00	19.00	15.50

Appendix C.2   Conversion from Diopters to Millimeters of Radius (for index of refraction of 1.3375).

Diopters	Radius	Diopters	Radius	Diopters	Radius	Diopters	Radius
37.25	9.06	41.25	8.18	45.25	7.46	49.25	6.85
37.50	9.00	41.50	8.13	45.50	7.42	49.50	6.83
37.75	8.94	41.75	8.08	45.75	7.38	49.75	6.78
38.00	8.88	42.00	8.04	46.00	7.34	50.00	6.75
38.25	8.82	42.25	7.99	46.25	7.30	50.25	6.72
38.50	8.77	42.50	7.94	46.50	7.26	50.50	6.68
38.75	8.71	42.75	7.90	46.75	7.22	50.75	6.65
39.00	8.65	43.00	7.85	47.00	7.18	51.00	6.62
39.25	8.60	43.25	7.80	47.25	7.14	51.25	6.59
39.50	8.54	43.50	7.76	47.50	7.11	51.50	6.55
39.75	8.49	43.75	7.71	47.75	7.07	51.75	6.52
40.00	8.44	44.00	7.67	48.00	7.03	52.00	6.49
40.25	8.39	44.25	7.63	48.25	6.97	52.25	6.46
40.50	8.33	44.50	7.58	48.50	6.96	52.50	6.43
40.75	8.28	44.75	7.54	48.75	6.92	52.75	6.40
41.00	8.23	45.00	7.50	49.00	6.89	53.00	6.37

Glossary

aberration See *chromatic aberration; coma; curvature of image; distortion; oblique astigmatism; spherical aberration.*

AC/A ratio The ratio of accommodative convergence to accommodation; in determining the AC/A ratio, accommodation may be expressed either as the accommodative stimulus or the accommodative response.

> **calculated AC/A ratio** The clinically determined AC/A ratio, based on the difference between the values of a patient's distance phoria and near phoria; calculated by means of the formula
>
> $$\frac{AC}{A} = \frac{15 - \text{physiological exophoria}}{2.5},$$
>
> where 15 = convergence required at 40cm; 2.5 = stimulus to accommodation at 40cm; and physiological exophoria = the extent to which the phoria taken at 40cm is more exo (or less eso) than the phoria taken at 6m.

> **gradient AC/A ratio** The clinically determined AC/A ratio, based on the difference between the value of the phoria taken at 40cm through the subjective lenses and the phoria taken at 40cm through the subjective lenses combined with +1.00D.

> **response AC/A ratio** The AC/A ratio determined by means of a haploscope and optometer system, in which it is possible to measure the state of the patient's accommodation; specifically, the ratio between accommodative convergence and the accommodative response.

> **stimulus AC/A ratio** The AC/A ratio determined clinically (using either the calculated or the gradient method) in which it is not possible to measure the state of the patient's accommodation; specifically, the ratio between accommoda-tive convergence and the accommodative stimulus.

> **lag of accommodation** Accommodation beyond the plane of regard, usually specified in diopters.

> **mechanism of accommodation** When the ciliary muscle contracts, acting as a sphincter muscle, it releases the tension on the zonular fibers, allowing the elastic lens capsule to increase its curvature and, therefore, allowing the lens to become thicker and more nearly spherical.

> **near-point of accommodation** The nearest object for which an image point will be formed on the retina of an emmetropic or uncorrected ametropic eye.

> **range of accommodation** The linear distance between the far-point of accommodation and the near-point of accommodation of the eye.

accommodative esotropia Esotropia occur-ring as a result of uncorrected hyperopia, due to the convergence that accompanies the accommodation that is necessary to compensate for the hyperopia.

accommodative micropsia A decrease in the size of the retinal image occurring with accommo-dation.

Adie's tonic pupil A unilaterally dilated pupil having little or no reaction to light but a sluggish reaction to near stimulation; a benign condition due to a lesion of the ciliary ganglion, requiring no treat-ment.

accommodation The ability of the eye to focus clearly for objects at various distances.

> **amplitude of accommodation** The dioptric value of the near-point of accommodation of the eye less the dioptric value of the far-point of accommodation (with the dioptric value of the far-

point of accommodation for a hyperopic eye being considered negative).

far-point of accommodation The farthest object point for which an image point will be formed on the retina of an emmetropic or uncorrected ametropic eye.

amaurosis fugax A temporary loss of vision, due to a condition such as carotid artery occlusive disease or temporal arteritis.

amaurotic eye A blind eye.

amaurotic pupil The pupil of an amaurotic eye (having no light perception), having no direct pupillary reflex but contracting consenually when the normal fellow eye is stimulated by light.

amblyopia condition in which lowered visual acuity exists, even with the best corrective lenses, without obvious cause.

functional amblyopia Amblyopia, usually unilateral, in which no organic lesion exists, such as strabismic or refractive amblyopia.

hysterical amblyopia Amblyopia of neurotic or psychotic origin.

organic amblyopia Amblyopia due to a lesion or other abnormality in the eye or the visual pathway.

refractive amblyopia Amblyopia due to uncorrected anisometropia or astigmatism.

strabismic amblyopia Amblyopia associated with, and thought to be due to, strabismus.

toxic amblyopia Amblyopia due to endogenous or exogenous poisoning.

ametropia A refractive condition other than emmetropia (a refractive anomaly) in which, with accommodation relaxed, parallel rays of light fail to converge to a sharp focus on the retina.

anesthetics, topical When instilled into the conjuctival sac, these agents act by reducing the permeability of the nerve cell membrane to sodium ions, blocking nerve conduction so the nerve action potential does not occur. Examples are cocaine, proparacaine, benoxinate, and tetracaine. The most commonly used is proparacaine (Ophthaine, Ophthetic, Alcaine) because the possibility of adverse effects is small.

angle lambda The angle, subtended at the center of the entrance pupil of the eye, between the pupillary axis and the line of sight.

aniridia Absence of the iris, occurring as an autosomal dominant inherited trait.

aniseikonia A difference in the sizes or shapes of the retinal images for the two eyes, usually accompanying anisometropia or astigmatism.

anisometropia The condition in which the refractive state differs for the two eyes.

anomalous retinal correspondence In strabismus, a condition that exists during binocular vision in which an off-foveal point in the retina of the deviating eye is associated with (and has the same visual direction as) the fovea of the fixing eye.

antimetropia The condition in which the eye is myopic and the other is hyperopic.

aphakia The condition resulting when the crystalline lens has been removed because of a cataract. A strong convex lens is required (in the form of a spectacle lens, contact lens, or intraocular lens) to compensate for the loss of refracting power of the crystalline lens.

Argyll Robertson's pupil A pupil (in an eye that is not amaurotic) that fails to react to light but constricts on convergence, due to neurosyphilis.

asthenopia A feeling of fatigue, discomfort, or pain localized in or about the eyes or thought to be associated with the use of the eyes. Also called *eyestrain.*

astigmatic chart A chart designed for subjective measurement of astigmatism while the eye is fogged with sufficient plus lens power to place the entire conoid of Sturm in front of the retina. The chart consists of single or triple, radially oriented lines (the clock-dial chart) or perpendicular sets of lines (the rotating *T*) that may be rotated into any meridian.

astigmatism A refractive anomaly in which the eye's optical system is incapable of forming a point image for a point object, because the refracting power of the eye's optical system varies from one meridian to another.

against-the-rule astigmatism Astigmatism in which the refractive power of the eye is greater in the horizontal meridian than in the vertical meridian.

compound astigmatism Astigmatism in which, with accommodation relaxed, both focal lines are located in front of the retina (compound myopic astigmatism) or behind the retina (compound hyperopic astigmatism).

corneal astigmatism Astigmatism due to meridional variation in refracting power of the anterior surface of the cornea, as measured by the keratometer.

internal astigmatism Astigmatism due to meridional variation in refracting power of the posterior surface of the cornea, to the tilting of the crystaline lens with respect to the optic axis of the eye, and possibly to other factors.

irregular astigmatism Astigmatism in which the two principal meridians of the eye are not at right angles to one another.

mixed astimatism Astigmatism in which, with accommodation relaxed, one focal line is located in front of the retina and the other behind the retina.

refractive astigmatism The total astigmatism of the eye, as measured by objective or subjective refraction.

simple astigmatism Astigmatism in which, with accommodation relaxed, one focal line is located on the retina and the other is located in front of the retina (simple myopic astigmatism) or behind the retina (simple hyperopic astigmatism).

with-the-rule astigmatism Astigmatism in which the refracting power of the eye is greater in the vertical meridian than in the horizontal meridian.

balancing test A test of subjective refraction designed to balance the accommodative states of the two eyes.

base in to blur, break, and recovery See *negative fusional vergence test.*

base out to blur, break, and recovery See *positive fusional vergence test.*

bichrome test A test of subjective refraction making use of a chart having a red background on one side and a green background on the other side, taking advantage of the chromatic aberration of the eye. In undercorrected myopia or overcorrected hyperopia, the letters on the red background will appear to be more distinct; in overcorrected myopia or undercorrected hyperopia, the letters on the green background will appear to be more distinct. In emmetropia or in adequately corrected myopia or hyperopia, the letters on the red and green backgrounds will appear to be equally distinct.

binocular refraction A subjective refraction procedure in which the peripheral portions of the test chart are seen binocularly (providing a peripheral fusion lock), and the central portions are seen monocularly.

binocular vision syndrome An anomaly of binocular vision identified on the basis of distance and near phoria findings and resulting in predictable patient symptoms: convergence insufficiency, convergence excess, divergence insufficiency, divergence excess, and "false" convergence insufficiency.

biomicroscope An instrument designed for detailed examination of ocular tissue, particularly of the anterior segment of the eye, having a bright focal source of light with a slit of variable width and height, and a binocular microscope provided with variable magnification. Also called a *slit lamp.*

blepharitis An inflammatory process affecting the lid margins, involving the lash follicles or the openings of the Meibomian glands.

seborrheic blepharitis Blepharitis in which numerous small scales, or dandruff, may be seen clinging to the lid margins, commonly accompanied by dandruff of the scalp.

ulcerative blepharitis Blepharitis in which ulcerated areas are found along the lid margins, leading to loss of eyelashes. Caused by a bacterial infection, the most common being staphylococcus.

blood pressure The pressure of the blood in the walls of the arteries, dependent on the strength of the heart action, the elasticity of the arterial walls, and the blood volume and viscosity.

diastolic pressure The arterial pressure during ventricular diastole (dilitation).

mean arterial pressure The pressure that drives the blood through the arterial tree, equal to the product of the cardiac output and the peripheral vascular resistance.

systolic pressure The arterial pressure during ventricular systole (contraction).

blur circle A circular image formed on the retina resulting from an object point whose image is formed in front of or behind the retina.

carotoid artery occlusive disease Stenosis (narrowing) or occlusion of the internal carotid artery due to the deposition of atheromatous plaques, leading to complaints of transient loss of vision (amaurosis fugax) and to possible closure of the central retinal artery.

cataract An opacity in the crystalline lens that interferes with vision.

aftercataract An opacity present after cataract surgery in which an extracapsular operation has been done (removal of the lens, leaving the lens capsule in the eye).

congenital cataract A cataract present at birth or developing during childhood.

cortical cataract A cataract involving the cortex, or outer portion, of the crystalline lens, usually starting as radially oriented, wedge-shaped opacities visible only with a large or dilated pupil. Also called *cuneiform cataract*.

nuclear cataract A cataract involving the nucleus, or inner portion, of the crystalline lens, appearing with the slit lamp as a yellowing of the nucleus.

posterior subcapsular cataract A cataract involving the subcapsular portion of the posterior cortex, causing a golden or iridescent appearance of the posterior capsule as seen with the slit lamp.

senile cataract A cataract occurring with advanced age, either as a cortical cataract, a nuclear cataract, or a posterior subcapsular cataract.

chalazion A chronic granulomatous infection of a Meibomian gland.

choroiditis A usually chronic (but sometimes acute) inflammation of the choroid. Also called *posterior uveitis*.

chromatic aberration An aberration resulting when white light is incident on an optical system, in which light of different wavelengths is focused at different points along the optic axis.

ciliary body A portion of the middle coat, or uvea, of the eye, bordered anteiorly by the iris and posteriorly by the choroid, having the functions of formation of aqueous humor (by the ciliary epithelium) and accommodation (by the ciliary muscle).

ciliary muscle A portion of the ciliary body composed of smooth muscle tissue, which performs the function of accommodation by relieving the tension of the zonular fibers.

coloboma A sector-shaped absence of tissue, due to failure of the fetal fissure to close completely. A coloboma may involve the iris, the choroid, or the optic nerve.

coma An aberration of a large-aperture optical system, in which rays of light from an off-axial object point entering the periphery of the optical system are refracted to a greater or lesser extent than rays entering the system paraxially, resulting in a comma-shaped image.

complete problem list The second component of a problem-oriented record system, consisting of a numbered and titled list that includes every problem the patient has or has had. The complete problem list serves as an index to the patient's record and is kept in the front of the record (e.g., on the left-hand side of a mania folder).

computer-assisted refractors Computer-assisted instruments designed for either objective or subjective automatic refraction.

objective computer-assisted refractors Instruments making use of infrared light, which are examiner-objective as well as patient-objective, making use of optical principles such as those of the retinoscope, the lensometer, and Scheiner's disk.

subjective computer-assisted refractors Instruments designed for automatic subjective refraction making use of variable-focus lenses (Humphrey Vision Analyzer) or an optometer system (American Optical SR–IV).

confrontation fields A visual field screening procedure in which the examiner sits opposite the patient and uses a finger, a wand, or other test object to estimate the peripheral limits of the patient's visual field.

conjunctivitis An inflammation of the conjunctiva.

allergic conjunctivitis Conjunctivitis due to an antigen-antibody reaction, characterized by itching and a watery discharge.

atopic conjunctivitis A mild, nonspecific form of allergic conjunctivitis, occurring in association with allergic rhinitis, involving itching, tearing, and redness of the eyes and edema of the bulbar conjunctiva. Also known as *hay fever conjunctivitis*.

bacterial conjunctivitis Conjunctivitis due to a bacterial infection, characterized by irritation and redness of the eyes, a mucopurulent discharge, and complaints of the eyelids sticking together in the morning.

epidemic keratoconjunctivitis A highly contagious form of viral conjunctivitis, beginning as an acute follicular conjunctis with pain, injection, and tearing, with later occurrence of subepithelial opacities.

keratoconjunctivitis sicca Keratoconjunctivitis due to an absolute or partial deficiency in aqueous tear production, characterized by a burning or foreign body sensation, a scanty marginal tear strip, and excess debris in the tear film. Also called *aqueous tear defiency*.

vernal conjunctivitis Allergic conjunctivitis occurring mainly in the spring and summer months, characterized by extreme itching and a stringy or ropy discharge. In the palpebral form, giant cobblestone papillae are found in the upper tarsal conjunctiva; in the limbal form, thickened, gelatinous opacifications occur in the bulbar conjunctiva surrounding the limbus.

viral conjunctivitis Conjunctivitis caused by a virus.

conoid of Sturm Imagery formed along the optic axis of a cylindrical refracting element, consisting of a primary focal line, a circle of least confusion, and a secondary focal line. Also called *interval of Sturm.*

contact lens A correcting lens that is fitted on the cornea and in some cases extends onto the sclera.

gas-permeable contact lens A rigid contact lens that is oxygen permeable, due to the inclusion of silicone or other materials.

hard contact lens A rigid contact lens, containing little or no water, typically made of polymethyl methacrylate.

hydrogel contact lens A soft, flexible contact lens made of a material having a high water content (usually approximately 40 percent or more). Also called a *soft contact lens.*

contour interaction A phenomenon responsible for the fact that an amblyopic patient may achieve poorer visual acuity if several lines of letters or a single line of letters is presented than if a single letter is presented. Also called the *crowding phenomenon.*

contraction A visual field defect, usually a peripheral field defect, in which the area of the visual field is totally blind to all stimuli.

hemianoptic contraction A contraction defect involving one-half of the visual field, being either *homonymous* (involving either the right or left fields for both eyes) or *heteronymous* (involving either the nasal fields or temporal fields for both eyes). A hemianoptic contraction is called a *hemianopsia.*

peripheral contraction A contraction involving all or a part of the periphery of the visual field.

quadrant contraction A contraction involving a quadrant of the visual field.

sector contraction A contraction involving a sector (less than a quadrant) of the visual field.

contrast sensitivity test A visual perception test in which both spatial frequency (roughly equivalent to letter size in visual acuity testing) and contrast are varied.

convergence excess A binocular vision syndrome in which there is orthophoria or near-orthophoria at 6m and a high esophoria at 40cm, typically resulting in complaints of headaches and other symptoms of asthenopia accompanying prolonged close work.

convergence insufficiency A binocular vision syndrome in which there is orthophoria or near-orthophoria at 6m and a high exophoria at 40cm, resulting in complaints of fatigue, drowsiness, or even diplopia accompanying prolonged close work.

cornea The transparent anterior portion of the fibrous coat of the eyeball, serving as the first refractive medium of the eye.

corneal reflex test A test for strabismus in which the patient fixates a penlight or other light source and the examiner notes the positions of the reflections formed by the two corneas. Also called the *Hirschberg test.*

corresponding retinal points Pairs of points, one on each retina, having the same visual direction and represented at the same area in the visual cortex.

cover test A clinical test in which each eye is covered, by means of an occluder, to determine the presence of a phoria or a tropia.

alternating cover test A clinical test in which the two eyes are alternately covered by means of an occluder. Any deviation of the eye just uncovered indicates the presence of either a phoria or a tropia.

unilateral cover test A clinical test in which each eye is covered, but binocular fixation is allowed between the occlusion of one eye and occlusion of the other. Any deviation of the uncovered eye indicates the presence of a tropia.

cranial arteritis See *temporal arteritis.*

criteria for prescribing prism

Percival's criterion This criterion states that the point of zero demand should fall in the middle third of the total fusion range, without regard to the phoria.

Sheard's criterion This criterion states that for comfortable binocular vision, the fusional vergence reserve should be at least twice the fusional vergence demand.

crossed-cylinder test at near A subjective test, performed (either monocularly or binocularly) at a distance of 40cm while the patient wears his subjective lenses and a crossed cylinder with its minus axis at 90 degrees. Beginning with sufficient fogging lens power, the examiner reduces plus lens power until the patient reports that the vertical and horizontal lines are equally distinct. On a nonpresbyope this test may be considered to indicate the lag of accommodation; on a presbyope it may be used to determine the tentative addition.

crystalline lens   The lens located within the eye, which acts as a refracting medium and also is responsible for the change in focus, or accommodation, of the eye.

curvature of image   An aberration of a small-aperture optical system occurring when oblique astigmatism has been corrected, in which the image points corresponding to a plane object surface lie on a curved surface.

cyclitis   A chronic or acute inflammation of the ciliary body. If the inflammation involves the pars plana of the ciliary body, it is called *pars planitis.*

cycloplegic agents   Agents that act by antagonizing the muscarinic action of acetylcholine, by blocking its action at structures innervated by postganglionic parasympathetic nerve fibers. These agents paralyze the constrictor pupillae as well as the ciliary muscle, thereby causing mydriasis as well as cycloplegia.

   atropine   A naturally occurring alkaloid derived from the deadly nightshade plant, belladonna, which provides cycloplegia lasting from 7–10 days and mydriasis lasting for as long as 2 weeks.

   cyclopentolate (*Cyclogyl*)   A short-duration cycloplegic agent, providing cycloplegia in from 30–45 minutes (using one drop of 1 percent solution), which persists as long as 24 hours.

   homatropine   A semisynthetic alkaloid that acts as a cycloplegic agent, producing cyloplegia in from 45–60 minutes, with the cycloplegic effect lasting several days.

   tropicamide (*Mydriacyl*)   A short-duration, weak cycloplegic agent, providing cycloplegia within about 30 minutes (with from two to four drops of 1 percent solution), persisting only for 2–6 hours.

cycloplegic refraction   Refraction in which the ciliary muscle has been temporarily paralyzed by the use of a cycloplegic agent. In cases of latent hyperopia or pseudomyopia, more plus (or less minus) power is found in cycloplegic refraction than in noncycloplegic refraction.

cylindrical lens   A lens whose refracting power varies from a maximum in one principal meridian to a minimum in the opposite principal meridian, the two principal meridians being at right angles.

defined data base   The first component of a problem-oriented record system, consisting of a problem-oriented history together with all of the tests of eye health, refraction, and binocular vision that are appropriate for the patient in question.

delayed subjective   An overfogging procedure done after completion of the examination routine. Leaving the plus-lens-to-blur finding in the refractor, the patient's attention is called to a block of letters at 6m, and a refractive end point is determined by reducing lens power binocularly until best visual acuity is obtained.

depression   A visual field defect involving an area of the visual field that is blind to some stimuli but not to others. To detect a depression, at least two stimuli (of varying size or intensity) must be used.

depressor   An ocular muscle that depresses the eye when the eye makes a downward movement starting from a position of gaze in either the right or left field.

   left-hand depressor   An ocular muscle responsible for depressing the eye when a downward movement is made starting from a position of gaze in the left field: the left inferior rectus or the right superior oblique.

   right-hand depressor   An ocular muscle responsible for depressing the eye when a downward movement is made starting from a position of gaze in the right field: the right inferior rectus or the left superior oblique.

depth of field   The extent to which an object (such as a line of letters on a visual acuity chart) may be moved toward or away from an observer's eye, beginning with the position where the image is sharply focused on the retina and still appears to be acceptably clear, with no change in accommodation.

depth of focus   The extent to which the optical image of the eye may be located in front of or behind the retina and still appear to be acceptably clear (on the basis of a criterion such as a line of letters on a visual acuity chart), with no change in accommodation.

dichromat   A person who requires only two primary colors to match any given color stimulus. In a red-green mix to match a given yellow, the dichromat will accept any mixture of red and green stimuli as long as the patient can vary the brightness of the yellow stimulus.

deuteranope A dichromat who is green-deficient, lacking the green-absorbing pigment chlorolabe.

protanope A dichromat who is red-deficient, lacking the red-absorbing pigment erythrolabe.

tritanope A dichromat who is blue-deficient, lacking the blue-absorbing pigment cyanolabe.

diopter The unit used to designate the refracting power of a lens, equal to the reciprocal of the focal length (expressed in meters) of the lens. Used also as a unit of vergence of light: when used in this manner it is equal to the reciprocal of the distance along the optic axis from the light source (expressed in meters) to the point in question.

diplopia The occurrence of double vision.

binocular diplopia Diplopia in which one image is seen by one eye and the other image is seen by the other eye.

crossed diplopia Diplopia occurring in an exo deviation, in which the image seen by the right eye is perceived as being to the left of the image seen by the left eye.

monocular diplopia Diplopia in which two images are seen by one eye.

physiological diplopia Double vision occurring due to the fact that an object is located in front of or behind the horopter; such images are formed on noncorresponding retinal points and outside Panum's fusional areas.

uncrossed diplopia Diplopia occurring in an eso deviation, in which the image seen by the right eye is perceived as being to the right of the image seen by the left eye.

diplopia field test A test in which the patient wears a red lens on one eye and a green lens on the other, and is asked to report the presence of diplopia when a penlight is placed in various fields of gaze.

dissociated phoria See *phoria*.

dissociation The elimination of all stimuli to fusion, with the result that the visual axes of the eyes will assume the phoria position (e.g., by occluding one eye or by placing a strong prism in front of one eye).

distortion An aberration of an optical system that occurs if a stop, or aperture, is placed at some distance in front of or behind the optical system, occurring because the only rays from an off-axial object point that can be included in the image are those entering the periphery of the system.

divergence excess A binocular vision syndrome in which there is a high exophoria at 6m and a lower exophoria or even esophoria at 40cm, possibly resulting in symptoms of eyestrain and diplopia accompanying prolonged distance vision tasks such as driving an automobile or watching television.

divergence insufficiency A binocular vision syndrome in which there is esophoria at both 6m and 40cm, resulting in complaints of headaches and other symptoms of asthenopia accompanying both distance and near vision.

eccentric fixation In strabismus, a condition that exists during both monocular and binocular vision in which an off-foveal point in the retina of the deviating eye is used for fixation.

ectropion A turning outward (eversion) of the lower eyelid, usually occurring in an older individual, allowing the tears to overflow the eyelid and run down the check (epiphora).

electrodiagnostic procedures Objective procedures used in the diagnosis of ocular disease.

electro-oculogram Measurement of the potential difference between the cornea and the back of the eyeball, both in dark adaptation and in light adaptation, by having the patient fixate back and forth between two fixation points (about 40 degrees apart) with electrodes placed at the inner canthus of one eye and the outer canthus of the other eye.

electroretinogram The mass response of the retina when the whole retina is subjected to an intense flash of light, while an electrode is placed on the cornea with the aid of a contact lens, and a second electrode is placed on the face or forehead.

visually evoked response (VER) The recording of a potential which is indicative of cortical activity while the patient views an oscillating checkerboard or striped pattern with an electrode placed on the scalp near the occipital protuberance. The recording of the VER while the patient looks through lenses of various powers has been advocated as a method of measurement of refractive error, because the VER amplitude is depressed by defocus.

elevator An ocular muscle that elevates the eye when the eye makes an upward movement starting from a position of gaze in either the right or left field.

left-hand elevator An ocular muscle responsible for elevating the eye when the eye makes an upward movement starting from a position of gaze in the left field; the left superior rectus or the right inferior oblique.

right-hand elevator An ocular muscle responsible for elevating the eye when the eye makes an upward movement starting from a position of gaze in the right field; the right superior rectus or the left inferior oblique.

emmetropia The normal refractive state of the eye in which, with accommodation relaxed, parallel rays of light will converge to a sharp focus on the retina.

emmetropization A process that operates to produce a greater frequency of emmetropia than would be expected to occur on the basis of chance.

  emmetropization mechanism A mechanism that operates to bring about and maintain a state of emmetropization. As the eyeball increases in axial length, emmetropia may be brought about or maintained by a reduction in the refracting power of the cornea, a reduction in the refracting power of the crystalline lens, or an increase in the depth of the anterior chamber.

entropion A turning inward (inversion) of the lower eyelid, usually occurring in an older individual, sometimes allowing the lashes to rub the cornea (trichiasis).

epicanthus A condition in which one or both of the inner canthal areas is covered by a fold of skin.

exophthalmometer An instrument designed to measure the amount of protrusion, or exophthalmia, of each eye relative to the outer orbital margin.

extinction phenomenon In visual field testing, if stimuli are presented in both the left and right halves of the visual field, hemianoptic field defects may be detected that would escape detection in ordinary field examination. The presence of the stimulus in the intact side of the visual field will "extinguish" the stimulus in the defective field.

eyestrain See *asthenopia.*

fixation disparity Underconvergence or over-convergence of the eyes with respect to the plane of regard, expressed as exo fixation disparity (underconvergence) or eso fixation disparity (overconvergence).

focal points Two points located on the axis of an optical system such that rays of light passing through the primary focal point, *F*, will leave the system as parallel rays, and rays entering the system parallel to the optic axis will be refracted such that they will pass through the secondary focal point, *F′*.

fogging principle In subjective refraction, the use of sufficient plus lens power to place the image of a fixation target (such as a line of letters) in front of the retina to prevent the patient from accommodating.

follicles Localized areas of lymphoid hyperplasia, appearing as white or gray elevations in the upper or lower tarsal conjunctiva, which may be accompanied by inflammation (folliculosis) or may occur in association with some forms of allergic, viral, or bacterial conjunctivitis.

fovea centralis A small pit or depression in the retina in the center of the macula lutea, containing no rods but only cones, each cone being connected to only one retinal ganglion cell; the point of most acute vision.

fundus The internal surface of a hollow organ; when applied to the eye, the retina, choroid, optic nerve, and blood vessels as seen with the ophthalmoscope.

fusion See *sensory fusion; motor fusion.*

fusional vergence demand The amount and direction of fusional vergence required to compensate for a patient's phoria. Positive fusional vergence compensates for an exophoria, and negative fusional vergence compensates for an esophoria.

fusional vergence reserve The amount and direction of fusional vergence held in reserve for a patient who has a phoria. Positive fusional vergence is the reserve of interest in exophoria, and negative fusional vergence is the reserve of interest in esophoria.

giant cell arteritis See *temporal arteritis.*

glaucoma An ocular disease characterized by an elevation in the intraocular pressure, which causes damage to optic nerve fibers entering the optic nerve, leading to loss of vision.

  angle-closure glaucoma Glaucoma occurring as a result of closure of the anterior chamber angle.

  congenital glaucoma Glaucoma occurring at birth or early in life, usually due to a malformation of the anterior chamber angle. Also called "hydrophthalmos" and "buphthalmos."

  open-angle glaucoma A slowly progressive form of glaucoma in which the anterior chamber angle remains open, apparently due to a decreased outflow of aqueous through the trabecular meshwork.

pigmentary glaucoma Glaucoma in which the spaces in the trabecular network have become blocked by uveal pigment.

primary glaucoma Glaucoma not due to a preexisting ocular disease.

secondary glaucoma Glaucoma due to a preexisting ocular disease.

gonioscope An instrument designed for observation of the anterior chamber angle of the eye. Such an instrument is required because light reflected from the anterior chamber angle normally is totally internally reflected by the anterior surface of the cornea.

haplopia Single vision.

haploscope A research instrument making use of mirrors for presenting various stimuli to accommodation and to convergence and measuring the accommodative response.

headache Pain in or around the head or face.

cluster headache A severe, burning, boring, unilateral headache, occurring in the temporal region, often accompanied by ipsilateral lacrimation and nasal congestion, occurring usually at night, usually affecting middle-aged men. Also called *histamine cephalalgia*.

eyestrain headache A headache due to an uncorrected refractive error or binocular vision anomaly, typically occurring in the brow region, but also occurring in the occipital and neck regions.

histamine cephalalgia See *headache, cluster*.

hypertension headache Headache due to hypertension (high blood pressure), usually a severe headache occurring early in the morning and disappearing at some time during the day.

migraine headache See *migraine*.

muscular contraction headache Considered to be the most common form of headache, tending to occur in the forehead, the vertex, or in the occipital area or the back of the neck, considered by some to be psychogenic in origin. Also called *tension headache*.

nasal sinusitis headache Pain accompanying acute nasal sinusitis, most often involving the region of the frontal sinus and being most pronounced when stooping down.

temporal arteritis headache Headache accompanying temporal arteritis (cranial arteritis), associated with a general feeling of malaise and loss of appetite, scalp tenderness (particularly when combing the hair). The patient may have a history of transient loss of vision.

tension headache See *headache, muscular contraction*.

tic douloureux See *headache, trigeminal neuralgia*.

trigeminal neuralgia An extremely sharp, piercing, knifelike pain, in the facial region, of sudden onset, due to the inflammation of any of the three divisions of the trigeminal nerve. The pain can be brought on when the patient touches a specific region of the face (the trigger zone). The pain is so severe that the patient may live in a constant state of fear, dreading the occurrence of the next attack. Also called *tic douloureux*.

heterophoria See *phoria*.

heterotropia See *tropia*.

high blood pressure See *hypertension*.

Hirschberg's test See *corneal reflex test*.

hordeolum An infection of a lash follicle, also called a *stye*. An internal hordeolum is an infection of a Meibomian gland.

Horner's syndrome Miosis, ptosis, and apparent enophthalmos, due to a lesion in the sympathetic pathway to the dilator of the pupil. In congenital cases, heterochromia irides may also be present. An absence of facial sweating may also occur.

horopter For any fixation point, the horopter is an imaginary surface containing all object points that form images on pairs of corresponding retinal points.

Hutchinson's pupil A fixed, dilated pupil, usually unilateral, due to a central nervous system lesion that compresses the optic nerve.

hypermetropia See *hyperopia*.

hyperopia A refractive anomaly in which, with accommodation relaxed, parallel rays of light converge to a focus behind the retina.

absolute hyperopia The amount of hyperopia that cannot be compensated for by accommodation.

axial hyperopia Hyperopia due to the axial length of the eye being less than that of the schematic emmetropic eye.

facultative hyperopia The amount of hyperopia that can be compensated for by accommodation.

latent hyperopia The amount of hyperopia that is compensated for by accommodation due to hypertonicity of the ciliary muscle and, therefore, may not be discovered in a routine subjective refraction.

manifest hyperopia The amount of hyperopia that is not compensated for by accommodation and, therefore, is measured in a routine subjective refraction.

refractive hyperopia Hyperopia due to the refractive power of the eye's optical system being less than that of the schematic emmetropic eye.

hypertension An elevation in either systolic or diastolic blood pressure, or both. Normal systolic blood pressure is considered to be below 140mmHg, borderline systolic blood pressure is between 140 and 160mmHg, and elevated systolic blood pressure is 160mmHg or above. Normal diastolic pressure is below 90mmHg, borderline diastolic pressure is between 90 and 95mmHg, and elevated diastolic pressure is 95mmHg or above.

illumination, methods of Methods of adjusting the illumination and observation systems of the slit lamp used to observe the various structures of the eye.

direct illumination Method of illumination in which the slit beam and the microscope are both focused sharply on the structure to be observed. With a wide slit a transparent structure (such as the cornea) can be observed as a three-dimensional structure known as a *parallelopiped*; with a narrow slit, an "optical section" can be observed; and with a small, round (or square) aperture, a "conical beam" can be obtained.

indirect illumination The beam is focused on a structure located adjacent to the structure to be observed by the microscope, and the area is observed somewhat in a shadow, by scattered light.

oscillation A variation of indirect illumination in which the microscope is kept in focus on the structure to be observed and the beam is oscillated back and forth, alternately resulting in direct and indirect illumination.

retroillumination A method of illumination in which the slit-lamp beam is focused on a structure behind (or beyond) the structure to be observed. Also called *transillumination*.

sclerotic scatter A method of illumination in which a slit of medium width is directed toward the limbus from a wide angle, illuminating the cornea by internal reflection and causing an opacity in the cornea to be visible due to local scattering of light.

specular reflection A method of illumination in which the source and the microscope are placed at equal angles from the normal to the corneal surface, so the image of the source will be observed; particularly useful for observing the corneal endothelium.

split-limbal method A method of illumination resembling sclerotic scatter but with the slit-lamp beam splitting the limbal area; designed for observation of central corneal clouding in a hard contact lens wearer.

initial treatment plans The third component of a problem-oriented record system, each numbered and titled treatment plan corresponding to a problem in the complete problem list. Each initial treatment plan includes three parts: more information concerning diagnostic workup and management, therapy, and patient education.

interpupillary distance (PD) The distance between the centers of a patient's pupils, as measured by a millimeter ruler or other instrumentation.

intraocular pressure The pressure within the eye, occurring as a result of the constant formation and drainage of the aqueous humor.

iritis A chronic or acute inflammation of the iris. Also called *anterior uveitis*.

isometropia The condition in which the refractive state is the same for the two eyes.

Jackson's crossed cylinder A lens having a plus cylinder ground on one side and a minus cylinder ground on the other side at an axis 90 degrees from that of the plus cylinder; used for refining the cylinder axis and power in the absence of fogging lenses.

keratitis An inflammation of the cornea.

corneal ulcer A deep form of keratitis, caused by any of a variety of bacteria, viruses, and fungi. The most severe bacterial ulcers are caused by *Pseudomonas aeruginosa* and *Streptococcus pneumoniae*; the most severe viral ulcers are caused by *Herpesvirus hominus*.

superficial keratitis A form of keratitis affecting mainly the superficial layers of the cornea, caused by any of a number of microorganisms, by antigenantibody reactions, or by factors such as exposure and interruption of sensory nerve supply to the cornea.

keratoconus A protrusion and thinning of the apical portion of the cornea; of obscure etiology, beginning during the teenage years and slowly progressing (with periods of remission) throughout life. Adequate optical correction is usually possible only with contact lenses.

keratometer An optical instrument designed to measure the radius of curvature of the cornea, making use of a doubling system to measure the size of the image of an illuminated object—known as a *mire*—reflected from the cornea's anterior surface.

Kruckenberg's spindle A vertically elongated, spindle-shaped deposition of uveal pigment on the corneal endothelium, indicating that pigment may be present in the trabecular meshwork.

laser refraction A method of subjective refraction in which the patient observes the speckle pattern produced by a laser and reports the direction of movement of the pattern. To measure astigmatism, the speckle pattern must be rotated in either four or six meridians.

light-near dissociation The pupil fails to react to light but constricts upon convergence. If caused by neurosyphilis, this is called the *Argyll Robertson pupil.*

lipid abnormality A qualitative change in the lipid secretion of the Meibomian glands, due to chronic blepharitis, causing dry spot formation in the precorneal film.

macula lutea A shallow depression in the retina near the posterior pole of the eye, about the size of the optic disk; a pigmented area (yellow spot) containing the fovea centralis.

manifest refraction Refraction in which a cycloplegic agent is not used.

Marcus Gunn pupil A pupil anomaly due to a conduction defect of the optic nerve, detected by the swinging flashlight test. When the pupil of the defective eye is illuminated, both pupils dilate, but both pupils constrict when the pupil of the normal eye is illuminated. Also called *afferent pupillary defect.*

metamorphopsia A visual phenomenon in which objects appear to be distorted in terms of size or shape.

meter angle A unit of measurement of convergence of the eyes, equal to the amount of convergence required to fixate an object located at a distance of 1m from the midpoint of a line joining the centers of rotation of the eyes. Meter angles of convergence can be converted to prism diopters of convergence by multiplying by the patient's interpupillary distance expressed in centimeters.

migraine A headache in which the pain is confined to one side of the head. Caused by the dilitation and congestion of branches of the external carotid and meningeal arteries.

   classic migraine A symptom complex beginning with a visual aura in the form of a "scintillating scotoma" in one side of the visual field, followed by a unilateral headache accompanied by a feeling of nausea.

   common migraine A migraine headache in which the visual aura does not appear, nausea being the predominant symptom.

monochromat A person who requires only one primary color to match any given color stimulus. The condition is also known as *achromatopsia*.

   cone monochromat A monochromat having foveal cones and, therefore, possibly having normal visual acuity. Also called an *atypical monochromat.*

   rod monochromat A monochromat having no foveal cones and, therefore, having poor visual acuity. Also called a *typical monochromat.*

motor fusion Movements of the eyes made in response to retinal disparity stimuli, in order to maintain single binocular vision.

movements of the eyes

   conjugate movements Eye movements in which both eyes move in the same direction (to the right, to the left, upward, or downward). Also called *version movements.*

   disjunctive movements Eye movements in which the eyes move toward each other (convergence) or away from each other (divergence). Also called *vergence movements.*

   following movement A slow conjugate movement, made for the purpose of keeping the image of a moving object on or near the fovea or for the purpose of keeping the image of a stationary object on or near the fovea as the head moves. Also called a *pursuit movement.*

   saccadic movement A fast, abrupt conjugate movement occurring as a voluntary refixation movement, as an involuntary or random movement, or in other situations including pursuit movements faster than 45 degrees per second.

mucin deficiency A deficiency in the production of mucin by the goblet cells of the conjunctiva, leading to an abnormally short precorneal film breakup time.

muscae volitantes Vitreous floaters (flying gnats) seen by patients having a partially liquefied vitreous, having the appearance of spots, strings, cobwebs, or rings.

mydriatic agents Agents that dilate the pupil, either by sympathomimetic or antimuscarinic activity.

> **antimuscarinic agents** Agents that antagonize the muscarinic action of acetylcholine by blocking its action on structures innervated by postganglionic parasympathetic nerve fibers, acting as cycloplegic agents as well as mydriatic agents. Examples are cyclopentolate (Cyclogyl) and tropicamide (Mydriacyl).
>
> **sympathomimetic agents** Agents that directly or indirectly stimulate the dilator pupillae of the iris, mimicking the action of the sympathetic division of the autonomic nervous system, examples of which are phenylephrine (Neosynephrine) and hydroxyamphetamine (Paradrine). Phenylephrine is available in both 10 and 2.5 percent solutions, but because of possible adverse cardiovascular effects with the 10 percent solution, the 2.5 percent solution is recommended.

myopia A refractive anomaly in which, with accommodation relaxed, parallel rays of light converge to a focus in front of the retina.

> **acquired myopia** Myopia acquired during life usually considered to begin during childhood. Because few cases of myopia are congenital, the great majority of cases of myopia are acquired.
>
> **axial myopia** Myopia due to the axial length of the eye being greater than that of the schematic emmetropic eye.
>
> **night myopia** Myopia occurring in low illumination, due to insufficient stimulus to the eye's accommodative mechanism and to the spherical aberration that occurs due to increased pupil size.
>
> **progressive myopia** A gradual increase in myopia occurring with age, usually leveling off in the late teen years or early 20s.
>
> **pseudomyopia** A reversible form of myopia due to spasm of the ciliary muscle.
>
> **refractive myopia** Myopia due to the refractive power of the eye's optical system being greater than that of the schematic emmetropic eye.

negative fusional vergence test A binocular vision test conducted at either 6m or 40cm, in which the patient views a vertical line of 20/20 letters while base-in prism power is gradually increased in front of each eye until the patient reports that the letters are blurred, and then that two lines of letters are seen. Prism power is then reduced until the patient reports that only one line of letters is seen.

nodal points Two points located on the axis of an optical system such that an incident ray directed toward the primary nodal point, N, leaves the system as though it passed through the secondary nodal point, N', with its direction unchanged.

nystagmus A repetitive, rhythmic, involuntary (usually conjugate) movement of the eyes, either having equal velocity and amplitude in both directions or having a slow movement in one direction and a fast movement in the other.

> **caloric nystagmus** A form of physiological, vestibular nystagmus typically induced by introducing either hot or cold water into the ear by means of a syringe.
>
> **central nystagmus** Pathological nystagmus, jerky in nature, of central origin, due to a lesion of the vestibular nucleus or nerve.
>
> **end-point nystagmus** Nystagmus occurring at the extremes of fixation.
>
> **jerky nystagmus** Either physiological or pathological nystagmus having a fast movement in one direction and a slow movement in the other.
>
> **micronystagmus** Minute nystagmus movements made during ordinary fixation; a form of physiological nystagmus.
>
> **ocular nystagmus** Pathological nystagmus of ocular origin, usually pendular in nature.
>
> **optokinetic nystagmus** Physiological nystagmus induced by attempting to fixate objects traversing the visual field, as when viewing a rotating drum having alternating black and white stripes.
>
> **pathological nystagmus** Nystagmus due to a pathological process, which may be of central, vestibular, or ocular origin.
>
> **pendular nystagmus** Either physiological or pathological nystagmus having movements of equal velocity and amplitude in both directions.
>
> **physiological nystagmus** Nystagmus of physiological origin; usually a jerky nystagmus, such as caloric, optokinetic, or rotational nystagmus.
>
> **rotational nystagmus** Physiological nystagmus induced by rotation, as when sitting on a rotating stool; a jerky nystagmus.
>
> **vestibular nystagmus** A pathological form of nystagmus, jerky in nature, due to a vestibular or labyrinthine lesion.

oblique astigmatism An aberration of a small-aperture optical system in which rays entering the system obliquely (from an off-axial object point) form an astigmatic beam, resulting in two focal lines at right angles to one another rather than a point image.

oblique illumination A method of examining the anterior segment of the eye, in which an ocular structure is illuminated from an oblique angle and inspected with or without magnification.

ophthalmodynamometer An instrument designed to measure the relative pressure within the ophthalmic artery. The instrument exerts pressure on the sclera, raising the intraocular pressure, and the examiner notes the pressure reading when the central artery of the retina begins to collapse. The intraocular pressure then equals or slightly exceeds the ophthalmic artery pressure.

ophthalmophakometer An optical instrument designed to measure the radii of curvature and the thickness of the crystalline lens, making use of a doubling system.

ophthalmoscope An instrument designed for the examination of the interior of the eye, having an illumination system involving a light source, lenses, and a prism or a mirror, and an observation system involving a peephole and a system of lenses.
  direct ophthalmoscope An ophthalmoscope that provides an upright image of the structure under observation, with a magnification of about 15 × and a field of view of about 6.5 degrees.
  indirect ophthalmoscope An ophthalmoscope that provides an inverted image of the structure under observation, with a magnification of 2 to 5× and a field of view of about 25 or 30 degrees. Indirect ophthalmoscopes are available as a monocular indirect ophthalmoscope (having an upright image due to a reinverting system) and a binocular indirect ophthalmoscope that provides intense illumination with stereoscopic vision.

optical image of the eye The image formed by the optical system of the eye. It is clearly focused, and it may or may not coincide with the retina.

optic disk The point of entry of the retinal ganglion cell fibers into the optic nerve, nasal to the posterior pole of the eye, visible with the ophthalmoscope as a vertically oval area white in color against the pinkish background of the fundus.

optometric records, problem-oriented A system of patient record keeping consisting of four basic components: the defined data base, complete problem list, initial treatment plans, and progress notes.

orthokeratology A method of fitting contact lenses for the purpose of reducing the wearer's refractive error.

Panum's fusional area An area in the retina of one eye such that simultaneous stimulation of any point in the area and a specific point in the retina of the other eye will result in a unitary percept.

papillae Flat-topped elevations in the upper tarsal conjunctiva containing blood vessels and having a smooth, velvety appearance, present in some forms of allergic conjunctivitis.

papilledema An elevation of the optic nerve head due to increased intracranial pressure.

papillitis Inflammation of the optic nerve within the eye, as seen by means of the ophthalmoscope. Also called *optic neuritis.*

patient profile In a problem-oriented record system, information concerning the patient, including birthplace, occupation, marital status, hobbies and special interests, and other items.

perimeter An arc-shaped or hemispherical surface designed to plot the peripheral visual field at a distance of 33cm.

perimetry Visual field plotting (either central or peripheral fields).
  kinetic perimetry The usual method of perimetry, in which a test object of a given size and intensity is moved in the visual field to determine the extent of the field or to determine the presence of scotomata within the visual field.
  static perimetry The presentation of a stimulus in a given area of the visual field, presented at several illumination levels in a stepwise fashion until a a response is illicited. The procedure is repeated for other stimuli, also at predetermined positions.

permeability The product of diffusivity (D) and solubility (k).

phi movement test An alternating cover test in which the patient is instructed to report the direction of movement of the fixated object. Movement in the same direction as the fixated object indicates exophoria, while movement in the opposite direction indicates esophoria.

phoria A latent deviation of the visual axes of the two eyes; a deviation brought about by eliminating all stimuli to fusion. Also called *heterophoria* and *dissociated phoria.*

associated phoria   The determination of the amount of prism power (base-in, base-out, base-up, or base-down) necessary to eliminate fixation disparity while peripheral fusion is operating.

dissociated phoria   A phoria test in which fusion is interrupted by the use of a prism or other means. See also *phoria.*

esophoria   A latent deviation of the visual axes of the two eyes in which the visual axis of one eye deviates inward with respect to the other, when all stimuli to fusion have been eliminated.

exophoria   A latent deviation of the visual axes of the two eyes in which the visual axis of one eye deviates outward with respect to the other, when all stimuli to fusion have been eliminated.

hyperphoria   A latent deviation of the visual axes of the two eyes in which the visual axis of one eye deviates upward with respect to the other, when all stimuli to fusion have been eliminated. Also called *vertical phoria.*

orthophoria   A condition in which the visual axes of the two eyes remain parallel when all stimuli to fusion have been eliminated.

phoria position   The position that the visual axes take with respect to one another in the absence of stimuli to fusion. For distance fixation, the visual axes are usually slightly divergent.

phoropter   See *refractor.*

pinguecula   A benign, elevated, yellowish white mass of tissue located on the bulbar conjuctiva either nasal or temporal to the cornea (usually nasal), consisting of a deposition of amorphous hyaline substance in areas of degenerative elastic tissue.

position of rest   The position taken by the visual axes in the absence of stimuli to fusion.

anatomical position of rest   The position taken by the visual axes in the absence of neuro-muscular control, as in death.

physiological position of rest   The position that the visual axes take with respect to one another in the presence of tonic convergence stimuli; also called the *fusion-free position* and the *phoria position.* For distance fixation, the visual axes are usually slightly divergent.

positive fusional vergence test   A binocular vision test conducted at either 6m or 40cm, in which the patient views a vertical line of 20/20 letters while base-out prism power is gradually increased in front of each eye until the patient reports that the letters are blurred and then that two lines of letters are seen. Prism power is then reduced until the patient reports that only one line of letters is seen.

presbyopia   The refractive condition that occurs when the near point of accommodation has receded to the point that near work is difficult or impossible without the use of corrective lenses. Presbyopia is usually considered to be present when the amplitude of accommodation has decreased to 5.00D or less.

absolute presbyopia   Presbyopia in which the amplitude of accommodation is reduced to zero.

principal planes   Two planes located perpendicular to the axis of an optical system such that rays of incident light entering the optical system may be considered as refracted by a single, thin lens located at the primary principal plane, and rays of light leaving the optical system may be considered as refracted by a single, thin lens located at the secondary principal plane. The primary and secondary principal points, P and P', are the points where the principal planes cross the optic axis.

prism   An optical element whose surfaces are angled with respect to one another in order to produce a given amount of deviation of incident light.

horizontal prism   A prism whose base-apex meridian is oriented horizontally; either a base-in prism or a base-out prism.

vertical prism   A prism whose base-apex meridian is oriented vertically; either a base-up prism or a base-down prism.

prism adaptation   A phenomenon in which a patient's phoria increases as a result of wearing prism, usually by the amount of the prism worn. This is thought to occur only for those patients whose symptoms did not justify the original prescription of prism.

prism diopter   A unit of tangent measurement (rather than arc measurement) used to specify convergence of the eyes, equal to a tangent displacement of 1cm at a distance of 1m from the midpoint of a line joining the centers of rotation of the eyes.

problem-oriented optometric records   See *optometric records.*

progress notes   The fourth component of a problem-oriented record system, forming the final step in the feedback loop. Each progress note is a narrative note, numbered and titled to correspond with a problem in the complete problem list. Each progress note includes four components: symptomatic, objective, assessment, and plan.

pseudoisochromatic plate A test plate designed to detect color vision anomalies, having numbers or other symbols made up of dots that may vary in both hue and brightness.

pterygium A triangular fold of opaque, vascularized tissue extending from the nasal or temporal bulbar conjunctiva (usually nasal) onto the cornea, most prevalent in individuals who spend much time outdoors in sunny, dusty, or windswept environments.

pupillary escape Dilation of both pupils when the pupil of the defective eye is illuminated during the swinging flashlight test; a manifestation of the Marcus Gunn pupil.

Purkinje images Images formed by reflection from the anterior and posterior surfaces of the cornea and from the anterior and posterior surfaces of the lens.

refractometer An optical instrument designed for the purpose of objectively determining the refractive state of the eyes, based on the principle of the retinoscope, the ophthalmoscope, or the lensometer. These instruments are patient-objective but examiner-subjective.

refractor An instrument designed for refraction and phorometry, equipped with spherical and cylindrical lenses, prisms, and the various accessories necessary for the performance of refraction and binocular vision testing. Also called a *phoropter*.

relative accommodation tests Clinical tests in which the stimulus to accommodation is varied by the use of plus or minus lenses, while the stimulus to convergence remains unchanged.

negative relative accommodation At a distance of 40cm, plus lens power is added to the subjective lenses, 0.25D at a time, until the patient reports that the 20/20 letters are blurred. Also called the *plus-lens-to-blur test*.

positive relative accommodation At a distance of 40cm, minus lens power is added to the subjective lenses, 0.25D at a time, until the patient reports that the 20/20 letters are blurred. Also called the *minus-lens-to-blur test*.

retinal detachment A condition in which the sensory retina has become detached from the pigment epithelium, the latter remaining attached to the choroid.

retinal disparity The situation occurring when an object point stimulates noncorresponding (disparate) retinal points.

retinal image The image formed on the retina by the eye's optical system. It may be sharply focused or blurred.

retinoscope An instrument designed for objective refraction. The illumination system consists of a source of light, condensing lenses, and a semisilvered mirror that reflects light into the patient's eye; the observation system consists of a peephole through which the examiner observes the retinoscope reflex seen in the plane of the pupil of the patient's eye.

spot retinoscope A retinoscope whose beam is circular in shape.

streak retinoscope A retinoscope whose beam is an oblong streak, which can be rotated into various meridians.

retinoscopy The determination of the refractive state of the eye by means of a retinoscope.

dynamic retinoscopy Retinoscopy with the patient's accommodation in play; usually done while a patient accommodates on letters, words, or pictures at a distance of 40 or 50cm.

static retinoscopy Retinoscopy with the patient's accommodation relaxed; done while the patient fixates on a target at a distance of 6m.

retrobulbar optic neuritis Inflammation of the optic nerve behind the eye, where it cannot be seen by ophthalmoscopy.

Scheiner's disk A double-aperture pupil placed in the light path of an optical instrument, causing a double image to be formed if the instrument is not in focus.

scotoma An area of partial or complete blindness within an area of normal or relatively normal visual field.

absolute scotoma A scotoma that is blind to all stimuli. The physiological blind spot is an example of an absolute scotoma.

negative scotoma A scotoma of which the person is not aware. The physiological blind spot is an example of a negative scotoma.

positive scotoma A scotoma of which the person is aware. The visual aura occurring in migraine is an example of a positive scotoma.

relative scotoma A scotoma involving an area of the visual field that is blind to some stimuli but not to others.

sensory fusion The process by means of which visual stimuli imaged on the two retinas are combined into a single percept; also known as *unification*.

slit lamp See *biomicroscope*.

Snellen acuity chart A visual acuity chart having letters of various sizes constructed in such a way that the width of a stroke equals the width of a gap, and such that each letter is 5 units high and 4 units wide.

Snellen fraction A representation of visual acuity in the form of a fraction, whose numerator is the testing distance (expressed in feet or in meters) and whose denominator is the distance at which a normal eye could see the smallest letter read.

specular microscope An instrument that permits a detailed examination of the corneal endothelium, requiring an anesthetic and applanating an area of the cornea measuring approximately 1mm × 1mm.

spherical aberration An aberration of a large-aperture optical system, in which rays of light from an axial object point entering the periphery of the optical system are refracted to a greater or lesser extent than rays entering the system paraxially.

spherical lens A lens whose refracting power is uniform in all meridians.

sphygmomanometer An instrument for measurement of blood pressure.

squint See *tropia*.

step-along method A method of making optical computations in which vergence of light is calculated separately for each surface impinged on by light, rather than making use of a formula.

stereopsis The perception of three-dimensional depth or solidity, occurring as a result of the stimulation of noncorresponding (disparate) retinal points.

strabismus See *tropia*.

suppression A phenomenon in which there is a cortical inhibition of the information arriving from specific regions of the retina of the deviating eye of a strabismic patient.

swinging flashlight test A test of the pupillary light reflexes, in which a penlight is used to alternately illuminate the pupil of each eye, being swung back and forth from one eye to the other; designed to detect a Marcus Gunn pupil.

tangent screen A flat, black felt screen, mounted on a roller or on a stiff backing, used to plot the central visual field at a distance of either 1 or 2m.

temporal arteritis An inflammation of the cranial arteries, and in particular the temporal arteries, in which giant cells are found in the inflammatory exudate, and which can cause closure of the central artery of the retina. Also called *cranial arteritis* and *giant cell arteritis*.

tonic pupil See *Adie's tonic pupil*.

tonometry A procedure for measurement of the pressure within the eye (intraocular pressure).
  applanation tonometry The measurement of the intraocular pressure by flattening (applanating) the cornea. With the Goldmann tonometer, the intraocular pressure is determined on the basis of the amount of pressure that must be applied by the tonometer to flatten a corneal area of a predetermined size.
  indentation tonometry The measurement of the intraocular pressure by determining the amount of indentation of the tonometer probe brought about by a specific weight (usually 5.5g).

transmissivity For a contact lens, the transmissivity of a gas is equal to the permeability divided by the thickness of the lens, or transmissivity = Dk/L.

trichromat A person having normal color vision, who requires three primary colors to match any given color stimulus.
  anomalous trichromat A person who requires three primary colors to match any given color stimulus, but who will match a given color stimulus with different proportions of the three primaries than will a normal trichromat.
  deuteranomalous trichromat A person who requires an excessive amount of green in a red-green mixture to match a standard yellow stimulus.
  protanomalous trichromat A person who requires an excessive amount of red in a red-green mixture to match a standard yellow stimulus.

tropia A manifest deviation of the visual axes of the two eyes; a deviation occurring when stimuli to fusion are operating. Also called *heterotropia*, *strabismus*, and *squint*.
  alternating tropia A tropia that may be manifest in either of the two eyes.
  concomitant tropia A tropia in which the angle of deviation is the same in all directions of gaze.

constant tropia A tropia occurring at all times.

esotropia A tropia in which the visual axis of one eye deviates inward.

extropia A tropia in which the visual axis of one eye deviates outward.

hypertropia A tropia in which the visual axis of one eye deviates upward.

hypotropia A tropia in which the visual axis of one eye deviates downward.

incomitant tropia A tropia in which the angle of deviation is not the same in all directions of gaze.

paralytic tropia A tropia occurring due to paralysis of a nerve or a muscle.

periodic tropia A tropia that occurs at only one testing distance.

unilateral tropia A tropia that is manifested in only one eye.

Turville infinity balance A method of binocular refraction making use of a mirror having a 3cm-wide septum, with the result that the right eye sees only the right side of the chart, and the left eye sees only the left side of the chart. The test can also be done without a mirror if a septum is placed approximately halfway between the patient and the chart or projector screen.

uveitis A chronic or acute inflammation of the uveal tract (the iris, ciliary body, or choroid).

vergence movements Disjunctive movements of the eyes, in which the visual axes move toward (convergence) or away from (divergence) one another.

accommodative convergence Convergence that accompanies accommodation.

fusional vergence Vergence (convergence or divergence) stimulated by retinal disparity, resulting in the avoidance of diplopia; also called *reflex vergence* and *disparity vergence.*

proximal convergence Convergence due to the awareness of nearness; also called *psychic convergence* and *voluntary convergence.*

tonic convergence Convergence due to the basic tonicity of the extraocular muscles; it is responsible, in part, for the distance phoria.

vertical fusional vergence test A binocular vision test conducted at either 6m or 40cm, in which the patient views a horizontal line of 20/20 letters while base-down prism (to test supravergence) or base-up prism (to test infravergence) is gradually increased in front of one eye until the patient reports that two lines of letters are seen. Prism power is then reduced until the patient reports that only one line of letters is seen.

visual acuity The resolving power of the eye, or the ability to see two separate objects as separate. The normal eye can resolve two objects as separate (with adequate illumination and contrast) if they are separated by an angular distance of 1 minute of arc.

decimal acuity The representation of visual acuity according to the decimal system, in which the resolution of the gap of 1 minute of arc in width represents visual acuity of 1.0.

English acuity The representation of visual acuity according to the English system of measurement, in which the resolution of a gap of 1 minute arc in width represents visual acuity of 20/20.

metric acuity The representation of visual acuity according to the metric system of measurement, in which the resolution of a gap of 1 minute of arc in width represents visual acuity of 6/6.

percentage acuity The representation of visual acuity in terms of a percentage, in which the resolution of a gap of 1 minute of arc in width represents visual acuity of 100 percent.

References

ABEL, C., and HOFSTETTER, H., Class Notes on Graphical Analysis, School of Optometry, Indiana University, undated.

ABRAHAM, S. V., Control of Myopia with Tropicamide, *J. Ped. Ophthal.*, Vol. 3, pp. 10–22, 1966.

ABRAMS, B. S., and SCHMAKEL, J. G., Second Generation C.A.B. Fitting, *Cont. Lens Forum*, pp. 39–55, May 1980.

ADAMS, A. J., Axial Length Elongation, Not Corneal Curvature, As a Basis of Adult Onset Myopia, *Amer. J. Optom.*, Vol. 64, pp. 150–152, 1987.

ADLER, F. H., *Physiology of the Eye*, 4th ed., St. Louis, Mosby, 1965.

AFANADOR, A. J., The EOG Ratio and Its Evaluation of Retinal Function, *J. Amer. Optom. Assoc.*, Vol. 40, pp. 1149–1156, 1977.

ALLANSMITH, M. R., Vernal Conjunctivitis, Vol. 4, Ch. 9, *Clinical Ophthalmology*, T. D. Duane, Editor, Hagerstown, Md., Harper & Row, 1978.

ALLANSMITH, M. R.; KORB, D. R.; GREINER, J. V.; HENRIQUEZ, A. S.; SIMON, M. A.; and FINNEMORE, V. M., Giant Papillary Conjunctivitis in Contact Lens Wearers, *Amer. J. Ophthal.*, Vol. 83, pp. 697–708, 1977.

ALVAREZ, L. W., Development of Variable Focus Lenses and a New Refractor, *J. Amer. Optom. Assoc.*, Vol. 49, pp. 24–30, 1978.

AMERICAN OPTICAL CORP., *A Compact Guide to Understanding the Executive Lens*, Southbridge, Mass., 1975.

ANONYMOUS, The Adjustment to Aphakia, *Amer. J. Ophthal.*, Vol. 35, pp. 118–122, 1952.

ANSTICE, J., Astigmatism: Its Components and Their Changes with Age. *Amer. J. Optom.*, Vol. 48, pp. 1001–1008, 1971.

AOA News, July 1, 1980.

AOA News, Sept. 1, 1981.

APELL, R. J., Clinical Application of Bell Retinoscopy, *J. Amer. Optom. Assoc.*, Vol. 46, pp. 1023–1027, 1975.

APPLEGATE, R. A., and MASSOF, R. W., Changes in Contrast Sensitivity Function Induced by Contact Lens Wear, *Amer. J. Optom.*, Vol. 52, pp. 840–846, 1975.

ARDEN, G. B., The Importance of Measuring Contrast Sensitivity in Cases of Visual Disturbance, *Brit. J. Ophthal.*, Vol. 62, pp. 198–209, 1978.

ARDEN, G. B., and GUCUKOGLU, A. G., Grating Test of Contrast Sensitivity in Patients with Retrobulbar Neuritis, *Arch. Ophthal.*, Vol. 96, pp. 1626–1629, 1978.

ARDEN, G. B., and JACOBSON, J. J., A Simple Grating Test for Contrast Sensitivity: Preliminary Results Indicate Value in Screening for Glaucoma, *Invest. Ophthal. Vis. Sci.*, Vol. 17, pp. 23–32, 1978.

ARMALY, M. F., and SAYEGH, R. E., The Cup-Disc Ratio: The Findings of Tonometry and Tonography in the Normal Eye, *Arch. Ophthal.*, Vol. 82, p. 191, 1969.

ARONS, I. J., Contact Lenses in the 80s: An International Overview, *Cont. Lens Forum*, pp. 21–25, July 1981.

BAILEY, I. L., New "Expaned Field" Bioptic Systems, *Optom. Monthly*, pp. 981–984, Oct. 1978a.

BAILEY, I. L., Refracting Low-Vision Patients, *Optom. Monthly*, pp. 519–523, May 1978b.

BAILEY, I. L. Specification of Nearpoint Performance, *Optom. Monthly*, pp. 895–898, Sept. 1978c.

BAILEY, I. L., Taking Case Histories of Low Vision Patients: The Key to Success, *Optom. Monthly*, pp. 294–297, March 1978d.

BAILEY, I. L., Telescopes: Their Use in Low Vision, *Optom. Monthly*, pp. 634–638, 1978e.

BAILEY, I. L., Centering High-Addition Spectacle Lenses, *Optom. Monthly*, pp. 523–527, July 1979.

BAILEY, I. L., Combining Hand Magnifiers with Spectacle Additions, *Optom. Monthly*, pp. 458–461, July 1980a.

BAILEY, I. L., Designation of Visual Acuity in Logarithmic Units, *Optom. Monthly*, pp. 53–57, 1980b.

BAILEY, I. L., Afocal Telescopes, *Optom. Monthly*, pp. 17–20, Nov. 1981.

BAILEY, N. J., Possible Factors in the Control of Myopia with Contact Lenses, *Contacto*, Sept., pp. 114–117, 1958.

BAILEY, N. J., Contact Lens Coating: The Effect on Service Life, *J. Amer. Optom Assoc.*, Vol. 46, pp. 214–218, 1975a.

BAILEY, N. J., Inspection of Hydrogel Lenses, *Inter. Cont. Lens Clin.*, Vol. 2, No. 1, pp. 42–47, 1975b.

BAILEY, N. J., Update Report 1981, *Cont. Lens Forum*, pp. 19–25, Feb. 1981.

BALDWIN, W. R., *Some Relationships Between Ocular, Anthropometric and Refractive Variables in Myopia*, Ph.D. dissertation, Indiana University, Aug. 1964.

BALDWIN, W. R., Clinical Research and Procedures in Refraction, in *Synopsis of the Refractive State of the Eye, A Symposium*. Minneapolis, Burgess, 1967.

BALDWIN, W. R., and MILLS, D., A Longitudinal Study of Corneal Astigmatism and Total Astigmatism, *Amer. J. Optom*, Vol. 58, pp. 206–211, 1981.

BALDWIN, W. R., and STOVER, W. B., Observations of Laser Standing Wave Patterns to Determine Refractive Status, *Amer. J. Optom.*, Vol. 45, pp. 143–151, 1968.

BALDWIN, W. R.; WEST, D.; JOLLY, J.; and RIED, W., Effects of Contact Lenses on Refractive Corneal and Axial Length Changes in Young Myopes, *Amer. J. Optom.*, Vol. 46, pp. 903–911, 1969.

BALLIET, R.; CLAY, A.; and BLOOD, K., The Training of Visual Acuity in Myopia, *J. Amer. Optom. Assoc.*, Vol. 53, pp. 719–724, 1982.

BANKS, M. S., Infant Refraction and Accommodation. *Inter. Ophthal. Clin.*, Vol. 20, No. 1, pp. 205–232, 1980.

BANNON, R. E., The Use of Cycloplegics in Refraction, *Amer. J. Optom.*, Vol. 24, pp. 513–568, 1947.

BANNON, R. E., Recent Developments in Techniques for Measuring Astigmatism, *Amer. J. Optom.*, Vol. 35, pp. 353–359, 1958.

BANNON, R. E., Binocular Refraction: A Survey of Various Techniques, *Optom. Weekly*, Vol. 56, pp. 25–31, Aug. 5, 1965.

BANNON, R. E., A New Automated Subjective Optometer, *Amer. J. Optom.*, Vol. 54, pp. 433–438, 1977.

BANNON, R. E., and WALSH, R., On Astigmatism, Parts 1 and 2, *Amer. J. Optom.*, Vol. 22, pp. 101–111, 162–179, 1945.

BARR, J. T., Silicone Lenses Are Elastic and Permeable, *Rev. Optom.*, pp. 59–62, April 1981.

BARR, J. T., and SCHOESSLER, J. P., Corneal Endothelia: Response to Rigid Contact Lenses, *Amer. J. Optom.*, Vol. 57, pp. 267–274, 1980.

BARRAQUER, J. I., Refraction Experimental Surgery, *Contacto*, Vol. 8, pp. 8–11, 1964.

BARSTOW, R., *How to Succeed in Optometry*, 2nd ed., Chicago, Illinois College of Optometry Press, 1959.

BATES, W. H., *Perfect Sight Without Glasses*, New York, Central Fixation Pub. Co., 1920.

BECHTOLD, E. W., The Aberrations of Ophthalmic Lenses, *Amer. J. Optom.*, Vol. 35, pp. 10–24, 1958.

BEHRENDT, T., Fluorescein Angiography, Vol. 3, Ch. 4, in *Clinical Ophthalmology*, T. D. Duane, Editor, Hagerstown, Md., Harper & Row, 1976.

BENJAMIN, W. J., and HILL, R. M., Ultra-Thins: An Oxygen Update, *Cont. Lens Forum*, pp. 43–45, Jan. 1979.

BENJAMIN, W. J., and SIMONS, M. H., Extended Wear of Rigid Contact Lenses in Aphakia, a Preliminary Report. *Inter. Cont. Lens Clin.*, Vol. 11, pp. 44–57, 1984.

BENNETT, A. G., *Optics of Contact Lenses*, Assoc. of Dispensing Opticians, London, 1956.

BERNSTEIN, I. H., and BRODRICK, J., Contrast Sensitivities Through Spectacles and Soft Contact Lenses. *Amer. J. Optom.*, Vol. 58, pp. 309–313, 1981.

BERMAN, P. E.; LEVINGER, S. I.; MASSOTH, N. A.; GALLAGHER, D.; KALMAR, K.; POS, L.; and WESTERVELD, M., The Effectiveness of Biofeedback Visual Training As a Viable Method of Treatment and Reduction of Myopia, *J. Optom. Vis. Devel.*, 1985.

BIEBER, J. C., Why Nearpoint Retinoscopy with Children? *Optom. Weekly*, pp. 54–57, Jan. 17; and pp. 78–81, Jan. 24, 1974.

BIER, N., *Contact Lens Routine and Practice*, 2nd ed., London, Butterworths, 1957.

BLUM, H. L.; PETERS, H. B.; and BETTMAN, J. W., *Vision Screening for Elementary Schools, The Orinda Study*, Berkeley, University of California Press, 1959.

BOBIER, C. W., and SIVAK, J. G., Chromoretinoscopy, *Vis. Res.*, Vol. 18, p. 24, 1978.

BOBIER, C. W., and SIVAK, J. G., Chromoretinoscopy and Its Instrumentation, *Amer. J. Optom.*, Vol. 47, pp. 106–108, 1980.

BOLTZ, R. L., Visual Acuity in Amblyopia: Measurement of Visual Acuity in Infants and Children, *Texas Optom.*, Vol. 37, pp. 7–9, July 1981.

BOLTZ, R. L., Lecture given at University of Houston, Continuing education course, Houston, Tex., Jan. 17, 1982.

BORISH, I. M., Comments on a Delayed Subjective Test, *Amer. J. Optom.*, Vol. 22, pp. 433–436, 1945.

BORISH, I. M., *Clinical Refraction*, 3rd ed., Chicago, Professional Press, 1970.

BORISH, I. M., Refraction Techniques, continuing education course, University of Waterloo, Waterloo, Ontario, Canada, 1972.

BORISH, I. M., The Borish Nearpoint Chart, *J. Amer. Optom. Assoc.*, Vol. 49, pp. 41–44, 1978.

BORISH, I. M., Fitting Bifocal Contact Lenses, lecture at the University of Houston, Houston, Tex., Oct. 1985.

BORISH, I. M.; HITZMAN, S. A.; and BROOKMAN, K. E., Double masked Study of Progressive Addition Lenses, *J. Amer. Optom. Assoc.*, Vol. 51, pp. 533–540.

BORISH, I. M.; HITZMAN, S. A.; and BROOKMAN, K. E., Double masked Study of Progressive Addition Lenses, *J. Amer. Optom. Assoc.*, Vol. 51, pp. 933–943, 1980.

BORLEY, W. E., and TANNER, O. R., Use of Scleral Resection in High Myopia: Report of a Case, *Amer. J. Ophthal.*, Vol. 28, pp. 517–520, 1964.

BOTT, A. G., Lecture given at University of Auckland, Auckland, New Zealand, Jan. 1965.

BROCKHURST, R. J., Modern Indirect Ophthalmoscopy, *Amer. J. Ophthal.*, Vol. 41, pp. 265–272, 1956.

BRODSTEIN, R. S.; BRODSTEIN, D. E.; OLSON, R. J.; HUNT, S. C.; and WILLIAMS, R. R., The Treatment of Myopia with Atropine and Bifocals, *Ophthal.*, Vol. 91, pp. 1373–1379, 1984.

BROOKS, C. W., Streak Retinoscopy Technique, *Optom. Weekly*, Vol. 66, pp. 502–505, June 5, 1975.

BROOKS, C. W., Absorptive Lenses, Part 5: The Photochromics, *Optom. Monthly*, pp. 955–958, 1978.

BROWN, B., and GARNER, L. F., Effects of Luminance on Contrast Sensitivity in Senile Macular Degeneration, *Amer. J. Optom.*, Vol. 60, pp. 788–793, 1983.

BROWN, N., The Changes in Lens Curvature with Age, *Exp. Eye Res.*, Vol. 19, pp. 175–183, 1974.

BRUNGARDT, T. F., A Fast, Accurate and Practical Measurement of the Secondary Curve Radius, *J. Amer. Optom. Assoc.*, Vol. 34, p. 131, 1962a.

BRUNGARDT, T. F., Lecture given at Southwest Contact Lens Congress, Oklahoma City, 1962b.

BRUNGARDT, T. F., Reliability of Keratometer Readings, *Amer. J. Optom.*, Vol. 46, pp. 686–691, 1969.

BRUNGARDT, T. F., Determining the Problem Patient Early, *Optom. Weekly*, Feb. 3, 1972.

BRUNGARDT, T. F., and POTTER, E., Adaptation to Corneal Contact Lenses, *Amer. J. Optom.*, Vol. 49, pp. 41–49, 1972.

BURDE, R. M., The Extraocular Muscles, Ch. 5, Pt. 1, in *Adler's Physiology of the Eye*, R. A. Moses, Editor, St. Louis, Mosby, 1975.

CARTER, D. B., Studies in Fixation Disparity: Historical Review, *Amer. J. Optom.*, Vol. 34, pp. 320–329, 1957.

CARTER, D. B., Effects of Prolonged Wearing of Prism, *Amer. J. Optom.*, Vol. 40, pp. 265–273, 1963.

CARTER, D. B., Fixation Disparity and Heterophoria Following Prolonged Wearing of Prisms, *Amer. J. Optom.*, Vol. 42, pp. 141–152, 1965.

CARTER, D. B. (ed.), *Interdisciplinary Approaches to Learning Disorders*, Chilton, Philadelphia, 1970.

CARTER, D. B., *Optometric Examination*, Multimedia Center, School of Optometry, University of California, 1973.

CARTER, D. B., Parameters of Fixation Disparity, *Amer. J. Optom.*, Vol. 57, pp. 610–617, 1980.

CARTER, D. B., Personal communication, 1981.

CARTER, J. H., Some Variations in Methodology for Crossed Cylinder Astigmatic Tests, *Optom. Monthly*, Vol. 72, pp. 15–19, Feb. 1981.

CASSIN, B., Strabismus and Learning Disabilities, *Amer. Orthopt. J.*, Vol. 25, pp. 38–45, 1976.

CAVELLERANO, A.; GUTNER, R.; and GARSTEN, M., Indirect Biomicroscopy Techniques, *J. Amer. Optom. Assoc.*, Vol. 57, pp. 755–758, 1986.

CHANG, F. W., Pharmacology of Mydriasis for Modern Optometric Procedures, *J. Amer. Optom. Assoc.*, Vol. 48, pp. 1365–1368, 1977.

CHARLES, A. M.; CALLENDER, M.; and GROSVENOR, T., Efficacy of Chemical Asepticizing System for Soft Contact Lenses, *Amer. J. Optom.*, Vol. 50, pp. 777–781, 1973.

CHASE, W. W., Infrared Radiation Transmission of Photochromic Lenses, *Optom. Weekly*, pp. 1070–1074, Nov. 6, 1975.

CLARK, B. A. J., A Survey of Optical Properties of Sunglasses, *Austral. J. Optom.*, Vol. 51, pp. 150–162, 1968.

CLARK, B. A. J., Color in Sunglass Lenses, *Amer. J. Optom.*, Vol. 46, pp. 825–840, 1969.

COCKBURN, D. M., Prevalence and Significance of Narrow Anterior Chamber Angles in Optometric Practice, *Amer. J. Optom.*, Vol. 58, pp. 171–175, 1981.

COGAN, D. M., Vascularization of the Cornea, *Trans. Amer. Ophthal. Soc.*, Vol. 46, p. 457, 1948.

COGAN, D. M., and KINSEY, V. E., Hydration Properties of the Whole Cornea, *Arch. Ophthal.*, Vol. 28, p. 449, 1942.

COHEN, A. I., The Retina and Optic Nerve, Ch. 14, in *Adler's Physiology of the Eye*, R. A. Moses, Editor, 6th ed., St. Louis, Mosby, 1975.

COLENBRANDER, A., Principles of Ophthalmoscopy, Vol. 1, Ch. 63, in *Clinical Ophthalmology*, T. D. Duane, Editor, Hagerstown, Md., Harper & Row, 1979.

COLLIN, H. B., Lymphatic Drainage of I^{131} Albumin from the Vascularized Cornea, *Invest. Ophthal.*, Vol. 9, p. 146, 1970.

COMERFORD, J. P., Vision Evaluation Using Contrast Sensitivity Functions, *Amer. J. Optom.*, Vol. 60, pp. 394–398, 1983.

COOK, R. C., and GLASSCOCK, R. E., Refractive and Ocular Findings in the Newborn, *Amer. J. Ophthal.*, Vol. 34, pp. 1407–1413, 1951.

CRAWFORD, H. E., and HAMMAR, R. E., Racial Analysis of Ocular Deformaties in Schools of Hawaii, *Hawaii Med. J.*, Vol. 9, pp. 90–93, 1949.

CRISWELL, M. H., and GOSS, D. A. Myopia Development in Nonhuman Primates—A Literature Review. *Amer. J. Optom.*, Vol. 60, pp. 250–268, 1983.

CROSS, A. J., *Dynamic Skiametry in Theory and Practice*, New York, Cross Optical Co., 1911.

CURTIN, B. J., *The Myopias, Basic Science and Clinical Management*, Philadelphia, Harper & Row, 1985.

CURTIN, B. J., and KARLIN, D. B., Axial Length Measurements and Fundus Changes of the Myopic Eye, *Amer. J. Ophthal.*, Vol. 71, pp. 42–53, 1971.

CULLEN, A. P., Fluorescein Angiography of the Ocular Fundus, *Amer. J. Optom.*, Vol. 56, pp. 592–596, 1979.

DAVIES, P. H. O., *The Actions and Uses of Ophthalmic Drugs*, London, Barrie and Jenkins, 1972.

DAVIS, H. E., The CSI Crofilcon A: A Membrane Lens for Aphakic Extended Wear. *J. Amer. Optom. Assoc.*, Vol. 51, pp. 217–220, 1980.

DAVIS, J. K., Aspheric lenses: What's Possible and What Isn't. *Rev. Optom.* Vol. 115, pp. 68–74, May 1978.

DAWSON, C. R., Follicular Conjunctivitis, Vol. 4, Ch. 7, in *Clinical Ophthalmology*, T. D. Duane, Editor, Hagerstown, Md., Harper & Row, 1979.

DeCARLE, J., Extended Wear Gaining Ground. *Cont. Lens Forum*, pp. 31–41, Sept. 1979.

DICKINSON, F. and HALL, C., *An Introduction to the Prescribing and Fitting of Contact Lenses*, London, Hammond, Hammond and Co., 1946.

DICKINSON, F., The Value of Microlenses in Progressive Myopia, *Optician*, March, pp. 263–264, 1957.

DICKINSON, F., Lecture given at a University of Waterloo, Waterloo, Ontario, Canada, Feb. 1971.

DOBSON, V.; FULTON, A.; and SEBRIS, S. L., Cycloplegic Refractions of Infants and Young Children: The Axis of Astigmatism, *Inves. Ophthal. Vis. Sci.*, Vol. 25, pp. 83–87, 1984.

DOGGART, J. H., *Ocular Signs in Slit-Lamp Microscopy*, London, Henry Kimpton, 1948.

DONDERS, F. C., *On the Anomalies of Accommodation and Refraction of the Eye*, London, New Sydenham Society, 1864 (reprinted by Milford House, Boston, 1972).

DOUGAL, J.; HOEFT, W. W.; and DOWALIBY, P., Speaking Up for the Spot Retinoscope, or Flash vs. Streak, *Optom. Monthly*, Vol. 71, pp. 259–262, April 1980.

DREWS, L. C., Ophthalmological Head Pain, Ch. 52, in *Headache: Diagnosis and Treatment*, R. E. Ryan, St. Louis, Mosby, 1954.

DUANE, T. D., Editor, *Clinical Ophthalmology*, Hagerstown, Md., Harper & Row, Vol. 3, 1976.

DUKE-ELDER, S., *Textbook of Ophthalmology*, Vol. 4, St. Louis, Mosby, 1949.

DUKE-ELDER, S., *System of Ophthalmology*, Vol. 5, St. Louis, Mosby, 1970.

DWYER, W. O.; GRANATA, D.; BOSSIN, R.; and ANDREAS, S. R., Validity of the Laser Refraction Technique for Determining Spherical Error in Different Refractive Groups, *Amer. J. Optom.*, Vol. 50, pp. 222–225, 1973.

DWYER, W. O.; KENT, P.; POWELL, J.; McELVAIN, R. M.; and REDMOND, J., Reliability of the Laser Refraction Technique for Different Refractive Groups, *Amer. J. Optom.*, Vol. 49, pp. 929–931, 1972.

EAMES, T. H., Comparison of Eye Conditions Among 1,000 Reading Failures, 500 Ophthalmic Patients and 150 Unselected Children, *Amer. J. Ophthal.*, Vol. 31, pp. 713–717, 1948.

EFRON, N., and CARNEY, L. G., Oxygen Levels Beneath the Closed Eyelids, *Invest. Ophthal. Vis. Sci.*, Vol. 18, pp. 93–95, 1979.

EL BAYADI, G., New Method of Slit-Lamp Micro-ophthalmoscopy, *Brit. J. Ophthal.*, Vol. 37, pp. 625–628, 1953.

ELLIS, P. P., *Ocular Therapeutics and Pharmacology*, St. Louis, Mosby, 1977.

EMSLEY, H. H., *Visual Optics*, 5th ed., London, Hatton Press, 1953.

ENOCH, J. M., A Spectacle-Contact Lens Combination Used as a Reverse Galilean Telescope in Unilateral Aphakia, *Amer. J. Optom.*, Vol. 45, pp. 231–240, 1968.

ENOCH, J. M., Personal communication, 1971.

ERICKSON, P., Mathematical Model for Predicting Dioptric Effects of Optical Parameter Changes in the Eye, *Amer. J. Optom.*, Vol. 59, pp. 226–233, 1982.

ERICKSON, P., Theoretical Binocular Depth of Field in Monovision (abstract), *Amer. J. Optom.*, Vol. 64, p. 51P, 1987.

ESKRIDGE, J. B., The Raubitschek Astigmatism Test, *Amer. J. Optom.*, Vol. 35, pp. 238–247, 1958.

ESPINDA, S. D., Color Vision Deficiency: A Learning Disability? *J. Learn. Dis.*, Vol. 6, pp. 163–166, 1973.

EWALT, H. W. JR., The Baltimore Myopia Control Project, *J. Amer. Optom. Assoc.*, Vol. 17, pp. 167–185, 1946.

FAIRMAID, J. A., The Constancy of Corneal Curvature, *Brit. J. Physiol. Opt.*, Vol. 16, pp. 2–23, 1959.

FALASCA, N. A., and PANARIELLO, G. Corneal Infiltrates Induced by Contact Lenses, *Inter. Cont. Lens Clin.*, pp. 28–32, July/Aug. 1981.

FANNIN, T., Personal communication, 1962.

FANNIN, T., and GROSVENOR, T., *Clinical Optics*, Boston, Butterworths, 1987.

FATT, I., Oxygen Supply Under a Gas Permeable Hard Lens, *Cont. Lens Forum*, April 1979.

FATT, I.; FREEMAN, R. D.; and LIN, D., Oxygen Tension Distribution in the Cornea: A Re-examination, *Exp. Eye Res.*, Vol. 18, pp. 357–365, 1964.

FAYE, E. E., *Clinical Low Vision*, Boston, Little, Brown, 1976.

FELDMAN, G. L., Clinical Application of Corneal Physiology, *Contact Lens Medical Seminar*, Vol. 1, Springfield, Ill., Thomas, 1970.

FELDMAN, G., Basic Considerations for Extended Wear of Ultra-Thin Hydrogel Lenses, *Inter. Cont. Lens Clin.*, Vol. 4, No. 4, pp. 44–51, 1977.

FELDMAN, G., Annual Review of Contact Lenses, Continuing education program, University of Houston, Houston, Tex., Feb. 1979.

FELDMAN, G., Annual Review of Contact Lenses, Continuing education program, University of Houston, Houston, Tex., Feb. 1980.

FELDMAN, G. L., and SAMPSON, W., Physiology of Hard and Soft Contact Lens Wear, *Cont. Lens Med. Bul.*, Vol. 3, pp. 14–18, 1970.

FICHMAN, S.; BAKER, V. V.; and HORTON, H. R., Iatrogenic Red Eyes in Soft Contact Lens Wearers, *Inter. Cont. Lens Clin.*, pp. 20–24, Sept./Oct. 1978.

FINCHAM, E. F., The Mechanism of Accommodation, Mon. Supp. 8, *Brit. J. Ophthal.*, London, Putman, 1937.

FISHER, E. J., Hydrophilic Contact Lenses, *Can. J. Optom.*, Vol. 29, pp. 139–144, 1968.

FITZGERALD, J. K., The Silicone Lens That Works, *Cont. Lens Forum*, pp. 43–50, June 1981.

FLEDELIUS, H. C., Changes in Refraction and Eye Size During Adolescence, with Special Reference to Low Birth Weight, *Doc. Ophthal. Proc.*, Series 28, Third International Conference on Myopia, H. C. Fledelius, P. H. Alsbirk, and E. Goldschmidt, Editors, The Hague, Dr. W. Junk Publishers, 1981.

FLEDELIUS, H. C., Is Myopia Getting More Frequent? A Cross-Sectional Study of 1416 Danes Aged 16 Years +, *Acta. Ophthal.*, Vol. 61, pp. 545–559, 1983.

FLETCHER, M. C., and BRANDON, S., Myopia of Prematurity, *Amer. J. Ophthal.*, Vol. 40, pp. 474–481, 1955.

FLOM, M. C., On the Relationship Between Accommodation and Accommodative Convergence, Part 3: Effects of Orthoptics, *Amer. J. Optom.*, Vol. 37, pp. 619–632, 1960.

FLOM, M. C., Treatment of Binocular Anomalies of Vision, Ch. 7, *Vision of Children*, M. J. Hirsch and R. E. Wick, Editors, Philadelphia, Chilton, 1963.

FLOM, M. C., New Concepts in Visual Acuity, *Optom. Weekly*, Vol. 57, No. 28, pp. 63–68, 1966.

FLOM, M. C., and TAKAHASHI, E., The AC/A Ratio and Undercorrected Myopia, *Amer. J. Optom.*, Vol. 39, pp. 305–312, 1962.

FOWLER, S. A., and ALLANSMITH, M. R., Evolution of Soft Contact Lens Coatings, *Arch. Ophthal.*, Vol. 98, pp. 95–99, 1980.

FOWLER, S. A.; GREINER, J. V.; and ALLANSMITH, M. R., Soft Contact Lenses from Patients with Giant Papillary Conjunctivitis, *Amer. J. Ophthal.*, Vol. 88, pp. 1057–1061, 1979.

FRANCIS, L., *The Relationship of Eye Anomalies and Reading Ability*, Ann Arbor, Mich., University Microfilms, 1973.

FRANCOIS, J., *Heredity in Ophthalmology*, St. Louis, Mosby, 1961.

FRANCOIS, J., and GOES, F., Comparative Study of Ultrasonic Biometry of Emmetropes and Myopes, with Special Regard to Heredity of Myopia, in *Ophthalmic Ultrasound*, Ch. 19, K. Gitter, A. Keeney, L. Sarin, and D. Meyer, Editors, St. Louis, Mosby, pp. 165–180, 1969.

FRANCOIS, J., and GOES, F., Echographic Study of the Lens-Thickness As a Function of the Axial Eye Length in Emmetropic Eyes of the Same Age, in *Ultrasonographia Medica*, J. Bock and K. Ossoing, Editors, Vienna, Verlag der Weiner Med. Akad., pp. 473, 515, 1971.

FREIBERG, J., Deposition of Calcium Carbonate and Calcium Phosphate on Hydrophilic Contact Lenses, *Inter. Cont. Lens Clin.*, pp. 63–70, July/Aug. 1977.

FREIS, E. D., The Treatment of Hypertension, *Hypertension Manual*, J. H. Laragh, Editor, New York, Yorke Medical Books, 1974.

FRY, G. A., An Experimental Analysis of the Accommodation Convergence Relation, *Amer. J. Optom.*, Vol. 11, pp. 64–76, 1937.

FRY, G. A., Fundamental Variables in the Relationship Between Accommodation and Convergence, *Optom. Weekly*, March 18 and March 25, 1943 (reprinted in *Optom. Weekly*, pp. 21–25, Sept. 3, 1964).

FULTON, A. B.; HANSEN, R. M.; and PETERSEN, R. A., The Relation of Myopia and Astigmatism in Developing Eyes, *Ophthalmol.*, Vol. 89, pp. 298–302, 1982.

FYODOROV, S. N., and DURNEV, V. V., Operation of Dosaged Dissection of Corneal Circular Ligament in Cases of Myopia of Mild Degree, *Ann. Ophthal.*, Vol. 12, pp. 1885–1890, 1979.

GALLAWAY, M.; PEARL, S. M.; WINKELSTEIN, A. M.; and SCHEIMAN, M., Biofeedback Training of Visual Acuity and Myopia: A Pilot Study, *Amer. J. Optom.*, Vol. 64, pp. 62–71, 1987.

GARNER, L. F.; GROSVENOR, T.; KINNEAR, R. F.; McKELLAR, M.; KLINGER, J.; and HOVENDER, M., The Prevalence of Myopia in Melanesian School Children in Vanuatu (abstract), *Amer. J. Optom.*, Vol. 63, p. 63P, 1986.

GARNER, L. F.; KINNEAR, R. F.; KLINGER, J. D.; and McKELLAR, M. J., Prevalence of Myopia in School Children in Vanuatu, *Acta Ophthal.*, Vol. 63, pp. 323–326, 1985.

GARNETT, B. D., and WELLS, G. A., Reliability of Power Measurements of Toric Soft Contact Lenses, *Amer. J. Optom.*, Vol. 60, pp. 794–797, 1983.

GARSTON, M., and CAVALLERANO, A., Binocular Indirect Ophthalmoscopy, *Rev. Optom.*, pp. 49–57, Feb. 1980.

GARSTON, M. J., A Closer Look at Diagnostic Drugs for Optometric Use, *J. Amer. Optom. Assoc.*, Vol. 46, pp. 39–43, 1975.

GENTSCH, L. W., and GOODWIN, H. E., A Comparison of Methods of Determination of Binocular Refractive Balance, *Amer. J. Optom.*, Vol. 43, pp. 653–663, 1966.

GESSELL, A.; ILG, F. L.; and BULLIS, G. E., *Vision: Its Development in Infant and Child*, New York, Hoeber, 1949.

GIGLIO, E., and SHERMAN, J., Ophthalmic Ultrasound as a Diagnostic Tool, *J. Amer. Optom. Assoc.*, Vol. 50, pp. 73–78, 1979.

GILES, G. H., *Practice of Orthoptics*, 2nd ed., London, Hammond, 1949.

GILES, G. H., *The Principles and Practice of Refraction and Allied Subjects*, Philadelphia, Chilton, 1965.

GIMBEL, H. V., The Control of Myopia with Atropine, *Can. J. Ophthal.*, Vol. 8, pp. 527–532, 1973.

GINSBERG, A. P., A New Contrast Sensitivity Vision Test Chart, *Amer. J. Optom.*, Vol. 61, pp. 403–407, 1984.

GLASER, J. S., Neuro-ophthalmologic Examination: General Considerations and Special Techniques, Vol. 2, Ch. 2, in *Clinical Ophthalmology*, T. D. Duane, Editor, Hagerstown, Md., Harper & Row, 1979.

GLEISS, J., and PAU, H., Die Entwicklung der Refraction vor der Geburt, *Klin. Mbl. Augenheilk*, Vol. 121, pp. 440–445, 1952.

GLOVER, H.; BIRD, S.; and LAP, M., Performance of Amblyopic Children on Printed Contrast Sensitivity Test Charts, *Amer. J. Optom.*, Vol. 64, pp. 361–366, 1987.

GOLD, S. M., and ORENSTEIN, J., Surfactant Cleaners vs. the Enzyme Cleaner, *Cont. Lens Forum*, pp. 39–41, Jan. 1980.

GOLDBERG, J. B., The Hype for Rigid Gas Permeable Contact Lenses (guest editorial), *J. Amer. Optom. Assoc.*, Vol. 57, p. 172, 1986.

GOLDSCHMIDT, E., On the Etiology of Myopia, an Epidemiological Study, Suppl. 98, *Acta Ophthal.*, Copenhagen, Munksgaard, 1968.

GOLDSCHMIDT, E., Refraction in the Newborn, *Acta Ophthal.*, Vol. 47, pp. 570–578, 1969.

GOLDSCHMIDT, E.; JENSEN, H.; MARUSHAK, D.; and OSTERGAARD, E. Can Timolol Maleate Reduce the Progression of Myopia? (abstract). *Acta Ophthal.* Suppl. 173, vol. 63, p. 90, 1985.

GOMBOS, G. M., *Handbook of Ophthalmologic Emergencies*, 2nd ed., Flushing, N.Y., Med. Exam. Pub. Co., 1977.

GOSS, D., Overcorrection of Myopia as a Possible Means of Reducing Its Rate of Progression, *Amer. J. Optom.* Vol. 61, pp. 85–93, 1964.

GOSS, D. A., Refractive Status and Premature Birth, *Optom. Monthly*, Mar., pp. 109–111, 1985.

GOSS, D. A., Effect of Bifocal Lenses on the Rate of Childhood Myopia Progression, *Amer. J. Optom.*, Vol. 63, pp. 135–141, 1986.

GOSS, D. A., and CRISWELL, M. H., Myopia Development in Experimental Animals—A Literature Review, *Amer. J. Optom.*, Vol. 58, pp. 859–869, 1981.

GOSS, D. A., and ERICKSON, P., Meridional Corneal Components of Myopia Progression in Young Adults and Children, *Amer. J. Optom.*, Vol. 64, pp. 475–481, 1987.

GOSS, D. A.; ERICKSON, P.; and COX, D. V., Prevalence and Pattern of Adult Myopia Progression in a General Optometric Practice Population, *Amer. J. Optom.*, Vol. 62, pp. 470–477, 1985.

GOSS, D. A., and WINKLER, R. L., Progression of Myopia in Youth: Age of Cessation, *Amer. J. Optom.*, Vol. 60, pp. 651–658, 1983.

GRAHAM, R., The Evolution of Contact Lenses, *Amer. J. Optom.*, Vol. 36, pp. 55–72, 1959.

GRAY, L. G., Fundamentals of Gonioscopy, *Rev. of Optom.*, pp. 51–60, Oct. 1977; and pp. 47–55, July 1978.

GREENE, P. R., Mechanical Considerations in Myopia: Relative Effects of Accommodation, Convergence, Intraocular Pressure, and Extraocular Muscles, *Amer. J. Optom.*, Vol. 57, pp. 902–914, 1980.

GREENE, P. R., Myopia and the Extraocular Muscles, *Doc. Ophthal. Proc.*, Series 28, Third International Conference on Myopia, H. C. Fledelius, P. H. Alsbirk, and E. Goldschmidt, Editors, The Hague, Dr. W. Junk Publishers, 1981.

GREENBERG, D. A., Basic Evaluation of Exophthalmos, *J. Amer. Optom. Assoc.*, Vol. 48, pp. 1431–1437, 1977.

GREENBERGER, M. H., A Chlorhexidine-free Chemical Regimen for Hydrophilic Contact Lenses, *Inter. Cont. Lens Clin.*, pp. 13–15, Jan./Feb. 1981.

GREENSPAN, S. B., Behavioral Effects of Children's Nearpoint Lenses, *J. Amer. Optom. Assoc.*, Vol. 46, pp. 1031–1037, 1975.

GREY, C. P., Changes in Contrast Sensitivity During the First Hour of Soft Lens Wear, *Amer. J. Optom.*, Vol. 63, pp. 702–707, 1986.

GRIFFIN, J. R., *Binocular Anomalies: Procedures for Vision Therapy*, Chicago, Professional Press, 1976.

GROLMAN, B., Binocular Refraction: A New System, *New Engl. J. Optom.*, pp. 118–129, May 1966.

GROSVENOR, T., Clinical Use of the Keratometer in Evaluating the Corneal Contour, *Amer. J. Optom.*, Vol. 38, pp. 237–246, 1961.

GROSVENOR, T., *Contact Lens Theory and Practice*, Chicago, Professional Press, 1963.

GROSVENOR, T., The Visual Status of New Zealand's Maoris: A Preliminary Report, *Amer. J. Optom.*, Vol. 42, pp. 593–605, 1965.

GROSVENOR, T., Refractive State, Intelligence Test Scores, and Academic Ability, *Amer. J. Optom.*, Vol. 47, pp. 355–361, 1970a.

GROSVENOR, T., Refractive Error Distribution in New Zealand's Polynesian and European Children, *Amer. J. Optom.*, Vol. 47, pp. 673–679, 1970b.

GROSVENOR, T., *Contemporary Contact Lens Practice*, Chicago, Professional Press, 1972a.

GROSVENOR, T., Visual Acuity, Astigmatism, and Soft Contact Lenses, *Amer. J. Optom.*, Vol. 49, pp. 407–412, 1972b.

GROSVENOR, T., Changes in Corneal Curvature and Subjective Refraction of Soft Contact Lens Wearers, *Amer. J. Optom.*, Vol. 52, pp. 405–413, 1975a.

GROSVENOR, T., Graphical Analysis of Optometric Findings, *Optom. Weekly*, pp. 747–749, Aug. 21, 1975b.

GROSVENOR, T., Interpretation of Graphical Findings, *Optom. Weekly*, pp. 775–778, Aug. 28, 1975c.

GROSVENOR, T., Binocular Vision Syndromes, *Optom. Weekly*, pp. 803–808, Sept. 4, 1975d.

GROSVENOR, T., Field of View of the Contact Lens Wearer, *Optom. Weekly*, Feb. 12, 1976a.

GROSVENOR, T., Aberrations of Ophthalmic Lenses, Part 2, *Optom. Weekly*, April 29, 1976b.

GROSVENOR, T., Aberrations of Ophthalmic Lenses, Part 3, *Optom. Weekly*, May 3, 1976c.

GROSVENOR, T., Ophthalmic Lens Design, *Optom. Weekly*, May 13, 1976d.

GROSVENOR, T., Effects of Depth of Focus and Proximal Convergence on the Zone of Clear Single Binocular Vision, *Optom. Weekly*, July 15, 1976e.

GROSVENOR, T., Relative Spectacle Magnification and Retinal Image Size in Axial and Refractive Ametropia, *Optom. Weekly*, Nov. 27, 1976f.

GROSVENOR, T., What Causes Astigmatism? *J. Amer. Optom. Assoc.*, Vol. 47, pp. 926–933, 1976g.

GROSVENOR, T., Refractive Anomalies of the Eye, Part II: A Survey of Adult Refractive Changes, *Optom. Weekly*, Vol. 68, pp. 24–25, Jan. 6, 1977a.

GROSVENOR, T., A Longitudinal Study of Refractive Changes Between Ages 20 and 40, Part 1: Mean Changes and Distribution Curves, *Optom. Weekly*, Vol. 68, pp. 386–389, April 14, 1977b.

GROSVENOR, T., A Longitudinal Study of Refractive Changes Between Ages 20 and 40, Part 4: Statistical Analysis of Data, *Optom. Monthly*, Vol. 68, 1977c.

GROSVENOR, T., A Longitudinal Study of Refractive Changes Between Ages 20 and 40, Part 5: Changes in Astigmatism, *Optom. Monthly*, Vol. 68, pp. 475–478, May 1977d.

GROSVENOR, T., The Relationship Between Refractive Error and Scores on the Minnesota Multiphasic Personality Inventory, Paper presented at the Third International Myopia Congress, Copenhagen, August 1980a.

GROSVENOR, T., Can Myopia Be Controlled? Part 2: The Bates System of Eye Exercises, *Optom. Monthly*, Vol. 71, pp. 545–549, Sept. 1980b.

GROSVENOR, T., *A Biometric Study of the Presbyopic Eye*, Third International Symposium on Presbyopia, Vol. 2, pp. 85–93, Essilor International, 1985.

GROSVENOR, T., A Review and a Suggested Classification System for Myopia on the Basis of Age-Related Prevalence and Age of Onset, *Amer. J. Optom.*, Vol. 64, pp. 545–555, 1987a.

GROSVENOR, T., Decrease in Axial Length with Age: An Emmetropizing Mechanism for the Adult Eye? *Amer. J. Optom.*, Vol. 64, pp. 657–663, 1987b.

GROSVENOR, T.; PERRIGIN, D. M.; PERRIGIN, J.; MOOREHEAD, A.; and LAMB, M., A Comparison of Cycloplegic and Non-Cycloplegic Refractive Findings on a Group of Young Adults, *Texas Optom.*, pp. 7–8, Dec. 1983, and pp. 8–11, Jan. 1984.

GROSVENOR, T.; PERRIGIN, D. M.; and PERRIGIN, J. Three-Way Comparison of Retinoscopy, Subjective, and Dioptron Nova Refractive Findings, *Amer. J. Optom.*, Vol. 62, pp. 63–65, 1985a.

GROSVENOR, T.; PERRIGIN, J.; and PERRIGIN, D. M., Comparison of American Optical SR-IV Refractive Data with Clinical Refractive Data on a Group of Myopic Children, *Amer. J. Optom.*, Vol. 60, pp. 224–235, 1983.

GROSVENOR, T.; MASLOVITZ, B.; PERRIGIN, D. M.; and PERRIGIN, J., The Houston Myopia Control Study: A Preliminary Report of the Patient Care Team, *J. Amer. Optom. Assoc.*, Vol. 56, pp. 636–643, 1985b.

GROSVENOR, T.; PERRIGIN, D. M.; PERRIGIN, J.; and MASLOVITZ, B., Houston Myopia Control Study: Randomized Clinical Trial, Part II: Final Report by the Patient Care Team, *Amer. J. Optom.*, Vol. 64, pp. 482–498, 1987.

GROSVENOR, T.; QUINTERO, S.; and PERRIGIN, D. M., Predicting Refractive Astigmatism, a Suggested Simplification of Javal's Rule, In press, *Amer. J. Optom.*, 1988.

GULLSTRAND, A., The Cornea, App. 2, Pt. 1, in *Treatise on Physiological Optics*, H. Helmholtz, Editor, New York, Opt. Soc. of America, 1924.

GUTNER, R. K., Slit Lamp Photodocumentation, *Amer. J. Optom.*, Vol. 56, pp. 559–562, 1979.

GWAIZDA, J.; SCHEIMAN, M.; MOHINDRA, I.; and HELD, R., Astigmatism in Children: Changes in Axis and Amount from Birth to Six Years, *Inves. Ophthal. Vis. Sci.*, Vol. 25, pp. 88–92, 1984.

HAINE, C. L., Personal communication, St. Louis, Mo., 1981.

HAINE, C. L.; LONG, W. F.; and READING, R. W., Laser Meridional Refractometry: A Preliminary Report, *Optom. Weekly*, Vol. 64, pp. 1064–1067, 1973.

HAINE, C. L.; LONG, W. F.; and READING, R. W., Laser Meridional Refractometry, *Amer. J. Optom.*, Vol. 53, p. 194, 1976.

HALLAK, J., Reflections on Retinoscopy, *Amer. J. Optom.*, Vol. 53, pp. 224–228, 1976.

HANNA, C., and O'BRIEN, J., Cell Production and Migration in the Epithelial Layers of the Cornea, *Arch. Ophthal.*, Vol. 64, pp. 536–539, 1960.

HARRINGTON, D. O., *The Visual Fields*, 4th ed., St. Louis, Mosby, 1976.

HARRIS, J. E., Transport of Fluid from the Cornea, in *Transparency of the Cornea*, S. Duke-Elder, Editor, Oxford, Blackwell's, 1960.

HARRIS, M. G., Continuing education lecture, Annual Meeting of American Academy of Optometry, Dec. 11, 1981.

HARRIS, M. G.; GALE, B.; GANSEL, K.; and SLETTE, C., Flexure and Residual Astigmatism with Paraperm O_2 and Boston

II Lenses on Toric Corneas, *Amer. J. Optom.*, Vol. 64, pp. 269–273, 1987.

HARRIS, M. G., and CHU, C. S., The Effect of Contact Lens Thickness and Corneal Toricity on Flexure and Residual Astigmatism, *Amer. J. Optom.*, Vol. 49, pp. 304–307, 1972.

HARRIS, M. G., and MANDELL, R. B., Contact Lens Adaptation: Osmotic Theory, *Amer. J. Optom.*, Vol. 46, pp. 196–202, 1969.

HARTSTEIN, J., Corneal Warping Due to Contact Lenses, *Amer. J. Ophthal.*, Vol. 60, pp. 1103–1104, 1965.

HARTSTEIN, J., and BECKER, B., Research into the Pathogenesis of Keratoconus, *Arch. Ophthal.*, Vol. 84, pp. 728–729, 1970.

HARWOOD, L., A Unique Method of Subjective Refraction in Which No Lenses are Near the Patient, Paper presented at Annual Meeting of the American Academy of Optometry, Dec. 1974.

HAYASHI, T., and FATT, I., A Lubrication Model of Tear Exchange Under a Contact Lens, *Amer. J. Optom.*, Vol. 53, pp. 101–103, 1976.

HAZLETT, R. D., Central Corneal Clouding, *J. Amer. Optom. Assoc.*, Vol. 40, pp. 268–275, 1969.

HEATH, G. G., The Use of Graphical Analysis in Visual Training, *Amer. J. Optom.*, Vol. 36, pp. 337–350, 1959.

HEATH, G. G., Color Vision, Ch. 12, in *Vision of Children*, M. J. Hirsch and R. E. Wick, Editors, Philadelphia, Chilton, 1963.

HELMHOLTZ, H. VON, *Treatise on Physiological Optics*, Vol. 1, New York. Opt. Soc. of America, 1924.

HENKIND, P., and CHAMBERS, J. K., Arterial Occlusive Disease of the Retina, Vol. 3, Ch. 14, in *Clinical Opthalmology*, T. D. Duane, Editor, Hagerstown, Md., Harper & Row, 1979.

HENRY, V. A.; BENNETT, E. S.; and FORREST, J. F., Clinical Investigation of the Papaperm EW Rigid Gas-Permeable Contact Lens, *Amer. J. Optom.*, Vol. 64, pp. 313–320, 1987.

HERING, E., Der Raumsinn und die Bewegrungender Auges, in Hermann and Ludimar, *Handbuch der Physiologie 3* (Part 1), 1879 (cited by Ogle, 1950).

HERRNHEISER, J., Die Refractionsentwicklung des Menschlichen Auges, *Zeitscrift für Heilkunde*, Vol. 13, pp. 342–377, 1892 (cited by Hirsch, 1963b).

HESS, R. F., and HOWELL, E. R., The Threshold Contrast Sensitivity Function in Strabismic Amblyopia: Evidence for a Two-Type Classification, *Vis. Res.*, Vol. 17, pp. 1049–1055, 1977.

HILL, J. F., Comparison of Computerized Refraction with Standard Refractive Technique, *Optom. Weekly*, pp. 1279–1282, Dec. 27, 1973.

HILL, J. F., Diurnal Variations in Corneal Curvature After Wearing Flexible (HEMA) Contact Lenses, *Amer. J. Optom.*, Vol. 31, pp. 56–60, 1974.

HILL, R. M., Hydrogel Lens Design: The Thick and Thin of It, *Proceedings of the Second National Symposium on Soft Contact Lenses*, Amsterdam, Excerpta Medica, 1975.

HILL, R. M., Behind the Closed Lid, *Inter. Cont. Lens Clin.*, Vol. 4, No. 1, pp. 68–70, 1977a.

HILL, R. M., C. A. B.: A Practical Lens Option? *J. Amer. Optom. Assoc.*, Vol. 48, pp. 387–389, 1977b.

HILL, R. M., Oxygen Permeable Contact Lenses: How Convinced Is the Cornea? *Inter. Cont. Lens Clin.*, Vol. 4, No. 2, pp. 34–36, 1977c.

HILL, R. M., Extended Wear: Closing the Gap, *Cont. Lens Forum*, pp. 67–69, Dec. 1979.

HILL, R. M., and FATT, I., Oxygen Deprivation of the Cornea by Contact Lenses and Lid Closure, *Amer. J. Optom.*, Vol. 41, pp. 678–687, 1964a.

HILL, R. M., and FATT, I., Oxygen Measurements under a Contact Lens, *Amer. J. Optom.*, Vol. 41, pp. 382–397, 1964b.

HILL, R. M., and JEPPE, W. A., Hydrogels: Is a Pump Still Necessary? *Inter. Cont. Lens Clin.*, Vol. 2, No. 4, pp. 27–29, 1975.

HILL, R. M., and MAUGER, T. F., Oxygen Update: Hydrophilics, *Inter. Cont. Lens Clin.*, pp. 47–49, Sept./Oct. 1980.

HILL, R. M., and MAUGER, T. F., Oxygen Update: Nonhydrophilics; *Inter. Cont. Lens Clin.*, pp. 17–20, Jan./Feb. 1981.

HIRSCH, M. J., Relation of Visual Acuity to Myopia, *Arch. Ophthal.*, Vol. 34, pp. 418–421, 1945.

HIRSCH, M. J., An Analysis of Inhomegeneity of Myopia in Adults, *Amer. J. Optom*, Vol. 11, pp. 562–571, 1950.

HIRSCH, M. J., The Changes in Refraction Between the Ages of 5 and 14—Theoretical and Practical Considerations, *Amer. J. Optom.*, Vol. 29, pp. 445–459, 1952.

HIRSCH, M. J., The Relationship Between School Achievement and Visual Anomalies, *Amer. J. Optom.*, Vol. 33, pp. 262–270, 1955.

HIRSCH, M. J., Changes in Refractive State After the Age of 45, *Amer. J. Optom.*, Vol. 35, pp. 229–237, 1958.

HIRSCH, M. J., The Relationship Between Refractive State and Intelligence Test Scores, *Amer. J. Optom.*, Vol. 36, pp. 12–20, 1959a.

HIRSCH, M. J., Changes in Astigmatism After the Age of 40, *Amer. J. Optom.*, Vol. 36, pp. 395–405, 1959b.

HIRSCH, M. J., A Longitudinal Study of Refractive State of Children During the First Six Years of School: A Preliminary Report on the Ojai Study, *Amer. J. Optom.*, Vol. 38, pp. 564–571, 1961.

HIRSCH, M. J., Changes in Astigmatism During the First Eight Grades of School: An Interim Report from the Ojai Longitudinal Study, *Amer. J. Optom.*, Vol. 40, pp. 127–132, 1963a.

HIRSCH, M. J., The Refraction of Children, Ch. 5, in *Vision of Children*, M. J. Hirsch and R. E. Wick, Editors, Philadelphia, Chilton, 1963b.

HIRSCH, M. J., Predictability of Refraction at Age 14 on the Basis of Testing at Age 6: Interim Report on the Ojai Longitudinal Study of Refraction, *Amer. J. Optom.*, Vol. 41, pp. 567–573, 1964.

HIRSCH, M. J., Anisometropia: A Preliminary Report of the Ojai Longitudinal Study, *Amer. J. Optom.*, Vol. 44, pp. 581–585, 1967.

HIRSCH, M. J., Lecture given at the Annual Conference of the New Zealand Optometrical Association, Wairaki, New Zealand, Oct. 1969.

HIRSCH, M. J., What You Wanted to Know About Myopia but Never Dared Ask, *Can. J. Optom.*, Vol. 34, pp. 54–56, 1972.

HIRSCH, M. J., and DITMARS, D. L., Refraction of Young Myopes and Their Parents: A Re-analysis, *Amer. J. Optom.*, Vol. 46, pp. 30–32, 1969.

HIRSCH, M. J., and WEYMOUTH, F. W., Notes on Ametropia: A Further Analysis of Stenstrom's Data, *Amer. J. Optom.*, Vol. 24, pp. 601–608, 1947.

HITZMAN, S. A., and MYERS, C. O., Comparison of the Acceptance of Progressive Addition Multifocal vs. a Standard Multifocal Lens Design, *J. Amer. Optom. Assoc.*, Vol. 56, pp. 706–710, 1985.

HODOS, W., and KUENZEL, W. J., Retinal-Image Degradation Produces Ocular Enlargement in Chicks, *Invest. Ophthal. Vis. Sci.*, Vol. 25, pp. 652–659, 1984.

HOFSTETTER, H. W., The Zone of Clear Single Binocular Vision, *Amer. J. Optom.*, Vol. 22, pp. 361–365, 1945.

HOFSTETTER, H. W., *Optometry: Professional, Economic and Legal Aspects*, St. Louis, Mosby, 1948.

HOFSTETTER, H. W., Aims in Optometric Evaluation, *J. Amer. Optom. Assoc.*, Vol. 22, p. 270, 1950.

HOFSTETTER, H. W., Emmetropization: Biological Process or Mathematical Artifact? *Amer. J. Optom.*, Vol. 46, pp. 447–450, 1969.

HOFSTETTER, H. W., and GRAHAM, R., Leanardo and Contact Lenses, *Amer. J. Optom.*, Vol. 30, pp. 41–45, 1953.

HOLDEN, B. A.; ZANTOS, S. G.; and JACOBS, K. J., The Holden-Zantos Technique for Endothelial and High Magnification Slit Lamp Photography, Rochester, N.Y., Bausch & Lomb Soft Lens International, 1978.

HOLLY, F. J., Formation and Stability of the Tear Film, *Inter. Ophthal. Clin.*, Vol. 13, No. 1, pp. 73–96, 1973.

HOLLY, F. J., and LEMP, M. A., Surface Chemistry of the Tearfilm: Implications for Dry Eye Syndromes, Contact Lenses and Ophthalmic Polymers, *Cont. Lens Soc. Amer. J.*, Vol. 5, April 1971.

HOPKINS, G. A., and LYLE, W. M., Potential Systemic Side Effects of Six Common Ophthalmic Drugs, *J. Amer. Optom. Assoc.*, Vol. 48, pp. 1241–1245, 1977.

HOWLAND, C., and SAYLES, N., Photorefractive Measurements of Astigmatism in Infants and Young Children, *Invest. Ophthal. Vis. Sci.*, Vol. 25, pp. 93–102, 1984.

HUBEL, D., WEISEL, T. N. and RAVIOLA, E., Myopia and Eye Enlargement after Neonatal Lid Fusion in Monkeys, *Nature*, Vol. 266, pp. 485–488, 1977.

HUMPHREY, W. E., A New and Unique Type of Lens Surface Used to Generate Variable Cylinder Lens Power, paper presented at the Annual Meeting of the American Academy of Optometry, Dec. 1974.

HUMPHRISS, D., and WOODRUFF, E. W., Refraction by Immediate Contrast, *Optom. Weekly*, Vol. 53, pp. 2171–2175, 1962.

HURST, J. W., How Does One Develop a Defined Data Base? Who Collects the Data? Ch. 6, in *The Problem-Oriented System*, J. W. Hurst and H. K. Walker, Editors, Baltimore, Williams & Wilkins, 1972.

HURTES, R., Evolution of Ophthalmic Photography, *Inter. Ophthal. Clin.*, Vol. 16, No. 2, pp. 1–22, 1976.

HUTCHISON, J. C., *Hypertension: A Practical Guide to Therapy*, Flushing, N.Y., Med. Exam. Pub. Co. (undated).

JACKSON, E., Norms of Refraction, *JAMA*, Vol. 98, pp. 132–137, 1932.

JAFFE, N. S., *The Vitreous in Clinical Ophthalmology*, St. Louis, Mosby, 1969.

JAKUS, M., The Fine Structure of the Human Cornea. *The Structure of the Eye*, G. Smelser, Editor, New York, Academic Press, 1961.

JAKUS, M., *Ocular Fine Structure*, London, Churchill, 1964.

JALIE, M., *The Principles of Ophthalmic Lenses*, 2nd ed., London, Assoc. of Dispensing Opticians, 1974.

JANOFF, L. E., Hard Contacts: Some Problem Cases, *Cont. Lens Forum*, Vol. 1, pp. 46–53, 1976.

JAUREGUI, M. J., and POLSE, K. A., Mydriatic Effect Using Phenylephrine and Proparacaine, *Amer. J. Optom.*, Vol. 51, pp. 545–549, 1974.

JENSEN, H., Prevention of Myopia Progression, the Role of Pharmaceutical Agents, Myopia Workshop, Copenhagen, June 1987.

JOHNSON, C. A., and KELTNER, J. L., Automated Suprathreshold Static Perimetry, *Amer. J. Ophthal.*, Vol. 89, pp. 731–741, 1980a.

JOHNSON, C. A., and KELTNER, J. L., Comparative Evaluation of the Autofield-1, DFA–120 and Fieldmaster Model 101–PR Automated Perimeters, *Ophthalmology*, Vol. 87, pp. 777–784, 1980b.

JONES, L. T., Anatomy of the Tear System, *Inter. Ophthal. Clin.*, Vol. 13, pp. 3–22, 1973.

JOSE, R. T.; BROWNING, R. A.; and BRILLIANT, R. L., Low Vision in Primary Care Optometry, *Texas Optom.*, Jan. 1982.

JOSEPHSON, J. E., and CAFFERY, B., Bifocal Hydrogel Lenses: An Overview, *J. Amer. Optom. Assoc.*, Vol. 57, pp. 190–195, 1986.

KANNEL, W. B.; GORDON, T.; and SCHWARTZ, M. J., Systolic Versus Diastolic Blood Pressure and Risk of Coronary Heart Disease: The Framingham Study, *Amer. J. Cardiol.*, Vol. 27, pp. 335–346, 1971.

KEECH, P. M., The Effect of Cycloplegia on the Determination of Refractive Error by the Ophthalmetron, *Amer. J. Optom.*, Vol. 56, pp. 228–230, 1979.

KELLER, J. T., An Optical Evaluation of Book Retinoscopy, *J. Amer. Optom.*, Assoc., pp. 483–487, 1977.

KELLY, C. E., *Visual Screening and Child Development*, Dept. of Psychology, North Carolina State College, Raleigh, N.C., 1957.

KELLY, S. A., and TOMLINSON, A., Effect of Repeated Testing on Contrast Sensitivity, *Amer. J. Optom.*, Vol. 64, pp. 241–245, 1987.

KELLY, T.; CHATFIELD, C.; and TUSTIN, C., Clinical Assessment of the Arrest of Myopia, *Brit. J. Ophthal.*, Vol. 59, pp. 529–538, 1975.

KELLY, T. S., Myopia or Expansion Glaucoma, *Doc. Ophthal. Proc*, Series 28, Third International Conference on Myopia, H. C. Fledelius, P. H. Alsbirk, and E. Goldschmidt, Editors, The Hague, Dr. W. Junk Publishers, 1981.

KELLY, T. S., Bifocals and Contacts in Myopia Control, *Optician*, June 24, pp. 19–25, 1983.

KELTNER, J. L., and JOHNSON, C. A., Comparative Material on Automated and Semiautomated Perimeters—1985, *Ophthalmol.*, Instrument and Book Supplement, pp. 34–57, 1984.

KEMPH, G. A.; COLLINS, S. D.; and JARMAN, B. L., *Refractive Errors in the Eyes of Children as Determined by Retinoscopic Examination with a Cycloplegic*, Public Health Bulletin No. 182, Washington D.C., U.S. Government Printing Office, 1928.

KERNS, R. L., Research in Orthokeratology, *J. Amer. Optom. Assoc.*, Vol. 47, pp. 1047–1051, 1275–1285, 1505–1515, 1976; Vol. 48, pp. 227–238, 345–359, 1134–1147, 1541–1543, 1977; Vol. 49, pp. 308–314, 1978.

KIRKENDALL, W. M.; BURTON, A. C.; EPSTEIN, F. H.; and FREIS, E. D., *Recommendation for Human Blood Pressure Measurement by Sphygmomanometers*, Amer. Heart Assoc., 1967.

KLEIN, P., Use of Hyper-Thin, Low Water Content Hydrophilic Lenses for Extended Wear, *Amer. J. Optom*, Vol. 60, pp. 783–787, 1983.

KLEINSTEIN, R. N., Contrast Sensitivity, *Optom. Monthly*, Vol. 72, pp. 38–40, April 1981.

KNOLL, H. A., Measuring Ametropia with a Gas Laser: A Preliminary Report, *Amer. J. Optom.*, Vol. 43, pp. 415–418, 1966.

KNOLL, H. A.; MOHRMAN, R.; and MAIER, W. F., Automatic Objective Refraction in an Office Practice, *Amer. J. Optom.*, Vol. 47, pp. 644–649, 1970.

KO, L. S., The Problem of Myopia in Taiwan, *J. Korean Ophthal. Soc.*, Vol. 25, pp. 591–604, 1984.

KOETTING, R. A., Advantages of Contact Lens Fitting Early in Aphakia, *Austr. J. Optom.*, Vol. 49, pp. 209–213, 1966.

KOETTING, R. A.; ACKERMAN, D. H.; and KOETTING, R. R., An Evaluation of the Cavitron Autorefractor 7 with Contact Lenses and Non-Contact Lens Wearing Patients, *J. Amer. Optom. Assoc.*, Vol. 54, pp. 115–118, 1983.

KOTOW, M.; HOLDEN, B. A.; and GRANT, T., The Value of Regular Replacement of Low Water Content Contact Lenses for Extended Wear, *J. Amer. Optom. Assoc.*, Vol. 58, pp. 461–464, 1987.

KORB, D. R., and EXFORD, J. M., The Phenomenon of Central Corneal Clouding, *J. Amer. Optom. Assoc.*, Vol. 39, pp. 223–230, 1968.

KORB, D. R., and KORB, J. M., Corneal Staining prior to Contact Lens Wearing, *J. Amer. Optom. Assoc.*, Vol. 41, pp. 228–233, 1970a.

KORB, D. R., and KORB, J. M., A New Concept in Contact Lens Design, *J. Amer. Optom. Assoc.*, Vol. 41, pp. 1023–1024, 1970b.

KORB, D. R.; RICHMOND, P. R.; and HERMAN, J. P., Physiological Response of the Cornea to Hydrogel Lenses before and after Cataract Extraction, *J. Amer. Optom. Assoc.*, Vol. 51, pp. 267–270, 1980.

KORS, K., and PETERS, H. B., Absorption Characteristics of Selected Commercially Available Ophthalmic Lenses, *Amer. J. Optom.*, Vol. 49, pp. 727–735, 1972.

KRATZ, L. D., and FLOM, M. C., The Humphrey Vision Analyzer: Reliability and Validity of Refractive Error Measures, *Amer. J. Optom.*, Vol. 54, pp. 653–659, 1977.

KREZANOSKI, J., What Are the Implications of Dirty Soft Contact Lenses? *Inter. Cont. Lens Clin.*, pp. 57–60, March/April 1977.

KRONFELD, P. C., The Early Ophthalmoscopic Diagnosis of Glaucoma, *J. Amer. Optom. Assoc.*, Vol. 23, pp. 156–159, 1951.

KRUGER, P. B., Changes in Fundus Reflex with Increased Cognitive Processing, *Amer. J. Optom.*, Vol. 54, pp. 445–451, 1977.

LAATIKAINEN, L., and ERKKILA, H., Refractive Errors and Other Ocular Findings in School Children, *Acta Ophthal.*, Vol. 58, pp. 129–136, 1980.

LARAGH, J. H., Evaluation and Care of the Hypertensive Patient, in *Hypertension Manual*, J. H. Laragh, Editor, New York, Yorke Medical Books, 1974.

LAST, R. J., *Eugene Wolff's Anatomy of the Eye and Orbit*, 6th ed., Philadelphia, Saunders, 1968.

LEE, A., and SARVER, D. S., The Gel Lens: Transferred Corneal Toricity as a Function of Lens Thickness, *Amer. J. Optom.*, Vol. 49, pp. 35–40, 1972.

LEIGHTON, D. A., and TOMLINSON, A., Changes in Axial Length and Other Dimensions of the Eyeball with Increasing Age, *Acta Ophthal.*, Vol. 50, pp. 815–826, 1972.

LEMP, M. A., Break-up of the Tear Film, *Inter. Ophthal. Clin.*, Vol. 13, pp. 97–102, 1973.

LEMP, M. A., Tear Deficiencies, Vol. 4, Ch. 14, in *Clinical Ophthalmology*, T. D. Duane, Editor, Hagerstown, Md., Harper & Row, 1980.

LEMP, M. A., and HOLLY, F. J., Recent Advances in Ocular Surface Chemistry, *Amer. J. Optom.*, Vol. 47, pp. 669–672, 1970.

LENNERSTRAND, G., and LUNDH, B. L., Improvement of Contrast Sensitivity from Treatment for Amblyopia, *Acta Ophthal.*, Vol. 58, pp. 292–294, 1980.

LESSER, S. K., *Introduction to Modern Analytical Optometry*, Duncan, Okla., Optometric Extension Program, 1969.

LEVENE, J. R., *Clinical Refraction and Visual Science*, Woburn, Mass., Butterworth, 1977.

LEVY, B., Rigid Gas-Permeable Lenses for Extended Wear—A 1-Year Clinical Evaluation, *Amer. J. Optom.*, Vol. 62, pp. 889–894, 1985.

LICHTER, P. R., Gonioscopy, Vol. 3, Ch. 44, in *Clinical Ophthalmology*, T. D. Duane, Editor, Hagerstown, Md., Harper & Row, 1976.

LIN, L. L.; CHEN, C.; HUNG, P.; and KO, L., Nation-Wide Survey of Myopia Among Schoolchildren in Taiwan, Myopia Workshop, Copenhagen, June 1987.

LINKSZ, A., and BANNON, R. E., Aniseikonia and Refractive Problems, *Inter. Ophthal. Clin.*, Vol. 5, No. 2, pp. 513–534, 1965.

LONG, W. F., A Mathematical Analysis of Multi-Meridional Refractometry, *Amer. J. Optom.*, Vol. 51, pp. 260–263, 1974.

LONG, W. F., Prism in Ophthalmic Lenses, *Optom. Weekly*, pp. 13–17, Sept. 11, 1975a.

LONG, W. F., Decentration of Sphero-cylindric Lenses, *Optom. Weekly*, pp. 20–22, Sept. 18, 1975b.

LONG, W. F., Stenopaic Slit Refraction, *Optom. Weekly*, Vol. 66, pp. 1063–1066, 1975c.

LONG, W. F., Effectivity of Ophthalmic Lenses: Distance Correction, *Optom. Weekly*, pp. 37–42, Feb. 26, 1976a.

LONG, W. F., Effectivity of Ophthalmic Lenses: Near-point Correction, *Optom. Weekly*, pp. 50–53, March 4, 1976b.

LONG, W. F., Estimating Edge Thickness, *Optom. Weekly*, pp. 47–50, Nov. 4, 1976c.

LONG, W. F., A Simple System for External Ophthalmic Photography, *Can. J. Optom.*, Vol. 41, No. 2, pp. 67–98, 1979.

LONG, W. F., and WOO, G. C. S., Photometry for Clinicians, *Optom. Monthly*, Vol. 70, pp. 668–670, Sept. 1979.

LONG, W. F., *Ocular Photography*, Chicago, Professional Press, 1984.

LOSHIN, D. S., and BROWNING, R. A., Contrast Sensitivity in Albinotic Patients, *Amer. J. Optom.*, Vol. 60, pp. 158–166, 1983.

LOSHIN, D. S., and WHITE, J., Contrast Sensitivity, the Visual Rehabilitation of the Patient with Macular Degeneration, *Arch. Ophthal.*, Vol. 102, pp. 1301–1306, 1984.

LOWTHER, G. E., Comparing Corneal Thickness Changes with Silicon Resin Lenses to Changes with PMMA, CAB and Polycon Lenses, *Inter. Cont. Lens Clin.*, pp. 23–29, May/June, 1981a.

LOWTHER, G. E., Rigid Gas Permeable Lenses: Why Use PMMA Lenses? *Inter. Cont. Lens Clin.*, pp. 7–8, March/April 1981b.

LOWTHER, G. E.; HILBERT, J. A.; and KING, J. E., Appearance and Location of Hydrophilic Lens Deposits, *Inter. Cont. Lens Clin.*, pp. 30–34, March/April 1975.

LOWTHER, G. E., and HILL, R. M., Sensitivity Threshold of the Lower Lid Margin in the Course of Adaptation to Contact Lenses, *Amer. J. Optom.*, Vol. 45, pp. 587–594, 1968.

LUNDH, B., and LENNERSTRAND, G., Effects of Amblyopia Therapy on Contrast Sensitivity as Reflected in the Visuogram, *Acta Ophthal.*, Vol. 61, pp. 431–446, 1983.

LYLE, W. M., Changes in Corneal Astigmatism with Age, *Amer. J. Optom.*, Vol. 48, pp. 467–478, 1971.

LYLE, W. M.; GROSVENOR, T.; and DEAN, K. C., Corneal Astigmatism in Amerind Children, *Amer. J. Optom.*, Vol. 49, pp. 517–524, 1972.

MAINO, J. H.; CIBIS, G. W.; CRESS, P.; SPELLMAN, C. R.; and SHORES, R. E., Noncycloplegic vs. Cycloplegic Retinoscopy in Preschool Children, *Annals Ophthal.*, Vol. 16, pp. 880–882.

MALACARA, D., Measurement of Visual Refractive Defects with a Gas Laser, *Amer. J. Optom.*, Vol. 51, pp. 15–23, 1974.

MALIN, H. A., and KOHLER, J., Measuring Toric Rotation, *Cont. Lens Forum*, pp. 17–23, Oct. 1981.

MALLETT, R. F. J., The Investigation of Heterophoria at Near and a New Fixation Disparity Technique, *Optician*, pp. 547–551, Dec. 4; and pp. 574–580, Dec. 11, 1964.

MALLETT, R. F. J., A Fixation Disparity Test for Distance Use, *Optician*, pp. 1–3, July 8, 1966.

MANDELL, R. B., Myopia Control with Bifocal Correction, *Amer. J. Optom.*, Vol. 36, pp. 652–658, 1959.

MANDELL, R. B., Methods to Measure the Peripheral Corneal Curvature, Part 2: Geometric Construction and "Computers," *J. Amer. Optom. Assoc.*, Vol. 33, pp. 585–589, 1962.

MANDELL, R. B., Lecture given at Southwest Contact Lens Congress, Dallas, Tex., 1963.

MANDELL, R. B., New Thoughts on Gel Lenses, *Inter. Cont. Lens Clin.*, Vol. 1, pp. 32–35, 1974.

MANDELL, R. B., and ALLEN, M. J., The Causes of Bichrome Test Failure, *J. Amer. Optom. Assoc.*, Vol. 31, pp. 531–533, 1960.

MANDELL, R. B., and POLSE, K. A., Corneal Thickness Changes as a Contact Lens Fitting Index: Experimental Results and a Proposed Model, *Amer. J. Optom.*, Vol. 46, pp. 479–491, 1969.

MANDELL, R. B., and POLSE, K. A., Corneal Thickness Changes Accompanying Central Corneal Clouding, *Amer. J. Optom.*, Vol. 48, pp. 129–132, 1971.

MANN, W. A., History of Photography of the Eye, *Surv. Ophthal.*, Vol. 15, pp. 179–189, 1970.

MANTYJARVI, M., Incidence of Myopia in a Population of Finnish School Children, *Acta Ophthal.*, Vol. 61, pp. 417–423, 1983.

MARG, E., Computer-Assisted Eye Examination, Part 1: Computer-Actuated Eye Refractors, *Amer. J. Optom.*, Vol. 5, pp. 601–615, 1973.

MARG, E.; JOHNSON, D.; ANDERSON, K. W.; BAKER, R. L.; and NEROTH, C. C., Computer Assisted Eye Examination, Part 5: Preliminary Evaluation of Refractor III System for Subjective Examination, *Amer. J. Optom.*, Vol. 54, pp. 2–18, 1977.

MARG, E.; ANDERSON, K. W.; CHUNG, K. O.; and NEROTH, C. C., Computer Assisted Eye Examination, Part 6: Identification and Correction of Errors in the Refractor III System for Subjective Examination, *Amer. J. Optom.*, Vol. 55, pp. 249–266, 1978a.

MARG, E.; ANDERSON, K. W.; CHUNG, K. O.; and NEROTH, C. C., Computer Assisted Eye Examination, Part 7: Final Evaluation of the Refractor III System for Subjective Examination After Reducing Softwear and Hardwear Errors, *Amer. J. Optom.*, Vol. 55, pp. 317–330, 1978b.

MASCI, E., Sull'astigmatismo Oftalmometrico: Modificzioni Della Curvatura Corneale in Rapporto alla Attivita Palpebrale ed alla Rigidita Sclerale, *Bull. d' Oculist.*, Vol 44, pp. 755–763, 1965.

MAURICE, D. M., The Movement of Fluorescein in the Cornea, *Amer. J. Ophthal.*, Vol. 49, pp. 1011–1016, 1960a.

MAURICE, D. M., The Physics of Corneal Transparency, in *Transparency of the Cornea*, S. Duke-Elder, Editor, Oxford, Blackwell's, 1960b.

MAURICE, D. M., The Cornea, in *The Eye*, Davson, Editor, New York, Academic Press, 1962.

MAURICE, D. M., The Dynamics and Drainage of Tears, *Inter. Ophthal. Clin.*, Vol. 13, pp. 103–116, 1973.

MAURICE, D. M., and MUSHIN, A. S., Production of Myopia in Rabbits by Raised Body Temperature and Increased Intraocular Pressure, *Lancet*, pp. 1160–1162, 1966.

MAZOW, B., *Synopsis of Corneal Contact Lens Fitting for Optometrists*, Minneapolis, Burgess, 1962.

MCCORMACK, G., and MARG, E., Computer Assisted Eye Examination, Part 2: Visual Evoked Response Meridional Refractometry, *Amer. J. Optom.*, Vol. 50, pp. 889–903, 1973.

MCGILL, E., and ERICKSON, P., Stereopsis in Presbyopes Wearing Monovision and Simultaneous Vision Contact Lenses (abstract), *Amer. J. Optom.*, Vol. 64, p. 51P, 1987.

MEHR, E. B., and FREID, A. N., *Low Vision Care*, Chicago, Professional Press, 1975.

MILLODOT, M., A. Centenary of Retinoscopy, *J. Amer. Optom. Assoc.*, Vol. 44, pp. 1057–1059, 1973.

MILLODOT, M., *Dictionary of Optometry*, London, Butterworths, 1986.

MILLODOT, M., and O'LEARY, D., The Discrepancy between Retinoscopic and Subjective Measurements: Effect of Age, *Amer. J. Optom.*, Vol. 55, pp. 309–316, 1978.

MILLODOT, M., and RIGGS, L. A., Refraction Determined Electrophysiologically, *Arch. Ophthal.*, Vol. 84, pp. 272–278, 1970.

MITCHELL, D. W. A., *The Use of Drugs in Refraction*, London, Brit. Optical Assoc., 1959.

MITRA, S., and LAMBERTS, D. W., Contrast Sensitivity in Soft Lens Wearers, *Cont. Lens Intraoc. Lens Med. J.*, Vol. 7, pp. 315–322, 1981.

MOHINDRA, I., Comparisons of "Near Retinoscopy" and Subjective Refraction in Adults, *Amer. J. Optom.*, Vol. 54, pp. 319–322, 1977a.

MOHINDRA, I., A Non-cycloplegic Refraction Technique for Infants and Young Children, *J. Amer. Optom. Assoc.*, Vol. 48, pp. 518–523, 1977b.

MOHINDRA, I., Near Retinoscopy: An Objective Noncycloplegic Refraction Technique, *Optom. Monthly*, Vol. 71, pp. 28–31, Jan. 1980a.

MOHINDRA, I., Physiological Basis of Near Retinoscopy, *Optom. Monthly*, Vol. 71, pp. 97–99, Feb. 1980b.

MOHINDRA, I., and HELD, R., Refraction in Humans from Birth to 5 Years, *Doc. Ophthal. Proc*, Series 28, Third International Conference on Myopia, H. C. Fledelius, P. H. Alsbirk, and E. Goldschmidt, Editors, The Hague, Dr. W. Junk Publishers, 1981.

MOHINDRA, I., and MOLINARI, J. F., Near Retinoscopy and Cycloplegic Retinoscopy in Early Primary Grade School Children, *Amer. J. Optom.*, Vol. 56, pp. 34–38, 1979.

MOLINARI, J. F., and CAPLAN, L., Clinical Evaluation of Two Soft Lens Bifocals, *J. Amer. Optom. Assoc.*, Vol. 57, pp. 684–687, 1986.

MORELAND, J. D., Inert Pigments and the Variability of Anomoloscope Matches, *Amer. J. Optom.*, Vol. 49, pp. 735–741, 1972.

MORGAN, M. W., Analysis of Clinical Data, *Amer. J. Optom.*, Vol. 21, pp. 477–491, 1944a.

MORGAN, J. D., The Clinical Aspects of Accommodation and Convergence, *Amer. J. Optom.*, Vol. 21, pp. 301–313, 1944b.

MORGAN, M. W., The Turville Infinity Binocular Balance Test, *Amer. J. Optom.*, Vol. 26, pp. 231–239, 1949.

MORGAN, M. W., The Ciliary Body in Accommodation and Accommodative Convergence, *Amer. J. Optom.*, Vol. 31, pp. 219–229, 1954.

MORGAN, M. W., Changes in Refraction Over a Period of Twenty Years in a Nonvisually Selected Sample, *Amer. J. Optom.*, Vol. 35, pp. 281–299, 1958.

MORGAN, M. W. The Turville Infinity Binocular Balance Test, *J. Amer. Optom. Assoc.*, Vol. 31, pp. 447–450, 1960.

MORGAN, M. W., The Analysis of Clinical Data, *Optom. Weekly*, Sept. 2, 9, 1948 (reprinted in *Optom. Weekly*, Aug. 13, p. 20, 1964).

MORGAN, M. W., The Maddox Classification of Vergence Movements, *Amer. J. Optom.*, Vol. 57, pp. 537–539, 1980.

MORGAN, M. W., and PETERS, H. B., *The Optics of Ophthalmic Lenses*, Berkeley, Calif., University of California, 1948.

MORRISON, R. J., Contact Lenses and the Progression of Myopia, *Optom. Weekly*, Vol. 47, pp. 1487–1488, 1956.

MORRISON, R. J., Observations on Contact Lenses and the Progression of Myopia, *Contacto*, pp. 20–25, Jan. 1958.

MORRISON, R. J., The Use of Contact Lenses in Adolescent Myopic Patients, *Amer. J. Optom.*, Vol. 37, pp. 165–168, 1960.

MORRISON, R. J., Hydrophilic Contact Lenses, *J. Amer. Optom. Assoc.*, Vol. 37, pp. 211–218, 1966.

MOSES, R. A., *Adler's Physiology of the Eye*, 6th ed., St. Louis, Mosby, 1975.

MOSS, H. I., Corneal Contact Lenses and Myopia, *Optom. Weekly*, pp. 22–23, March 1966.

MYROWITZ, E.; PEARLMAN, P.; and GOLDBERG, H., A Case of Pseudomonas Keratitis in a Soft Contact Lens Wearer Using Contaminated Chemical Disinfecting Solution, *Cont. Lens*, pp. 337–338, Oct./Dec. 1981.

NATHAN, J.; CREWTHER, S. G.; CREWTHER, D. P.; and KIELY, P. M., Effects of Retinal Image Degradation on Ocular Growth in Cats, *Invest. Ophthal. Vis. Sci.*, Vol. 25, pp. 1300–1306, 1984.

NOLAN, J. A., Progress of Myopia and Contact Lenses, *Contacto*, Vol. 8, No. 1, pp. 25–26, 1964.

NOVER, A., *The Ocular Fundus: Methods of Examination and Typical Findings*, Philadelphia, Lea and Febiger, 1974.

OAKLEY, K. H., and YOUNG, F. A., Bifocal Control of Myopia, *Amer. J. Optom.*, Vol. 52, pp. 738–764, 1975.

O'DAY, D. M.; FEMAN, S. S.; and ELLIOTT, J. H., Visual Impairment Following Radial Keratotomy, a Cluster of Cases, *Ophthal.*, Vol. 93, pp. 319–326, 1986.

OGLE, K. N., *Researches in Binocular Vision*, Philadelphia, Saunders, 1950.

OGLE, K. N.; MARTINS, T. G.; and DYER, J. A., *Oculomotor Imbalance and Fixation Disparity*, Philadelphia, Lea and Febiger, 1967.

O'HARA, R., Lecture given at University of Houston continuing education course, Houston, Tex., Jan. 16, 1982.

O'NEAL M. R., and CONNON, T. R., *Refractive Error Change at the United States Air Force Academy—Class of 1985*, Ohio, Wright-Patterson Air Force Base, 1986.

OLIVER, B. M., Sparkling Spots and Random Diffraction, *Proc. I.E.E.E.*, Vol. 51, pp. 220–221, 1963.

OLSEN, O. J., External Ophthalmic Photography, *Amer. J. Optom.*, Vol. 56, pp. 548–557, 1979a.

OLSEN, O. J., Goniophotography, *Amer. J. Optom.*, Vol. 56, pp. 563–568, 1979b.

ONG, J.; HAMASAKI, D.; and MARG, E., The Amplitude of Accommodation in Presbyopia, *Amer. J. Optom.*, Vol. 33, p. 3, 1956.

OWSLEY, C.; SEKULER, R.; and SIESMEN, D., Contrast Sensitivity Throughout Adulthood, *Vis. Res.*, Vol. 23, pp. 689–699, 1983.

PARENT, De la Kératoscopie, Pratique et Théorie, *Recueil d'Ophthalmologie*, 2, pp. 65–87, 1890.

PARKS, M. M., Ocular Motility and Strabismus, Vol. 1, Ch. 1–20, in *Clinical Ophthalmology*, T. D. Duane, Editor, Hagerstown, Md., Harper & Row, 1979.

PASCAL, J., Role of the Unit of Accommodation, *Opt. J. Rev. Optom.*, pp. 35–36, Nov. 15, 1947.

PATELLA, V. M., and ARNESTY, M., Clinical Evaluation of the Humphrey Automatic Refractor: Preliminary Report, Humphrey Instruments, San Leandro, Calif., 1981.

PAYNE, C. R.; GRISHAM, J.; and THOMAS, K. L. A Clinical Evaluation of Fixation Disparity, *Amer. J. Optom.*, Vol. 51, pp. 88–90, 1980.

PENCE, N. A., Ophthalmodynamometry: The Technique, and Its Use in the Detection of Carotid Artery Occlusive Disease, *J. Amer. Optom. Assoc.*, Vol. 51, pp. 49–56, 1980.

PERCIVAL, A. S., *The Prescribing of Spectacles*, 3rd ed., New York, William Wood and Co., 1928.

PERKINS, E. S., Morbitity from Myopia, *Sightsaving Rev.*, pp. 12–19, Spring 1979.

PERRIGIN, D. M., Photography for Optometrists, Continuing education lecture, University of Houston, Houston, Tex., Nov. 1980.

PERRIGIN, D. M.; GROSVENOR, T.; and PERRIGIN, J., Comparison of Refractive Findings Obtained by the Bausch & Lomb IVEX and by Conventional Clinical Refraction, *Amer. J. Optom.*, Vol. 62, pp. 562–567, 1985.

PERRIGIN, D. M.; PERRIGIN, J.; and GROSVENOR, T., A Clinical Evaluation of the American Optical SR III Subjective Refractor, *Amer. J. Optom.*, Vol. 58, pp. 581–589, 1981.

PERRIGIN, J.; PERRIGIN, D. M.; GROSVENOR, T., A Comparison of Clinical Refraction Data Obtained by Three Examiners, *Amer. J. Optom.*, Vol. 59, pp. 515–519, 1982.

PERRIGIN, J.; QUINTERO, S.; PERRIGIN, D.; and GROSVENOR, T., The Use of Silicone-Acrylate Contact Lenses for the Control of Myopia: Results After One Year (abstract), *Amer. J. Optom. Physiol. Opt.*, Vol. 64, p. 12P, 1987.

PHEIFFER, C. H., Book Retinoscopy, *Amer. J. Optom.*, Vol. 32, pp. 540–545, 1955.

PHELPS, C. D., Examination and Functional Evaluation of the Crystalline Lens, Vol. 1, Ch. 72, in *Clinical Ophthalmology*, T. D. Duane, Editor, Hagerstown, Md., Harper & Row, 1976.

PHILLIPS, D. E.; McCARTER, G. S.; and DWYER, W. O., Validity of the Laser Refraction Technique for Meridional Measurement, *Amer. J. Optom.*, Vol. 53, pp. 447–450, 1976.

PHILLIPS, D. E.; STERLING, W.; and DWYER, W. O., Validity of the Laser Refraction Technique for Determining Cylinder Error, *Amer. J. Optom.*, Vol. 52, pp. 328–331, 1975.

PIRENNE, M. H., *Vision and the Eye*, London, Chapman & Hall, 1967.

PITTS, D. G., The Ocular Effects of Ultra-Violet Radiation, *Amer. J. Optom.*, Vol. 55, pp. 19–35, 1978.

PITTS, D. G.; CULLEN, A. P.; and HACKER, P. D., Ocular Effects of Near Ultraviolet Radiation, *Amer. J. Optom.*, Vol. 54, pp. 542–549, 1977.

POLSE, K. A., Contact Lens Fitting in Aphakia, *Amer. J. Optom.*, Vol. 46, pp. 213–219, 1969.

POLSE, K. A., Tear Flow Under Hydrogel Contact Lenses, *Invest. Ophthal. Vis. Sci.*, Vol. 18, pp. 409–413, 1979.

POLSE, K. A.; BRAND, R. J.; SCHWALBE, J. S.; VASTINE, D. W.; and KEENER, R. J., The Berkeley Orthokeratology Study. Part II: Efficacy and Duration, *Amer. J. Optom.*, Vol. 60, pp. 187–198, 1983.

POLSE, K. A., and MANDELL, R. B., Critical Oxygen Tension at the Corneal Surface, *Arch. Ophthal.*, Vol. 84, pp. 505–508, 1970.

POLSE, K. A., and MANDELL, R. B., Etiology of Corneal Striae Accompanying Hydrogel Lens Wear, *Invest. Ophthal.*, Vol. 15, pp. 553–556, 1976.

POLSE, K. A.; SARVER, M. D.; and HARRIS, M. G., Corneal Edema and Vertical Striae Accompanying the Wearing of Hydrogel Lenses, *Amer. J. Optom.*, Vol. 52, pp. 185–191, 1975.

POLSE, K. A.; SARVER, M. D.; RIVERA, R. K.; and BONANNO, J., Ocular and Visual Effects of Hard Gas-Permeable-Lens Extended Wear (abstract), *Amer. J. Optom.*, Vol. 63, pp. 5P–6P, 1986.

POST, R. H., Population Differences in Vision Acuity: A Review, with Speculative Notes on Selection Relaxation, *Eugenics Quart.*, Vol. 9, pp. 189–192, 1962.

POSTER, M. G., Hydrated Method of Determining Dioptral Power of a Hydrophilic Contact Lens, *J. Amer. Optom. Assoc.*, Vol. 42, p. 369, 1971.

QUINTERO, S., El Bayadi Indirect Biomicroscopy Technique, Unpublished course notes, University of Houston, Houston, Tex., 1986.

RAVIOLA, E., Experimental Myopia; Animal Experiments, Myopia Workshop, Copenhagen, 1987.

RAVIOLA, E., and WIESEL, T. N., Effect of Dark-Rearing on Experimental Myopia in Monkeys, *Invest. Ophthal. Vis. Sci.*, Vol. 17, pp. 485–488, 1978.

RAVIOLA, E., and WIESEL, T. N., An Animal Model of Myopia, *New Engl. J. Med.*, Vol. 312, pp. 1609–1615, 1985.

REBER, N., Visual Screening Program for Schools, *J. Amer. Optom. Assoc.*, Vol. 35, pp. 675–680, 1964.

REFOJO, M. F., *Encyclopedia of Polymer Science and Technology*, Suppl. No. 1, New York, John Wiley & Sons, 1976.

REFOJO, M. F., Mechanism of Gas Transport Through Contact Lenses, *J. Amer. Optom. Assoc.*, Vol. 50, pp. 285–287, 1979.

REFOJO, M. F., and HOLLY, F. S., Tear Protein Adsorption on Hydrogel: A Possible Cause of Contact Lens Allergy, *Cont. Lens*, pp. 23–25, Jan./March 1977.

REGAN, D., Rapid Objective Refraction Using Evoked Brain Potentials, *Invest. Ophthal.*, Vol. 12, pp. 669–673, 1973.

REINECKE, R. D., and SIMONS, K., A New Stereoscopic Test for Amblyopia Screening, *Amer. J. Ophthal.*, Vol. 78, pp. 714–721, 1974.

REMBA, M. J., Purging Soft Contacts, *Cont. Lens Forum*, pp. 56–61, Nov. 1979.

REMBA, M. J., Clinical Evaluation of the Tangent Streak, a Translating Bifocal Rigid Gas-Permeable Contact Lens (abstract), *Amer. J. Optom.*, Vol. 64, p. 5, 1987.

RENGSTORFF, R. H. A Study of Visual Acuity Loss After Contact Lens Wear, *Amer. J. Optom.*, Vol. 43, pp. 431–440, 1966a.

RENGSTORFF, R. H., Observed Effects of Cycloplegics on Refractive Findings, *J. Amer. Optom. Assoc.*, Vol. 37, p. 360, 1966b.

RENGSTORFF, R. H., Variations in Corneal Curvature Measurements: An After-Affect Observed with Habitual Wearers of Contact Lenses, *Amer. J. Optom.*, Vol. 44, pp. 45–51, 1967.

RENGSTORFF, R. H., Relationship Between Myopia and Corneal Curvature After Wearing Contact Lenses, *Amer. J. Optom.*, Vol. 46, pp. 357–362, 1969a.

RENGSTORFF, R. H. Studies of Corneal Curvature Changes after Wearing Contact Lenses, *J. Amer. Opt. Assoc.*, Vol. 40, pp. 298–299, 1969b.

RENGSTORFF, R. H., Diurnal Variations in Myopia After the Wearing of Contact Lenses, *Amer. J. Optom.*, Vol. 46, pp. 812–815, 1969c.

RENGSTORFF, R. H., Diurnal Variations in Corneal Curvature After the Wearing of Contact Lenses, *Amer. J. Optom.*, Vol. 48, pp. 239–244, 1971a.

RENGSTORFF, R. H., and ARNER, S., Refractive Changes in the Cornea: Mathematical Considerations, *Amer. J. Optom.*, Vol. 44, pp. 913–918, 1971b.

RENGSTORFF, R. H., Prevention and Treatment of Corneal Damage After Wearing Contact Lenses, *J. Amer. Optom. Assoc.*, Vol. 75, pp. 277–278, 1975.

RENGSTORFF, R. H., Corneal Refraction: Relative Effects of

Each Component, *J. Amer. Optom. Assoc.*, Vol. 56, pp. 218–219, 1985.

RENGSTORFF, R. H., and NILSSON, K. T., Long-Term Effects of Extended Wear Lenses: Changes in Refraction, Corneal Curvature, and Visual Acuity, *Amer. J. Optom.*, Vol. 62, pp. 66–68, 1985.

RICHARDS, O. W., A Literature Review of Retinoscopy, *Opt. J. Rev. Optom.*, pp. 69–73, May 1977.

RICHTER, S. J., and SHERMAN, J., Electro-Oculography, Dark Adaptometry, and Laser Interferometry, *J. Amer. Optom. Assoc.*, Vol. 50, pp. 101–104, 1979.

RIGDEN, J. D., and GORDEN, E. I., The Granularity of the Scattered Optical Laser Light, *Prod. I.E.E.E.*, Vol. 50, p. 2367, 1962.

RILEY, H. D.; DOYLE, D.; and FELTY, R. L., A Preliminary Study of Mercury Deposition Resulting in Spoilage of Soft Contact Lenses, *Inter. Cont. Lens Clin.*, pp. 34–40, Sept./Oct. 1981.

RILEY, H. D., and PRESSBURGER, K. G., An Unusual Case of Viral Keratoconjunctivitis After Short-Term Wear of Soft Contact Lenses, *Inter. Cont. Lens Clin.*, pp. 37–43, 1981.

ROBERTS, W. L., and BANFORD, R. D., Evaluation of Bifocal Correction Technique in Juvenile Myopia, *Optom. Weekly*, pp. 25–31, Sept. 21; pp. 21–30, Sept. 28; pp. 23–28, Oct. 5; pp. 27–34, Oct. 12; and pp. 19–26, Oct. 26, 1967.

ROGGENKAMP, J. R.; RICHARDSON, N. L.; KREBSBACH, J. B.; and YOLTON, R. L., The IVEX Refraction System: A Clinical Comparison, *J. Amer. Optom. Assoc.*, Vol. 56, pp. 532–536, 1985.

ROSE, A. H. T., Personal communication, Christchurch, New Zealand, 1964.

ROSEN, R. C.; SCHIFFMAN, H. R.; and MYERS, H., Behavioral Treatment of Myopia: Refractive Error and Acuity Changes in Relation to Axial Length and Intraocular Pressure, *Amer. J. Optom.*, Vol. 61, pp. 100–105, 1984.

ROSENBERG, R., Paper given at the annual meeting of the Amer. Acad. Optom., Orlando, Fla., 1981.

ROSNER, J., The Effectiveness of the Random Dot E Stereotest as a Preschool Vision Screening Instrument, *J. Amer. Optom. Assoc.*, Vol. 49, pp. 1121–1124, 1978.

ROSNER, J., and GRUBER, J., Differences in the Perceptual Skills Development of Young Myopes and Hyperopes, *Amer. J. Optom.*, Vol. 62, pp. 501–504, 1985.

ROSNER, J., and ROSNER, J., Comparison of Visual Characteristics in Children with and Without Learning Difficulties, *Amer. J. Optom.*, Vol. 64, pp. 531–533, 1987.

ROSSOW, B., and WESEMANN, W., Automatic Infrared Refractors—1985, *Ophthal.*, Instr. and Book Suppl., 1985.

ROUSE, M.; PECK, B.; and BEST, T., Researches in Fixation Disparity Parts 1 and 2, *Optom. Monthly*, Vol. 69, pp. 96–98, 1978; and Vol. 70, pp. 94–98, Jan. 1979.

RUBEN, M., Corneal Vascularization, in *Complications of Contact Lens Wear*, D. Miller and P. F. White, Editors, *Inter. Ophthal. Clin.*, Vol. 21, No. 2, 1981.

RUSHTON, Trans., Opth. Soc. U. K., Vol. 58, p. 136, 1938.

RUSHTON, W. A. H., Visual Pigments in Man, *Scientific American*, Nov. 1962.

RYAN, R. E., *Headache: Diagnosis and Treatment*, St. Louis, Mosby, 1954.

RYAN, V., Predicting Aniseikonia and Anisometropia, *Amer. J. Optom.*, Vol. 52, pp. 96–105, 1975.

SABISTON, D. W., The Association of Keratoconus, Dermatitis and Asthma, *Transaction N.Z. Cont. Lens Soc.*, Aug. 1965.

SALADIN, J. J., and SHEEDY, J. E., Population Study of Fixation Disparity, Heterophoria and Vergence, *Amer. J. Optom.*, Vol. 55, pp. 744–750, 1978.

SANDERS, T. L.; POLSE, K. A.; SARVER, M. D.; and HARRIS, M. G., Central and Peripheral Corneal Swelling Accompanying the Wearing of Bausch and Lomb Soflens Contact Lenses, *Amer. J. Optom.*, Vol. 52, pp. 393–397, 1975.

SARVER, M. D., Visual Correction With Contact Lenses, Ch. 23, in *Clinical Refraction*, 3rd ed., I. M. Borish, Editor, Chicago, Professional Press, 1970.

SARVER, M. D., Striate Corneal Lines among Patients Wearing Hydrophilic Contact Lenses, *Amer. J. Optom.*, Vol. 48, pp. 762–763, 1971.

SARVER, M. D., and HARRIS, M., Corneal Lenses and Spectacle Blur, *Amer. J. Optom.*, Vol. 44, pp. 316–318, 1967.

SARVER, M. D., and HARRIS, M. G., A Standard for Success in Wearing Contact Lenses, *Amer. J. Optom.*, Vol. 48, pp. 382–385, 1971.

SARVER, M. D.; KAME, R. T.; and WILLIAMS, C. E., A Bitoric Gas Permeable Hard Contact Lens with Spherical Power Effect, *J. Amer. Optom. Assoc.*, Vol. 56, pp. 184–189, 1985.

SATO, C., *The Causes of Acquired Myopia*, Tokyo, Kanehara Shuppan Co., 1957.

SATO, T.; AKIYAMA, K.; and SHIBATA, H., A New Surgical Approach to Myopia, *Amer. J. Ophthal.*, Vol. 36, pp. 823–829, 1953.

SCHANZLIN, D. J.; SANTOS, V. R.; WARING, G. O.; LYNN, M.; BOURQUE, L.; CANTILLO, N.; EDWARDS, M. A.; JUSTIN, N.; REINIG, J.; and ROSZKA-DUGGAN, V., Diurnal Change in Refraction, Corneal Curvature, Visual Acuity, and Intraocular Pressure After Radial Keratotomy in the PERK Study, *Ophthalmol.*, Vol. 93, pp. 167–175, 1986.

SCHAPERO, M., *Amblyopia*, Philadelphia, Chilton, 1971.

SCHAPERO, M., and HIRSCH, M. J., The Relationship of Refractive Error and Guilford-Martin Temperament Test Scores, *Amer. J. Optom.*, Vol. 29, pp. 32–36, 1952.

SCHEIE, H. G., and ALBERT, D. M., *Textbook of Ophthalmology*, 9th ed., Philadelphia, Saunders, 1977.

SCHNIDER, C.; ZABKIEWICZ, K.; TERRY, R.; LaHOOD, D.; and HOLDEN, B., Unusual Complications of RPG Extended Wear (abstract), *Amer. J. Optom.*, Vol. 63, pp. 35P–36P, 1986.

SCHOCK, S., Lecture given at University of Houston continuing education course, Houston, Tex., Jan. 16, 1982.

SCHOR, C., Fixation Disparity: A Steady State of Disparity-Induced Vergence, *Amer. J. Optom.*, Vol. 57, pp. 618–631, 1980.

SCHOR, C. and ERICKSON, P., Binocular Depth of Field in Monovision (abstract), *Amer. J. Optom.*, Vol. 64, p. 51P, 1987.

SCHWARTZ, B., Primary Open-Angle Glaucoma, Vol. 3, Ch. 52, in *Clinical Ophthalmology*, T. D. Duane, Editor, Hagerstown, Md., Harper & Row, 1980.

SCOTT, S., Photodocumentation Equipment: An Overview of Ophthalmic Photography Instrumentation, *Amer. J. Optom.*, Vol. 56, pp. 603–604, 1979.

SEKULER, R.; OWSLEY, C.; and HUTMAN, L., Assessing Spatial Vision of Older People, *Amer. J. Optom.*, Vol. 59, pp. 961–968, 1982.

SHAVER, W. W., A Photochromatic Glass with Ophthalmic Applications, *Amer. J. Optom.*, Vol. 46, pp. 339–346, 1969.

SHEARD, C., *Dynamic Skametry*, Chicago, Cleveland Press, 1920.

SHEARD, C., Accommodative or Physiological Exophoria with Comments on Prescribing of Prisms, *Amer. J. Physiol. Opt.*, Vol. 6, pp. 580–591, 1925 (reprinted in *The Sheard Volume*, Philadelphia, Chilton, 1957).

SHEARD, C., Zones of Ocular Comfort, *Amer. J. Optom.*, Vol. 7, pp. 9–25, 1930 (reprinted in abridged form in *The Sheard Volume*, Philadelphia, Chilton, 1957).

SHEEDY, J. E., Actual Measurement of Fixation Disparity and Its Use in Diagnosis and Treatment, *J. Amer. Optom. Assoc.*, Vol. 51, pp. 1079–1084, 1980a.

SHEEDY, J. E., Fixation Disparity Analysis of Oculomotor Imbalance, *Amer. J. Optom.*, Vol. 57, pp. 632–639, 1980b.

SHEEDY, J. E.; BURI, M.; BAILEY, I. L.; AZUS, J.; and BORISH, I. M., Optics of Progressive Addition Lenses, *Amer. J. Optom.*, Vol. 64, pp. 90–99, 1987.

SHEEDY, J. E., and SALADIN, J. J., Exophoria at Near in Presbyopia, *Amer. J. Optom.*, Vol. 52, pp. 474–481, 1975.

SHEEDY, J. E., and SALADIN, J. J., Phorias, Vergences and Fixation Disparity in Oculomotor Problems, *Amer. J. Optom.*, Vol. 54, pp. 474–478, 1977.

SHEEDY, J. E., and SALADIN, J. J., Association of Symptoms with Measures of Oculomotor Deficiencies, *Amer. J. Optom.*, Vol. 55, pp. 670–676, 1978.

SHEPARD, C. F., The Baltimore Project, *Optom. Weekly*, pp. 133–135, Jan. 1946.

SHICK, C. A., A Simple Mire Modification to Improve Keratometer Efficiency, *J. Amer. Optom. Assoc.*, Vol. 34, pp. 388–390, 1962.

SHIRMER, K. E., Corneal Sensitivity and Contact Lenses, *Brit. J. Optom.*, Vol. 47, pp. 493–495, 1963.

SHLAIFER, A., *Synopsis of Glaucoma for Optometrists*, Minneapolis, Burgess, 1959.

SHULTZ, L. B., Personality and Psychological Variables as Related to Refractive Errors, *Amer. J. Optom.*, Vol. 37, pp. 551–571, 1960.

SIEGFRIED, J., Electrodiagnosis: Its Potential in Your Practice, *Rev. Optom.*, Vol. 114, pp. 20–32, Dec. 1977.

SIMMONS, R. J., and DALLOW, R. L., Primary Angle-Closure Glaucoma, Vol. 3, Ch. 53, in *Clinical Ophthalmology*, T. D. Duane, Editor, Hagerstown, Md., Harper & Row, 1976.

SIVAK, J. G., and BOBIER, C. W., Accommodation and Chromatic Aberration in Young Children, *Invest. Ophthal. Vis. Sci.*, pp. 705–709, 1978.

SLATAPER, F. J., Age Norms in Refraction and Vision, *Arch. Ophthal.*, Vol. 43, pp. 466–481, 1950.

SLOAN, P. G., and POLSE, K. A., Preliminary Clinical Evaluation of the Dioptron, *Amer. J. Optom.*, Vol. 51, pp. 189–197, 1974.

SMELSER, G., and CHEN, D. K., Physiological Changes in Cornea Induced by Contact Lenses, *Arch. Ophthal.*, Vol. 53, pp. 676–679, 1955.

SMELSER, G., and OZANICS, V., Importance of Atmospheric Oxygen for Maintenance of the Optical Properties of the Human Cornea, *Science*, Vol. 115, p. 140, 1952.

SMITH, E. L.; McGUIRE, G. W.; and WATSON, J. T., Axial Lengths and Refractive Errors in Kittens Reared with an Optically Induced Anisometropia, *Invest. Ophthal. Vis. Sci.*, Vol. 19, pp. 1250–1255, 1980.

SMITH, J. L., *The Pupil* (monograph), J. L. Smith, Miami, Fla.

SMITH, J. L., *The Visual Fields*, Neuro-ophthalmology, Tape No. 3, J. L. Smith, Miami, Fla.

SMITH, J. L., *The Pupil*, Neuro-ophthalmology Tape No. 6, J. L. Smith, Miami, Fla.

SMITH, J. L., *Headaches*, Neuro-ophthalmology Tape No. 47, J. L. Smith, Miami, Fla.

SMITH, J. L., *Temporal Arteritis Management*, Neuro-ophthalmology Tape. No. 64, J. L. Smith, Miami, Fla.

SORSBY, A., *Ophthalmic Genetics*, 2nd ed., London, Butterworths, 1970.

SORSBY, A.; BENJAMIN, D.; DAVEY, J. B.; SHERIDAN, M.; and TANNER, J. M., *Emmetropia and Its Aberrations*, London, Her Majesty's Stationery Office, 1957.

SORSBY, A.; BENJAMIN, B.; and SHERIDAN, M., *Refraction and Growth of the Eye from the Age of Three*, London, Her Majesty's Stationery Office, 1961.

SORSBY, A., and LEARY, G. A., *A Longitudinal Study of*

Refraction and Its Components During Growth, London, Her Majesty's Stationery Office, 1970.

SORSBY, S.; SHERIDAN, M.; and LEARY, G. A., *Refraction: Its Components in Twins*, London, Her Majesty's Stationery Office, 1962.

SPAETH; G. L., Tonography and Tonometry, Vol. 3, Ch. 47, in *Clinical Ophthalmology*, T. D. Duane, Editor, Hagerstown, Md., Harper & Row, 1980.

SPOONER, J. D., *Ocular Anatomy*, London, Butterworths, 1957.

STARK, L.; KENYON, R. V.; KRISHNAN, V. V.; and CIUFFREDA, K. J., Disparity Vergence: A Proposed Name for a Dominant Component of Binocular Vergence Eye Movements, *Amer. J. Optom.*, Vol. 57, pp. 606–609, 1980.

STEIGER, A., *Die Entstehung der Sphärischen Refractionen des Menschlichen Auges*, Berlin, S. Karger, 1913.

STEIN, H.; BOYANER, D.; and DEMERS, J., Soft Contact Lens Care System Alternatives, *Inter. Cont. Lens Clin.*, pp. 11–16, July/Aug. 1981.

STEIN, H. A., and SLATT, B., Extended Wear Soft Contact Lenses in Perspective, *Inter. Cont. Lens Clin.*, Vol. 4, No. 5, pp. 35–40, 1977.

STENSTROM, S., Investigation of the Variation and the Correlation of the Optical Elements of the Human Eye, Trans. by D. Woolf, *Amer. J. Optom.*, Vol. 25, pp. 218–232, 1948.

STEVENS, GEORGE T., *A Treatise on the Motor Apparatus of the Eyes*, Philadelphia, F. A. Davis, 1906.

STEVENSON, R. W. W., Adhesion of Lenses During Extended Wear of the Boston "Equalens" (abstract), *Amer. J. Optom.*, Vol. 63, p. 37P, 1986.

STEWART, C. R., Functional Blinking and Corneal Lenses, *Amer. J. Optom.*, Vol. 45, 687–691, 1968.

STEWART, C. R., Lecture given at University of Houston continuing education course, Houston, Tex., Jan. 16, 1982.

STILES, W. S., and CRAWFORD, B. H., The Luminous Efficiency of Rays Entering the Eye Pupil at Different Points, *Proc. Royal Soc.* (London), Series B, 112, pp. 428–450, 1933.

STONE, J., Contact Lens Wear in the Young Myope, *Brit. J. Physiol. Opt.*, Vol. 28, pp. 90–134, 1973.

STONE, J., The Possible Influence of Contact Lenses on Myopia, *Brit. J. Physiol. Opt.*, Vol. 31, pp. 89–114, 1976.

STONE, J., and POWELL-CULLINGFORD, G., Myopia Control After Contact Lens Wear, *Brit. J. Physiol. Opt.*, Vol. 29, pp. 93–108, 1974.

STRAATSMA, B. R.; FOOS, R. Y.; and FEMAN, S. S., Degenerative Diseases of the Peripheral Retina, Vol. 3, Ch. 26, in *Clinical Ophthalmology*, T. D. Duane, Editor, Hagerstown, Md., Harper & Row, 1980.

STRAATSMA, B. R.; FOOS, R. Y.; and KREIGER, A. E., Rhegmatogenous Retinal Detachment, Vol. 3, Ch. 27, in *Clinical Ophthalmology*, T. D. Duane, Editor, Hagerstown, Md., Harper & Row, 1980.

STRANCH, L. A. W., Water-Absorbent CAB Lenses Combat Corneal Edema, *Rev. Optom.*, pp. 67–72, April 1981.

STREFF, J. W., and CLAUSSEN, V. E., Retinoscopy Measurement Differences as a Variable of Technique, *Amer. J. Optom.*, Vol. 48, pp. 671–676, 1971.

STRUGHOLD, H., The Sensitivity of the Cornea and Conjunctiva of the Human Eye and the Use of Contact Lenses, *Amer. J. Optom.*, Vol. 30, pp. 625–630, 1953.

SWARBRICK, H. A., and HOLDEN, B. A., RP Lens Binding—A Retrospective Analysis (abstract), *Amer. J. Optom.*, Vol. 63, p. 37P, 1986.

TAIT, E. F., Accommodative Convergence, *Amer. J. Ophthal.*, Vol. 34, pp. 1093–1107, 1951.

TAIT, E. F., A Quantitative System of Dynamic Skiametry, *Amer. J. Optom.*, Vol. 30, pp. 113–129, 1953.

TASMAN, W., The Vitreous, Vol. 3, Ch. 39, in *Clinical Ophthalmology*, T. D. Duane, Editor, Hagerstown, Md., Harper & Row, 1976.

TASSMAN, I. S., Frequency of Various Kinds of Refractive Errors, *Amer. J. Ophthal.*, Vol. 15, pp. 1044–1053, 1932.

TATE, G. W., *Principles of Quantitative Perimetry*, New York, Grune & Stratton, 1970.

TERRY, J. E., Mydriatic Angle-Closure Glaucoma: Mechanism, Evaluation and Reversal, *J. Amer. Optom. Assoc.*, Vol. 48, pp. 159–168, 1977.

THOMPSON, T., *Tyler's Quarterly Soft Contact Lens Guide*, Little Rock, March 1987.

TIACHAC, C. A., and PATELLA, V. M., A Comparison of Reading Add Values: Humphrey Vision Analyzer and Phoropter, *Optom. Monthly*, Vol. 70, pp. 602–606, Aug. 1979.

TRACHTMAN, J. N., Biofeedback of Accommodation to Reduce Functional Myopia: A Case Report, *Amer. J. Optom.*, Vol. 55, pp. 400–406, 1978.

TROOST, B. T., Migraine, Vol. 2, Ch. 19, in *Clinical Ophthalmology*, T. D. Duane, Editor, Hagerstown, Md., Harper & Row, 1978.

TSUDA, S.; TANAKA, K.; ANAN, N.; and YOSHIDA, K., Analysis of Surface Deposits and Effective Countermeasures, *Inter. Cont. Lens Clin.*, pp. 46–52, March/April 1981.

TURVILLE, A. E., *Outline of an Infinity Balance*, London, Raphael's, 1946.

Tyler's Quarterly Soft Contact Parameter Guide, Little Rock, AR, March 1987.

U.S. Department of Health, Education and Welfare, *Characteristics of Persons with Corrective Lenses*, Rockville, Md., HEW, 1974a.

U.S. Department of Health, Education and Welfare, *Refraction Status and Motility Defects of Persons 4–74 Years*, Hyattsville, Md., HEW, 1974b.

U.S. Department of Health, Education and Welfare, *Refraction Status and Motility Defects of Persons 4–74 Years, United States, 1971–1972*, HEW Publ. No. (PHS) 78–1654, Hyattsville, Md., 1978.

VAN ALPHEN, G. W. H. M., *On Emmetropia and Ametropia*, Supp. ad Ophthalogica, Vol. 142, Basel, Switzerland and New York, S. Karger, 1961.

VAN ALPHEN, G., Emmetropia and Ametropia, in *Refractive Anomalies of the Eye*, NINDB Monograph No. 5, pp. 29–34, Bethesda, Md, U.S. Department of Health, Education and Welfare, 1967.

VAN ALPHEN, G. W. H. M., Choroidal Stress and Emmetropization, *Vis. Res.*, Vol. 26, pp. 723–734, 1986.

VAN HERICK, W.; SHAFFER, R. N.; and SCHWARTZ, A., Estimation of Width of Angle of Anterior Chamber, *Amer. J. Ophthal.*, Vol. 68, pp. 626–629, 1969.

VAN HOVEN, R. C., Cycloplegia and the Accommodation-Convergence Relationship, *Amer. J. Optom.*, Vol. 36, pp. 22–39, 1959.

VAUGHAN, D., and ASBURY, T., *General Ophthalmology*, 8th ed., Los Altos, Calif., Lange, 1977.

VERBAKEN, J. H., and JOHNSTON, A. W., Clinical Contrast Sensitivity Testing; the Current Status, *Clin. Exper. Optom.*, Vol. 69, pp. 204–212, 1986a.

VERBAKEN, J. H., and JOHNSTON, A. W., Population Norms for Edge Contrast Sensitivity, *Amer. J. Optom.*, Vol. 63, pp. 724–732, 1986b.

VON NORDEN, G. K., and CRAWFORD, M. L. J., Lid Closure and Refractive Error in Macaque Monkeys, *Nature*, Vol. 272, pp. 53–54, March 2, 1978.

WALLMAN, J., and GOTTLIEB, M., Stroboscopic Illumination Protects Chicks Against Deprivation-Induced Myopia (abstract), *Amer. J. Optom.*, Vol. 64, p. 102P, 1987.

WALLMAN, J.; GOTTLIEB, M. D.; RAJARAM, V. V.; and FUGATE-WENTZEK, L. A., Local Retinal Regions Control Local Eye Growth and Myopia, *Science*, Vol. 23, pp. 73–77, July 3, 1987.

WALLMAN, J.; ROSENTHAL, D.; ADAMS, J. I.; TRACHTMAN, J. N.; and ROMAGNANO, L., Role of Accommodation and Developmental Aspects of Experimental Myopia in Chicks, *Doc. Ophthal. Proc.*, Series 28, Third International Conference on Myopia, H. C. Fledelius, P. H. Alsbirk, and E. Goldschmidt, Editors, The Hague, Dr. W. Junk Publishers, 1981.

WALLMAN, J.; TURKEL, J.; and TRACHTMAN, J., Extreme Myopia Produced by Modest Changes in Early Visual Experience, *Science*, Vol. 201, p. 1249, 1978.

WALSH, T. J., *Neuro-ophthalmology: Clinical Signs and Symptoms*, Philadelphia, Lea and Febiger, 1978.

WALTERS, J. W., Electrodiagnostics, *Texas Optom.*, pp. 7–10, Dec. 1981a.

WALTERS, J. W., Personal communication, Houston, Tex., 1981b.

WALTERS, J. W., Evaluation of Automated Perimeters, unpublished report, University of Houston, Houston, Tex., 1986.

WARING, G. O.; LYNN, M. J.; GELENDER, H.; LAIBSON, P. R.; LINDSTROM, R. L.; MYERS, W. D.; OBSTBAUM, S. A.; ROWSEY, J. J.; MCDONALD, M. B.; SCHANZLIN, D. J.; SPERDUTO, R. D.; and BOURQUE, L. B., Results of the Prospective Evaluation of Radial Keratotomy (PERK) Study One Year After Surgery, *Ophthal.*, Vol. 92, pp. 177–208, 1985.

WEALE, R., *The Aging Eye*, London, Lewis, 1963.

WEED, L. L., Medical Records that Guide and Teach, *New Engl. J. Med.*, Vol. 278, pp. 593–599, 652–657, 1968.

WEED, L. L., *Medical Records, Medical Education, and Patient Care: A Problem-Oriented Record as a Basic Tool*, Case Western Reserve University Press, 1969.

WEED, L. L., The Problem-Oriented Record, Ch. 5, in *The Problem-Oriented Record System*, J. W. Hurst and H. K. Walker, Editors, Baltimore, Williams & Wilkins, 1972.

WEISSMAN, B. A.; REMBA, M. J.; and FUGEDY, E., Results of the Extended Wear Contact Lens Survey of the Contact Lens Section of the American Optometric Association, *J. Amer. Optom. Assoc.*, Vol. 58, pp. 166–171, 1987.

WELSH, R., Contact Lenses in Aphakia, *Inter. Ophthal. Clin.*, Vol. 1, No. 2, pp. 401–440, 1961.

WELSH, R. C., Aphakia: Optical Considerations, *Amer. J. Optom.*, Vol. 48, pp. 852–856, 1971.

WESEMANN, W., and RASSOW, B., Automatic Infrared Refractors—A Comparative Study, *Amer. J. Optom.*, Vol. 64, pp. 627–638, 1987.

WEYMOUTH, F. W., and HIRSCH, M. J., History, Classification and Methods of Measurement of Myopia, Ch. 1 in *Researches in Refractive Error: Clinical Applications*, T.

Grosvenor and M. Flom, Editors, Boston, Butterworths, in press.

WHITE, J. W., The Screen Test and Its Modifications, *Amer. J. Ophthal.*, Vol. 29, pp. 156–160, 194, 1946.

WICHTERLE, O., and LIM, D., Hydrophilic Gels for Biological Use, *Nature*, Vol. 185, p. 4706, Jan. 1960.

WIBAUT, F., Über die Emmetropization und den Ursprung sphärischen Refractionsanomalien, Albert von Graefe's *Archif für Ophthalmologie*. Vol. 116, pp. 596–612, 1926 1963).

WIESEL, T. N., and RAVIOLA, E., Myopia and Eye Enlargement After Neonatal Lid Fusion in Monkeys, *Nature*, Vol. 233, pp. 66–68, March 3, 1977.

WIESEL, T. N., and RAVIOLA, E., Increase in Axial Length of the Macaque Monkey Eye After Corneal Opacification, *Invest. Ophthal. Vis. Sci.*, Vol. 18, pp. 1232–1236, 1979.

WILBUR, J. A., and BARROW, G. Hypertension: A Community Problem, in *Hypertension Manual*, J. J. Laragh, Editor, New York, Yorke Medical Books, pp. 711–742, 1974.

WILSON, G.; BELL, C.; and CHOTAI, S., The Effect of Lifting the Lids on Corneal Astigmatism, *Amer. J. Optom.*, Vol. 59, pp. 670–674, 1982.

WIXSON, R. J., The Relative Effects of Heredity and Environment upon the Refractive Errors of Identical Twins, Fraternal Twins, and Like-Sex Siblings, *Amer. J. Optom.*, Vol. 35, pp. 346–351, 1958.

WOLFF, E., *Anatomy of the Eye and Orbit*, 6th ed., R. J. Last, Editor, London, H. K. Lewis & Co., Ltd, 1968.

WOO, G. C., Contrast Sensitivity Function as a Diagnostic Tool in Low Vision, *Amer. J. Optom.*, Vol. 62, pp. 648–651, 1985.

WOO, G. C., and DALZIEL, C. C., A Pilot Study of Contrast Sensitivity Assessment of the CAM Treatment of Amblyopia, *Acta Ophthal.*, Vol. 59, pp. 35–37, 1981.

WOO, G. C., and LONG, W. F., Recommended Light Levels for Clinical Procedures, *Optom. Monthly*, Vol. 70, pp. 722–725, Oct. 1979.

WOO, G. C., and WOODRUFF, M. E., The AO SR III Subjective Refraction System, Comparison with Phoropter Measures, *Amer. J. Optom.*, Vol. 55, pp. 591–596, 1978.

WOODRUFF, M. E., Cross-Sectional Studies of Corneal and Astigmatic Characteristics of Children Between the Twenty-Fourth and Seventy-Second Month of Life, *Amer. J. Optom.*, Vol. 48, pp. 650–659, 1971.

WOODS, A. C., Report from the Wilmer Institute on the Results Obtained in the Treatment of Myopia by Visual Training, *Trans. Amer. Acad. Ophthal. and Otol.*, Vol. 49, pp. 37–65, 1945.

WORELL, B. E.; HIRSCH, M. J.; and MORGAN, M. W., An Evaluation of Prism Prescribed by Sheard's Criterion, *Amer. J. Optom.*, Vol. 48, pp. 373–376, 1971.

YATES, J. T.; HARRISON, J. M.; O'CONNOR, P. A.; and BALLENTINE, C., Contrast Sensitivity: Characteristics of a Large, Young, Adult Population, *Amer. J. Optom.*, Vol. 64, pp. 519–527, 1987.

YELLEN, M., and SHERMAN, J., Static vs. Dynamic Field Evaluation, with Emphasis on the Utility of the Friedman Field Analyzer, *J. Amer. Optom. Assoc.*, pp. 95–98, 1979.

YOUNG, F. A., The Effect of Restricted Visual Space on the Primate Eye, *Amer. J. Ophthal.*, Vol. 52, pp. 799–806, 1961.

YOUNG, F. A., Reading, Measures of Intelligence and Refractive Errors, *Amer. J. Optom.*, Vol. 40, pp. 257–264, 1963.

YOUNG, F. A., The Effect of Atropine on the Development of Myopia in Monkeys, *Amer. J. Optom.*, Vol. 42, pp. 439–449, 1965.

YOUNG, F. A., Animal Experimentation and Research in Refractive State, Ch. 4, in *Synopsis of the Refractive State of the Eye*, Vol. 5, M. J. Hirsch, Editor, Minneapolis, Burgess, 1967a.

YOUNG, F. A., Myopia and Personality, *Amer. J. Optom.*, Vol. 44, pp. 192–198, 1967b.

YOUNG, F. A., The Development and Control of Myopia in Human and Subhuman Primates, *Contacto*, Vol. 19, pp. 16–31, 1975.

YOUNG, F. A., The Nature and Control of Myopia, *J. Amer. Optom. Assoc.*, Vol. 48, pp. 451–457, 1977.

YOUNG, F. A., Intraocular Pressure Dynamics Associated with Accommodation, *Doc. Ophthal. Proc.*, Series 28, Third International Conference on Myopia, H. C. Fledelius, P. W. Alsbirk, and E. Goldschmidt, Editors, The Hague, Dr. W. Junk Publishers, 1981.

YOUNG, F. A.; BEATTIE, R. J.; NEWBY, F. J.; and SWINDAL, M. T., The Pullman Study: A Visual Survey of Pullman School Children, Parts 1 and 2, *Amer. J. Optom.*, Vol. 31, pp. 111–121, 192–203, 1954.

YOUNG, F. A., and LEARY, G. A., The Mechanism of Visual Accommodation and Its Role in Refraction (abstract), *Amer. J. Optom.*, Vol. 64, p. 10P, 1987.

YOUNG, F. A.; LEARY, G. A.; BALDWIN, W. R.; WEST, D. C.; BOX, R. A.; HARRIS, E.; and JOHNSON, C., The Transmission of Refractive Errors Within Eskimo Families, *Amer. J. Optom.*, Vol. 46, pp. 676–685.

YOUNG, F. A.; LEARY, G. A.; GROSVENOR, T.; MASLOVITZ, B.; PERRIGIN, D. M.; PERRIGIN, J.; and QUINTERO, S., Houston Myopia Control Study: A Randomized Clinical Trial, Part

I: Background and Design of the Study, *Amer. J. Optom.*, Vol. 62, pp. 605–613, 1985.

YOUNG, F. A.; SINGER, R. M.; and FOSTER, D., The Psychological Differentiation of Male Myopes and Nonmyopes, *Amer. J. Optom.*, Vol. 52, pp. 679–686, 1975.

ZABA, J. N., Color Deficiency, Optometry, and Education, *J. Amer. Optom. Assoc.*, Vol. 45, pp. 94–95, 1974.

ZABKIEWICZ, K.; TERRY, R.; HOLDEN, B. A.; and SCHNIDER, C., The Frequency of Rigid Lens Binding in Extended Wear Decreases with Time (abstract), *Amer. J. Optom.*, Vol. 64, pp. 110P, 1987.

ZANTOS, S. G., and HOLDEN, B. A., Transient Changes Soon After Wearing Soft Contact Lenses, *Amer. J. Optom.*, Vol. 54, pp. 856–858, 1977.

ZANTOS, S. G., and ZANTOS, P. O., Extended Wear Feasibility of Gas-Permeable Hard Lenses for Myopes, *Inter. Eyecare*, Vol. 1, pp. 66–75, June 1985.

Answers to Study Questions

Chapter 1

1. (a) Emmetropia is the normal refractive state of the eye. For an emmetropic eye with accommodation relaxed, parallel rays of light focus sharply on the retina. **(b)** Myopia is the condition in which, with accommodation relaxed, parallel rays of light converge to a focus in front of the retina. **(c)** Hyperopia is the condition in which, with accommodation relaxed, parallel rays of light converge to a focus behind the retina. **(d)** Astigmatism is a refractive condition in which the eye's optical system is incapable of forming a point image for a point object, because the refracting power of the optical system varies from one meridian to another. **(e)** Anisometropia is the condition in which the refraction differs (e.g., by 1.00D or more) for the two eyes. **(f)** Presbyopia is the condition that occurs when the near point of accommodation has receded to the point where it is difficult or impossible to accommodate sufficiently for reading or other close work.

2. The optical image is the clearly focused image formed by the optical system of the eye, which may or may not coincide with the retina; the retinal image is the image formed on the retina, which may be either sharply focused or blurred.

3. (a) 20/100; **(b)** 20/400; **(c)** 20/40; **(d)** 20/200; **(e)** 20/15.

4. (a) 9.00D; **(b)** 0.50D.

5. (a) $-1.00 +1.00 \times 90$; **(b)** $-1.00 +2.50 \times 80$; **(c)** $+3.50 -1.00 \times 165$; **(d)** $+1.00 -1.00 \times 100$.

6. The shape of the lens capsule, as described by Fincham, molds the lens substance, during accommodation, into a form in which the anterior surface is much more highly curved than would be possible otherwise.

7. (a) Front surface, 7.7mm; back surface, 6.8mm; **(b)** 3.6mm; **(c)** 24.0mm; **(d)** aqueous, 1.336; lens cortex, 1.386; lens nucleus, 1.406; vitreous, 1.336.

8. (a) -2.00D; **(b)** -10.00D; **(c)** $+5.00$D; **(d)** $+0.25$D.

9. (a) 0.01; **(b)** 1.2/120; **(c)** 4/400.

10. (a) $+2.50$D; **(b)** $+1.50$D.

11. (a) For a 5.00D uncorrected myope, the 2mm pupil resulting from bright illumination would increase the depth of focus of the eye and, therefore, would be expected to improve the visual acuity as compared with dim illumination with a 5mm pupil. **(b)** For a corrected 5.00D myope there would probably be little, if any, difference in acuity in the two situations.

12. (a) 2.00D; **(b)** none.

13. (a) Plano -0.50×180; **(b)** $+0.25 -0.50 \times 90$.

14. (a) -0.50×90; **(b)** -0.75×180; **(c)** -1.75×90; **(d)** -2.00×180; **(e)** -3.00×90.

15. -5.60D.

16. (a) $+1.00$D; **(b)** $+1.50$D.

17. (a) More; **(b)** less.

18. The front surface of the lens moves forward and increases markedly in curvature, while the back surface of the lens maintains its position and increases only slightly in curvature. Helmholtz proposed that, during accommodation, the ciliary muscle has the action of a sphincter muscle, causing the tension on the zonular fibers to be relaxed. This relaxation in tension allows the crystalline lens to assume a more highly curved (more spherical) form.

19. (a) Visual acuity falls off rapidly for off-foveal fixation, reaching 20/100 at about 10 degrees from the fovea and 20/200 at about 20 degrees from the fovea. **(b)** Reducing luminance very much below the "standard" luminance of 10 foot-lamberts (say, to 5

563

foot-lamberts or below) causes a considerable loss in visual acuity, but increasing luminance to 100 or even 1,000 foot-lamberts causes little improvement in acuity. **(c)** Visual acuity decreases with a decrease in contrast below approximately 90 percent.

20. **(a)** Simple myopic astigmatism lowers distance acuity but has relatively little effect on acuity for near work (depending on the amount of astigmatism) as long as the individual is able to accommodate. **(b)** Simple hyperopic astigmatism has little effect on either distance or near acuity as long as the individual has adequate accommodation (the effect on acuity being greater the greater the amount of astigmatism). **(c)** Mixed astigmatism may have relatively little effect on distance acuity if the circle of least confusion is on the retina, and near acuity may also be affected little if amplitude of accommodation is adequate.

Chapter 2

1. **(a)** Ages 65–74; **(b)** ages 12–17 years.

2. Sorsby found that the emmetropic eye shows a wide range of axial lengths, corneal powers, and lens powers, and found that the proportion of emmetropes in the general population was higher than would be expected on the basis of free association.

3. Cook and Glasscock found a wide distribution of refractive error for newborn babies, as compared with Herrnheiser's report that newborn babies had from 1.00 to 6.00D of hyperopia.

4. **(a)** Spherical refraction increased from an average of +0.18D at age 45 through 49 to approximately 1.00D at over the age of 75, with a marked increase in dispersion of refractive error with age. **(b)** Astigmatism increased an average of 1.00D in the against-the-rule direction between the ages of 40 and 80 years, or an average of 0.25D every 10 years.

5. The refractive error distribution curve was more peaked (leptokurtotic) than a normal distribution curve, and it was skewed toward myopia. This curve can be made to look more like a normal distribution curve by eliminating cases of myopia with degenerated fundi.

6. **(a)** Hyperopia in excess of 1.50D; **(b)** hyperopia between 0.50 and 1.50D; **(c)** a spherical refraction below +0.50D, particularly if against-the-rule astigmatism were present.

7. Van Alphen proposed that the ciliary body and choroid form an elastic envelope that limits the stretch of the sclera by counteracting part of the intraocular pressure, and that the macula provides

information to the brain indicating the required amount of stretch.

8. **(a)** Between the ages of about 20 and 40 years; **(b)** at ages 5–6; **(c)** during the school years.

9. **(a)** 5mm (from an average of 18mm at birth to 23mm at age 3); **(b)** 1mm.

10. **(a)** Holding axial length and anterior chamber depth constant, a correlation of +0.70 between corneal radius and refractive state can be accounted for by the fact that a flattening of the cornea leads to hyperopia; however, if axial length and anterior chamber depth are allowed to change, flattening of the cornea is associated with a lengthening of the eye and, therefore, an increase in myopia. **(b)** Holding all other variables constant, a correlation of +0.25 between anterior chamber depth and refractive state indicates that an increase in anterior chamber depth leads to hyperopia; however, if axial length and other variables are allowed to change, the increase in axial length that occurs with an increase in anterior chamber depth would lead to myopia.

11. A child who has uncorrected hyperopia must use an excessive amount of accommodation for reading or other close work. This excessive accommodation brings into play an excessive amount of accommodative convergence, causing the child to be esophoric, with the result that negative fusional vergence must be used to maintain single binocular vision. The constant use of negative fusional vergence results in headaches and other forms of asthenopia, often resulting in an aversion to reading and other close work. However, a child who is an uncorrected myope will have to use only a small amount of accommodation for reading, and only a small amount of accommodative convergence; therefore, high esophoria is not apt to occur, and the use of negative fusional vergence will not be necessary.

12. Fincham observed that when a 40-year-old subject (whose lens substance had been absorbed, leaving an empty lens capsule) tried to accommodate, a great change in the form of the lens capsule occurred. As a result of this, Fincham concluded that the ciliary muscle was very active in the absence of the lens substance.

13. Evidence includes **(a)** the fact that with-the-rule astigmatism tends to gradually decrease in amount, beyond the age of 40, apparently due to a decrease in the pressure exerted on the cornea by the tarsal plate of the upper lid; **(b)** the fact that wearers of hard contact lenses tend to develop with-the-rule astigmatism and even keratoconus, apparently due to the increased mechanical pressure on the horizontal meridian of the cornea; and **(c)** the prevalence of

large amounts of with-the-rule corneal astigmatism in American Indian children, apparently associated with factors such as changing living styles and changing diets.

14. Although myopes tend to have higher intelligence test scores than hyperopes on intelligence tests that require reading, there is no significant difference between scores made by myopes and by hyperopes on intelligence tests that do not require reading.

15. Tron found that all of the refractive components of the eye were normally distributed, with the exception of axial length.

16. (a) A child who may have been myopic or hyperopic at birth would typically be found to have about 0.50 to 1.00D of hyperopia by age 6, probably with a small amount of with-the-rule astigmatism. (b) During the school years, those children who do not become myopic tend to change in the direction of becoming less hyperopic as they grow older (although some will become more hyperopic and some will stay the same). (c) Between the ages of 20 and 45 years, most people will change little, but during the late 30s and early 40s, some will increase in hyperopia due to latent hyperopia becoming manifest; in addition, presbyopia becomes manifest by the age of 45. (d) Beyond age 45, presbyopia will increase in amount, leveling off at about the age of 55. While most people will become somewhat more hyperopic beyond the age of 45, a few will become myopic due to the presence of changes in the nucleus of the crystalline lens.

17. (a) Refraction may be either hyperopic or myopic at birth, but by the age of 6 the child will usually be found to have a small amount of hyperopia (possibly no more than 0.50D). (b) Myopia usually manifests itself at some time between the ages of 6 and 15 or 16, gradually increasing (at the rate of about 0.40 or 0.50D per year) during the school years. (c) The amount of myopia may stay about the same between the ages of 20 and 45, or it may increase slightly. (d) Presbyopia (usually beginning prior to the age of 45) will gradually increase in amount, leveling off at about age 55; myopia may be expected to decrease slightly (just as hyperopia would increase slightly) beyond age 55 unless nuclear lens changes occur.

18. For a trait to be normally distributed, it must be made up of a large number of independent variables. This situation does not apply to refractive error because the variables responsible for the refractive state of the eye (corneal refracting power, anterior chamber depth, lens refracting power, and axial length) are interdependent rather than independent variables.

19. The eye develops rapidly just prior to birth, with the axial length increasing and with both the cornea and the lens growing rapidly and decreasing in refracting power. If an infant is born during this period of rapid ocular development, myopia is likely to be present; but the myopia is likely to gradually disappear during the early months of life.

20. It is known that during adult life the cornea steepens somewhat, the anterior chamber becomes shallower, and the lens becomes steeper as cortical fibers are added with the passage of time. Sorsby's data (in which the axial length of the eye was calculated) can be interpreted as indicating that the eye becomes shorter with age. At least two A-scan ultrasonography studies have also shown that the eye becomes shorter with age. If this is the case, the shortening of the axial length would counteract the increase in refracting power of the cornea, anterior chamber, and lens, and thus act as an emmetropizing mechanism. At alternate (or perhaps additional) emmetropizing mechanism may be a change in the index of refraction of the lens with increasing age.

Chapter 3

1. Forms of visual deprivation other than lid-suturing, including opacification of the cornea and blurring of the retinal image by the use of a strong minus lens, have been found to cause the development of myopia in experimental animals. On the other hand, lid-sutured monkeys raised in the dark failed to develop myopia, showing that abnormal visual input must be present for myopia to develop.

2. If it is true that emmetropization occurs by virtue of a mechanism whereby the macula supplies information concerning focus to the brain and that the brain feeds this information to the choroid-ciliary body envelope that supplies the correct amount of stretch to maintain emmetropia, it is possible that if the eyes are habitually accommodated for near, the process of emmetropization would serve to move the refractive state of the eye in the direction of myopia.

3. A number of twin studies have shown a remarkable agreement in ocular refraction in identical twins as opposed to fraternal twins, siblings, or unrelated pairs; and additional studies have shown that myopic children tend to have myopic parents. Studies of animals have shown that myopia tends to occur when vision is restricted to a near environment; and a large number of population studies with humans have shown that people who engage in occupations requiring a large amount of near work tend to be myopic.

4. (a) It has been found by Goss et al. that myopia in young adults tends to be accompanied by an increase in corneal refracting power; (b) the fact that myopia is often preceded by "pseudomyopia" in which distance vision blurs after prolonged work has been

considered by some people to constitute evidence for an increase in refracting power of the lens being a cause of myopia; **(c)** there is overwhelming evidence (studies of Stenstrom, Sorsby et al., and others) that myopia occurring during childhood occurs because the lengthening of the eye has outpaced the ability of the flattening of the cornea and the lens to maintain the eye in an emmetropic state. There is also some evidence that a similar mechanism is responsible for myopia occurring in young adults.

5. The approximate prevalence of myopia in an industrialized society is **(a)** on the order of 25 percent at birth; **(b)** from 1–2 percent at ages 5–6; **(c)** increasing from about 20–30 percent during the decade from ages 20–30; **(d)** decreasing to below 20 percent between ages 40–50 due to many low myopes becoming emmetropic or hyperopic; **(e)** increasing beyond the age of 60 because of nuclear changes in the lens.

6. Wide differences in the prevalence of myopia have been reported in various population groups. Melanesians, Polynesians, and other isolated population groups primarily engaged in hunting and food-gathering have been found to have low prevalences of myopia, whereas members of industrialized population groups have much higher prevalences of myopia. It has been proposed that these population differences are due to a relaxation of natural selection pressure in industrialized societies; an alternate explanation is that myopia occurs as a direct result of concentrated near work.

7. **(a)** If a child becomes myopic at age 7, the condition tends to progress at a relatively rapid rate (more than 0.50D per year) for several years, reaching a relatively high degree by the time the progression "levels off" in the middle or late teen years; **(b)** if myopia does not appear until age 12 or beyond, it is likely to progress relatively slowly (less than 0.50D per year) and to remain at a relatively low level.

8. Possible etiological factors in myopia at various ages are: **(a)** in newborn infants myopia may be due to a lack of development of the eye (myopia of prematurity), in which case it may resolve into emmetropia or hyperopia during the early years of life, or it may be genetically determined, in which case it is usually due to the axial length being unusually long; **(b)** myopia occurring in primary schoolchildren may be genetically determined, environmentally determined (e.g., as a result of near work), or both genetic and environmental factors may be involved, but, in any case, the myopia occurs as a result of the increasing length of the eye not being compensated by corneal or lens flattening; **(c)** myopia occurring in young adults is thought to be more due to environmental

than genetic factors, and is possibly due to a combination of an increase in axial length and a slight steepening of the cornea; **(c)** myopia occurring in older adults is usually the result of an increase in the refracting power of the lens due to nuclear changes.

9. Van Alphen found that when the posterior sclera of a recently enucleated human eye is removed and the intraocular pressure is increased by inflating the eye, the ciliary body and choroid expand in an anterio-posterior direction, leading him to conclude that the tonus of the ciliary muscle determines the tension on the choroid, which ultimately determines the length of the eye.

10. It was proposed by Greene that an increase in intra-ocular pressure due to convergence exerts stress on the posterior sclera, causing it to weaken and stretch in the area of the posterior pole of the eye.

11. Congenital myopia tends to be of a higher degree than acquired myopia. Whereas some cases of congenital myopia are due to prematurity of the eye, others are thought to be genetically determined and due to axial elongation. Acquired myopia tends to be of greater degree the earlier it develops, and is considered to be due to axial elongaton that is not compensated by the cornea, anterior chamber depth, or the lens.

12. Levinsohn and others, who produced myopia in monkeys by placing them so that their eyes were directed downward, believe that the myopia occurred due to the dependent position of the eyes with regard to gravity. However, it is possible that the myopia was partially or entirely due to accommodation for the near distance or to deprivation as a result of a lack of contrast in the visual environment. For monkeys kept in restraining chairs with hoods, the myopia was due to either (or both) accommodating for a near distance or to deprivation resulting from a lack of contrast.

13. The results of three experiments conducted by Raviola and Wiesel pointed to different mechanisms for lid-suture myopia in the rhesus and stump-tail monkey. **(a)** It was found that when atropine was instilled daily into the lid-sutured eye, it prevented the development of myopia in the stump-tail monkey but not in the rhesus monkey, indicating that accommodation is responsible for lid-suture myopia in the stump-tail monkey but not in the rhesus monkey. **(b)** When the ciliary ganglion was removed from the orbit of a lid-sutured rhesus monkey, myopia developed, suggesting that accommodation was not involved in lid-suture myopia in the rhesus monkey but the myopia may be initiated by the retina itself. **(c)** Sectioning of both optic nerves was found to prevent the development of myopia in the lid-sutured, stump-tail monkey but not in the lid-sutured, rhesus monkey, indicating again that accommodation is necessary for the development of myopia in the lid-sutured, stump-tail monkey but that local (retinal) factors were responsible in the rhesus monkey.

14. (a) When plastic occluders depriving only the nasal or temporal retina were placed on newly hatched chicks, myopia and axial elongation were found to occur only for the deprived portions of the retina, causing Wallman et al. to conclude that myopia occurs because of a lack of sufficient retinal activity. **(b)** As evidence that myopia in humans may occur due to a lack of retinal activity, Wallman et al. noted that the printed page contains mainly small (high spatial frequency) features, has a restricted range of luminances, and is achromatic with the result that nonfoveal neurons, having large receptive fields, are not stimulated; therefore, this lack of local retinal activity might be responsible for eye elongation and myopia.

15. Visual training for the control of myopia. The Baltimore myopia study, conducted in 1944, demonstrated that visual training can improve visual acuity but that there was no evidence of a reduction in the amount of myopia. The majority of studies using biofeedback training for myopia control have shown an increase in visual acuity as a result of the training (which Gallaway et al. suggested may have been due to a learning effect in the measurement of visual acuity) but have not reported a reduction in the amount of myopia.

16. Bifocal lenses for the control of myopia. Several controlled studies making use of bifocal lenses for myopia control have been reported, but only that of Oakley and Young found a significant decrease in the rate of myopia progression of bifocal wearers. It was reported by Goss that bifocals tended to reduce the progression of myopia for subjects who had esophoria at near.

17. Contact lenses for juvenile myopia stabilization. The most decisive controlled study of this kind was the 5-year study reported by Stone et al., who found a significant difference in the progression of myopia for PMMA contact lens wearers, accompanied by a flattening of the cornea, as compared to spectacle wearers. At the end of the first year of the 3-year study of silicone-acrylate contact lenses, Perrigin et al. found that the lenses were causing a slight corneal flattening and that they tended to stabilize myopia progression.

18. Contact lenses for the reduction of myopia. In a controlled study, Kerns found that the fitting of contact lenses to "initiate" a reduction in myopia

tended to cause a decrease in myopia but an increase in with-the-rule astigmatism, with results varying widely from one subject to another, but that the reduction in myopia tended to disappear after lens wear was discontinued. Polse et al. also found that results due to orthokeratology were not permanent, reversing unless "retainer" lenses were worn for a part of each day.

19. Atropine and other pharmacological agents for myopia control. Atropine has been found to stabilize myopia progression, but all studies involving atropine have suffered a large drop-out rate because of the inconvenience of instilling the drops, the development of sensitivities to the atropine, and other problems. Studies making use of timolol mileate have shown that myopia tends to be stabilized for those subjects who show a decrease in intraocular pressure.

20. Surgical procedures. Scleral resection (to shorten a highly myopic eye), scleral reinforcement (to strengthen the sclera at the posterior pole), crystalline lens removal, and refractive keratoplasty (removing a slice of the cornea, freezing it, lathing it to the desired shape, and then putting it back on the eye) all have had only limited use. Radial keratotomy (making radial cuts in the cornea to weaken it and cause a flattening of the corneal apex) has gained popularity in recent years but tends to result in sensitivity to glare, variations in visual acuity and, in some cases, overcorrection or undercorrection resulting in anisometropia.

Chapter 4

1. (a) Corresponding retinal points are pairs of points, one on each retina, having the same visual direction and represented at the same area in the visual cortex. **(b)** For any fixation point, the horopter is an imaginary surface containing all object points that form images on pairs of corresponding retinal points.

2. (a) 3.00D; **(b)** 18Δ.

3. Fixated objects at about 20m and beyond have their images falling entirely within Panum's fusional areas, so no doubling of images will occur.

4. (a) Right medial rectus and left lateral rectus; **(b)** right lateral rectus and left medial rectus.

5. Convergence is the more highly developed function. In the near point of convergence test it is possible to converge the eyes as much as 60 degrees, while in the base-in prism test at 6m it is possible for the eyes to diverge only about 6 degrees.

6. Minus lenses may be used, or the subject may be

asked to fixate on an object at some distance closer than infinity (or, clinically, closer than 6m).

7. **(a)** The use of a prism (approximately 7Δ of vertical prism or approximately 15Δ of base-in prism placed before one eye); **(b)** the use of a Maddox rod in front of one eye; **(c)** the use of polarized (vectographic) targets and polarized spectacles; and **(d)** the use of a red lens in front of one eye and a green lens in front of the other eye, with red and green test objects.

8. Fusional vergence.

9. **(a)** Sensory fusion is the process by means of which visual stimuli imaged on the two retinas are combined into a single percept. **(b)** Motor fusion refers to movements of the eyes made in response to retinal disparity stimuli to maintain single binocular vision.

10. **(a)** Due to Panum's fusional areas, the horopter is a solid rather than a surface. **(b)** Because of Panum's fusional areas, physiological diplopia occurs only under extreme conditions, and it does not occur at all for objects farther than about 20m.

11. The stimulus AC/A ratio is the AC/A ratio as determined clinically, based on the accommodative stimulus (because there is no method of measuring the accommodative response). The response AC/A ratio is the AC/A ratio determined on the basis of the accommodative response, as measured by a haploscope and optometer.

12. **(a)** No movement is made. For example, in the lateral or vertical phoria test, a large amount of prism placed in front of one eye causes diplopia. **(b)** A fusional movement is made to keep the image of a fixated object on the fovea. For example, in the base-out-to-blur, break, and recovery test the introduction of a small amount of base-out prism in front of each eye will cause the eyes to make a positive fusional vergence movement.

13. Stereoscopic perception of depth occurs because the two eyes are separated in space, one eye viewing an object from a slightly different angle than the other, causing disparate retinal points to be stimulated. Because the monocular "picture painting" clues to the perception of depth are not based on a specific stimulus situation, it is thought that depth perception due to these clues must be acquired on the basis of experience.

14. Fusional vergence movements, due to the use of base-out prisms, may cause an object to first appear to be double, but the two objects (if not too far apart) suddenly move toward one another as if attracted by a magnetic force.

15. Fixation disparity. It differs from strabismus in that it involves only a tiny amount of underconvergence or overconvergence.

16. 0.50D; 4.00D.

17. Exophoria requires the use of positive fusional vergence, which is a well-developed function, while esophoria requires the use of negative fusional vergence, which is not a well-developed function. The constant use of negative fusional vergence may lead to headaches or other forms of asthenopia.

18. **(a)** The unilateral cover test, in which each eye is covered for a second or two and then uncovered. A movement of the uncovered eye in this test indicates the presence of strabismus (turning inward indicates exotropia, and turning outward indicates esotropia). **(b)** The corneal reflex test, in which the patient is instructed to look at a penlight or other source of light while the examiner views the corneal reflex in each eye while keeping his eye in line with the light source. If the corneal reflex for one eye is located temporalward to that for the other eye, the patient is esotropic; a nasalward displacement indicates that the patient is exotropic.

19. **(a)** The limit of positive fusional vergence has been reached, and accommodation (with accommodative vergence) is being used to maintain single binocular vision. **(b)** The limit of accommodative vergence has been reached, and the visual axes have returned to the phoria position. **(c)** The eyes have undergone a positive fusional vergence movement, bringing about single binocular vision.

20. **(a)** Saccadic movements can occur at speeds as fast as 400 degrees per second. **(b)** Following movements occur at a speed of about 30 degrees per second.

21. **(a)** Tonic convergence, due to the basic tonicity of the extraocular muscles—responsible, in part, for the distance phoria; **(b)** fusional vergence (convergence or divergence) stimulated by retinal disparity, resulting in the avoidance of diplopia; **(c)** accommodative convergence, accompanying accommodation; and **(d)** proximal convergence, due to the awareness of nearness.

22. **(a)** The eye fields in the frontal lobe of the brain (area 8); **(b)** the visual association area of the brain (area 19).

23. No. Because of a lag of accommodation, many people will employ less accommodation than that indicated by the stimulus.

24. In the anatomical position of rest (as in death), the visual axes are divergent; in the physiological position of rest (when tonic convergence stimuli are in operation), the visual axes are slightly divergent, but less divergent than in the anatomical position of rest.

25. (a) Positive fusional vergence demand is equal to the amount of the patient's exophoria. **(b)** Positive fusional vergence reserve is the base-out-to-blur finding.

26. (a) Suppression is a cortical inhibition of stimuli arriving from the deviating eye in the macular area (avoiding confusion) and in the peripheral area of the retina corresponding to the fixation area for the normal eye (avoiding diplopia). **(b)** Amblyopia apparently occurs as a result of long-continued suppression and involves a reduction in visual acuity of the deviating eye. **(c)** In eccentric fixation, an off-foveal point in the retina of the deviating eye is used for fixation (both in monocular and binocular vision). **(d)** In anomalous retinal correspondence, an off-foveal point in the retina of the deviated eye is associated, in consciousness, with the fovea of the fixing eye.

Chapter 5

1. (a) When present glasses or contact lenses were prescribed and, if glasses, when worn or, if contact lenses, how many hours per day worn; when glasses were first prescribed; any history of eye injury, disease, or operation. **(b)** Present state of health; recent illness; medications currently taken; most recent medical and dental examinations; presence of hypertension, diabetes, or other current disease. **(c)** Family history of sight-threatening conditions such as glaucoma, hypertension, and diabetes. **(d)** Chief complaint in patient's own words; additional complaints.

2. (a) Accompanies use of the eyes; **(b)** medium in intensity; **(c)** dull pain; **(d)** weeks' or months' duration; **(e)** possibly due to change in occupation, visual tasks, or lighting conditions; **(f)** brow region, around or behind eyes, or back of neck.

3. (a) Flaking or "dandruff" on lid margins indicates seborrheic blepharitis, while red, encrusted, inflamed areas at roots of lashes indicate ulcerative blepharitis. **(b)** Dandruff, associated with dandruff of scalp; bacterial infection. **(c)** Selenium sulfate (Selsun) or baby shampoo for both scalp and lid margins; antibacterial treatment.

4. Monocular diplopia due to astigmatism or keratoconus; binocular diplopia due to strabismus or a high phoria. Does double vision occur with one eye closed? Are the two images completely apart, or do they blend into one another? Is one image beside the other or above or below the other?

5. Diabetes would be expected to affect both eyes equally, but nuclear sclerosis usually begins earlier in one eye than the other.

6. (a) Blurred distance vision; **(b)** headaches or a feeling of eyestrain after reading or other close work; **(c)** blurred distance vision; eyestrain accompanying prolonged use of the eyes for distance or near tasks.

7. (a) The defined data base is a problem-oriented history together with appropriate tests of eye health, refraction, and binocular vision. **(b)** The complete problem list is a permanent list, including every problem the patient has or has had regarding vision (including vision-related health problems). **(c)** Initial treatment plans are numbered and titled plans, based on problems in the problem list, each plan including additional diagnostic workups, therapy, and patient education. **(d)** Progress notes are narrative notes recorded at progress visits, each progress note including four components: symptomatic, objective, assessment, and plan.

8. (a) Headache present on awakening in the morning, disappearing at some time during the day; **(b)** headache accompanied by tenderness of the scalp (particularly while combing hair), feeling of lassitude, possible transient loss of vision, and possible claudication of the jaw while chewing.

9. (a) Feeling of fatigue and possibly the occurrence of diplopia accompanying reading; **(b)** headache or other asthenopic symptoms accompanying reading; **(c)** symptoms of asthenopia accompanying distance as well as near vision; **(d)** diplopia accompanying distance vision, with one eye turning out occasionally.

10. (a) There will be a visual aura in the form of "shadows" or "heat waves" in the visual field, followed by a headache accompanied by nausea. **(b)** A visual aura is not present, nausea ("sick headache") being the most prominent symptom.

11. Likely causes are a corneal ulcer, anterior uveitis, or angle-closure glaucoma.

12. For a young or middle-aged adult, the most likely causes would be migraine or multiple sclerosis, while for older adults (beyond the age of 55 or 60), temporal arteritis and carotid artery occlusive disease should be considered as possible causes.

13. (a) More information concerning diagnostic workup and management, including plans for each diagnostic possibility; **(b)** therapy, including goals, end points, and contingency plans; **(c)** education of both the patient and the family.

14. Contact lens patients, visual training patients, and low-vision patients.

15. **(a)** Hyperopia; **(b)** the prescription of lenses to correct the hyperopia.

16. **(a)** Severe, boring headaches in the temporal region, possibly with ipsilateral lacrimation and nasal congestion; **(b)** pain in the forehead, vertical region of the head, or back of the neck, usually following a prolonged period of stress.

17. Headaches, diplopia, and other symptoms of eyestrain.

18. **(a)** Question the patient concerning the presence of a visual aura prior to the headache, and ask whether or not nausea accompanies the headache. **(b)** Ask the patient if the "shadow" changes shape or if it "comes and goes." **(c)** Ask about pain in the temporal region of the scalp, especially when combing the hair; also ask about a general feeling of malaise or loss of appetite and a closing or tightness of the upper jaw while eating. **(d)** Negative responses to the questions given in part (c) should heighten a suspicion of carotid artery occlusive disease in an older person who complains about temporary loss of vision.

19. **(a)** Allergic conjunctivitis, or a bacterial or viral infection; **(b)** conjunctivitis and blepharitis due to a bacterial infection; **(c)** foreign body (stimulation of the ophthalmic division of fifth cranial nerve), ectropion (in an older person), stenosis of the lacrimal drainage system (in an infant); **(d)** aqueous or mucin tear deficiency.

20. Few, if any, in an established case of strabismus. Complaint of double vision, for strabismus of recent onset.

Chapter 6

1. **(a)** 0.17D, 1.00Δ (both considered to be zero); **(b)** 2.50D, 15Δ.

2. A strabismic patient who has harmonious anomalous retinal correspondence will see no target movement in the alternating cover test, because the visual direction of an off-foveal point of the deviating eye is the same as that of the fovea of the fixing eye.

3. By glaucomatous changes in the optic disk as seen by the ophthalmoscope (high cup/disk ratio, "bean pot" profile of margin of cup) and visual field changes (nerve fiber-bundle scotomas).

4. **(a)** All colors will appear to be less vivid than for a normal observer, with the result that the child may have difficulties in naming pastel colors or very dark color tones. **(b)** Many color names will have little meaning for the child, since green, yellow, orange, red, and brown all look the same to him.

5. This can be done only when the near point of accommodation is measured while the patient wears lenses that correct the refractive error, and there is no assurance that this is the case.

6. Excessive room illumination may cause an increase in depth of focus (due to constriction of the pupils) that will result in erroneously high acuity findings in myopia and in absolute hyperopia; it will also tend to reduce contrast on the visual acuity chart.

7. Functional amblyopia may be missed if a single row of letters or a single letter is used.

8. Left exotropia.

9. **(a)** The point at which the initial tapping sound is heard for at least two consecutive beats; **(b)** the onset of a soft, muffled, "blowing" sound.

10. The lowest of the three readings is the most likely to be the correct reading, because most sources of inaccuracy (particularly anxiety on the part of the patient) tend to cause a reading to be abnormally high.

11. Systolic pressures between 140 and 160mmHg, and diastolic pressures between 90 and 95mmHg.

12. The Stycar and Sheridan-Gardiner tests.

13. **(a)** Right superior rectus or left inferior oblique; **(b)** left inferior oblique.

14. **(a)** Horner's syndrome; **(b)** Adie's tonic pupil; **(c)** Marcus Gunn pupil.

15. **(a)** Optic tract or optic radiations; **(b)** visual cortex; **(c)** optic chiasm.

16. Either esophoria or esotropia.

17. **(a)** 10/400; **(b)** 5/400; **(c)** 2/400.

18. One eye may lose fixation (turning outward), with no report of double vision, due to suppression.

19. **(a)** Approximately 0.5mm nasal to the center of the pupil; **(b)** eccentric fixation.

20. **(a)** Right superior rectus and left inferior oblique; **(b)** right inferior rectus and left superior oblique; **(c)** left superior rectus and right inferior oblique; **(d)** left inferior rectus and right superior oblique.

Chapter 7

1. (a) Specular reflection; (b) sclerotic scatter (or split limbal); (c) direct illumination with a conical beam; (d) direct illumination with a narrow beam; (e) retroillumination.

2. (a) Grade 4; (b) grade 2; (c) grade 4.

3. (a) The direct ophthalmoscope has greater magnification (15× as compared with 2 to 3×). (b) The indirect ophthalmoscope has a greater field of view (25 degrees as compared with 6.5 degrees).

4. (a) Downward; (b) to the right.

5. Cotton wool exudates.

6. Keratoconjunctivitis sicca (aqueous tear deficiency).

7. Keratic precipitates; hypopyon.

8. Ten seconds.

9. Drusen. The prognosis is good unless they occur in the macular area.

10. A dry eye. A qualitative change in the Meibomian gland secretion can cause a release of fatty acids, leading to almost instantaneous dry spot formation.

11. (a) Entropion; (b) trichiasis; (c) ectropion; (d) epiphora.

12. (a) 4.0×; (b) 2.5×.

13. (a) Type IV; (b) type I; (c) type III; (d) type II.

14. Lattice degeneration.

15. Senile macular degeneration.

16. 0.6.

17. Corneal guttata; Fuchs' dystrophy.

18. (a) Arteriolar sclerosis; (b) hypertension.

19. (a) Less than one-fourth; (b) one-fourth; (c) between one-fourth and one-half; (d) more than one-half.

20. (a) Papillae; (b) follicles.

21. (a) Side-effects of cocaine are drying and desquamation of the corneal epithelium; (b) the possibility of adverse effects due to proparacaine is very small, (c) benoxinate may have side-effects for patients having cardiac disease, thyroid disease, or allergies; (d) if it is accidentally introduced into the blood stream, tetracaine can cause nervous-system stimulation and cause convulsive activity and depression.

22. (a) To determine the anterior chamber angle width; (b) in the case of a Kruckenberg spindle, to inspect the trabeculum for pigment deposits; (c) to rule out the presence of blood vessels in the anterior chamber angle in cases of rubeosis irides; and (d) to rule out the possibility of angle recession following an injury in which an eye has been submitted to blunt trauma.

23. A scotoma or other visual field defect of a given angular size will result in a field defect twice as large on a 2m tangent screen as on a 1m tangent screen.

24. In static perimetry, a given stimulus is presented first at a low illumination level, and illumination is increased in steps until the patient reports that the stimulus is seen. This procedure is repeated for multiple stimuli in predetermined positions. Kinetic perimetry is the commonly used method in which a test object of a given size and intensity is used to determine the peripheral limits of the field of view or the presence of scotomata within the visual field.

25. The light brightness comparison test. If a light appears to be dimmer with one eye than the other, it is because of the presence of a conduction defect in the optic nerve; and a conduction defect in the optic nerve is also responsible for a positive result on the swinging flashlight test.

26. (a) Retinitis pigmentosa and other rod dystrophies; (b) a retinal pigment epithelium abnormality such as Best's disease.

27. (a) Adverse cardiovascular effects; (b) confusion, ataxia, hallucinations, speech difficulties, and convulsions; (c) few, if any, have been reported.

28. The slit lamp and the Hruby lens could be used for determining the presence of elevations or depressions in the retina or the optic nerve, including suspected macular detachment, macular degeneration, papillademe, and drusen of the optic disc, as well as for inspection of the vitreous for posterior detachment or other degenerative changes.

29. (a) The patient is seated in a dimly illuminated room to allow the pupils to dilate, and the fundus is illuminated with a dim infrared light; (b) with the 145-degree fundus camera, the camera objective must be in contact with the cornea.

30. (a) Because the wand is a stronger stimulus than the target; (b) a drooping upper lid is the most likely cause.

31. An optic nerve defect.

32. An iridectomy should be done to provide the aqueous with access to the anterior chamber angle.

33. By aiming every other stimulus at the blind spot.

34. A retinal problem.

35. The illumination of the patient's entire visual field is controlled; both the test object and background illumination are subject to accurate calibration. Testing is possible not only of the peripheral isopters but of the central and midperipheral portions of the visual field.

36. **(a)** The superior fundus; **(b)** inverted.

37. Using double stimulation, a hemianoptic field defect may be detected that would otherwise be missed, due to the extinction phenomenon; the stimulus on the sound side "extinguishing" the stimulus on the defective side.

38. By retesting distance visual acuity while directing sufficient light toward the eye to reduce the size of the pupil.

39. Pilocarpine-induced pupillary constriction tends to last longer than the mydriasis, and it is possible that the use of a miotic agent following the use of a cycloplegic or mydriatic agent may cause pupillary block.

40. By flipping the test target over to see if the patient reports that it disappears.

41. **(a)** A complaint of transient loss of vision in an older patient; **(b)** carotid artery insufficiency; **(c)** relative ophthalmic artery pressure; **(d)** one criterion is a difference in ophthalmodynamometry readings for the two eyes that is greater than 20 percent; a second criterion is a relative ophthalmic artery pressure that is less than 50 percent of the corresponding (systolic or diastolic) brachial artery pressure.

42. In some automated static perimeters, each light emitting diode is presented in what appears to the patient as a "black hole" in the white perimeter background, with the result that the patient knows where the stimuli will appear. One method of avoiding this problem is to have all LEDs constantly illuminated at a level equivalent to that of the perimeter's background; a second method is to cover the hole containing the LED with a translucent plastic sheet, which is transilluminated by the LED when it is lit.

43. A visual acuity chart only provides information concerning vision for high contrast and high-spatial frequency stimuli, whereas contrast sensitivity testing provides information about the visibility of stimuli having a range of contrasts and spatial frequencies. Many ocular disease processes have little effect on visual acuity but have pronounced effects on contrast sensitivity.

44. It has been shown that contrast sensitivity of normal subjects decreases with age throughout adult life, not only because of a reduction in pupil size and lenticular changes but apparently because of neural factors.

45. Contrast sensitivity testing has been shown to provide diagnostic information in glaucoma, optic nerve disease, macular degeneration, albinism, and amblyopia.

Chapter 8

1. **(a)** 8.04mm at 180, 7.76mm at 90; **(b)** with-the-rule astigmatism.

2. −1.37 × 180.

3. **(a)** Same direction; **(b)** same direction.

4. **(a)** Rotating the barrel of the keratometer so the plus signs rather than the minus signs are used for the finding in the vertical meridian; **(b)** modifying the keratometer mires for vernier alignment, as described by Shick.

5. The retinoscope reflex is not only very dim; it is larger than the patient's pupil, so the "edges" of the reflex cannot be seen as it moves back and forth, making the judgment of its direction of movement difficult or impossible.

6. A very steep keratometer finding of about 50.00D or more, or possibly off the keratometer scale.

7. The examiner may either use plus lenses or move the retinoscope backward while the patient fixates letters or other stimuli in a fixed position.

8. Lenses may be changed much more quickly than with the use of trial lenses; rotating prisms may be used; and tests involving large changes in lens power (such as the plus- and minus-to-blur tests) may be done easily.

9. **(a)** If a spherical hard contact lens is sufficiently rigid, it will retain its curvature while on the cornea and, therefore, will render the tear layer spherical, eliminating corneal astigmatism; if the lens flexes (bends) on the cornea, only a part of the corneal astigmatism will be eliminated. **(b)** A spherical soft contact lens will usually conform to the shape of the cornea; therefore, it will not eliminate corneal astigmatism.

10. **(a)** Opposite direction ("against" motion); **(b)** same direction ("with" motion).

11. Young children, who have trouble sitting still behind a refractor; presbyopic patients, for verification of bifocal addition; and invalids who must be refracted at home, in a hospital, or in a convalescent home.

12. **(a)** Too much plus; **(b)** too little plus; **(c)** too little plus.

13. Scoping off the patient's visual axis, failure to obtain a reversal, failure to locate the principal meridians; and failure to recognize scissors motion.

14. The Scheiner disk mechanism. This is a two-hole diaphragm that causes the image of the object (the mire) to double if the telescope is not focused on the image plane.

15. The examiner could measure the patient's near PD and add 4mm.

16. +2.00DS −1.25DC × 90.

17. **(a)** The findings are not reliable (poor repeatability), and the instrument may or may not be properly calibrated; **(b)** the findings are reliable, but the instrument is not correctly calibrated; **(c)** the findings are reliable, and the instrument is correctly calibrated.

18. Pediatric patients, vision screening programs, progress evaluations, and assessment of contact lens fit.

19. −1.00DS −1.00DC × 180.

20. Radical retinoscopy is static retinoscopy performed at an unusually close working distance. It is used in situations in which, due to opacities in the media, it is impossible to obtain a finding at the usual 50 or 67mm working distance.

21. **(a)** Bobier and Sivak found that subjects tended to overaccommodate for distance fixation (focusing for red light) and to underaccommodate for near fixation (focusing for green light). **(b)** They concluded that the eye uses its chromatic aberration to spare accommodation.

22. **(a)** Emmetropia; **(b)** 1.00D of hyperopia; **(c)** 1.00D of myopia.

23. **(a)** For children aged 4–6 years, subjects overaccommodated for distance fixation and underaccommodated for near fixation, just as adult subjects did. A younger group of subjects overaccommodated for both distance and near fixation, and for an even younger group of subjects, accommodative responses were found to be mixed. **(b)** These findings were interpreted as indicating that the focusing mechanism is not fully developed until the fourth year of life, at which time selective focusing is done in such a way as to spare accommodation.

24. **(1) (a)** −1.75DC × 90; **(b)** −1.50DC × 90. **(2) (a)** −0.50DC × 90; **(b)** −0.50DC × 90. **(3) (a)** −0.75DC × 180; **(b)** −0.50DC × 180. **(4) (a)** −2.62DC × 180; **(b)** −2.00DC × 180.

Chapter 9

1. *Fogging* is placing enough plus lens power in front of the eye so the patient is artificially myopic. If the patient is not fogged prior to beginning the subjective refraction, the patient may accommodate, therefore accepting too little plus power or too much minus power.

2. The patient is instructed to report which of the two lenses allows him or her to read farther down the chart.

3. The binocular balancing procedure is conducted for the purpose of balancing the state of accommodation for the two eyes. In a binocular refraction procedure, each eye is refracted in the presence of stimuli for peripheral fusion, but with the central portion of the test chart seen monocularly.

4. Tropicamide is considered inadequate for producing cycloplegia in children. For adults, from 2–4 drops of 1 percent tropicamide are required to produce cycloplegia, as compared with 1 drop of 1 percent cyclopentolate.

5. Assuming the minus axis is located in the 180-degree meridian: **(a)** +0.50DC × 90; −0.50DC × 180; **(b)** +0.50DS −1.00DC × 180; **(c)** −0.50DS +1.00DC × 90.

6. **(a)** 180 degrees; **(b)** 135 degrees.

7. If the patient accepts less cylinder power in the crossed-cylinder test than in retinoscopy or the astigmatic chart test, the crossed cylinder is removed and the patient is asked to report whether the letters become clearer as an additional −0.25D cylinder is added. If a second −0.25D cylinder is added, +0.25D sphere is added to maintain the spherical equivalent.

8. Plus lens power is reduced, 0.25D at a time, until the patient can read all of the 20/40 letters and only a few of the 20/30 letters.

9. With the crossed cylinder removed, the patient is instructed to watch a row of 20/20 or 20/15 letters and is asked to report when the letters begin to blur as the cylinder axis is slowly rotated first in one direction and then in the other. The correct axis will be the midpoint between the two positions where a blur is reported.

10. **(a)** The criterion is "maximum plus lens power for best visual acuity." **(b)** As each 0.25D of plus lens power is removed (or each 0.25D of minus power is added), the patient is instructed to read all additional letters possible while viewing a chart consisting of several lines of letters, until the criterion of "maximum plus lens power for best visual acuity" is achieved. **(c)** No. Although it is possible that the patient may notice that the letters appear smaller when too much minus lens power has been added (or too little plus lens power has been removed), the patient's response that the letters are getting smaller cannot be counted upon to insure that he is not overminused or underplussed.

11. The projector screen should be in virtual darkness except for the light from the projector; the projector should be in first-class condition, with clean optics, a properly adjusted mirror, and a clean filter; a highly aluminized projector screen should be used, angled for maximum reflection; and the projector should be matched with the line voltage.

12. It is appropriate to use this procedure whenever there is reason to believe that the patient's accommodation was not relaxed during the subjective examination. After completion of the plus-lens-to-blur test (at 40cm), the near-point card is moved away, the patient's attention is called to a block of letters at the 6m distance (ranging from about 20/40 to 20/15). As plus lens power is reduced binocularly, 0.25D at a time, the patient is asked to read all the letters possible with each change in lens power.

13. Both the vertical and horizontal focal lines are located in front of the retina, with the horizontal focal line closer to the retina than the vertical focal line.

14. The ointment must be instilled in the patient's eyes twice a day for 3 days; cycloplegia may last as long as 2 weeks; the ointment is poisonous and can cause death if taken by mouth; and complete cycloplegia could possibly cause an intermittent strabismus or high esophoria to become a constant convergent strabismus.

15. The bichrome test.

16. **(a)** Both focal lines are located on the retina (actually in the form of a point focus). **(b)** The vertical focal line is located in front of the retina, and the horizontal focal line is behind the retina. **(c)** The horizontal focal line is located in front of the retina, and the vertical focal line is behind the retina.

17. By first estimating the width of the anterior chamber angle, using the Van Herick slit-lamp technique, and instilling a cycloplegic agent only if the angle is a grade 3 or grade 4 angle.

18. **(a)** When a child having esotropia fails to accept plus lens power in routine refraction; and **(b)** when a patient is suspected of having latent hyperopia not uncovered by routine fogging techniques or by "overfogging" techniques such as the Borish delayed subjective.

19. With the patient binocularly viewing a block of letters at a 6m distance, **(a)** add +0.25D binocularly. The patient should report a slight blur of the 20/20 letters. **(b)** Add an additional +0.25D binocularly. The patient should now report that the 20/20 letters are badly blurred. **(c)** Add a third +0.25D binocularly. The patient should report that the 20/20 letters are completely blurred out. If the 20/20 letters completely blur out with less than +0.75D of added power, the patient is probably overminused or underplussed.

20. **(a)** Hyperopes (particularly children, on whom atropine was used) tended to accept somewhat more plus in cycloplegic refraction than in noncycloplegic refraction. **(b)** Myopes were about equally likely to accept either more minus or less minus in cycloplegic as compared with noncycloplegic refraction.

Chapter 10

1. The vertical phoria could be caused by a cerebral vascular accident.

2. No eye movements are made. The image of the row of letters simply moves across the retina of the patient's right eye while the letters are observed to move laterally in the visual field.

3. Supra 2/0 and infra 4/1.

4. With a high level of illumination, the depth of focus would be so great that the patient would have difficulty determining whether the vertical or horizontal lines of the cross grid were more distinct.

5. **(a)** 4.4/1; **(b)** 3/1.

6. **(a)** The associated phoria is determined by the amount of prism necessary to eliminate fixation disparity. **(b)** It differs from a dissociated phoria in that a dissociated phoria is measured while fusion has been interrupted, but an associated phoria is

measured while peripheral stimuli to fusion are present. An associated phoria is usually much less in amount than a dissociated phoria.

7. The push-up test would be expected to result in a higher finding, because the angular size of the letters increases as the test card is moved toward the eyes, with the result that the patient's task is to report a blur for larger letters than would be the case with the minus lens test at 40cm.

8. **(a)** While the prisms were worn, the phoria finding would be 7Δ of exophoria. **(b)** The positive fusional vergence reserve finding would be 15Δ base-out (blur finding).

9. When the alignment method is used, the patient may make fusional vergence movements. Such movements are not likely when the flash method is used.

10. When vertical prism power is slowly added in front of one eye, there is no change in the stimulus to accommodation.

11. **(a)** 20Δ; **(b)** 4Δ; **(c)** 8Δ.

12. **(a)** The lag of accommodation; **(b)** the tentative bifocal addition.

13. Because the calculated AC/A ratio involves phoria measurements taken at both 6m and 40cm, the calculated AC/A ratio includes the effects of proximal convergence. However, the gradient AC/A ratio involves two phoria findings taken at the same distance (40cm) and, therefore, does not include the effects of proximal convergence; hence, it is somewhat lower in value than the calculated AC/A ratio.

14. Negative fusional vergence is used to counteract the accommodative convergence.

15. **(a)** 8/1; **(b)** 6/1.

16. **(a)** A finding equal to the patient's amplitude of accommodation; **(b)** +2.50D

17. 2Δ base-down, left eye (or 2Δ base-up, right eye).

18. The resulting lag of accommodation will cause the phoria finding to be in error in the direction of too much exophoria or too little esophoria.

19. **(b)** The Borish near-point card.

20. **(a)** The slope indicates the rate of change of fixation disparity as prism power is changed, and it is usually low (less than 45 degrees) in asymptomatic patients.

(b) The y-intercept indicates the fixation disparity with no prism. **(c)** The x-intercept indicates the amount of prism required to eliminate fixation disparity (the associated phoria).

21. **(a)** Suppression of the left eye; **(b)** suppression of the right eye; **(c)** normal binocular vision; **(d)** diplopia.

22. **(a)** The child is deeply amblyopic; **(b)** the child may or may not be amblyopic.

23. **(a)** Harmonious anomalous retinal correspondence; **(b)** unharmonious anomalous retinal correspondence; **(c)** normal retinal correspondence; **(d)** paradoxical anomalous retinal correspondence.

24. The patient may localize the streak as being somewhat closer than the distance of the light source, so the phoria finding may be in error in the direction of too much esophoria or too little exophoria.

25. *Step 1:* responsible muscles are the right superior rectus, right inferior oblique, left inferior rectus, and left superior oblique. *Step 2:* responsible muscles are the right inferior oblique and the left inferior rectus. *Step 3:* the responsible muscle is the right inferior oblique.

Chapter 11

1. Small cylinders tend to be difficult to find, and the refractive end-point may be in error in the direction of too much minus or too little plus.

2. **(a)** Patient-subjective; **(b)** patient-subjective; **(c)** patient-objective; **(d)** patient-subjective; **(e)** patient-objective.

3. Optical innovations include the following. **(a)** Variable-focus spherical and cylindrical lenses consist of two elements shaped in such a way that they move laterally in the light path. **(b)** The lenses are in front of the projector instead of the patient's eyes, so an aerial image of the lenses is formed in front of the patient's eyes. **(c)** Astigmatism is measured by means of two variable-power crossed cylinders, one with principal meridians at 0 and 90 degrees and the other with principal meridians at 45 and 135 degrees, and with line targets oriented vertically and at 45 degrees. **(d)** There is a separate optical channel for each eye, without the need for Polaroids or septums.

4. The refraction is measured in each of either four or six preselected meridians, and the sphere power, cylinder power, and cylinder axis are determined by means of a computer program.

5. By the use of a rotating stenopaic slit.

6. (a) An optical system similar to that of a lensometer; (b) the principle of the retinoscope; (c) the optometer; (d) the Scheiner double-pupil.

7. The apical keratometer reading; the shape factor (related to eccentricity); the vertical displacement (height) of the corneal apex; and a "conformance" factor, which compares the cornea being measured to the normal cornea.

8. An advantage is that the objective end-point may be verified subjectively in a short period of time. The disadvantage is that, due to instrument accommodation and the lack of a method of balancing, it is not advisable to prescribe on the basis of the instrument's findings.

9. High-frequency ultrasound waves are emitted by a silicone transducer placed in contact with the eye. These waves pass through the media and are reflected backward, as "echos," at interfaces between the various media, are converted into an electrical potential by a piezoelectric crystal, and are displayed on an oscilloscope screen. Using velocity constants, the time taken of travel for each medium is converted to the appropriate axial distance.

10. In the routine practice of optometry, A-scan ultrasonography may be used (a) to determine whether a patient's anisometropia is mainly due to axial or refractive differences; and (b) in the management of spherical ametropia, to determine the extent to which the refractive error is axial or refractive, and to monitor axial length changes with time.

11. *Advantages:* the cost of the instrument may not be a problem in a large practice; patients are impressed with the up-to-date equipment; and the instrument can be operated by an assistant or technician, saving the practitioner time. *Disadvantages:* patients may depend more on impressive technician-operated equipment than on the knowledge and skill of the practitioner; and by not performing retinoscopy, the practitioner may miss many subtle clinical signs.

12. *Advantages:* as with an objective auto-refractor, the cost of a computer-assisted subjective refractor may be relatively small in a busy practice, and patients will be impressed that the latest equipment is being used; if operated by the practitioner, an adequate job of refracting may be done (but there is no evidence that the results would be superior to those obtained by conventional refraction). *Disadvantages:* with most instruments, a binocular balance cannot be done, and "instrument accommodation" may be a problem; the greatest disadvantage occurs when the instrument is operated by an assistant or a technician, causing the profession to "give away" the job of refraction.

Chapter 12

1. (a) Night myopia; and (b) a retinal receptor degeneration such as retinitis pigmentosa.

2. (a) The addition is determined on the basis of the patient having to use only one-half of the accommodative amplitude. (b) On the basis of the spherical lens power that makes the horizontal and vertical lines of the cross grid appear to be equally distinct. (c) On the basis of the spherical lens power that makes the plus-to-blur finding equal to or slightly greater than the minus-to-blur finding. (d) On the basis of the spherical lens power that places the patient's desired reading or working distance approximately at the midpoint of the range.

3. (a) (1) The distance phoria, (2) the AC/A ratio, (3) the amplitude of accommodation, (4) the range of positive fusional vergence, and (5) the range of negative fusional vergence; (b) (1) the origin of the graph, (2) the slope of the graph; (c) (1) the upper limit of the graph, (2) the right-hand limit of the graph, and (3) the left-hand limit of the graph.

4. (a) 4Δ base-in; (b) no prism is required.

5. The depth of focus causes the graph to fan out toward the top, because it has a tendency to widen the graph but widens it more for near findings than for distance findings.

6. (a) 6/1; (b) 2.4/1; (c) 8.4/1.

7. (a) Visual fatigue and drowsiness, and possibly diplopia, accompanying prolonged close work. (b) Orthophoria or near-orthophoria at 6m and a high exophoria at 40cm (indicating a low AC/A ratio), and possibly also a poor near point of convergence and a low base-out reserve at 40cm. (c) Base-out training is the treatment of choice, with base-in prism for near work as a second choice in the event that training is not successful.

8. The stimulus AC/A ratio (the clinical AC/A ratio) may be falsely low due to a lag of accommodation. In such a case, base-out training will often reduce the measured exophoria at 40cm and, therefore, appear to reduce the AC/A ratio. Although the response AC/A ratio (as measured by means of an optometer system) is usually considered to be inalterable, Flom found that the response AC/A ratio could be changed by training.

9. The best way to do this is to first have the patient look at the near-point card at 40cm through the lenses correcting near vision, then have the patient look at the distance chart through the same lenses (resulting in a report that the letters are blurred), and then

again at the near-point card (resulting in a report that the letters are again clear).

10. It causes the right-hand side of the graph to fan out toward the top.

11. **(a)** It is a process that operates to maintain approximate orthophoria for distance fixation and also maintains a near phoria somewhat in the exophoric range (or approximately orthophoria in the downgaze position). **(b)** If prism is prescribed for a patient who has not developed the fusion adaptation process, the patient is not likely to adapt to the prism.

12. **(a)** 2Δ base-out; **(b)** no prism is required.

13. **(a)** Headaches or other symptoms of asthenopia accompanying prolonged reading or other close work; **(b)** orthophoria or near orthophoria at 6m and a high esophoria at 40cm, indicating a high AC/A ratio. **(c)** The treatment of choice is the provision of added plus lens power for near work. A second possible form of treatment is base-out prism power for near work, and a third possibility (not often successful) is base-in training.

14. **(a)** It can be accounted for on the basis that before a full correction for the myopia was worn, the reduced accommodative demand at the reading distance resulted in a relative exophoria at that distance, requiring the use of positive relative convergence in order to maintain single binocular vision. This becomes conditioned with time, so when the myopia is fully corrected, the conditioned convergence remains in play, causing a change in the direction of esophoria. **(b)** This is not a matter of concern because the near phoria (along with the AC/A ratio) is found to return to its previous level within a short period.

15. The presence or absence of fixation disparity. The amount (and direction) of the prism that reduces the fixation disparity to zero is the prism to be prescribed.

16. The presbyope apparently has unrestricted use of accommodative convergence, which has the effect of reducing or eliminating the need for positive fusional vergence.

17. **(a)** The patient may complain of headaches or other forms of asthenopia accompanying distance or near visual tasks, or both; **(b)** a high esophoria at 6m and either a low or high esophoria at 40cm; **(c)** base-out prism, possibly in combination with added plus lens power at near (depending on the AC/A ratio).

18. If the patient has complaints (headaches, other forms of asthenopia, double vision, and so on) that can be accounted for by the phoria, prism adaptation is not likely to occur.

19. **(a)** If a patient having a Type I fixation disparity curve is symptomatic, the curve probably has a high slope (greater than 45 degrees), and training should be given. The training has the effect of reducing the slope of the curve. **(b)** A patient who has a Type II fixation disparity curve is usually esophoric, and either base-out prism or plus lens power for near work should be prescribed.

20. **(a)** The patient may complain of occasional diplopia at distance or may be told that one eye sometimes turns out. **(b)** A high exophoria at 6m and a lower exophoria or orthophoria at 40cm, indicating a high AC/A ratio. **(c)** Possible forms of treatment are (1) an overcorrection of minus power (or undercorrection of plus power) for distance vision, (2) base-in prism for distance only, or (3) base-in prism for both distance and near (depending on the amount of exophoria at near).

Chapter 13

1. Each lens must be decentered out 2.5mm.

2. 1Δ base-up, right eye.

3. Transverse chromatic aberration can cause a wearer of highly powered single vision lenses to see color fringes when looking through the edges of the lenses. Chromatic aberration is a property of the material of which the lens is made, and there is no material available that will eliminate it.

4. **(a)** A point-focal lens is a lens that is corrected for oblique astigmatism. **(b)** The oblique power of a point-focal lens is less than the axial power. **(c)** The consequence of this is that a hyperope, when viewing obliquely through the lens, can obtain clear vision by accommodating; for a myope, however, accommodating while viewing obliquely through the lens will only make vision more blurred.

5. By prescribing a plastic lens.

6. In axial ametropia, relative spectacle magnification is equal to $1/(1 + aF)$, where a is the distance between the primary focal plane of the eye and the secondary principal plane of the correcting lens. If the correcting lens is located such that its secondary principal plane coincides with the eye's primary focal plane (a distance of approximately 14mm from the cornea), relative spectacle magnification is equal to 1. Therefore, if one eye is emmetropic and the other eye has purely axial ametropia, spectacle lenses will result in a minimum of induced aniseikonia. If contact lenses rather than spectacle lenses were worn, the

value of *a* would be approximately 14mm, and this would result in a significant image size difference for the two eyes. For example, the relative spectacle magnification induced by a −5.00D contact lens would be 1.08 (or +8 percent), while the relative spectacle magnification induced by a +5.00D contact lens would be 0.93 (or −7 percent).

7. **(a)** Keratoconjunctivitis, which causes photophobia and itching of the eyes; **(b)** exposure to a point source of ultraviolet light, such as the sun, can cause a retinal burn. Exposure to an extended source can cause cataracts.

8. **(a)** It is the product of the power of the bifocal addition times the distance from the segment pole to the reading level. **(b)** In each case there is no segment-induced prismatic effect, because the segment pole coincides with the reading level.

9. In the Varilux 2 lens, the progressive corridor incorporates a change in power beginning at the top of the lens, whereas the Ultravue lens has a well-defined distance portion in the upper part of the lens with a relatively greater progression of power in the lower part of the lens. Unwanted astigmatism, therefore, is spread throughout both the upper and lower part of the Varilux 2 lens (with the exception of the narrow progressive corridor), whereas in the Ultravue lens the unwanted astigmatism is concentrated on either side of the wider progressive corridor at the lower part of the lens.

10. **(a)** The distance from the temporal edge of one segment to the nasal edge of the other is measured. **(b)** A vertical line is viewed through each lens while the lens is moved sideways until the position is found in which the vertical line does not deviate in passing through the dividing line between the distance and near portions of the lens. That position is marked, for each lens, and the distance between the two points is measured using a millimeter ruler.

11. 3Δ base-up, left eye.

12. One can be reasonably certain (but not positive) that a patient's ametropia is axial if it is in the amount of +4.00 or −4.00D or more. Refractive ametropia is sure to be present **(a)** when ametropia is due to a nuclear cataract, **(b)** when ametropia is due to aphakia; and **(c)** when ametropia is due to corneal astigmatism.

13. **(a)** Photochromic materials fail to effectively absorb infrared radiation. **(b)** The lenses return to their lightest state (highest transmittance) only after overnight fading.

14. In refractive ametropia, relative spectacle magnification is equal to $1/(1 - xF)$, where x is the distance from the secondary principal plane of the spectacle lens to the entrance pupil of the eye. Magnification, therefore, increases with increasing values of x; since the value of x will be at a minimum when a contact lens is worn, it follows that in purely refractive ametropia the relative spectacle magnification may be minimized by the use of a contact lens, and that if one eye is emmetropic and the other has refractive ametropia, a minimum of aniseikonia will be induced if a contact lens is worn on the ametropic eye. For example, the relative spectacle magnification for a −5.00D contact lens ($x = 3$mm) would be 0.99 (or −1 percent), while the relative spectacle magnification for a −5.00D spectacle lens ($x = 15$mm) would be 0.93 (or −7 percent).

15. For distance vision, because large eye movements (which involve viewing obliquely through the lens) are more often made during distance vision than during near vision.

16. By using a high-index material such as Hi-lite, by avoiding unusually large lens sizes and by using lens shapes not having sharp corners, and by placing most of the bevel in the front of the lens edge or using the "hide-a-bevel" technique.

17. Petzval's surface is a property of the correcting lens, and its radius of curvature is equal to −nf, whereas the far point sphere is a property of the eye and has a radius of curvature equal to $s - f$ (where s is the distance from the correcting lens to the center of rotation of the eye). Petzval's surface can coincide with the far point sphere only when $-nf = s - f$, and this will occur (if $s = 25$mm and if $n = 1.5$) only when the power of the correcting lens is −20.00D.

18. Distortion is a problem only for wearers of highly powered ophthalmic lenses. For example, wearers of aphakic lenses will experience pincushion distortion, and wearers of very strong minus lenses will experience barrel-shaped distortion. Distortion can be eliminated only by using very steep back surface curves.

19. Each lens will have to be decentered out 5mm.

20. Spherical aberration is a problem only for large-aperture optical systems, and it presents little problem with ophthalmic lenses because the pupil of the eye allows entrance of only a relatively small bundle of rays.

21. **(a)** Spectacle magnification is 1.124 (or +12.4 percent). **(b)** Spectacle magnification is 1.034 (or 3.4 percent).

22. The spectacle magnification formula can be written in the following form: SM = 1/(1 − xF), where x is the distance from the secondary principal plane of the spectacle lens to the entrance pupil of the eye, and F is the equivalent power of the lens. The value of x will be on the order of 3mm for a contact lens and 15mm for a spectacle lens. Inspection of the formula indicates that for negative values of F, the smaller the value of x, the smaller will be the value of the denominator of the fraction and, therefore, the greater will be the spectacle magnification. However, for positive values of F, the smaller the value of x, the greater the value of the denominator and, therefore, the smaller the spectacle magnification.

23. 0.6Δ base-in for each eye, or a total of 1.2Δ base-in.

24. Coma requires a large aperture, and the pupil is sufficiently small so that coma is not a problem with ophthalmic lens wearers. However, when coma is eliminated by the use of a small aperture, oblique astigmatism may be present.

25. (a) Petzval's surface is the image surface resulting from refraction by a lens, for an object of large extent. Its radius of curvature is equal to −nf, where n is the index of refraction of the glass, and f is the back focal length of the lens. (b) The sagittal and tangential image shells coincide with Petzval's surface. (c) It is a property of the refracting power of the lens, and for a lens of a given refracting power it cannot be changed.

26. Retinal image size is estimated to change at the rate of about 1.4 percent per diopter of lens power for refractive ametropia, and 0.25 percent per diopter of lens power for axial ametropia. The estimated percentage is not zero for axial ametropia, because most spectacle lenses have the back vertex located somewhat inside the primary focal plane of the eye; the less ametropic eye cannot be expected to have the optical characteristics of the schematic eye; and one cannot always be sure that the more ametropic eye has purely axial ametropia.

27. The intermediate segment should be placed so that the top of the lower segment is in the same position at which the top of a bifocal segment would be.

28. Image jump is the abrupt movement of the environment experienced by the bifocal wearer when the line of sight crosses the dividing line into the bifocal segment. It is determined by multiplying the power of the bifocal addition by the distance from the segment top to the segment pole. The Executive bifocal provides no image jump (since the segment top coincides with the segment pole). The Ultex A bifocal provides a large amount of jump.

29. (a) The far-point sphere is a surface traced out by the far-point of the eye when the eye changes fixation. (b) The far-point sphere is a property of the eye, and it cannot be changed.

30. Designers concentrate mainly on the correction of oblique astigmatism. When oblique astigmatism is fully corrected, the hyperope can obtain clear vision for oblique rays by accommodating slightly, and the myope can obtain clear vision for oblique rays if slightly overcorrected for axial rays. However, when curvature error is corrected at the expense of oblique astigmatism, no amount of accommodation will reduce the astigmatism for oblique rays.

31. (a) A round lens; (b) the frame PD should be equal to the patient's PD, so that no decentration is necessary; (c) −3.00 to −5.00D; (d) as close as possible.

Chapter 14

1. (a) −5.50D; (b) +6.59D.

2. (a) For the correction of internal astigmatism; (b) to provide a comfortable physical fit on a highly toric cornea.

3. (a) The macular field of view is greatly restricted, resulting in the roving ring scotoma and the "jack-in-the-box phenomenon." (b) This problem is solved when a contact lens is worn, because with a contact lens the macular field of view is limited only by the extent of the field of fixation (because a contact lens, unlike a spectacle lens, moves with the eye when the eye changes fixation).

4. From 3½–7 days.

5. (a) Diffusivity (D) and solubility (k): permeability = Dk. (b) Gas permeability increases exponentially with the water content of the lens. (c) The transmissivity of a contact lens is equal to the permeability of the material (Dk) divided by the thickness (L) of the lens: transmissivity = Dk/L.

6. (a) Wearing time (minimum of 8 hours per day), (b) comfort (only a slight lens awareness), (c) vision (no significant blur), (d) absence of ocular tissue changes, and (e) normal appearance of patient.

7. The position, blink lag, and lag on upward gaze may be evaluated with the slit lamp; in addition, the presence of air bubbles underneath the lens may be noted.

8. Lens coating with protein and calcium deposits, frequent lens replacement, edema, and corneal staining.

9. (a) A corneal steepening of approximately 0.50D; (b)

a corneal flattening of about 0.25D (compared with the prefitting curvature) after 1 year and about 0.62D after 2 years; **(c)** a flattening of the cornea (accompanied by a decrease in myopia) and unpredictable changes in astigmatism.

10. (a) 42.19D; **(b)** 61.25D.

11. It eliminates corneal astigmatism.

12. It fails to increase the peripheral field of vision but greatly increases the macular field of vision, because (due to the fact that the lens moves with the eye) the macular field is limited only by the extent of the field of fixation of the eye.

13. −5.00D.

14. By the process of tear pumping. With each blink, oxygenated tears are pumped undrrneath the lens and tears containing carbon dioxide are pumped out from under the lens. A PMMA lens has to be fitted in such a way that a reservoir of tears is available underneath the peripheral zone of the lens, and such that these tears will be pumped underneath the lens during the process of blinking. This requires that the lens lag downward after each blink. The patient should be instructed in correct blinking.

15. (a) Supplying adequate oxygen to the cornea and removing carbon dioxide, removal of keratinized epithelial cells from under the lens, keeping the cornea and the lens in a hydrated condition, providing a natural appearance for the wearer, providing optimum lens movement and positioning; keeping a clean anterior lens surface and providing an observable fluid flow beneath the lens. **(b)** Oxygen and carbon dioxide exchange; removal of keratinized epithelial cells from under the lens; maintaining clean lens surfaces, reducing the possibility of coating; reduced possibility of lens dehydration; and a possibility of extending the useful life of the lenses.

16. (a) 2 percent; **(b)** 5 percent; **(c)** 10 percent.

17. (a) Aphakia; **(b)** keratoconus; and **(c)** high myopia.

18. Base curve radius; secondary curve radius; peripheral curve (bevel) radius; overall diameter; optic zone diameter; power; center thickness; tint.

19. (a) A telescope protractor reticule; **(b)** a slit lamp with a rotatable lamp housing having a protractor scale; and **(c)** a trial frame and slit-lamp beam or the beam of a streak retinoscope.

20. (a) There should be a deep green ring all the way around the peripheral zone of the lens, with little or no fluorescein visible underneath the optical zone of the lens. **(b)** There will be a definite area of central touch, indicated by a lack of fluorescein, and a wide green ring underneath the peripheral zone of the lens. **(c)** There will be a pooling of fluorescein under the apical portion of the lens, a black ring of touch underneath the transition zone, and a green ring of pooling under the peripheral zone of the lens. **(d)** A "dog bone-" or "dumbbell-" shaped area of touch (horizontally oriented) will appear under the optical zone of the lens, with pooling of fluorescein above and below the area of touch and under the peripheral zone of the lens.

21. (a) Contact lenses for distance vision, with reading glasses or bifocals for near work; **(b)** monovision fitting (a contact lens is fitted on one eye for distance vision and on the other eye for near vision); and **(c)** bifocal contact lenses.

22. A keratometer finding taken with the lenses on should indicate **(a)** clear mire images, **(b)** the same amount (and axis) of corneal astigmatism as without the lens, and **(c)** no change in the appearance of the mire images between blinks.

23. Dry eye conditions; bullous keratopathy; corneal dystrophies, including Fuchs' dystrophy and anterior membrane dystrophies; some kinds of corneal ulcers; and some conditions resulting from corneal trauma.

24. (a) Excessive tearing may cause corneal edema because the decreased osmotic pressure of the tears causes water to move into the cornea. **(b)** Inadequate blinking can cause corneal edema as a result of corneal hypoxia.

25. Wearing time is gradually reduced (by ½ or 1 hour per day) to 8 or 9 hours per day before refitting. This will allow the patient to wear the lenses during the working day until the new lenses are fitted. If the patient has no wearable glasses, the first priority may be to order new glasses to be worn during the part of the day when the contact lenses are not worn.

26. Avascularity is due to the fact that corneal tissue is compact, not allowing blood vessels to enter it. Long-term hypoxia, accompanied by edema, can lead to corneal vascularization.

27. It has no effect on corneal astigmatism; that is, it does not correct or eliminate corneal astigmatism.

28. (a) More accommodation. **(b)** Newly presbyopic myopes may have little or no problem with close work while wearing glasses, but if they switch to contact lenses they may find that reading is difficult or impossible without reading glasses.

29. The high-plus spectacle lens necessary for an aphakic patient results in a large amount of "pin-cushion" distortion. Because distortion is due to the fact that the entrance pupil of the eye is at some distance behind the correcting lens, distortion can be reduced to a minimum if the patient wears a contact lens rather than a spectacle lens.

30. The patient can be given a mucomimetic tear substitute (such as Adsorbotear) and be instructed to put 1 or 2 drops in each eye several times a day for a week or longer, after which the breakup test is repeated.

31. Corneal edema caused by hydrogel lenses involves the entire extent of the cornea rather than just the central portion of the cornea, as with hard lenses. Whereas hard lens edema can be seen with the slit lamp because of the boundary between the edematous and nonedematous portions, hydrogel lens edema cannot easily be seen with the slit lamp because there is no boundary line. Hard lens edema results in steepening of the cornea, as determined by keratometry, whereas hydrogel lens edema possibly causes a very slight flattening (about 0.12D) of the cornea.

32. A spherocylindrical refraction should be done in order to determine how much uncorrected astigmatism is present, and an equivalent sphere (best sphere) refraction should be done to determine the acuity with the contact lens in spite of the astigmatism.

33. Keratometer findings, subjective refraction, visual acuity testing, and slit-lamp examination are done both before and after the initial wearing of lenses for a 3-hour period. If corneal steepening after 3 hours' wear is 0.37D or less, and if the increase in myopia is also 0.37D or less with no loss of acuity with the subjective refraction in place, the patient can be predicted to be a successful wearer. The extent of central corneal clouding after 3 hours' wear can also be used as a predictor of successful wear, with those wearers having the least edema (barely visible) being considered the most successful wearers.

34. Gas-permeable hard lenses differ from PMMA lenses in not being as structurally stable, with the result that they correct (or eliminate) less corneal astigmatism and may change in curvature with time. Lenses made of methyl methacrylate/silicone combination materials may be fitted like PMMA lenses, but CAB lenses must be fitted somewhat steeper than PMMA lenses to allow for subsequent flattening.

35. **(a)** If it is found that the lenses are fitting too tightly, looser lenses can be ordered. **(b)** If the lenses are found to be coated with materials originating from the tear film, the patient can be instructed in more effective lens-care procedures. **(c)** If the patient is found not to be blinking often enough or to be a partial blinker, the patient can be instructed in correct blinking.

36. The lens having the flattest base curve that will center on the cornea without causing discomfort.

37. The amount of refractive astigmatism. Corneal astigmatism presents no physical problem with hydrogel lenses (as it does with PMMA lenses), and because a hydrogel lens corrects little or no corneal astigmatism (and also corrects no internal astigmatism), one would expect that all or most of the refractive astigmatism would remain uncorrected with a hydrogel lens.

38. **(a)** A large amount of corneal edema may occur in the early morning hours, and an accumulation of debris may be found under the lens. **(b)** If no movement occurs with blinking, epithelial cells and other debris will become trapped underneath the lens.

39. **(a)** Nerve endings in the corneal epithelium and the lid margins must adapt to the presence of the lenses, and good blinking habits must be established. **(b)** Because hydrogel lenses require little or no adaptation of sensory nerves, adaptation to these lenses is mainly a matter of establishing good blinking habits.

40. If the patient desires glasses to wear during the evening hours after wearing contact lenses during the day, the most desirable procedure is to refract the patient in the late afternoon or early evening, after the lenses have been worn for 8 hours or more. If pronounced spectacle blur or distortion of the keratometer mire images is found to be present on lens removal, it may be necessary to wait 30 minutes or so before refracting the patient. In prescribing the spectacle lenses, small amounts of astigmatism may be neglected.

41. A mechanical system, such as Swirl-Clean, may be used to clean the lenses.

42. The argument in favor of using the papain enzyme cleaner is that even with routine cleaning of the lenses (using a surfactant cleaner) and overnight storage in the hydrating solution, protein materials from the tears may be deposited on the lenses. An argument against the use of the papain enzyme is that if the enzyme is not thoroughly removed from the lenses, chlorhexidine in the disinfecting solution will bind to the remaining protein, causing coating of the lenses.

43. Seven percent.

44. **(a)** The patient's symptoms can be described in terms of four stages: (1) minimal symptomatology, such as mucus in the corner of the eye on awakening; (2) mild blurring of vision and increased lens awareness; (3) increased mucous discharge, severe itching, and excessive lens movement; and (4) total loss of lens tolerance. **(b)** Giant cobblestone papillae are found on the tarsal conjunctiva on eversion of the upper lid. **(c)** Proteins adsorbing onto the lens surface are thought to be in a somewhat denatured state (especially if the lenses are boiled regularly). These proteins may desorb onto the tear film or tarsal conjunctiva acting as an antigen and resulting in the development of allergic conjunctivitis.

45. **(a)** To succeed with extended-wear of soft lenses, the patient should have a tear break-up time of 10–12 seconds; the tears should be free of mucus strands and other debris; there should be an absence of papillary hypertrophy; the patient should not have a history of allergies and should be willing to follow instructions. **(b)** The oxygen transmission of the lens must be high, either as a result of the lens material having a high water content or, for low and medium water content lenses, the lens must be very thin. **(c)** The lenses must be fitted in such a manner as to move freely on the eyes, in both the primary and upgaze positions.

46. Well-adapted monovision wearers may not make good soft bifocal wearers; low myopes and low hyperopes may not make good monovision wearers; patients who plan to wear the lenses only for social occasions may not be well motivated; pupil size should be in the 3.5–4.5mm range; there should be little or no uncorrected astigmatism.

47. **(a)** The patient must have equally good acuity for both eyes, with a minimum of uncorrected astigmatism; if refractive astigmatism is as high as 0.75D or more, gas-permeable hard lenses are usually preferable to spherical or toric soft lenses. **(b)** The dominant eye is normally fitted for distance vision, and the power of the near lens is determined in the same manner as for a bifocal add. **(c)** One of the major adaptation problems will be the result of night driving, when bright light sources may elicit diplopia.

48. Although experience with gas-permeable hard lenses for extended wear is limited, a potential advantage is that the lenses will have a longer useful life than soft lenses for extended wear. A disadvantage is that the lenses tend to cause corneal flattening and, for some patients, lens "binding" occurs.

Chapter 15

1. In the Bailey-Lovie chart, there is a constant size-progression ratio (5/4) from each row of letters to the next, each row has the same number of symbols, and there is a constant spacing between rows and between letters.

2. Visual acuity testing should be done at a distance of 5 feet so that the patient will be encouraged by achieving success.

3. **(a)** It determines the extent of intact retina available for magnification. **(b)** A large X can be taped to the tangent screen, and the patient is asked to fixate where the two limbs of the X come together.

4. If an afocal telescope is used at a distance closer than infinity, the divergence of the light rays entering the objective will be increased (on emerging from the eyepiece) by the square of the magnification of the telescope.

5. **(a)** The size of the print is indicated by the distance (in meters) at which lowercase letters (without ascenders or descenders) subtend 5 minutes of arc. **(b)** The patient can resolve one-M letter at a distance of 0.40m. **(c)** The patient can resolve three-M letters at a distance of 0.40m. **(d)** The patient can resolve two-M letters at a distance of 0.20m.

6. Large-print books provide a limited choice of reading material and a magnification of only 2–3× (with 18- to 24-point type). A patient requiring only 2× or 3× magnification can easily read normal print with a high-addition lens and will have a much greater choice of reading material.

7. **(a)** No more than about 3×; **(b)** magnifications as high as 10× or greater are available, but such high magnifications require close working distances (e.g., a reading distance of 2.5cm is required for a +40.00D lens).

8. It can be held against the patient's distance lens. This requires the patient to move in close to the print, with a high-addition lens.

9. When acuity is tested at 40cm using a chart in which acuity is designated in the M system, the power of the reading addition can be estimated by multiplying the M designation of the smallest print that the patient is able to read by +2.50D. The approximate reading distance will be the reciprocal of the power of the lens (expressed in meters). For a patient who can read 2M print at 40cm, the estimated addition is +5.00D; for a patient who can read 5M print at 40cm, the estimated addition is +12.50D.

10. The advantage of a telemicroscope for near vision is that for the same magnifying power, the telemicroscope provides the wearer with a greater working distance than the high-addition bifocal or reading lens. A disadvantage is its smaller field of view.

Index